M000250138

Primary Care of Native American Patients: Diagnosis, Therapy, and Epidemiology

Sponsored through an unrestricted educational grant by Ortho-McNeil Pharmaceutical, Inc., makers of

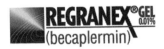

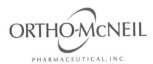

Primary Care of Native American Patients: Diagnosis, Therapy, and Epidemiology

Edited by

James M. Galloway, M.D., F.A.C.P., F.A.C.C.

Director, The Center for Native American Health and The Native American Cardiology Program, Indian Health Service and Arizona Health Sciences Center, Tucson; Assistant Clinical Professor of Public Health, The Arizona Prevention Center, and Assistant Professor of Clinical Medicine, University of Arizona College of Medicine, Tucson

Bruce W. Goldberg, M.D.

Associate Professor, Departments of Family Medicine and Public Health and Preventive Medicine, Oregon Health Sciences University School of Medicine, Portland

Joseph S. Alpert, M.D.

Robert S. and Irene P. Flinn Professor of Medicine and Head, Department of Medicine, University of Arizona College of Medicine, Tucson; Clinical Service Chief, Department of Medicine, University of Arizona Health Sciences Center, Tucson

Foreword by

Michael H. Trujillo, M.D., M.P.H., M.S.

Assistant Surgeon General and Director of Indian Health Service, Rockville, Maryland

With 65 Contributing Authors

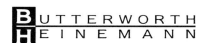

Boston   Oxford   Johannesburg   Melbourne   New Delhi   Singapore

Copyright © 1999 by Butterworth–Heinemann

 A member of the Reed Elsevier group

All rights reserved.

No part of this publication may be reproduced, stored in a retrieval system, or transmitted in any form or by any means, electronic, mechanical, photocopying, recording, or otherwise, without the prior written permission of the publisher.

Every effort has been made to ensure that the drug dosage schedules within this text are accurate and conform to standards accepted at time of publication. However, as treatment recommendations vary in the light of continuing research and clinical experience, the reader is advised to verify drug dosage schedules herein with information found on product information sheets. This is especially true in cases of new or infrequently used drugs.

Recognizing the importance of preserving what has been written, Butterworth–Heinemann prints its books on acid-free paper whenever possible.

 Butterworth–Heinemann supports the efforts of American Forests and the Global ReLeaf program in its campaign for the betterment of trees, forests, and our environment.

Note: The opinions expressed in this document are those of the authors and do not necessarily represent those of the Indian Health Service or the editors.

Library of Congress Cataloging-in-Publication Data

Primary care of Native American patients: diagnosis, therapy, and
  epidemiology / [edited by] James M. Galloway, Bruce W.
  Goldberg, Joseph S. Alpert; foreword by Michael H. Trujillo.
        p.   cm.
     Includes bibliographical references and index.
     ISBN 0-7506-9989-2
     1. Indians of North America--Medical care. 2. Indians of North
  America--Diseases. 3. Indians of North America--Health and hygiene.
  4. United States. Indian Health Service. I. Galloway, James M.
  (James Malcolm), 1953-   . II. Goldberg, Bruce W. III. Alpert,
  Joseph S.
     [DNLM: 1. United States. Indian Health Service. 2. Health
  Services, Indigenous--United States. 3. Primary Health Care-
  -methods--United States. 4. Indians, North American--United States.
  5. Health Services Needs and Demand--United States. WA 305P952
  1999]
  RA448.5.I5P75 1999
  362,1'089'97073--dc21
  DNLM/DLC
  for Library of Congress   98-29285
                                                                       CIP

British Library Cataloguing-in-Publication Data
A catalogue record for this book is available from the British Library.

The publisher offers special discounts on bulk orders of this book.
For information, please contact:

Manager of Special Sales
Butterworth–Heinemann
225 Wildwood Avenue
Woburn, MA 01801-2041
Tel: 781-904-2500
Fax: 781-904-2620

For information on all Butterworth–Heinemann publications available,
contact our World Wide Web home page at: http://www.bh.com

10 9 8 7 6 5 4 3 2 1

Printed in the United States of America

*To the Native American people who have enriched us
with their culture, wisdom, and friendship*

Contents

Contributing Authors

Joseph S. Alpert, M.D.
Robert S. and Irene P. Flinn Professor of Medicine and Head, Department of Medicine, University of Arizona College of Medicine, Tucson; Clinical Service Chief, Department of Medicine, University of Arizona Health Sciences Center, Tucson

L. Roderick Anderson, M.D.
Cerebrovascular Fellow, Department of Neurology, University of Arizona Health Sciences Center, Tucson

Ann Andonyan, M.D.
Resident, Department of Emergency Medicine, Thomas Jefferson University, Philadelphia

N. Burton Attico, M.D., M.P.H., F.A.C.O.G.
Director, Maternal Child Health Program, Phoenix Area Indian Health Service; Assistant Chief, Department of Obstetrics and Gynecology, Phoenix Area Medical Center

Sardar Ijlal Babar, M.D.
Fellow, Pulmonary/Critical Care, University of Arizona College of Medicine and University of Arizona Health Sciences Center, Tucson

Michael Biernoff, M.D.
Chief, Behavioral Health Program, Albuquerque Indian Health Service; Clinical Assistant Professor of Psychiatry, University of New Mexico School of Medicine, Albuquerque

Ora Botwinick, M.D.
Clinical Assistant Professor of Family Medicine, Oregon Health Sciences University School of Medicine, Portland

George Brenneman, M.D.
Associate Director, Center for American Indian and Alaskan Native Health, Department of International Health, Johns Hopkins University School of Hygiene and Public Health, Baltimore; Joint Appointment in Pediatrics, Johns Hopkins University School of Medicine, Baltimore

Eric A. Brody, M.D.
Assistant Professor of Clinical Medicine, University Heart Center, and Associate Director, Native American Cardiology Program, Indian Health Service, University of Arizona Health Sciences Center, Tucson

James E. Cheek, M.D., M.P.H.
Principal Epidemiologist for Infectious Diseases, Division of Community and Environmental Health, Indian Health Service Headquarters West, Albuquerque, New Mexico; Clinical Assistant Professor of Family and Community Medicine, University of New Mexico School of Medicine, Albuquerque

Kelly R. Chrestman, Ph.D.
Clinical Psychologist, Behavioral Health Services, Hopi Guidance Center, Second Mesa, Arizona; Clinical Psychologist, Department of Behavioral Health, Keams Canyon Hospital, Indian Health Service, Keams Canyon, Arizona

Nathaniel Cobb, M.D.
Director, Cancer Prevention and Control Program, Indian Health Service, Albuquerque, New Mexico; Clinical Assistant Professor of Family and Community Medicine, University of New Mexico School of Medicine, Albuquerque

Larry D. Crook, M.D., F.A.C.P.
Chief of Internal Medicine, Gallup Indian Medical Center, Gallup, New Mexico

Thomas E. Crow, M.S.E.H.
Principal Environmental Consultant, Division of Community and Environmental Health, Indian Health Service, Rockville, Maryland

Mario Cruz, M.D.
Assistant Clinical Professor, Department of Psychiatry, University of Arizona College of Medicine, Tucson; Associate Head of Clinical Services, Department of Psychiatry, Arizona Health Sciences Center, Tucson

Theresa Cullen, M.D.
Medical Director, Sells Indian Health Service Hospital, Sells, Arizona

Eugene Dannels, D.P.M., F.A.C.F.A.S.
Senior Podiatry Consultant, Indian Health Service, Phoenix; Chairman, American Podiatric Medical Association Committee on Indian Health; Chairman, Council of Indian Health Podiatrists; Chief, Department of Podiatry, Phoenix Indian Medical Center

Don J. Davis, M.P.H.
Director, Phoenix Area Indian Health Service

James M. Galloway, M.D., F.A.C.P., F.A.C.C.
Director, The Center for Native American Health and The Native American Cardiology Program, Indian Health Service and Arizona Health Sciences Center, Tucson; Assistant Clinical Professor of Public Health, The Arizona Prevention Center, and Assistant Professor of Clinical Medicine, University of Arizona College of Medicine, Tucson

Bruce W. Goldberg, M.D.
Associate Professor, Departments of Family Medicine and Public Health and Preventive Medicine, Oregon Health Sciences University School of Medicine, Portland

Deborah L. Goldsmith, M.D.
Assistant Professor of Clinical Medicine, Department of Internal Medicine and Infectious Disease, University of Arizona College of Medicine and University of Arizona Medical Center, Tucson

David C. Grossman, M.D., M.P.H.
Associate Professor of Pediatrics, Adjunct Associate Professor of Health Services, and Co-Director, Harborview Injury Prevention and Research Center, University of Washington School of Medicine, Seattle

Eric Henley, M.D., M.P.H.
Assistant Professor of Family and Community Medicine, University of Illinois College of Medicine, Rockford

Walter B. Hollow, M.D., M.S.
Director, Native American Center of Excellence, University of Washington School of Medicine, Seattle; Clinical Associate Professor, Department of Family Medicine and Minority Affairs Program, University of Washington School of Medicine, Seattle; Family Practice, Group Health Cooperative of Puget Sound, Northgate Clinic, Seattle

Barbara V. Howard, Ph.D.
President, Medlantic Research Institute, Washington, D.C.

Wm. James Howard, M.D.
Senior Vice President and Medical Director, Department of Medical Affairs, and Lipid Disease/Disorder Specialist, Washington Hospital Center, Washington, D.C.; Professor of Medicine, George Washington University School of Medicine and Health Sciences, Washington, D.C.

Diana C. Hu, M.D.
Acting Maternal Child Health Consultant, Navajo Area Indian Health Service, Department of Pediatrics, Tuba City Indian Medical Center, Tuba City, Arizona

Jonathan Vilasier Iralu, M.D.
Navajo Area Indian Health Service Infectious Diseases Consultant, Department of Internal Medicine, Gallup Indian Medical Center, Gallup, New Mexico

Amit Karmakar, M.D.
Fellow, Pulmonary/Critical Care, University of Arizona College of Medicine and University of Arizona Health Sciences Center, Tucson

David Kessler, M.D.
Clinical Director, Zuni Comprehensive Community Health Center, Zuni, New Mexico; Assistant Clinical Professor of Pediatrics, University of New Mexico School of Medicine, Albuquerque

Mary P. Koss, Ph.D.
Professor of Public Health, Family and Community Medicine, Psychiatry, and Psychology, Arizona Prevention Center, University of Arizona College of Medicine, Tucson; Active Staff, Department of Psychiatry, University of Arizona Health Sciences Center, Tucson

Jonathan Krakoff, M.D.
Staff Internist, Whiteriver Indian Health Service Hospital, Whiteriver, Arizona; Adjunct Assistant Clinical Professor of Medicine, Columbia University College of Physicians and Surgeons, New York

Jean A. Kunkel-Thomas, M.D.
Electromyography/Neuromuscular Fellow, Department of Neurology, University of Arizona Health Sciences Center, Tucson

David M. Labiner, M.D.
Associate Professor of Neurology and Director, Arizona Comprehensive Epilepsy Program, University of Arizona Health Sciences Center, Tucson

Norman Levine, M.D.
Professor of Medicine (Dermatology), University of Arizona College of Medicine, Tucson; Chief of Dermatology, University of Arizona Health Sciences Center, Tucson

Carol S. Locust, Ph.D.
Director of Training, Native American Research and Training Center, University of Arizona College of Medicine, Tucson

Ana Mariá López, M.D., M.P.H.
Clinical Assistant Professor of Medicine and Pathology, Arizona Cancer Center, Department of Internal Medicine, University of Arizona Health Sciences Center, Tucson

William W. Lunt, M.D.
Clinical Fellow, Department of Gastroenterology, University of Arizona Health Sciences Center, Tucson

Anthony A. Marfin, M.D., M.P.H.
Deputy State Epidemiologist, Oregon Health Division, Portland

Melvina McCabe, M.D.
Associate Professor of Family and Community Medicine and Director, Family Medicine Geriatrics Program, University of New Mexico School of Medicine, Albuquerque

Dorothy J. Meyer, C.N.M., M.P.H.
Maternal Child Health Consultant, Phoenix Area Indian Health Service

Andrew S. Narva, M.D.
Director, Kidney Disease Program, Indian Health Service, Albuquerque, New Mexico; Assistant Clinical Professor of Medicine, University of New Mexico School of Medicine, Albuquerque

John F. Neale III, D.D.S., M.P.H.
Chief of Dental Services, Fort Duchesne Indian Health Center, Fort Duchesne, Utah

Mona A. Polacca, M.S.W.
Research Specialist, Senior Arizona Prevention Center, University of Arizona Health Sciences Center, Tucson

Raymond Reid, M.D.
Research Associate, Department of International Health, Johns Hopkins University School of Medicine, Baltimore; Physician and Clinical Researcher, Whiteriver Indian Health Service Hospital, Whiteriver, Arizona

David C. Robbins, M.D.
Director of Research for Atherosclerosis and Diabetes, Penn Medical Laboratory, Medlantic Research Institute, Washington, D.C.; Senior Attending Physician, Department of Medicine, Washington Hospital Center, Washington, D.C.

Yvette Roubideaux, M.D., M.P.H.
Senior Fellow in Indian Health, Native American Center of Excellence, University of Washington School of Medicine, Seattle

Richard E. Sampliner, M.D.
Professor of Medicine, University of Arizona College of Medicine, Tucson; Chief of Gastroenterology, University of Arizona Health Sciences Center and Tucson Veterans Affairs Medical Center, Tucson

Richard M. Schwend, M.D.
Assistant Professor of Orthopaedic Surgery, University at Buffalo School of Medicine and Biomedical Sciences, Buffalo, New York; Children's Orthopaedic Surgeon, Children's Hospital of Buffalo, Buffalo, New York

Jeffrey M. Sippel, M.D.
Fellow, Pulmonary Medicine, Pulmonary and Critical Care Division, Oregon Health Sciences University School of Medicine, Portland

Linda S. Snyder, M.D.
Assistant Professor of Clinical Medicine, Pulmonary and Critical Care Medicine Section, University of Arizona College of Medicine and University of Arizona Health Sciences Center, Tucson

Bruce Tempest, M.D.
Former Chief of Internal Medicine, Gallup Indian Medical Center, Gallup, New Mexico

Nicolette I. Teufel, Ph.D.
Research Assistant Professor, Arizona Prevention Center, University of Arizona College of Medicine, Tucson

Marc S. Traeger, M.D.
Staff Physician, Whiteriver Indian Health Service Hospital, Whiteriver, Arizona

Michael L. Tutt, M.D.
Director of Native American Studies and Assistant Professor of Clinical Medicine, University of Arizona Health Sciences Center, Tucson

W. Craig Vanderwagen, M.D.
Associate Clinical Professor of Family Practice, Uniformed Services University of the Health Sciences, F. Edward Hébert School of Medicine, Bethesda, Maryland

Bridget T. Walsh, D.O.
Assistant Professor of Clinical Medicine and Director of Clinical Research Unit, University of Arizona College of Medicine, Tucson

Alan G. Waxman, M.D., M.P.H.
Senior Clinician for Obstetrics and Gynecology, Indian Health Service, U.S. Public Health Service, Rockville, Maryland; Obstetrician/Gynecologist, Gallup Indian Medical Center, Gallup, New Mexico

Colleen Williams, P.A.-C.
Adolescent Health Specialist, Tuba City Indian Medical Center, Tuba City, Arizona

Charlton A. Wilson, M.D.
Director, Diabetes Center of Excellence and Deputy Chief, Department of Medicine, Phoenix Indian Medical Center

Joseph F. Wilson, M.D.
Former Surgeon, Alaska Native Medical Center, Anchorage

Darcy Hunt Wolsey, M.P.H.
Staff Epidemiologist, Division of Community and Environmental Health, Indian Health Service Headquarters, Albuquerque, New Mexico

David E. Yocum, M.D.
Professor of Medicine and Director, Arizona Arthritis Center, University of Arizona College of Medicine, Tucson

David A. Yost, M.D.
Clinical Instructor of Family and Community Medicine, University of Arizona College of Medicine, Tucson; Clinical Director, Whiteriver U.S. Public Health Service Hospital, Whiteriver, Arizona

T. Kue Young, M.D., Ph.D.
Professor of Community Health Sciences, University of Manitoba Faculty of Medicine, Winnipeg, Manitoba, Canada

Foreword

When I was confirmed as the director of the Indian Health Service in April 1994, I knew that the Indian health care system would change significantly as it entered a new era. The Indian Health Service, an agency of the U.S. Department of Health and Human Services, provides a health care delivery system for American Indians and Alaska Natives. In addition to the agency's direct care delivery system, tribes also administer and deliver their own health programs, contributing to a partnership between the agency and Indian people. A portion of the Indian health care system of services is delivered through urban Indian health programs. Through the federal, tribal, and urban delivery options, a comprehensive health program is provided to American Indian and Alaska Native people.

What does an Indian health care system mean for a health care provider or a health administrator? Through this handbook, you will learn what it has meant to the most dedicated of clinical providers and seasoned administrators. The successes are hard earned and the rewards, professional and personal, are worthwhile. The successes in Indian health are a tribute to the professional and personal responsibility of providers and administrators who serve and have served Indian people. The dedication that is revealed in these written pages reflects the kind of opportunities that you may experience by participating in a public health partnership such as the Indian health care system.

The Indian Health Service is unique among the Public Health Service agencies within the department. There is a special government-to-government relationship between the U.S. government and the tribal governments of the people the Indian Health Service serves and for whom it advocates. The federal responsibility to provide a comprehensive health care program for American Indians and Alaska Natives resulted from obligations initially assumed by the federal government through treaties with Indian nations in exchange for land, mineral rights, and much more. Another unique characteristic is the direct involvement of the people it serves in the management of the agency. The Indian Health Service's mission states that the opportunity must be provided for maximum tribal involvement in developing and managing programs. The agency has facilitated processes to involve tribes in the agency's budget development, the design of health programs and interventions, and organizational restructuring.

The Indian Health Service has experienced political, budgetary, and programmatic changes. To respond to the changes, the tribal/urban/Indian Health Service partnership must collaborate with other federal agencies, colleges and universities, international organizations, private organizations, and state-administered services and programs. The collaboration and interaction that result will help cultivate new audiences with interest in the dynamics of the Indian health care system. New audiences and partnerships may lead to creating and supporting new ways of addressing Indian health issues.

Politically, the change reflects an improvement of the executive branch's internal management of the government's unique legal relationship with tribal governments. As a result of President Clinton's memorandum to the heads of executive departments and agencies directing them to consult with tribal governments before taking actions that affect them, the Department of Health and Human Services issued in August 1997 its policy on consultation with tribes and Indian organizations. The consultation practice of the Indian Health Service was formalized in a written policy, issued in September 1997, requiring consultation with tribal governments on the agency's program policies and activities.

Budgetary changes have affected the Indian Health Service as well as other federal agencies. All agencies are experiencing the pressures of restricted funding, decreased administrative budgets, unfunded costs, and government downsizing. Unique to the Indian Health Service budget is the transfer of funding amounts to tribal governments that have chosen to administer their own health programs. In addition, as the responsibility for administering federal programs is transferred to the states, the funding stream itself is changing and states now receive federal funds directly. The challenge for our tribal and urban partners is how to access those resources appropriately and directly. This challenge creates the opportunity to collaborate with states and to increase the understanding of many people about Indian health needs and the successes of Indian programs.

Programmatically, the agency operates a health services delivery system designed to provide preventive, curative, rehabilitative, and environmental services. We have significant program areas that should be addressed in a more collaborative way, extending beyond the agency, urban Indian health programs, and tribal partnerships. These areas include diabetes and its complications, continuing increases in heart disease and cancer rates, and alcohol and substance abuse, especially among youth. At the community level, we should collaborate on addressing conditions that contribute to injuries, violence, abuse, and poor living environments that include substandard housing, unclean water, and exposure to sewage.

As the director, I began initiatives for program areas that need special emphasis. One of my initiatives emphasizes the alliance of traditional and modern medicine practices between community traditional healers and Indian Health Service health care providers. The Elder Care Initiative addresses the variety of elder services available from tribal, local, state, and federal programs. This initiative is designed to collect information from all these sources on their elder programs, resources, and other initiatives. When the American Indian and Alaska Native elder population doubled in the period from 1980 to 1990, their health needs shifted from acute and infectious diseases to chronic and degenerative diseases, thus requiring a different mix of services and resources. The Indian Children and Youth Initiative was expanded and proposed as an initiative for the President's Domestic Policy Council. The proposal was accepted and resulted in the American Indian and Alaska Native Children and Adolescents Initiative. This government-wide initiative promotes a multiagency approach so that youth can live healthier and happier lives in Indian communities. This initiative encompasses the physical, mental, social, environmental, economic, cultural, and spiritual well-being of Indian youth.

If this handbook is your introduction to the Indian health care system, I hope that it will inspire you to pursue an association with our partnership. We invite you to consider serving in a partnership that promotes listening as a path to mutual respect, dignity, and harmony.

Michael H. Trujillo

Preface

One evening in the late 1980s, the idea for this text was conceived on the Zuni Reservation in northwest New Mexico. Our original idea was to create a small handbook that would be helpful to physicians and medical students newly arrived at an Indian Health Service facility. Over the years, as we discussed and worked on the outline of this text, it expanded both with respect to the number of topics covered and the level of detail. The final text now includes 46 chapters ranging in topics from the interface between a Western-trained physician and his or her Native American healing counterpart to the impact and care of diabetes mellitus in Native Americans.

We have tried to focus each chapter on the specific characteristics of the presentation and management of illnesses in Native Americans. Much of the standard pathophysiology, history, physical examination, and laboratory data are not included because this information is readily available in well-known textbooks of medicine. Rather, we present material that takes up where standard texts leave off with respect to Native American patients. We include chapters on the organization of health care for Native Americans and a variety of psychosocial aspects of health care in this environment because we believe that this information will be helpful to the newly arrived health care provider in a Native American health facility.

We dedicate this book to the many Native American patients for whom we have cared over the years; countless individuals who have given us as much or more than we gave them. All of the authors' honoraria derived from the sale of this text are being donated to a college scholarship fund for Native Americans through the Center for Native American Health at the University of Arizona.

J.M.G.
B.W.G.
J.S.A.

Acknowledgments

We gratefully acknowledge the tireless dedication and hard work of our coordinator and good friend, Mr. Joshua Gormally, as well as the staff of The Center for Native American Health and The Native American Cardiology Program for their efforts in the successful completion of this text.

J.M.G.
B.W.G.
J.S.A.

Primary Care of Native American Patients: Diagnosis, Therapy, and Epidemiology

Part I
Epidemiology and Health Care Delivery

Chapter 1

Health Care for Alaska Natives and Native Americans: Historical Perspective

Don J. Davis

To understand the history of health care for Alaska Natives and Native Americans, it is necessary to know the historic relationships between Indian tribes and the U.S. federal government.

Before the arrival of Northern Europeans on the North American continent, the indigenous people occupied the entire expanse of land between the Atlantic and Pacific Oceans. The tribes located along the eastern seaboard, the midwest and central plains, and the southwestern and the northwestern segments of the United States differed in origins and structure. Despite these differences, all tribes exhibited the same basic concepts of natural harmony and spiritual integrity. Although there were occasional confrontations between various tribal members, there is no historic evidence of total supremacy of any one group, nor is there evidence of any significant major conflicts.

As the colonies were formed and then unified into "United States," any tribal claims to land were ignored. Despite the reputed purchase of the New York area for a few beads and trinkets, the land was generally considered to be "there for the taking" and "first come, final owner," and the white settlers' perspective became the law of the land. In spite of the fact that the United States "purchased" land from other entities (e.g., the Louisiana purchase from France, the purchase of Alaska from Russia, the Gadsden purchase from Mexico), no effort was made to purchase land from American Indian tribes. Tribes, however, consider their treaties to be the original health maintenance organizations, or prepaid health (and education) insurance. The exchange of their land as payment for perpetual health care and education was and remains a bargain for the United States of America.

With the increase in nonindigenous populations came the need for more land. As the settlers pushed westward, the American Indians were generally pushed ahead, frequently with the assistance of the armies of the United States or the "territories." Resolutions to the conflicts have many forgettable instances of injustices and broken promises. It is enough to say that the position taken by the United States was to sign "treaties" with many of the tribal governments. Although these treaties were frequently ignored and modified, especially as they related to land boundaries of the so-called reservations, they still formed the basis of safety for the people migrating westward and endless segregation of Native American people.

Enforcement of the treaties' boundaries was generally left to the U.S. Army, as was the provision of other components of the treaties. Common language in the treaties stated that education and health care would be provided "as long as the grass grows and the rivers flow." The army was also given the assignment to provide health care to the American Indian people under their surveillance. Needless to say, health care for Native Americans was not one of the priorities of the U.S. Army at this time.

As the United States became more understanding of the difficulties in the administration of Indian programs promised by treaty, the Bureau of Indian Affairs (BIA) was formed, and health care programs for Native Americans became the responsibility of this bureau within the Department of the Interior. The BIA built clinics and hospitals, and the health care provided improved somewhat over the very meager services rendered by the army. In 1954 the federal government decided to transfer the provision of health care from the BIA to the Public Health Service, and in 1955 the Indian Health Service (IHS) was established as the entity to carry out this assignment.

The budgets appropriated for Indian health care are generally considered to be authorized by the Snyder Act of 1920. This legislation states that health care for Indian people will be financed as Congress "from time to time" appropriated funds. In the early days of the IHS, these funds amounted to barely enough to provide health care in the format established by the BIA. One difference was the involvement of the U.S. Public Health Service in the administering of health care, which led to significant improvement in the health of and health care provided to

American Indian people, even though funding remained scant.

With the admission of Alaska as a state in 1959, several Alaska Native tribes eventually received the benefits provided to Native Americans.

The 1960s were a time of significant improvement in the health of the beneficiaries of the IHS. The life expectancy for an Indian baby in 1955, when the IHS was organized, was approximately 60 years, compared to the current life expectancy of approximately 74 years.[1] By far, the greatest problem in 1955 was infectious disease. Although some effort was made to treat these conditions, more work was focused on prevention as standard sanitation practices were brought to the reservations. For 15 years, the IHS struggled to provide liquid and solid waste facilities and potable water. Evidence of this effort was present on the Navajo Reservation, where in 1960 it was estimated that no Navajo family traveled more than 10 miles for potable water (personal communication, Theodore J. Redding, 1986). (An innovative carrying system had been developed previously in which families were provided with caissons from World War II that helped in keeping the water relatively safe for a longer period than previously.) With a tremendous effort concentrated on drilling "shallow wells," the distance necessary for a family to obtain potable water decreased to less than 2 miles during the next 4 years. This effort has not diminished over the years, and today one of the requirements for all new housing projects on reservation land is to have the Office of Environmental Health and Engineering of the IHS approve the project and provide support in furnishing potable water and waste disposal.

Another of the original initiatives of the IHS was to improve the immunization status of Indian children. Previously, immunization records were often incomplete and the status of community immunity was only estimated. During the mid-1970s, the IHS concentrated on evaluating and improving this situation. Consequently, the immunization rate of children currently living on reservation lands is better than any other identified group of children and generally is greater than 90% (J.S. Takehara, National IHS Immunization Coordinator, quarterly report to IHS director for first quarter, Fiscal Year 1998).

After achieving a decrease in the number of cases of infant diarrhea, facilitated by improved sanitation, and an increase in the number of immunized children, the IHS turned its attention to major treatable infectious diseases. Tuberculosis clinics were held in even the smallest settlements, and treatment was meticulously administered and monitored by public health nurses. Education and treatment efforts paid off, with a reduction in age-adjusted tuberculosis death rates per 100,000 population from 57.9 in 1955 to 2.2 in 1991. This is a reduction of 96% in the rate of Indian patients dying from tuberculosis.[2] Trachoma, an infection of the conjunctiva and cornea causing extensive blindness in Indian people in the southwest,

presented an interesting challenge. Teams were formed to travel throughout the region providing education on the treatment and prevention of this very contagious infection. Treatment was provided, and follow-up visits verified the effectiveness of the therapy. Today, trachoma is seldom seen on reservations.

It is interesting that an Indian person at age 25 years in 1955 could expect to live almost as long as the same person at the same age today. Furthermore, the difference in life expectancy at age 5 years has changed relatively little in the past 40 years. It has become evident that health and wellness should be emphasized to Indian people in association with pregnancy, gestation, delivery, and early childhood. Prenatal clinics have been established throughout Indian country and been well publicized. The number of nonhospital deliveries has declined dramatically, and today an Alaska Native or Native American pregnant woman has just as good a chance of delivering a healthy baby as any identified group of women in the United States. There is still some improvement necessary before the same can be said about the first year of life, and the health of infants 1–12 months old is a current emphasis of Indian health programs.

The mid-1960s to the mid-1980s seemed to be the "golden years" for the IHS. With few exceptions, the IHS grew by constructing a large number of hospital and clinic facilities and an infrastructure to support this rapid expansion. Communities were identified as the focus of attention and the term *community-oriented primary care* became a national definition of the best rural, or frontier, medical care available, and that care was delivered by the IHS.

The 1990s have seen interesting developments in the organization of health care for Alaska Natives and Native Americans. After statutory changes in the late 1980s, tribal governments became more interested in operating their own health care delivery systems. Individual tribes and tribal (or village) consortiums took over the administration of health programs for their members. Provisions within the Indian Self Determination and Education Act, with amendments, permitted tribes the opportunity to shape their delivery systems to meet their self-identified needs. In the process of this transformation, administrative funds were made available to tribes to fulfill needs that did not require the involvement of a federal employee. In accepting these responsibilities, the tribes were funded with money previously used to pay IHS administrative personnel. Of necessity, the IHS was redesigned and transformed into a partnership between the federal program, tribes, and urban programs.

The decade of the 1990s has demonstrated that Native American people now experience the same chronic health problems as the rest of the American population. Once problems related to infectious diseases were essentially overcome, chronic diseases and lifestyle diseases made their presence known. Type 2 diabetes mellitus, obesity, heart disease, high blood pressure, and cancer have became significant concerns. As medical interventions became more sophisticated, the IHS found the expensive technological advances in the field of medicine difficult to develop internally and looked around for outside alliances. Therefore, the IHS established practical relationships that allow cooperative work with other federal programs (veteran's hospitals and military facilities), public programs (medical schools and university hospitals), and private programs (Mayo Clinic and others). It was with this intent—to provide the best continuum of care—that the IHS Native American Cardiology program was instituted. This program uses a traveling ambulatory staff, providing consultants and follow-up care at the local facility, with inpatient procedures being performed at the University of Arizona and Tucson Veteran's Administration hospitals by the same IHS staff.

The future seems to be clear for smaller reservation-based care delivery systems. Small, rural hospitals cannot maintain the sophisticated technology required by many of today's therapies. Therefore, reservations with less than a 10,000-member patient base will be hard pressed to maintain facilities. Working with nearby non-Indian communities may help provide support for these operations. Indeed, with the growth in technology and managed care and the tremendous increase in the chronic diseases treated on an outpatient basis, it is difficult to see any other alternative. Clearly, the changes in the Indian and general U.S. health care field will continue to bring dramatic changes to the delivery of health care to Indian people. Although sometimes painful, these changes allow Indian people the opportunity to create an improved health care system.

Many of the problems confronting the beneficiaries of the IHS are the same that people all over the world confront: conditions relating to lifestyle (e.g., obesity, diabetes, heart disease, high blood pressure, alcoholism, substance abuse, and acquired immunodeficiency syndrome) and other conditions related to aging (e.g., long-term care, dementia, arthritis, multisystem failure). By doing what is possible to intervene in these conditions and placing primary emphasis on wellness and healthy lives, the outlook for improving the length and quality of life remains encouraging.

References

1. Indian Health Service. Chart Series Book. Washington, DC: U.S. Department of Health and Human Services, Public Health Service, Health Resources and Planning, Evaluation, and Legislation, Program Statistics Branch, 1985;20.
2. Indian Health Service. Trends in Indian Health. Washington, DC: U.S. Department of Health and Human Services, Public Health Service, Indian Health Service, Office of Planning, Evaluation, and Legislation, Division of Program Statistics, 1995;72,77.

Chapter 2

Epidemiologic Patterns of Morbidity and Mortality

Darcy Hunt Wolsey and James E. Cheek

The health status of American Indians (AIs) and Alaska Natives (ANs) in the United States has improved dramatically since the mid 1950s. However, the mortality and morbidity in this population remains markedly different from that of other populations. Overall rates of death are significantly higher than those of the general U.S. population. In 1991–1993, the age-adjusted mortality rate for AIs was 732.2 per 100,000, 43% higher than the U.S. all races rate of 504.5 for 1992.[1] Poor socioeconomic conditions, lack of education, cultural barriers to good health, and other factors contribute to a health status of AIs and ANs that continues to lag behind that of other Americans.[2, 3]

Complete information on the health of AIs often is not available, accurate, or representative. Although national and state surveys and census data often include AIs, results may be severely biased due to racial misclassification on death certificates and health records.[4, 5] The Indian Health Service (IHS) maintains health information for the IHS service population (the number of AIs and ANs identified to be eligible for IHS services, or approximately 1.43 million people), which comprises approximately 60% of all Indians living in the United States, and the IHS user population (the number of AIs and ANs who are eligible and actually use IHS services, or approximately 1.2 million people).[6] Due to known underreporting and racial misclassification, three IHS areas—California, Oklahoma, and Portland—are often not included in overall rate comparisons.

This chapter provides comparisons of morbidity and mortality among AIs, ANs, and the U.S. all races or white population. Historic patterns are mentioned briefly, with emphasis on changes since 1960. Leading causes of death, as well as leading causes of morbidity, for AIs and ANs and the U.S. general population are discussed. Information is based on IHS national data and more localized studies done throughout the United States. Due to regional differences in patterns of diseases, localized studies often may not be generalized to the Indian population as a whole.

Historical Patterns

There is little information about the health of AIs and ANs in the centuries before contact with Europeans. The population of Native Americans in the continental United States was small and dispersed over an immense geographic area. Archaeologic evidence suggests illnesses, such as osteomyelitis, syphilis, tuberculosis (TB), metabolic bone diseases, tumors, and arthritis, may have been important causes of morbidity and mortality.[7]

After contact with Europeans, the patterns of mortality reflect the introduction of novel pathogens into naive, susceptible populations. Massive epidemics were described by early European settlers in which entire communities or tribes became extinct in a matter of months. The principal infectious agents were measles, smallpox, and TB.[8]

More recently, AIs and ANs have developed chronic disease conditions closely associated with the acculturation process.[9] Despite improvements in preventing mortality associated with infectious diseases, many AI and AN communities continue to have significant morbidity from infectious agents. With the current classification of diseases primarily by organ system, many infectious diseases are classified as chronic diseases despite their infectious etiologies (e.g., endocarditis is classified as a disease of the cardiovascular system).[10] Furthermore, although mortality has decreased markedly since 1960, many disease-specific mortality rates remain elevated disproportionately compared to non-Indians (Figure 2-1). For example, although the number of deaths attributable to TB has declined dramatically among AIs and ANs, the overall mortality rate due to TB continues to be almost five times that of the U.S. mortality rate.

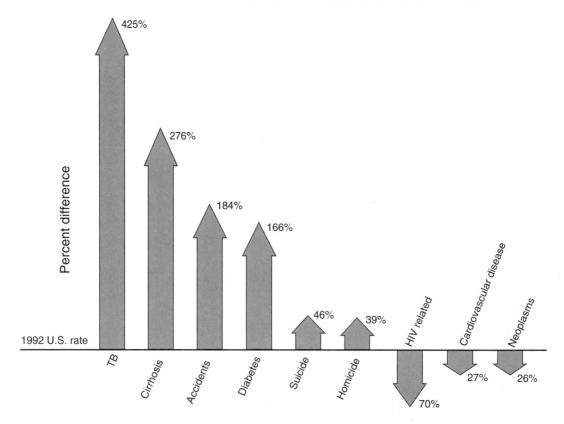

Figure 2-1. The percentage difference between the 1991–1993 mortality rates for all Indian Health Service areas compared to the U.S. all races rates for 1992. (HIV = human immunodeficiency virus; TB = tuberculosis.) (Adapted from Trends in Indian Health, 1996. Washington, DC: U.S. Department of Health and Human Services, Indian Health Service, Office of Planning, Evaluation, and Legislation, Division of Program Statistics, 1996.)

Mortality Patterns

The ranking of causes of death is similar among AIs, ANs, and the U.S. general population (Table 2-1).[1, 6] Heart disease, malignant neoplasms, and accidents are the top three leading causes of death for both AIs and ANs and the general population. However, AIs and ANs experience comparatively lower rates for both heart disease and cancer but a much higher rate for accidental deaths. In addition, diabetes, the fourth leading cause of death for AIs and ANs, is only eighth for the general population, accounting for less than 2% of all U.S. deaths.[6, 11] Three of the leading four causes of death for both AIs and ANs and the U.S. all races were chronic diseases.

Heart Disease

Historically, AIs and ANs have had lower rates of heart disease compared to the U.S. general population. Heart disease has now become the leading cause of death in AI and AN men and women, and rates appear to be increasing in some groups.[12, 13] IHS data for 1991–1993 attrib-

uted 21.9% of all deaths in this population to heart disease. When Portland, California, and Oklahoma IHS areas are excluded, the rate of 132.4 per 100,000 increases to 143.3 per 100,000, which is not significantly different from the U.S. all races rate of 144.3 for 1992.[1, 6]

As with diabetes, cardiovascular disease (CVD) mortality rates and the prevalence of risk factors related to CVD vary greatly among different tribes and regions. In general, southwestern Indian tribes have low rates of heart disease (84.2 per 100,000), whereas Indians in the Northern Plains have rates as high or higher than overall U.S. rates (230.0 per 100,000).[1, 13] Differences in CVD rates may be attributed in part to variations in the prevalence of diabetes and CVD risk factors among AIs and ANs. type 2 diabetes is estimated to increase the risk of CVD by two to four times.[14] The relationship of diabetes to CVD and associated cardiovascular risk factors has been studied in several tribes. CVD, the leading cause of mortality in diabetics, occurs twice as frequently in diabetic than in nondiabetic subjects.[12] A study of CVD in Navajos found that diabetics had a fivefold greater risk of heart disease than nondiabetics; women and middle-aged

Table 2-1. Leading Causes of Death for American Indians (1991–1993, all Indian Heath Service Areas) and the U.S. Population (1992)

Population Group	Causes of Death	Rate/100,000
American Indians/ Alaska Natives	Heart disease	132.4
	Malignant neoplasms	98.8
	Accidents	83.4
	Diabetes mellitus	31.7
	Chronic liver disease and cirrhosis	30.1
	Cerebrovascular disease	25.3
	Pneumonia and influenza	19.2
	Suicide	16.2
	Chronic obstructive pulmonary disease	14.8
	Homicide	14.6
	Human immunodeficiency virus infection	2.7
United States all races	Heart disease	144.3
	Malignant neoplasms	133.1
	Accidents	29.4
	Cerebrovascular disease	26.2
	Chronic obstructive pulmonary disease	19.9
	Pneumonia and influenza	12.7
	Human immunodeficiency virus infection	12.6
	Diabetes mellitus	11.9
	Suicide	11.1
	Homicide	10.5
	Chronic liver disease and cirrhosis	8.0

Source: Adapted from Trends in Indian Health, 1996. Washington, DC: U.S. Department of Health and Human Services, Indian Health Service, Office of Planning, Evaluation, and Legislation, Division of Program Statistics, 1997.

diabetics of both sexes had the greatest increase in risk.[14] In addition to diabetes, rates of obesity have increased dramatically since the 1960s in some tribes.[12] Smoking patterns, dietary habits, and genetic background may also contribute to the increasing rates of heart disease among AIs and ANs, as well as the regional variation of the disease throughout the United States.[13]

Cancer

For the first time, in 1991–1993, malignant neoplasms replaced accidents as the second leading cause of death for AIs and ANs. The age-adjusted mortality rate for the IHS service population, excluding Portland, California, and Oklahoma IHS areas, is 113.4 per 100,000, which is 15% less than the U.S. all races rate of 133.1.[1] The rank order of the five leading causes of cancer mortality are similar for AIs and ANs and the U.S. all races population; however, AI and AN rates are generally lower.[15]

Although cancer mortality for AIs and ANs is lower than for the U.S. white population for the most common neoplasms, cancer remains a significant cause of death in this population.[16] In addition, several forms of neoplasms occur at rates much higher than in the U.S. all races population in some locations.[15] Regional variation may be dramatic; for example, ANs have some of the highest mortality rates for nasopharyngeal, kidney, salivary gland, liver, gallbladder, gastric, and esophageal cancers described among AIs and ANs.[17,18] Excess deaths from gallbladder cancer, especially among women, have also been described among Indians throughout the United States. Gastric cancer mortality rates are high among some southwestern tribes, with rates nearly twice those in the U.S. all races population.[15] Excess cervical cancer mortality is seen in varying degrees for all regions studied.[15]

Although incidence rates of most cancers are lower in AIs and ANs compared to the U.S. white population, cancer survival rates tend to be comparatively poor. A study of Montana and New Mexico/Arizona AIs found cancer survival rates for all cancers combined to be significantly lower than comparable survival rates for U.S. whites. In particular, estimated 3-year survival rates for prostate, cervical, and breast cancer were at least one-third lower. The disparities in survival are thought to be related to a higher prevalence of advanced disease at the time of diagnosis, as well as increased likelihood of not receiving treatment.[19]

Accidental Deaths

Although the age-adjusted accident death rate for AIs and ANs decreased by 56% between 1972 and 1993, the current rate—83.4 per 100,000 for the IHS service area—is nearly triple the U.S. all races rate of 29.4 per 100,000 for 1992.[6] Accidents are the third leading cause of death for all IHS areas, accounting for 14.7% of all deaths in this population. In Navajo, Albuquerque, and Alaska IHS areas, accidents are the leading cause of death.[1] In reviewing age-specific mortality rates, Indian men have rates more than three times greater than women for the ages of 25–54 years and 65–74 years. Injury is the leading cause of death for people ages 1–44 years, accounting for 63% of all deaths in that age group.[6] Forty percent of all accidental deaths are from motor vehicle accidents, with homicide and suicide second, each with 13%[20] (see Intentional Injuries: Suicides and Homicides).

Injuries are the second leading cause of hospitalization at IHS facilities. Trends in injury morbidity and mortality, however, differ by IHS area with respect to rate of injuries and the most prevalent types of injuries. Motor vehicle accidents are the leading cause of hospitalization due to injuries in all areas except Alaska, where drowning is the leading cause.[20] A study in New Mexico found that excessive cold or exposure was a leading cause of death among AI men and women. These conditions were not among the 10 leading causes of death for Hispanics or non-Hispanic whites studied in the state of New Mexico.[21]

AIs and ANs may be at increased risk for accidental injuries for several reasons. This population is younger than the total U.S. population. Young persons are at higher risk for injury because they are more likely to engage in risky behaviors. Furthermore, alcohol plays a major role in injury mortality. A study in New Mexico found that 55–65% of all motor vehicle accidents involved alcohol consumption. Because the possession and sale of alcohol is prohibited in many Native American communities, many people must travel to drink alcohol.[21, 22]

Diabetes

Diabetes, once a rare disease in AIs, has now become epidemic. The majority of cases of diabetes in AIs are type 2 or non–insulin-dependent diabetes mellitus (NIDDM).[23, 24] AIs have higher rates of diabetes than all other U.S. ethnic groups, with an estimated overall prevalence for 1987 of 8.9%.[24] The Strong Heart Study found that more than two-thirds of those aged 45–74 years living in Arizona and one-third of men and 40% of women living in Oklahoma and South and North Dakota had diabetes.[13] Diabetes was the fourth leading cause of death for AIs in the years 1991–1993,[6] and complications from the disease contribute to several other leading causes of death, including heart disease and cerebrovascular disease.[24] All IHS areas have rates greater than the U.S. rate. The 1991–1993 age-adjusted diabetes mortality rate of 31.7 per 100,000 for the entire IHS service population was 2.7 times greater than the U.S. all races rate of 11.9.[1, 6]

Once thought to be a "benign" disease in the Indian population, NIDDM exacts a heavy toll on AI health in the United States.[24] Chronic complications, such as end-stage renal disease (ESRD), retinopathy, cerebrovascular disease, amputations, and heart disease, occur at high rates.[24] Studies show that diabetic nephropathy resulting in ESRD occurs in AIs at approximately six times the rate of the U.S. white population.[24, 25] Available data on the Pima and some Oklahoma tribes show excess rates of retinopathy;[25] 50–70% of diabetics among Hopi, Navajo, and Oklahoma tribes were diagnosed with retinopathy.[7] More than 85% of IHS hospitalizations for lower-extremity amputations between 1982 and 1987 carried a diabetes code.[24] Amputation rates in the Pima Indians were 3.7 times greater than overall rates compiled for six surrounding states.[25]

The elevated prevalence of NIDDM in AIs is considered to be related to drastic changes in lifestyle or "west-

ernization" of these Indian communities. These changes include a diet higher in total calories and fat but lower in fiber, along with a less active lifestyle.[13, 25] In addition, some researchers hypothesize that many AIs and ANs are genetically adapted for surviving prolonged periods of famine with a "thrifty gene," which has become maladaptive with modern dietary habits.[8]

Cerebrovascular Disease

Currently, cerebrovascular disease is the sixth leading cause of death among AIs, ranking fourth among women and eighth among men. For the years 1991–1993, the age-adjusted stroke mortality rate was 25.3 per 100,000, a rate similar to the U.S. all races rate of 26.2 for 1992. When excluding Portland, California, and Oklahoma IHS areas, the rate is 29.0, a rate 11% higher than the U.S. rate.[1] In reports from 32 reservation states from 1985 to 1987, the death rate from cerebrovascular disease in AIs and ANs at ages 45–64 years was 35.4 per 100,000, the same as the U.S. all races rate. At age 65 years and older, however, the rate for AIs and ANs was only 296.5 per 100,000, 30% lower than the U.S. all races rate.[26]

Diabetes also plays a major role in the development of cerebrovascular disease among American Indians. Studies in the Navajo population indicate that the risk of stroke increases tenfold for diabetic patients compared to nondiabetics. Nearly one-third of the diabetics in the study population were afflicted with cerebrovascular disease. In addition, diabetic women may be at even greater risk than men, as suggested by a complete absence of cerebrovascular disease in women without diabetes.[14]

Chronic Liver Disease

AIs and ANs have rates of chronic liver disease and cirrhosis that are nearly three times that of the U.S. all races rate (30.1 per 100,000 and 8.0 per 100,000, respectively). Chronic liver disease accounts for 4.4% of all mortality and is the fifth leading cause of death for AIs and ANs of all ages and the second leading cause of death for AIs and ANs ages 24–44 years.[1, 6] Women account for almost half of cirrhosis deaths among Indians compared to blacks and whites, in whom women accounted for only one-third of cirrhosis deaths.[27]

Alcohol-related mortality, including alcoholic liver disease, cirrhosis, and end-stage liver disease, is 4.7 times that of the U.S. all races rate.[6] The high incidence of chronic liver disease is most likely related to the prevalence of alcohol abuse and, in some locations, chronic hepatitis B infections.

Pneumonia and Influenza

Since 1955, mortality related to pneumonia and influenza among AIs and ANs has decreased by 82%.[28] Nevertheless, the AI and AN mortality rate due to pneumonia and influenza of 19.2 per 100,000 is still 1.5 times higher than the rates reported for the U.S. general population (12.7 per 100,000).[6] From 1980–1986, pneumonia caused more deaths in AIs and ANs than any other respiratory disease, including cancer. AI men are more affected by the disease, with a male to female ratio for pneumonia of 1.4 compared to 1.0 for the U.S. general population.[29]

Although *Haemophilus influenzae* and pneumococcus are common etiologic agents, viral agents are also responsible for epidemics of respiratory infections. Respiratory infections appear to be more frequent among AIs and ANs, especially in children younger than 2 years of age, than in the general population. A large number of risk factors for acute respiratory infections have been identified, including outdoor air pollution, smoking, crowded living, poor nutrition, indoor air pollution (especially from cooking and heating with gas stoves and wood-burning stoves), psychosocial stress, weather conditions, and low socioeconomic status.[7]

Intentional Injuries: Suicide and Homicide

From 1972–1974 to 1991–1993, suicide and homicide death rates have substantially declined among AIs and ANs (23% and 40%, respectively). However, current rates are still noticeably higher in the Indian population compared to the U.S. general population.[6] In 1991–1993, the age-adjusted suicide mortality rate for the IHS service area population was 89% higher than the U.S. all races rate of 11.1 per 100,000. Four IHS areas—Alaska, Aberdeen, Albuquerque, and Billings—reported rates that were more than double the U.S. rate.[1] Suicides among AIs and ANs follow different trends compared to the U.S. general population. Suicide rates vary among tribes, with higher rates occurring on reservations where alcoholism, homicides, and other related behaviors are more frequent. Suicide also appears to be more frequent among urban than rural Indians. In contrast to the U.S. non-Indian population, in which suicide rates increase steadily with age, the bulk of AI and AN suicides is concentrated in people age 35 years and younger.[8] The differences noted in the age-specific suicide death rates between AIs and ANs and others is not completely understood. Possible factors include poverty, drug and alcohol abuse, unemployment, and cultural conflict.[30] Studies have reported that alcohol is involved in 50–75% of all traumatic deaths and suicides.[21,31]

Homicide rates are similar to those of suicide, with the IHS reporting an age-adjusted mortality rate of 14.6 per 100,000 in 1991–1993. The rate for U.S. all races was 10.5 per 100,000 and only 6.1 among U.S. whites.[6] AI and AN men are significantly more likely to die from a homicide or suicide. Indian men ages 15–44 years have suicide rates five times greater and homicide rates three to six times higher compared to AI and AN women in the same age group.[6]

In addition to significant levels of mortality, suicide and homicide attempts are the leading causes of injury hospitalization among AIs and ANs. From 1981–1985, homicide (by means other than firearms) was the leading cause of injury hospitalization for men ages 15–44 years at IHS facilities. Suicide (by means other than firearms) was the leading injury cause for women ages 25–34 years.[20]

Tuberculosis

Although certainly not eliminated, TB has declined dramatically since the mid-1950s.[32] Between 1955 and 1981, the tuberculosis incidence rate among AIs (excluding ANs) dropped from 563.2 per 100,000 to 50.9, an average annual decline of 8.8%.[33] Since 1970, the age-adjusted death rates for AIs have also seen an 80% decrease; nevertheless, the Indian rate for 1991–1993 of 2.1 per 100,000 population is still 5.3 times the U.S. all races rate of 0.4 for 1992.[6] The median age of AI and AN persons with TB is 45 years, substantially lower than the median age of 60 years reported for non-Hispanic whites in the United States.[34] In 1990, 9% of TB cases among AIs and ANs occurred in persons younger than 15 years of age, indicating that transmission, rather than reactivation of latent infection among previously infected individuals, continues to occur in this population.[34]

AI and AN rates for new cases of TB are also substantially higher than in the U.S. general population. In 1995, the rate for new cases among AIs and ANs was 20.2, 2.3 times the U.S. rate of 8.7. Alaska's rate of 57.0 is 6.5 times greater than the U.S. rate—the highest for all IHS areas.[1] Unlike other populations in the United States, in which increases in TB are attributed to the human immunodeficiency virus (HIV) epidemic, there does not appear to be a strong association between acquired immunodeficiency syndrome (AIDS) and TB among AIs and ANs.[34] The continued increase in diabetes prevalence, a recognized risk factor for TB, may contribute to the disproportionate rate of TB in AIs compared to the U.S. general population.[35]

Human Immunodeficiency Virus

Although AIs and ANs historically have been affected disproportionately by infectious disease epidemics, rates of deaths from HIV infection among AIs and ANs (2.7 per 100,000) are substantially lower than rates for the U.S. all races population (12.6 per 100,000).[6] Current reports, however, may underestimate AIDS cases in AIs and ANs due to racial misclassification, as well as to the cultural barriers to obtaining testing, especially in small rural communities.[36,37] One study found that only 9% of AI and AN AIDS patients were diagnosed at an IHS facility. Even in states with a high percentage of AIs and ANs served by the IHS (Alaska, Arizona, New Mexico, and Oklahoma), only

43% of AIDS patients were diagnosed in an IHS facility.[37] Alternatively, the prevalence of HIV infection may be low in many AI and AN populations as a result of their relative isolation from infected non-Indian populations.

Despite low reported HIV rates among AIs, evidence suggests an increase in the incidence of the disease. A seroprevalence study conducted in 1989–1991 at 58 IHS-affiliated facilities found in three of the largely rural states that third-trimester/perinatal AI and AN patients had seropositivity rates that were four to eight times higher than had been found for childbearing women of all races in the same states.[36] Rates for urban AI and AN male patients with sexually transmitted diseases (STDs) were similar to HIV rates observed for all races in other STD surveys in western U.S. cities. The study estimated that approximately 2,700 AIs and ANs were infected with HIV by January 1992. Rates observed in the study may have exceeded what might have been expected from the largely rural locations surveyed, as well as the reported low rates of HIV infection among Indians.[37]

Risk factors for HIV among AIs and ANs also differ from other ethnic groups.[37] A smaller proportion (53%) of cases were attributed to homosexual or bisexual contact for AIs and ANs compared to whites (76%), but a higher proportion compared to blacks (35%) or Hispanics (39%). The proportion of AI and AN cases attributed to intravenous drug use among women and heterosexual men (16%) was greater than for whites (8%) but less than for blacks (38%) and Hispanics (39%). Overall, one-third of cases had risk factors associated with intravenous drug use.

The rate of reported AIDS cases in AIs and ANs has been relatively low, but studies show HIV has entered this population and cases are being diagnosed more rapidly than in any other racial or ethnic group. AIs and ANs showed the greatest increase in diagnosed AIDS cases of any racial group between 1989 and 1990. AIs had a 23.1% increase in cases compared with Hispanics at 13.3%, blacks with a 12.0% increase, whites with a 2.5% increase, and Asian/Pacific Islanders with a 8.8% decrease.[37] Elevated rates of STD infections, history of alcohol and drug use among youth, and the effects of long-term unemployment and poverty reflect an increased risk for HIV infection among AI and AN populations.[36] Once HIV is introduced into an AI or AN community, it may spread rapidly.

Morbidity Patterns

Although a great deal of morbidity is associated with the diseases discussed in the preceding sections, major causes of morbidity among AIs and ANs are infectious diseases, many of which occur much more frequently among AIs and ANs than in neighboring non-AI/AN communities.[7] AI and AN communities continue to experience adverse health effects related to infectious diseases such as TB, STDs, and diarrheal diseases. In addition, some AI and AN populations have experienced the introduction of emerging infections such as hantavirus pulmonary syndrome (HPS), *Helicobacter pylori*, and antimicrobial-resistant strains of common pathogens.

Foodborne and Diarrheal Diseases

Diarrheal diseases continue to appear at higher rates in AI communities compared to the U.S. general population. *Shigella* is a widespread cause of diarrheal illness on AI reservations, with outbreaks common and complicated by the emergence of antimicrobial-resistant strains of *Shigella* species.[38] All common *Shigella* species except *Shigella dysenteriae* have caused community-wide outbreaks since 1990. The IHS reports *Shigella* rates for inpatient hospital visits that are eight times higher than the U.S. inpatient rate of 0.2 per 10,000. Outpatient visits related to *Shigella* for the IHS were 37.6 per 10,000. No comparison data were available for outpatient visits for the U.S. general population.[38] In addition, *Shigella* is more often isolated from cases of diarrheal illness for AIs compared to the U.S. general population (T.K. Welty, unpublished report, 1986). Isolation rates for AIs were 15.3 per 100,000 isolates versus 4.7 per 100,000 for the U.S. general population.[39] Other frequent causes of diarrheal disease include *Campylobacter* and *Salmonella*. *Escherichia coli* has also been reported in some areas; however, many facilities are not routinely testing for the disease (personal communication, R.F. Fulgham, Navajo Area IHS, 1997). Less frequent, but nevertheless more common than in non-AN populations, is botulism, often associated with traditional AN fermented foods.[40]

The high rates of enteric disease can be attributed to crowded living conditions, poverty, and the shared responsibility of caring for preschool children throughout the extended family.[41] In addition, many families living on reservations do not have access to running water. Twenty percent or more of households on some reservations must haul water from a source outside their homes and store it in containers within their homes. Due to lack of abundant water, containers that allow hands to contact the water, and the inconvenience of washing hands, enteric diseases, such as shigellosis, are easily spread within households. Hauling water has been associated with the spread of *Shigella* among family members during outbreaks of the disease on reservations in the southwest (R.F. Fulgham, unpublished report, 1995). Family drinking water frequently becomes contaminated, leading to localized clusters of illness among members of the extended family (Wolsey, unpublished data).

Hepatitis A

Before the implementation of hepatitis A virus (HAV) vaccination, this disease caused large outbreaks, cycling every

5–7 years in most AI and AN communities. The overall incidence of HAV among AIs and ANs in 1992 was 10 times the rate for the U.S. white population (Cheek, unpublished data). Incidence rates of HAV in South Dakota communities have exceeded non-Indian rates by 33 times from 1990–1994 (92.6 compared to 2.8 per 100,000 per year).[41] A study of Navajo schoolchildren found prevalence rates of HAV antibodies of 70.1%, with higher rates in children at higher grade levels. This is the highest reported prevalence rate for any subpopulation of children in the United States.[42] With the introduction of HAV vaccine in 1995, AI and AN communities using the vaccine, both for routine vaccinations and containment of outbreaks, have seen remarkable reductions in incidence of this disease.[43, 44] Because of frequent outbreaks and high levels of endemic transmission, the U.S. Public Health Service Advisory Committee on Immunization Practices (ACIP) recommends that routine HAV vaccination of all 2-year-old children should be instituted for AI and AN populations.[41] In some Indian communities, implementation is currently underway, with all children ages 2–18 years of age being vaccinated (Cheek, unpublished data).

Since implementation of universal vaccination for hepatitis B virus (HBV), incidence rates among AIs and ANs have decreased remarkably. Before use of the vaccine, HBV was relatively uncommon among AIs in the contiguous United States. Seroprevalence rates among the Navajo and Sioux were reported at 1–2% compared to the crude prevalence rate of HBV infection of 5% in the U.S. general population.[45] Studies in ANs, however, showed high prevalence rates of HBV infection.[46] A seroprevalence study among ANs found an overall total seropositivity of 13.8%.[46] The total percentage of both males and females positive for HBV increases with increasing age.[46] Chronic carriage of HBV is a risk factor in the development of several diseases, including hepatocellular carcinoma; chronic active hepatitis, with or without cirrhosis; chronic glomerulonephritis; and essential mixed cryoglobulinemia.[47] In Alaska, hepatocellular carcinoma was the most commonly occurring sequelae among carriers, accounting for 57% of fatal neoplasms and 22% of all deaths. In the noncarrier AN population, hepatocellular carcinoma accounted for only approximately 2% of cancer-related deaths.[47]

Although rates of HBV for most Indian communities are relatively low, AIs and ANs are still at increased risk based on crowded living conditions and environmental conditions. In addition, an outbreak of HBV in an AI community from intravenous drug use has been reported.[45] Vaccination of children and adolescents is imperative in these communities.

Sexually Transmitted Diseases

Many AI and AN populations experience disproportionate morbidity associated with STDs.[48] Although morbidity related to gonorrhea declined from 1985 to 1988, a study from 1984–1988 of 13 states with high AI populations found gonorrhea rates of 501 per 100,000, a rate two times higher than the rate for non-Indians in the same states and 1.4 times higher than the U.S. all races rate of 349 per 100,000. Syphilis rates in the same 13 states were comparable between AIs and the U.S. general population (12.9 and 13.3 per 100,000, respectively), but compared to non-natives in the same states, AIs had more than twice the rate of disease.[48]

Surveillance data suggest that many AI and AN populations have a high prevalence of genital *Chlamydia* infections. A study in a remote Alaskan area found that 23% of all women receiving a pelvic examination for any reason tested positive for *C. trachomatis*. This rate is several times higher than the 3–5% rate previously reported among women presenting for routine care in other U.S. studies at that time.[49] More recent *Chlamydia* positivity rates obtained from surveillance data range from 2.3% to 5.6% of all *Chlamydia* tests,[50] which are similar to percentages reported by family planning clinics in the United States.[51]

Human papillomavirus (HPV) may be found frequently in some populations. A study found 10.9% of ANs seeking routine gynecologic care were positive for any HPV genotype compared to 11% found for women presenting at a STD clinic in Seattle.[52] A study from New Mexico, however, found rates of 5.8% among AIs—lower than the reported 9.2% for Hispanics and 13.4% for whites.[53] AI and AN women have a high incidence of cervical cancer, which has been linked to HPV infection.[54]

Haemophilus influenzae *Type B*

H. influenzae type B (Hib) disease has almost disappeared since widespread use of vaccination.[55] Before the introduction of the vaccine, Hib disease was documented to occur five to 10 times more in various tribes than in the general U.S. population.[56] Studies in ANs revealed an incidence of invasive Hib disease of 74.4 per 100,000 population per year compared to a non-Native rate of only 14.2.[57] In children younger than age 5 years, the incidence among Eskimos in southwest Alaska was 705 cases per 100,000 per year—the highest reported in any racial group. This compares to a rate of 37 cases per 100,000 children for the continental United States.[58] Since immunization was licensed in 1987, the incidence of invasive Hib disease in U.S. children younger than 5 years declined by 96%, with only 86 cases of Hib identified in 1995. Of those cases, five (6%) were in AIs or ANs.[55] High immunization rates are imperative to control this disease, especially among AI and AN populations that have a history of high Hib infection rates.

Zoonotic Diseases

Although some zoonotic diseases occur more often in AIs than in non-Indians, there is no evidence of increased susceptibility to infection, morbidity, or mortality from these diseases. AIs may be disproportionately represented among zoonotic diseases in the United States because they frequently reside in rural areas, living in close proximity to vector or carrier species of animals. Increases in incidence of human cases typically reflect changes in population density of carrier species or increased incidence in vector species. For example, the number of plague cases on the Navajo Reservation each year appears to be proportionate to the scope and intensity of plague in animal populations.[59]

Plague

Bubonic plague is a rare disease among humans in the United States, yet a disproportionate number of cases have occurred among AIs.[59] Plague cases averaged only one or two per year in the United States until 1965, when an outbreak of seven cases occurred on the Navajo Reservation. From 1977 to 1987, an average of 19 cases of plague per year were reported in the United States.[60] From 1950 to 1991, 29% of all cases were among AIs; of those, Navajos composed 79% of the AI cases.[60]

Hantavirus Pulmonary Syndrome

In May 1993, physicians in the Four Corners area of the southwestern United States became aware of a previously unrecognized illness that caused severe respiratory decompensation and cardiovascular collapse. Early in the outbreak, the disease, now called hantavirus pulmonary syndrome (HPS), had a 50–75% mortality rate and most noticeably affected the Navajo people.[61] Since the initial outbreak (January 1993 to July 1997), 132 cases have been identified in 28 states, with only 29 occurring in the Four Corners area. Seventy-four percent of the HPS cases have been in non-Indians compared to only 23% in AIs (unpublished data, Centers for Disease Control). The incidence rate remains disproportionately high for AIs compared to all other racial groups. Although cases in AIs have substantially declined since the outbreak of 1993, AI populations, particularly in the southwestern United States, are still considered an at-risk population. The viruses are transmitted to humans primarily by inhalation of aerosols generated from saliva, urine, and feces of rodents.[62] The ecological location and structure of many homes may make people living in these areas more likely to be in contact with rodents.

Echinococcosis (Hydatid Disease)

AIs living in Arizona and New Mexico and ANs are at increased risk of echinococcosis.[63–65] AIs experience echinococcosis attack rates much higher than non-Indian populations of Arizona and New Mexico. AIs accounted for 87.5% of the echinococcosis cases but represented less than 6% of the total population.[63] Echinococcosis granulosa infection is most common in the southwest.[64] Widespread ownership of sheep and dogs, home butchering, proximity of dogs to persons, and the Spartan living conditions increase opportunities for exposure of AIs in the southwest.[63]

Echinococcosis multilocularis is endemic in the coastal regions of northwestern Alaska. Dogs, especially when kept in close proximity to the home, are risk factors associated with transmission of E. multilocularis in the Eskimo population.[65] Mortality associated with the disease is high. In Alaska, of the first 33 patients diagnosed, 63% died. Surgical resection of the lesion can cure the disease, but the lesion in most individuals presenting with clinical symptoms is no longer resectable because of its extension in the liver and invasion of surrounding organs.[65]

Conclusion

Mortality trends for AIs and ANs have changed dramatically since the 1950s when the IHS became part of the Public Health Service. Substantial decreases in overall mortality rates have been documented, along with a shift in disease patterns from infectious diseases to chronic diseases. Although the improvements in AI and AN health in such a short time are remarkable, inequalities between Indians and the U.S. general population still remain. Indians in the United States continue to experience overall higher mortality rates. In addition, diseases that have been historically lower among AIs and ANs, such as lung cancer and cardiovascular disease, have nearly equaled, or even surpassed in some communities, those of the U.S. general population.

Although significant differences exist in morbidity and mortality trends among tribes in different geographic areas, many overall similarities remain. Heart disease, malignant neoplasms, and accidents are the three leading causes of death for all areas; however, the magnitude and ranking of these diseases may vary among tribes. The rate of diabetes, a significant cause of morbidity and mortality among Indians of the southwest, continues to increase, even in populations with historically low rates of disease. In addition, infectious diseases, although not a significant cause of mortality among AIs and ANs, continue to cause high rates of morbidity in most populations.

Patterns of morbidity and mortality among AIs and ANs are similar to those seen in other indigenous populations throughout the world. For example, the indigenous populations of Australia have death rates that are two to eight times higher compared to non-Aboriginal rates. They also experience growing numbers of noncommunicable diseases, particularly CVD and diabetes, although there has been little decline in infectious disease morbidity. CVDs have become the leading cause of death among Australian Aborigines, followed by deaths due to injury and poisoning. Similar to AIs and ANs, Aborigines experience high rates of diabetes, with 30% of the adult population diagnosed with the disease.[66] The similarities in health status between two indigenous populations a world apart undoubtedly reflect similarities in the drastic changes both have experienced as they have become more integrated into a dominant culture much different from their traditional past.

Today, AI and AN health is affected by a complex mixture of social issues, including poverty, unemployment, diet, and lifestyle. Substantial future declines in mortality rates for AIs and ANs will no longer be attained by vaccinations and medications but must involve changes in lifestyle behaviors influenced and supported by health care institutions and, most important, by the tribal community in general.

References

1. Indian Health Service. Regional Differences in Indian Health, 1996. Washington, DC: U.S. Department of Health and Human Services, Indian Health Service, Office of Planning, Evaluation, and Legislation, Division of Program Statistics, 1996.
2. Joe JR. The health of American Indian and Alaska Native women. J Am Med Womens Assoc 1996;51:141–145.
3. Kimball EH, Goldberg HI, Oberle MW. The prevalence of selected risk factors for chronic disease among American Indians in Washington State. Public Health Rep 1996;111:264–271.
4. Sugarman JR, Soderberg R, Gordon JE, Rivara FP. Racial misclassification of American Indians: its effect on injury rates in Oregon, 1989–1990. Am J Public Health 1993;86:681–684.
5. Frost F, Tollerstrup K, Ross A, et al. Correctness of racial coding of American Indians and Alaska Natives on the Washington state death certificate. Am J Prev Med 1994;10:290–294.
6. Indian Health Service. Trends in Indian Health, 1996. Washington, DC: U.S. Department of Health and Human Services, Indian Health Service, Office of Planning, Evaluation, and Legislation, Division of Program Statistics, 1997.
7. Young TK. The Health of Native Americans: Towards a Biocultural Epidemiology. New York: Oxford University Press, 1994.
8. Sievers ML, Fisher JR. Diseases of North American Indians. In HR Rothschid (ed), Biocultural Aspects of Disease. New York: Academic Press, 1981;191–252.
9. Rhoades ER. American Indians and Alaska Natives—overview of the population. Public Health Rep 1996;111(Suppl 2):49–50.
10. Pinner RW, Teutsch SM, Simonsen L, et al. Trends in infectious diseases mortality in the United States. JAMA 1996;275:189–193.
11. Wallace RB. Prevention of Chronic Illness. In JM Last, RB Wallace (eds), Public Health and Preventive Medicine. Norwalk, CT: Appleton & Lange, 1992;806.
12. Ellis JL, Campos-Outcalt D. Cardiovascular disease risk factors in Native Americans: A literature review. Am J Prev Med 1994;10:295–307.
13. Welty TK, Lee ET, Yeh J, et al. Cardiovascular disease risk factors among American Indians: The Strong Heart Study. Am J Epidemiol 1995;142:269–287.
14. Hoy W, Light A, Megill D. Cardiovascular disease in Navajo Indians with type 2 diabetes. Public Health Rep 1995;110:87–94.
15. Paisano R, Cobb N. Cancer Mortality Among American Indians and Alaska Natives in the United States: Regional Differences in Indian Health. Rockville, MD: Indian Health Service, 1997.
16. Hampton JW. The Heterogeneity of Cancer in Native American Populations. In LA Jones (ed), Minorities and Cancer. New York: Springer-Verlag, 1989;45–53.
17. Lanier AP, Blot WJ, Bender TR, Fraumeni JF Jr. Cancer in Alaskan Indians, Eskimos, and Aleuts. J Natl Cancer Inst 1980;65:1157–1159.
18. Lanier AP, Bulkow LR, Ireland B. Cancer in Alaskan Indians, Eskimos, and Aleuts, 1969–83: implications for etiology and control. Public Health Rep 1989;104:658–664.
19. Bleed DM, Risser DR, Sperry S, et al. Cancer incidence and survival among American Indians registered for Indian Health Service care in Montana, 1982–1987. J Natl Cancer Inst 1992;84:1500–1505.
20. Smith RJ. Injuries among American Indians and Alaska Natives. IHS Primary Care Provider 1990;15:1145–1147.
21. Sewell CM, Becker TM, Wiggins CL, et al. Injury mortality in New Mexico's American Indians, Hispanics and non-Hispanic whites, 1958–1982. West J Med 1989;150:708–713.
22. Gallaher MM, Fleming DW, Berger LR, Sewell CM. Pedestrian and hypothermia deaths among Native Americans in New Mexico, between bar and home. JAMA 1992;267:1345–1348.
23. Schraer CD, Adler AI, Mayer AM, et al. Diabetes complications and mortality among Alaska Natives: 8 years of observation. Diabetes Care 1997;20:314–321.
24. Gohdes D, Kaufman S, Valway S. Diabetes in American Indians: an overview. Diabetes Care 1993;16(Suppl):239–243.
25. Carter JS, Pugh JA, Monterrosa A. Non-insulin-dependent diabetes mellitus in minorities in the United States. Ann Intern Med 1996;125:221–232.
26. Gillum RF. The epidemiology of stroke in Native Americans. Stroke 1995;26:514–521.
27. Johnson S. Cirrhosis mortality among American Indian women: rates and ratio, 1975–1976. Curr Alcohol 1979;7:455–463.
28. Rhoades ER, Hammond J, Welty TK, et al. The Indian burden of illness and future health interventions. Public Health Rep 1987;102:361–368.
29. Rhoades ER. The major respiratory diseases of American Indians. Am Rev Respir Dis 1990;141:595–600.
30. Ogden M, Spector MI, Hill CA Jr. Suicides and homicides among Indians. Pub Health Rep 1970;85:75–80.
31. Shore JH. American Indian Suicide—Fact and Fantasy. Psychiatry 1975;38:86–91.
32. Paulsen HJ. Tuberculosis in the Native American: indigenous or introduced? Rev Infect Dis 1987;9:1180–1186.

33. Rieder HL. Tuberculosis among American Indians of the contiguous United States. Pub Health Rep 1989; 104:653–657.

34. Sugarman J. Tuberculosis among American Indians and Alaska Natives, 1985–1990. IHS Primary Care Provider 1991;16:186–190.

35. Centers for Disease Control and Prevention. Tuberculosis among American Indians and Alaskan Natives—United States, 1985. MMWR Morb Mortal Wkly Rep 1987;36:493–495.

36. Conway GA, Ambrose TJ, Chase E, et al. Prevalence of HIV and AIDS in American Indians and Alaska Natives. IHS Primary Care Provider 1992;17:65–70.

37. Metler R, Conway GA, Stehr-Green J. AIDS Surveillance among American Indians and Alaska Natives. Am J Public Health 1991;81:1469–1471.

38. Griffin PM, et al. Emergence of highly trimethoprim-sulfamethoxazole-resistant *Shigella* in a Native American population: An epidemiologic study. Am J Epidemiol 1989;129:1042–1051.

39. Blaser MJ, Pollard RA, Feldman RA. *Shigella* infections in the United States, 1974–1980. J Infect Dis 1983;147:771–775.

40. Shaffer N, et al. Botulism among Alaska Natives. The role of changing food preparation and consumption practices. West J Med 1990;153:390–393.

41. Welty TK, et al. Guidelines for prevention and control of hepatitis A in American Indian and Alaska Native communities. South Dakota J Med 1996;49:317–322.

42. Williams R. Prevalence of hepatitis A virus antibody among Navajo school children. Am J Public Health 1986;76:282–283.

43. McMahon BJ, et al. A program to control an outbreak of hepatitis A in Alaska by using an inactivated hepatitis A vaccine. Arch Pediatr Adolesc Med 1996;150:733–739.

44. Magnus PD. Containment of a community-wide hepatitis A outbreak using hepatitis A vaccine. IHS Primary Care Provider 1996;21:117–118.

45. Centers for Disease Control and Prevention. Hepatitis B and injecting-drug use among American Indians—Montana, 1989. MMWR Morb Mortal Wkly Rep 1992; 41:13–14.

46. McMahon BJ, Schoenberg S, Bulkow L, et al. Seroprevalence of hepatitis B viral markers in 52,000 Alaska Natives. Am J Epidemiol 1993;138:544–549.

47. McMahon BJ, Alberts SR, Wainwright RB, et al. Hepatitis B-related sequelae: prospective study in 1,400 hepatitis B surface antigen-positive Alaska Native carriers. Arch Intern Med 1990;150:1051–1054.

48. Toomey KE, Oberschelp AG, Greenspan JR. Sexually transmitted diseases and Native Americans: trends in reported gonorrhea and syphilis morbidity, 1984–88. Public Health Rep 1989;104:566–572.

49. Toomey KE, Rafferty MP, Stamm WE. Unrecognized high prevalence of *Chlamydia trachomatis* cervical infection in an isolated Alaskan Eskimo population. JAMA 1987;258:53–56.

50. Wolsey DH, Shelby LK, Cheek JE. *Chlamydia* rates in the IHS. IHS Primary Care Provider 1998;23:5–6.

51. Centers for Disease Control and Prevention. *Chlamydia trachomatis* genital infections—U.S., 1995. MMWR Morb Mortal Wkly Rep 1997;46:193–198.

52. Kiviat NB, Koutsky LA, Paavvonen JA, et al. Prevalence of genital papillomavirus infection. J Infect Dis.

53. Davidson M, Schnitzer PG, Bulkow LR, et al. The prevalence of cervical infection with human papillomaviruses and cervical dysplasia in Alaska Native women. J Infect Dis 1994;169:792–800.

54. Kenney JW. Ethnic differences in risk factors associated with genital human papillomavirus infections. J Adv Nursing 1996;23:1221–1227.

55. Centers for Disease Control and Prevention. Progress toward elimination of *Haemophilus influenzae* type b disease among infants and children—United States, 1987–1995. MMWR Morb Mortal Wkly Rep 1996;45: 901–906.

56. Santosham M, Rivin B, Wolff M, et al. Prevention of *Haemophilus influenzae* type b infections in Apache and Navajo children. J Infect Dis 1992;165(Suppl):144–150.

57. Ward JI, Lum MKW, Hall DB, et al. Invasive *Haemophilus influenzae* type b disease in Alaska: background epidemiology for a vaccine efficacy trial. J Infect Dis 1986;153:17–25.

58. Mendelman PM, Smith AL. *Haemophilus Influenzae*. In RD Feigin, JD Cherry (eds), Textbook of Pediatric Infectious Diseases. Philadelphia: Saunders, 1992; 1127.

59. Centers for Disease Control and Prevention. Plague—United States, 1992. MMWR Morb Mortal Wkly Rep 1992;41:787–790.

60. Barnes AM, Quan TJ, Beard ML, Maupin GO. Plague in American Indians, 1956–1987. MMWR Morb Mortal Wkly Rep 1988;37:11–16.

61. Simpson SQ, Jones PW, Davies, PDO, Cushing A. Social impact of respiratory infections. Chest 1995;108: 63–69.

62. Khan AS, Khabbaz RF, Armstrong LR, et al. Hantavirus pulmonary syndrome: the first 100 cases. J Infect Dis 1996;173:1297–1303.

63. Schantz PM. Echinococcosis in American Indians living in Arizona and New Mexico. Am J Epidemiol 1977;106:370–379.

64. Schantz PM, von Reyn CF, Weltz T, et al. Epidemiologic investigation of echinococcosis in American Indians living in Arizona and New Mexico. Am J Trop Med Hyg 1977;26:121–126.

65. Stehr-Green JK, Stehr-Green PA, Schantz PM, et al. Risk factors for infection with *Echinococcus multilocularis* in Alaska. Am J Trop Med Hyg 1988;38:380–385.

66. Bhatia K, Anderson P. An overview of Aboriginal and Torres Strait Islander health: present status and future trends. Canberra, Australia: Aboriginal and Torres Strait Islander Health Unit, Australian Institute of Health and Welfare, 1995.

Chapter 3
Overview of Health Programs for Canadian Aboriginal Peoples

Carol S. Locust

The major source of information included in this chapter is the *Report of the Royal Commission on Aboriginal Peoples* (1996), Volumes 1–5. Chapter 3 of Volume 3 focused on health and healing issues, which are addressed here. Volume 3 was the responsibility of Chief Justice Brian Dickson. The volume contained mandates of social and cultural dimensions and included social, cultural, and educational issues. The Royal Commission believed that all three issues had extensive impact on the health of indigenous people. Whereas each province had its own bit of health information, the Canadian federal government had all the bits of information, and spelled it out in comprehensive form in the commission's report. Other information resources were used in this chapter where appropriate.

Terminology

Non-Canadians should be aware of Canadian terminology; therefore, a brief introduction to the terms used here is in order. For example, the indigenous people of Canada are called both *indigenous* and *Aboriginal*. *Aboriginal* is always capitalized and refers, in the general sense, to organic political and cultural entities, not so-called racial characteristics. Peoples of Aboriginal origin are referred to as *Aboriginal people*. The term *First Nations* is used similarly to the terms *American Indian* and *Native American* used in the United States and refers to "registered" or "status Indians." *Inuit* refers to the people once called *Eskimos* who are also "registered." The term *Metis* refers to a distinct Aboriginal people whose early ancestors were of mixed heritage and who associate themselves with a culture that is distinctly Metis.[1] The nation of Canada includes islands, peninsulas, and contiguous continental lands divided into 12 provinces and territories: Newfoundland, Prince Edward Island, Nova Scotia, New Brunswick, Quebec,

Ontario, Manitoba, Saskatchewan, Alberta, British Columbia, Northwest Territories, and Yukon.[2] The Canadian federal government has direct responsibility only for First Nations people who are status (registered) and Inuit. Metis and nonstatus First Nations people fall under the jurisdictions of provinces or territories. Federal responsibility is directly linked to agreements made years ago with bands and nations. In general, federal responsibilities have included public and community health, medical services, and outpost services, whereas provinces and territories have provided hospital services.

Historic Review of Aboriginal Health in Canada

An estimate of the number of indigenous populations within the boundaries of what is now Canada was placed at 500,000 before European contact in the early 1400s. A census estimate of the Aboriginal population in 1871 was 102,000.[3] Before non-Aboriginal people came to the land, the inhabitants of (now) Canada had illnesses treated by practitioners of traditional medicine with indigenous plant medicines and rituals. After most of the traditional healing methods were banned as "witchcraft" and access to medicinal plants was denied, the health of indigenous people failed miserably.[4] From the end of the nineteenth century to the middle of the twentieth century, health care was provided first by an assortment of semiprofessionally trained Royal Canadian Mounted Police (RCMP), missionaries, and officers and later by a number of nurses and doctors employed by the federal government. In 1930, the first on-reserve nursing station was opened, and by 1950 the Department of National Health and Welfare operated 33 nursing stations, 65 health centers, and 18 small regional hospitals for registered Aboriginals and Inuits.[5]

Health Issues

The problem of providing Aboriginal health services has been a broad issue and has included trying to provide equitable programs and services even though the responsibility for services for all Aboriginal people has been divided between federal and provincial or territorial governments.[6] In 1986, the Canadian federal government introduced a community health demonstration program (CHDP) that served 31 areas. The problem was that although the Federal Government provided these CHDPs, only seven of the programs focused on "transfer," another government policy that had also been introduced. Meanwhile, initiatives to introduce Aboriginal control of health care were put on hold. Of course, First Nations objected, and in 1987 the CHDP, with all its faults, was over.

In 1987, the government tried to reduce its financial responsibility for First Nations and Inuit health care.[7] At issue was the provision of noninsured health benefits such as prescription drugs and eyeglasses.[8] The ensuing debate grew to include all aspects of federal policy of health care for Aboriginal people, which led to the health transfer policy. The health transfer policy is quite complicated as it is linked with land claims and self-government and is further complicated by the federal government's efforts to shed responsibility for direct services to Aboriginal peoples. Transfer included (1) community development, (2) continuing special responsibility of the federal government for the health and well-being of First Nations people and Inuits, and (3) the essential contributions of all elements of the Canadian health systems, whether federal, provincial, territorial, or municipal; Aboriginal or non-Aboriginal; public or private. Before the policy was completed, however, transfer itself had already begun. By 1989, 58 pretransfer initiatives involving 212 First Nations communities were underway, and by March 1996, 141 First Nations communities had assumed administrative responsibility for health care service, with another 237 First Nations communities involved in the pretransfer process (see Health Transfer Policy).[9]

Although Canada is often referred to as the ideal place to live because of its quality of life, there are two realities in the nation. One is for most Canadians; the other is for its Aboriginal peoples. The statistics on the first inhabitants of what is now Canada are much like the statistics for most indigenous populations who have undergone colonization: inadequate nutrition; substandard housing and sanitation; unemployment and poverty; discrimination and racism; violence; inappropriate or absent services; high rates of physical, social, and emotional illness and injury; disability; and premature death.[10, 11] To this list Goleman[12] would add "epidemic depression."

All peoples of the world who undergo colonization tend to experience three stages of health and illness patterns as they become more urbanized and industrialized. The first stage is marked by famine, high rates of infectious disease, and high death rates, especially among infants and children. The second is marked by declining rates of infectious disease and rapid population growth. The third stage is marked by the rise of chronic and degenerative diseases.[13] Canadian Aboriginal people appear to be between the second and third stages, and despite the extension of medical and social services in some form to every Aboriginal community, Aboriginal people still experience unacceptable rates of illness and distress.[14]

Infectious diseases, such as smallpox, diphtheria, polio, measles, mumps, and rubella, have declined, but tuberculosis and human immunodeficiency virus are on the rise.[15] As a whole, infectious diseases have given way to chronic diseases, such as cardiovascular disease, cancer, metabolic disorders, respiratory and digestive diseases, and especially diabetes.[16]

Diabetes has often been the result of diet changes caused by colonization. These changes came about in two ways. First, colonization created contamination of waterways, pollution of air and land, and restriction of Aboriginal peoples from traditional methods of food gathering. Second, the Aboriginal people had to adapt to new foods of the colonizers as their source of nutrition. These two situations created Aboriginal dependency on welfare payments to purchase food, and the payments were insufficient for providing adequate nutrition. Thus, improper food intake led to the rise of diabetes in Aboriginal people.[17]

Disability among Aboriginal people in 1991 was 31%—more than twice the national average.[18] Aboriginals with disabilities face inaccessible buildings such as schools, band offices, churches, homes, places of community activity, arenas, meeting halls, and sites for recreation. The choice of staying with the band or leaving to seek services away from relatives, friends, and familiar surroundings is a difficult one.[19]

Inuit children have especially high rates of otitis media. As many as 80% of Inuit children show evidence of current infection or scarring. In one community, one child in 10 had permanent hearing loss, and in another community one child in five was found to be at least partly deaf.[20]

Among researchers studying addictions, depressive and suicidal behaviors, family violence, and other social pathologies, there is endless argument about their causes. Aboriginal people have no doubt about the cause; they say that the destruction of their ways of life, including multifaceted rupture of their spiritual ties to the land, is a major factor.[21, 22] Other factors are poor nutrition, poverty, stress, poor housing, guilt over cultural losses, grief (individual or collective) over Aboriginal spiritual and cultural losses, and powerlessness to help oneself or others.[23] Continuing research may shed light on the causes of other alarming statistics: Indigenous males die from motor vehicle accidents at three times the national male rate. Other accidents occur 50% more often, death from fire is twice the national rate, drowning is six times the national average, suicide is 3½ times greater, and poisoning of Aboriginal males is twice the national rate of non-Aboriginal averages.[24]

The National Native Alcohol and Drug Abuse Program provides 400 communities with alcohol prevention and treatment centers, 51 regional residential centers, and basic training to prepare Aboriginal staff to deliver most of these services.[25]

Rekindling of spiritual and social traditions of Aboriginal people is one way to restore health and respect for cultures.[26] Research indicates that several other factors are probably more significant than public care systems, however, such as improved economic conditions; enhanced social, psychological, and spiritual well-being; improved environmental conditions; and research on the role of genetic inheritance in such diseases as diabetes, heart disease, alcoholism, and other chronic and degenerative diseases.[27]

Health Transfer Policy

The Indian Health Transfer Policy was announced in 1986 by Health and Welfare Canada (now called Health Canada), Medical Services Branch, Indian and Northern Health Services Directorate. Its origin, however, was much earlier and occurred within the context of historical conflicts between the federal government and Canada's indigenous populations. In 1969, Prime Minister Pierre Trudeau introduced a "White Paper" that advocated assimilation of Aboriginal people by diminishing and devaluing the special legal and constitutional status inherent in the treaties with Aboriginal groups.[28] Aboriginal Canadians rejected the White Paper.[29] Another Indian health policy was established in 1979 in an attempt to achieve better levels of health in Indian communities through greater involvement from community members.[29] The Indian health transfer policy was designed in 1986 to make that program workable.

The transfer required a process that (1) stayed inside the budget, (2) slowly shifted responsibility to indigenous communities, and (3) set up federal block grants for provinces to use to administer the programs.[29]

The health transfer policy has the following 12 goals[30]:

1. To operate within current legislation.
2. To be optional but available to communities within provincial boundaries.
3. To permit health program control to be taken on at a pace determined by community needs and management capacity.
4. To include resources for community health programs currently delivered by Health Canada, with the exception of noninsured health services. Some noninsured health services are now being negotiated in some transfer agreements.
5. To enable communities to design health programs to meet their needs and to allocate funds according to community health priorities, provided that mandatory program requirements are met and capital funds are used for capital purposes only.
6. To provide resources for ongoing health management structures at the community level.
7. To permit multiyear agreements, not exceeding 5 years, that would be subject to annual appropriations with defined methods for annual price and volume adjustments.
8. To allow communities to retain unspent balances for health-related purposes and place on communities the responsibility to eliminate deficits.
9. To transfer to communities all movable capital assets associated with operating the health services included in the transfer agreement.
10. To require annual comprehensive financial program audits and schedule evaluation of the transfer process at specified intervals.
11. To implement new financial and program mechanisms to define the accountability of Chiefs and Councils to the community and to the Minister of Health Canada and also the accountability of the Minister of Health Canada to the Parliament. These mechanisms are needed to ensure responsible financial management and overall program results.
12. To provide a mechanism for intervention in the event of a health emergency or the inability of a community to meet its financial or health program commitments.

The programs and services eligible for transfer are nursing, community health representatives, health education, nutrition, dental therapy, medical and dental service and dental assistants, environmental health services, alcohol and drug abuse programs, home nursing, mental health, solvent abuse, and the program "Brighter Futures." Additional options and other alternatives are open for discussion to transfer.[29]

Despite the inherent problems in transferring federal responsibility and funds to provinces, it does have worth in that indigenous communities and bands will be able to direct their own services. Although federal monetary responsibility shrinks, however, federal jurisdiction over programs does not.[29] Another problem is that the initial budget will be less than provincial funding was in 1996. Also, the block funds are for 5-year periods, in which there are no budget changes. The budget[31] was written to save $1.9 billion in 1998–1999 by cost-cutting strategies. The savings for health care between 1996 to 1999 will be $40 million, and $103 million for Indian and Northern Affairs.

The Royal Commission on Aboriginal Health believes that the inherent rights of Aboriginal self-government are recognized and affirmed in section 35(1) of the Constitution Act of 1982. However, it will take time for both sides (Aboriginal and non-Aboriginal people) to recognize the full implication of partnership. Many Aboriginal people are unsure about transfer. Some think it might be a step toward termination of indigenous rights and services, whereas others say that although the transfer does give indigenous people responsibility for programs, their accountability to and dependence on the federal government remains unchanged. Also, in light of the intended cutbacks in federal spending, some think it is a continuation of the federal government's historic strategy to effect spending cutbacks to First Nations. Funding cycles of 5 years in block funding arrangements suggest that there are reasons to fear that downsizing of programs before transfer will reduce the funds that are actually transferred.[29]

The current paradigm shift in health care confirms the resonance between biomedical research and Aboriginal philosophies of health and healing. The new strategy calls for a reorganization of health and social service delivery through a system of healing centers and lodges under Aboriginal control, an Aboriginal human resources development strategy, the adaptation of mainstream services, training and professional systems to affirm the participation of Aboriginal people, and initiation of an infrastructure to address the pressing problems related to clean water, safe waste management, and adequate housing. The healing centers and lodges will benefit from federal, provincial, and territorial government collaborations with Aboriginal nations, organizations, or communities. The healing centers will provide direct services; referral and access to specialist services; will be part of a network of healing lodges that provide residential services oriented to family and community healing; will provide health and social services in culturally appropriate forms; and will make the network available to First Nations, Inuit, and Metis communities in rural and urban settings on an equitable basis.[32]

Conclusion

Canadian Aboriginal peoples exist with third, second, and first world country health statistics. Third world conditions of famine, infectious diseases, and early death still exist in remote territories. Second world statistics of declining rates of infectious diseases and rapid population increase are prevalent, but first world conditions of rising chronic and degenerative diseases are epidemic. Chronic diseases, such as cardiovascular disease, cancer, metabolic disorders, respiratory and digestive diseases, and diabetes, are decimating the Aboriginal populations of Canada nationwide. Health professionals working with Canadian Aboriginal peoples must necessarily be concerned with the broader implications of health, including social, cultural, economic, and educational issues, and the

overriding concerns of epidemic depression related to grief, loss, anger, and helplessness. These are very complex issues, especially with respect to federal and provincial jurisdictions, provincial regionalization and federal transfer, and status vs. nonstatus and Metis benefits. The transfer process itself with "status" groups is very complicated; there are several ways in which transfer can take place and each is quite individualized. Also, continual changes are being made to both the health transfer process for the status groups and regionalization in each of the provinces and territories. Thus, a comprehensive definition of *transfer* is very difficult. The bottom line is that provincial and federal governments both are trying to get out of the business of providing services. There does appear to be an answer, however: a multifaceted network of programs, in each Aboriginal community—possibly the healing centers—developed and run by Aboriginal people that would address all of the preceding issues.

During the National Health Forum of 1997,[33] the establishment of an Aboriginal Health Institute was proposed to specifically address the preceding issues. The institute would focus on health issues, serve as a support network for Aboriginal health workers in communities, perform and advocate an evidence-based approach in health research to meet the needs of Aboriginal peoples through improved health information, and would, perhaps most important, assist in the sharing of information within and outside of Aboriginal communities.

In its report, the Royal Commission revealed a federal plan—transfer—that would address all the issues, perhaps using the Aboriginal Health Institute as the vehicle with healing centers as community locations. However one looks at the task, it is as awesome as it is magnificent—both intimidating and costly. If healing of body, mind, and spirit of the Aboriginal peoples of Canada is not accomplished, and accomplished quickly, the twenty-first century may see them vanish.

References

1. Canadian Government. Report of the Royal Commission on Aboriginal Peoples. Minister of Supply and Services, Ottawa. Vol. 1, p. xii. Hereafter, RRCAP.
2. Canadian Government. Finance Department. Getting Government Right Budget Chart Book. 1996, pp. 1–15. http//www.fin.gc.ca/budget96/binbe/binb8e.html.
3. RRCAP, Vol. 1, p. 13.
4. RRCAP, Vol. 3, p. 112.
5. RRCAP, Vol. 3, p. 114.
6. RRCAP, Vol. 3, p. 151.
7. RRCAP, Vol. 3, p. 117.
8. RRCAP, Vol. 3, p. 151.
9. RRCAP, Vol. 3, p. 117.
10. RRCAP, Vol. 3, p. 107.

11. Duran E, Duran B. Native American Postcolonial Psychology. Albany, NY: State University of New York Press, 1995;101.
12. Goleman D. Emotional Intelligence. New York: Bantam Books, 1997;240.
13. RRCAP, Vol. 3, p. 125.
14. RRCAP, Vol. 3, p. 119.
15. RRCAP, Vol. 3, p. 137.
16. RRCAP, Vol. 3, pp. 143–146.
17. RRCAP, Vol. 3, p. 147.
18. RRCAP, Vol. 3, pp. 148–119.
19. RRCAP, Vol. 3, p. 150.
20. RRCAP, Vol. 3, p. 151.
21. RRCAP, Vol. 3, p. 195.
22. Davis R, Zannis M. The Genocide Machine in Canada: The Pacification of the North. Montreal: Black Rose Books, 1973;179.
23. RRCAP, Vol. 3, p. 131.
24. RRCAP, Vol. 3, p. 153.
25. RRCAP, Vol. 3, p. 161.
26. RRCAP, Vol. 3, p. 213.
27. RRCAP, Vol. 3, p. 216.
28. Angus M. And the Last Shall Be First. Toronto: NC Press Ltd, 1990;38.
29. Misener M. The Transfer Policy in First Nations communities: what does it mean for outpost nursing? Outpost Horizons 1997;2:7, 9, 11.
30. Canadian Government. Health Canada. Health Services Branch. Ottawa, 1995;16–17.
31. Canadian Government. Finance Department. Budget Chart Sheet for Action to Get Government Right Program. Ottawa, 1996;1–5.
32. RRCAP, Vol. 3, p. 247.
33. Canadian Government. National Forum on Health 1997. The Need For an Aboriginal Health Institute in Canada: Report of the Meeting. Ottawa, 1997;1–8.

Chapter 4

The Native American Population: Origins, Distribution, and Diversity

T. Kue Young

The origins and evolution of the indigenous populations of the Americas are steeped in controversy and uncertainty. The weight of the archaeologic, genetic, and anthropologic evidence points to an Asiatic origin, which is not in serious dispute in the scientific community.[1] This view, however, is challenged by some traditionalist Native Americans who maintain a literal interpretation of creationist legends that they had been in the Americas since time immemorial. A considerable diversity of opinions exists within the scientific community with respect to the date of the migration, the number of waves of migrations, the points of entry, and the time required to populate the entire land mass from the Arctic slope of Alaska to the tip of South America.

At the time of the arrival of Europeans—Norsemen in the northeast during the eleventh century and Italo-Iberian explorers in the late fifteenth century in central America—the Native American population already consisted of a large number of linguistic and cultural entities and had differentiated into social structures that ranged from egalitarian nomadic hunter-gatherers to highly stratified empires with aristocracies and slaves. Native Americans migrated to and settled in ecologically diverse habitats from the frozen tundra in the far north to the hot, dry desert in the southwest.

Genetic and Cultural Diversity

Physical anthropologists in the nineteenth and early twentieth centuries devoted considerable energy to describing and measuring various physical traits among Native Americans—for example, hair color, texture, and distribution; cranial and facial dimensions; anthropometric indices; epicanthic folds; skin pigmentation; dermatoglyphic patterns; and dental morphology. The development of modern biochemical genetics led to the recognition of a variety of inherited biochemical traits, the

distribution of which has been used to delineate the divergence and affinity between populations. Examples include the inactivation of the drug isoniazid, the ability to taste phenylthiocarbamide, the presence of enzyme variants, and the capacity to secrete specific chemicals in the urine and saliva. A large body of data has also been accumulated on polymorphisms of blood groups and other genetic markers, such as HLA and serum proteins, which can be used to determine the "relatedness" between Native Americans and the other races, and among Native Americans.[2]

Native American languages offer some clues to the genetic relationship of the different population groups. Whereas language per se is not inherited (although most of us do learn our mother tongue from genetically related family members), the process of genetic differentiation is akin to that of linguistic differentiation as a people migrates into and populates new lands. There are hundreds of mutually unintelligible Native American languages in North America, which can be grouped into larger families. There is, however, no agreement among linguists on the precise number and classification of distinct Native American languages. One radical scheme proposed that all Amerindian languages were ultimately derived from three stocks: Amerind, Na-Dene, and Aleut-Eskimo, corresponding to three separate migrations from North Asia.[3]

Cultural anthropologists have divided Native American populations into culture areas, which are contiguous geographic regions and reflect the shared ecological habitat, subsistence pattern, social organization, and religious beliefs and practices of the inhabitants. According to the authoritative handbook series on Native Americans published by the Smithsonian Institution, there are 10 culture areas in North America: arctic, subarctic, northwest coast, great basin, California, plateau, plains, southwest, southeast, and northeast.[4]

The arctic culture area, stretching across the top of the continent, is characterized by the treeless tundra and is inhabited by the Eskimo/Inuit and Aleuts, who subsisted on fishing and hunting of sea mammals (seals, walruses, whales) along the coast and caribou hunting in the interior.

The subarctic, which extends from the interior of Alaska to the Atlantic coast, is dominated by the boreal forest. Athapaskan and Algonkian Indians lived as nomadic hunters of large game such as moose and caribou and fished from the large number of lakes and rivers.

On the northwest coast, from southern Alaska to Oregon, the mild climate and bountiful coastal resources, particularly salmon, supported a large number of socially complex, sedentary villages of the Haidan, Tsimshian, Tlingit, Salishan, and Wakashan speaking peoples.

The plateau culture area in inland British Columbia, Washington, and Idaho was inhabited by Salishan and Kutenaian speakers, who fished salmon from the inland rivers.

The northeast encompasses the woodlands around the Great Lakes, the St. Lawrence River valley, and the Atlantic seaboard. Horticulture, especially of maize, beans, and pumpkins, was developed by various Iroquoian and Algonkian tribes. The Iroquoians also instituted the largest political units north of Mexico.

In the southeast, mostly Muskogean speakers lived in a rich, fertile region that once supported the Mississippian culture, with its huge temple mounds and large, cultivated fields.

The grassy plains occupy the central part of the continent, where Siouans and Caddoans hunted buffalo, a lifestyle that was fundamentally altered by the introduction of horses by the Spaniards.

The arid and dry great basin, which includes all of Nevada, Utah, and surrounding areas, was inhabited mainly by tribes belonging to the Uto-Aztecan language family. They led a rather precarious existence by gathering nuts, digging for wild vegetables, and hunting small game.

Although much of the southwest is dry desert, villages were founded along streams by people of the Uto-Aztecan and Yuman language families, who were probably descendants of the highly developed agricultural society of the Mogollon and Anasazi cultures. Around the tenth century, the Athapaskans (represented by the Navajo and Apache), who had retained their ancestral languages but adopted the culture of surrounding tribes, migrated from northern Canada and Alaska.

The diverse peoples of the California culture area led a settled village life and had the densest population north of Mexico, although they did not practice agriculture. Their main food was prepared from pounding acorns into meal.

The indigenous cultures of Native Americans were drastically reshaped by the arrival of Europeans, often referred to as *contact*. Although individual tribes differ in their experience, they follow a general pattern. Early contact occurred either directly with explorers, traders, and missionaries, or indirectly with goods traded through neighboring tribes. This was soon superseded by a period of displacement by, and conflict with, new settlers, often accompanied by epidemics and warfare. Ultimately, Native Americans came under the domination of the United States and Canadian governments and were incorporated into the modern economy.[5, 6]

Historical Change

The size of the Native American population in North America before the arrival of Europeans will never be known accurately, although estimates abound. These range from approximately 1 million to as high as 18 million.[7] What is not in dispute is that after contact, most groups experienced a decline in population, the result of depressed fertility and increased mortality from epidemics of introduced diseases, starvation, and warfare. Historic demographer Russell Thornton estimated the population in the area that was to become the 48 states; from about 5 million inhabitants at the beginning of the sixteenth century, the Native American population was halved approximately every 100 years and reached its lowest point toward the end of the nineteenth century, when they numbered less than 5% of the population at contact.[8]

At the beginning of the twentieth century, the Native American population began to recover, with the birth rate eventually overtaking the death rate. It was also in the 1900s that the United States and Canadian national censuses began to tally the number of Native Americans, making it possible to track the growth of this population. At the beginning of the century, just under 400,000 Native Americans were identified in the two countries. This number grew to 550,000 at mid-century, and to just under 2 million in the 1980s.[7] Although there are methodologic problems with enumeration and identification, the increase has been phenomenal and can be attributed to improving health status and the assurance of basic economic security.

Present Population Distribution

United States

According to the 1990 U.S. Census, there were approximately 1.96 million Native Americans in the United States—approximately 0.8% of the total population of the country.[9, 10] Approximately 22% of Native Americans lived on reservations and tribal trust lands, 10% in tribal jurisdiction areas in Oklahoma, 3% in tribal designated areas in other states, and 2% in Alaska Native villages. The 10 largest reservations accounted for almost 50% of the population of all reservation Indians. They are, in descending order of population size: the Navajo Reservation, with

143,400 people located in the border regions of Arizona, Utah, and New Mexico; the Pine Ridge, South Dakota, Reservation (Oglala Sioux), with 11,200; and various reservations with populations in the 7,000–10,000 range (Fort Apache, Gila River, Papago, San Carlos, Zuni Pueblo, and the Hopi reservations in Arizona; and the Rosebud, South Dakota, and Blackfeet, Montana, reservations).

The Native American population in the United States has become increasingly urbanized. In 1990, 51% of the population lived in metropolitan areas. The 10 metropolitan areas with the largest Native population were, in descending order: Tulsa, Oklahoma (48,000); Oklahoma City, Oklahoma (46,000); Los Angeles-Long Beach, California (44,000); Phoenix, Arizona (38,000); Seattle-Tacoma, Washington (33,000); Riverside-San Bernadino, California (26,000); New York City, New York (25,000); Minneapolis-St Paul, Minnesota (23,000); San Diego, California (22,000); and San Francisco-Oakland, California (21,000).

The present distribution of Native Americans reflects the consequences of the historic "opening up" of the country for settlement. In 1990, more than half of the Native American population lived in six Western states: Oklahoma (252,000), California (242,000), Arizona (204,000), New Mexico (134,000), Alaska (86,000), and Washington (81,000). Only three states among the top 10 states with the largest Native American populations are east of the Mississippi River: North Carolina (80,000), New York (63,000), and Michigan (56,000).

Canada

According to the 1991 Census, just more than 1 million Canadians claimed some Aboriginal (the preferred term in Canada) origins—approximately 4% of the country's population.[11, 12] Among the million Aboriginal people, 481,000 reported exclusive Aboriginal origins, while 522,000 had mixed Aboriginal and non-Aboriginal origins. Among those with exclusive Aboriginal origin, 78% were North American Indians (the preferred term is now *First Nations*), 6% Inuit, and 16% Metis. Metis are the descendants of European-Indian mixed marriages, particularly in the west, and are recognized by the Canadian Constitution as a culturally distinct Aboriginal group.

Aboriginal people were the majority in only one jurisdiction—the Northwest Territories, where they accounted for 62% of the population. The Yukon had the second largest proportion, with 23%. In the provinces, Aboriginals represented approximately 10% of the population of Manitoba and Saskatchewan, approximately 6% in Alberta and British Columbia, but only 2% in central and eastern Canada. Within the Aboriginal population itself, almost one in four resided in the largest province, Ontario.

More than half of the Aboriginal population lived in urban areas. Winnipeg and Montreal each had approximately 45,000 Aboriginal residents, Vancouver and Edmonton with 43,000 each, Toronto 40,000, Ottawa-Hull 31,000, and Calgary 24,000. In terms of the proportion of the total population in each metropolitan area, however, Aboriginal people constituted a large and highly visible minority in the cities of western Canada: approximately 7% in Winnipeg, Regina, and Saskatoon and 5% in Edmonton.

According to the Department of Indian Affairs, which maintains an Indian Register containing Aboriginal people with legally recognized Indian status, there were 512,000 "registered Indians" in Canada, less than 60% of whom resided in an Indian reserve. Canadian *reserves* are generally much smaller in population than *reservations* in the United States (note the slight difference in terminology). Only three reserves had populations exceeding 5,000: Kahnawake (Mohawk) in Quebec, Six Nations in Ontario, and the Blood reserve in Alberta.

Conclusion

Native American populations have a long history that predates the arrival of Europeans. They are genetically and culturally diverse and adapted to the wide-ranging ecological habitats across the continent. After initial depopulation as a result of imported diseases and economic displacement, the population has steadily recovered from its lowest point at the beginning of the twentieth century. Today, there are approximately 3 million Americans and Canadians who report some Native ancestry—approximately 1% of the total population of the two countries. The unique health needs of this minority population require special knowledge and understanding by health care providers—a task that this book is intended to achieve.

References

1. Fagan BM. The Great Journey: The Peopling of Ancient America. New York: Thames and Hudson, 1987.
2. Cavollo-Sforza LL, Menozzi P, Piazza A. The History and Geography of Human Genes. Princeton, NJ: Princeton University Press, 1994.
3. Greenberg JH, Turner CG, Zegura SL. The settlement of the Americas: a comparison of the linguistic, dental and genetic evidence. Current Anthropology 1986;27: 447–497.
4. Sturtevant WC (ed). Handbook of North American Indians. Washington, DC: Smithsonian Institution, 1978–1990 [20 volumes projected, nine volumes already published].
5. Trigger BG, Washburn WE (eds). The Cambridge History of the Native Peoples of the Americas. Vol 1. North America. New York: Cambridge University Press, 1996.
6. Waldram JB, Herring DA, Young TK. Aboriginal Health in Canada: Historical, Cultural and Epidemio-

logical Perspectives. Toronto: University of Toronto Press, 1995.

7. Verano JW, Ubelaker DH (eds). Disease and Demography in the Americas. Washington, DC: Smithsonian Institution Press, 1992.

8. Thornton R. American Indian Holocaust and Survival: A Population History Since 1942. Norman, OK: University of Oklahoma Press, 1987.

9. Sandefur GD, Rindfuss RR, Barney Cohen (eds). Changing Numbers, Changing Needs: American Indian Demography and Public Health. Washington, DC: National Academy Press, 1996.

10. U.S. Bureau of the Census. We the First Americans. Washington, DC: Racial Statistics Branch, Population Division, 1993.

11. Young TK. The Health of Native Americans: Towards a Biocultural Epidemiology. New York: Oxford University Press, 1994.

12. Statistics Canada. Profile of Canada's Aboriginal Population. Ottawa: Statistics Canada, 1995.

Chapter 5

Public Health, Prevention, and Primary Care in American Indian and Alaska Native Communities

W. Craig Vanderwagen

The prevention of illness in American Indian (AI) and Alaska Native (AN) communities has been a significant element of federal, tribal, and urban Indian health policy and practice throughout the twentieth century. Prevention will continue to be a central focus of health activities well into the twenty-first century, if not longer. Prevention efforts may in fact become the primary focus of health activities in AI and AN communities as the communities take greater control of health delivery programs and resources.

The major prevention efforts of the twentieth century in AI and AN communities were designed and provided as part of a holistic approach to health care. This approach resonates with traditional community values held by the population served. These efforts reflect the commonly held goal in federal, tribal, and urban Indian programs to elevate the health status of AIs and ANs to the highest possible level. This chapter briefly reviews the historic and intellectual basis for prevention efforts in AI and AN communities as delivered through federal and tribal health programs. It describes some outcomes of these efforts and examines the contemporary and future prevention challenges confronting these communities.

The historic approach to health service delivery by federal programs may be characterized as a system of community-oriented primary care programs. This approach can be further described as the delivery of clinical medicine and other health services guided by epidemiologic and social examination of the environment of patients and their communities. In this model, the determination of health resource investment and individual provider effort is not simply targeted to the health conditions that present as individual patient encounters. Assessment is the cornerstone on which health delivery choices are made. This approach to assessment should include the measurement of the total patient population to be served, evaluation of the health needs of that population, and a description of the resources available or required to address these health needs.[1]

Accordingly, the individual providers work with a broader set of health workers and community members to identify health goals, plan, and implement programs of health services that integrate facility-based clinical care activities with strong community-based prevention efforts. The clinical providers, community health workers, and community members are bound to a common set of goals for the health activity and have definable roles in achieving these goals.[2] The effort made by Indian communities to reduce infant mortality is instructive because it was accomplished with great success.

During the 1940s and 1950s, the infant mortality rates of AI and AN communities were two- and threefold the infant mortality rates in the general U.S. population. In 1955, for example, aggregate infant mortality in Indian communities was reported as 62.7 deaths per 1,000 live births compared to a rate in the U.S. general population of 26.4 deaths per 1,000 live births.[3] This was in large measure attributable to the impact of infectious diseases.

Of particular concern was dehydration associated with gastroenteritis in very early childhood. Pediatricians, public health professionals, and parents were greatly troubled by this situation. Assessment of the factors causing these circumstances and identification of potential solutions to the problems were conducted in a variety of Indian communities. Waterborne diseases were identified as a common cause of the problem. Vaccine-preventable diseases were also noted to be a common cause of illness. Early intervention through simple home-based fluid therapies was also noted to be potentially life saving once a child was observed to have gastroenteritis.

Action plans were designed and implemented on a number of fronts. Pediatricians developed effective approaches to oral rehydration therapy that could be used by parents in home settings. Parents were informed about the early signs of disease and how they could provide early treatment at home. This approach gave greater control to the family and often meant that a child seen by the pediatrician did not need heroic resuscitation efforts to survive. Community and public health sector advocacy for access to clean water and the safe handling of sewage resulted in funding of programs to install water and sewer systems previously unavailable to most AI and AN communities. The communities were also provided extensive information about the prevention of many childhood illnesses through implementation of an effective program of well-child care and childhood immunization. The communities have accepted and supported widespread outreach activities to ensure that children are appropriately immunized.

This example illustrates the integration of community prevention and clinical service that characterizes community-oriented primary care. It also illustrates the categories or types of prevention activities that have been used in Indian communities. The prevention efforts may be primary, secondary, or tertiary in nature depending on the health issue and the resources available.

Primary prevention services include immunization or the provision of safe water designed to prevent occurrence of the adverse health conditions. Secondary prevention efforts target the prevention of sequelae of a disease once the disease has been diagnosed. Rehydration approaches to gastroenteritis and diarrhea exemplify secondary prevention. Tertiary prevention is aimed at ameliorating the end-stage or end-organ effects of a disease and ensuring survival, such as cardiac resuscitation in extreme dehydration.

Another feature of this effort and success was the development of local capacity to address the health problem. Technical skills were needed at the community level both in the form of pediatric staff and sanitation engineering. Programmatic skills were also needed to design and implement a comprehensive water and sewage-handling system as well as a system of maternal and child health care. Financial and management skills were needed to ensure that new water systems would be adequately financed and installed. Finally, political skills were needed to bring about the commitment of the community and congressional leadership to fund these activities. Many community members were educated and given leadership roles for addressing this challenge. Other skills were imported until local community members were able to assume these roles.[1,2]

It can be seen from these descriptions that there is a distinct overlap between community-based primary prevention and the clinical treatment efforts of providers. Indeed, there is a continuum of prevention activity that engages all aspects of the health team. The common goal is the elevation of the health status of the population.

This approach was predicated on assessment of health status. Assessment allows all individuals involved to identify the scope of the health issues and identify options in managing these problems. The sources of information for this assessment are many and can be quite complex. The information sources must be defined and appropriately maintained if a successful health outcome is expected.[4]

The first and most critical sources of information are community perceptions of what the problems are. These are reflected in the issues brought to community political leadership and the health managers in the community. The information may be supported by other information sources, or it may be idiosyncratic. An example of such information may be complaints about poor dump management because disposable diapers are being blown out of a solid waste site into someone's yard. Although this does not appear to be a measurable data point, it must be addressed or community confidence in the health system and political leadership will be compromised.

Another more measurable pool of information arises from the workload and morbidity data of the health providers. This would be typified by the number of visits to a particular type of provider (e.g., dentist, pharmacist, or physician) or the types of diagnoses recorded at a clinic (e.g., upper respiratory illness, well-child care, or diabetes). This data pool informs the community about the events that drive the daily demand for health care. This information does not inform about the causes of life-threatening disease that burden the community, and it is limited to the segments of the population that use a particular source of care. It does, however, provide information on illness or disease that motivates people to seek care.

The most frequently used information for the assessment of health status is vital events (birth and death) data. These data are provided through states for all Indian people irrespective of source of health care. Thus, it is not limited to those in a community who may use a particular clinic. There are shortcomings in the use of these data in that numerous studies have indicated that underreporting of Indian deaths is quite common. Notwithstanding, the foundations of epidemiology are in the reporting and analysis of birth and death events.

Taken together, this information on health status can be most useful in targeting services and interventions as noted in the preceding paragraphs and used in measuring progress. Using these strategies, the programs funded by the Indian Health Service (IHS) have made significant changes in the health status of Indian people in the last half of the twentieth century. Infant mortality declined by 60% between 1972 and 1974 and 1991 and 1993 (IHS uses 3-year averages to adjust for a smaller population).[3] Deaths due to selected diseases have declined significantly as well. Deaths due to unintentional injuries have declined by 56% in the same period. Deaths due to tuberculosis declined by 80%, and deaths due to gastroenteric diseases declined by 76%. Life expectancy has increased from 63.5 years to 73.2 years in this period. The result has been a rapidly expanding population of AIs and ANs and a rapidly changing set of health problems.

The issues affecting this population are changing along two dimensions. One dimension is the change in health problems of the population. The second is the instability of resources for health services that confronts Indian communities. The first issue is one of focus and the other is one of tools available to address the issues. Both will have significant impact on the future health status of AI and AN people.

The diseases that cause death among this population have shifted to lifestyle-related illnesses. No longer are infectious diseases the primary concern. The leading causes of death now are associated with preventable risk factors such as diet and exercise control, tobacco use, motor vehicle accidents, and diseases not preventable by vaccine. A review by Golaz et al. revealed that lifestyle choices of individuals regarding diet, exercise, tobacco use, alcohol use, use of firearms, and automobile safety contributed to 40% of all deaths.[5] This is reflected in the increasing percentage of Indian deaths associated with heart disease, cancers of various types, and various forms of violence (both intentional and unintentional).

The target population for intervention has changed as well. Whereas excess infant mortality was a major factor in shortened life expectancy, premature deaths are now occurring predominantly in adolescents and young adults. In addition, lifestyle behaviors developing in this age group may have devastating effects in the future. For example, the IHS dental program conducted an oral health survey in 1991 that revealed, among other things, that 40% of individuals seeking dental care between the ages of 20 and 34 years reported that they were regular tobacco users.[6] Clearly, interventions to prevent illness should account for this age group.

This shift in disease patterns is also important because there was a lower cost for the public health interventions associated with the decline of vaccine-preventable diseases and other interventions that reduced infant mortality and deaths related to infectious diseases. The emerging disease patterns are associated with very high costs for treatment, and in many diseases, there are no proven primary prevention interventions. The Indian communities will be embarking on a search for primary prevention interventions that are effective and chart new terrain, which is a costly venture.

In the past, for example, public health nurses could seek out and immunize children relatively inexpensively. Today, public health nurses and community health representatives need to identify families at risk for diabetes and other lifestyle diseases. Then, working with the families, they must implement a lifelong prevention effort that may involve constant diet and exercise management and monitoring. This is not an inexpensive investment, and there is no guarantee that it will prevent illness. It is also difficult to maintain community enthusiasm, support, and sustained effort since the "payoff" will only be known 20 years later, given the nature of the disease. This is in contrast to efforts to reduce infant mortality rates; reductions in infant deaths are measurable within months or a few years rather than decades.

Other health issues, such as intentional violence-related morbidity and mortality, are not amenable to patient-driven health solutions. The roots of such "health" problems are in economic adversity or poor social conditions. The strategies for improving health status require engagement of a wider variety of community resources. This would include engagement of the educational, law enforcement, and judicial resources of the community. It would also require full engagement of any financial expertise available to the community (e.g., banking and investment firms).[7]

Health care providers must assume a strong role in such issues. There is a belief that because there is no medical solution, it must be addressed by others in the community. However, health care providers are the front-line managers of the sequelae of these social failures. The advocacy that health care workers can provide and the energy and successful experience with team building in the community to address these issues demand engagement by the providers. Again, the model interface of clinical care concerns and community public health principles must be used if the outcome is to be successful.

Assessment information must be provided to the stakeholders at the community and national levels. Policy options for local and national action must be clarified. Finally, local capacity to address the issues must be built and stabilized to ensure that health issues are addressed. This strategy has brought about significant improvements in the health of AIs and ANs and holds the potential for continued elevation of the health status of this unique and important population.

References

1. Institute of Medicine, Committee on the Future of Public Health. The Future of Public Health. Washington, DC: National Academy Press, 1988.
2. Clark EG, Leavell HR. Preventive Medicine for the Doctor in His Community (3rd ed). New York: McGraw-Hill, 1965.
3. Indian Health Service. Trends in Indian Health, 1996. Washington, DC: U.S. Department of Health and Human Services, Indian Health Service, Office of Planning, Evaluation, and Legislation, Division of Program Statistics, 1997.
4. Feinstein AR. Clinical Judgement. Huntington, NY: Robert Kreiger Publishing, 1967.
5. Golaz A, Paisano R, Cobb N. Preventable Causes of Death Among Native Americans: A Tool for Setting Priorities for Public Health Action. Unpublished, 1997.
6. Indian Health Service Dental Program. The Oral Health of Native Americans. Albuquerque, NM: U.S. Department of Health and Human Services, Indian Health Service, 1994.
7. Indian Health Service. Profile of the State of Indian Children and Youth. Silver Spring, MD: Support Services International, 1997.

Chapter 6
Traditional Indian Medicine

Walter B. Hollow

In pre-Columbian times, traditional Indian medicine (TIM) was a health care system that met the physical, mental, and spiritual health needs of Indian people (Figure 6-1). European contact with Indians in the Americas and the subsequent establishment of the U.S. government affected TIM in many ways.

In the early contact period, TIM was openly practiced by Indians and was their sole source of health care. In 1887, the U.S. Congress passed the Dawes' Act, making it illegal for Indians to practice TIM. TIM was covertly practiced by Indian people from 1887 until 1978, when the Indian Religious Freedom Act made it legal for Indians to use TIM. But most western practitioners are unaware of Indian patients who currently use TIM but who may still be reluctant to disclose that information to their western practitioner. Currently, TIM holds a place of high respect among tribes throughout the United States. The majority of the nation's 2 million Indians, both on and off reservations, consult traditional healers for their health problems.

Clinical Implications of Traditional Indian Medicine

Why should primary care physicians be aware of TIM and Indian patients who use it? It is well known that one-third of all Americans use some form of alternative medicine,[1] and there are data to document Indians' increasing use of TIM. For instance, Guyette confirmed that 74% of urban Indian alcoholics preferred a health care system that included TIM.[2] Fuchs and Bashshur reported that one-third of the Indian patients in San Francisco using an urban Indian clinic used TIM.[3] Marebella et al. reported that 38% of the urban Indians of Milwaukee regularly see a TIM healer, and of those who do not, 86% would consider seeing one in the future.[4] There are no surveys documenting reservation Indian use of TIM. Estimates of the Indian Health Service (IHS), however, range from 70% to 90% depending on which tribal group is being considered.[5] Substantial TIM use rates have thus been established for Indians who are also using western allopathic medicine for their health problems.

How are clinical outcomes affected by Indian patients using both TIM and modern western medicine (MWM) for their health care problems? What is the impact—positive or negative—of TIM in this setting of clinical outcome measures? There are no studies available that address this issue. Given the current mistrust Indian people have toward scientific research, secondary to their historic maltreatment, the breaking of treaties, and the western scientific labeling of TIM as "savage" and "uncivilized," it will be some time before these data are seen, if ever.

Positive Implications

There are some data demonstrating that a traditional Indian lifestyle does import a potential positive outcome. There is some evidence of decreased injury and suicide rates among populations of Indians who are "more traditional."[6, 7] Homicide rates were also shown to be decreased among plains, plateau, and southwest tribes among their "more traditional" members.[8, 9]

There is evidence that alcohol sobriety rates are higher among populations of Indians who have a stake in their cultural ways—that is, they are "more traditional."[10, 11] Alcohol treatment programs with TIM incorporated in the treatment process also show increased sobriety rates.[12]

In spite of the lack of prospective outcome study data, there are data from case studies that demonstrate the positive effect of TIM when coupled with MWM. For instance, Couleham described three case studies showing how Navajo TIM led to successful health outcomes because it dealt with needs of sick Navajos when MWM

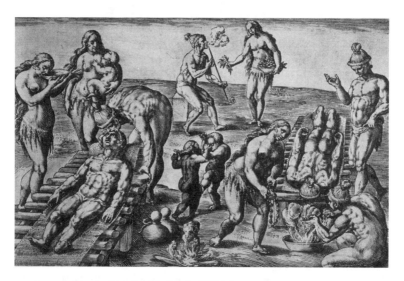

Figure 6-1. This engraving was done by Theodore de Bry in 1590 of a watercolor painting by French artist Jacques le Moyne de Morgues of the Florida Indians in 1564. This scene is the first illustration of early contact with traditional Indian medicine. Although the illustration shows several medical procedures common for this tribe occurring at once, keep in mind that the ceremonial aspect is not depicted here, and it is doubtful that all of these would occur simultaneously but rather separately. le Moyne's original description of the engraving is as follows:

They build a bench long enough and wide enough for the sick person, and he is laid upon it, either on his back or on his stomach. This depends upon the nature of his illness. Then cutting the skin of his forehead with a sharp shell, they suck the blood with their own mouths, spitting it out into an earthen jar or a gourd. Women who are nursing or are pregnant come and drink this blood, especially if it is that of a strong young man. They believe that drinking it makes their milk better and their children stronger, healthier, and more active.

For the sick, whom they lay face downward, a fire of hot coals is prepared, onto which seeds are thrown. The sick man inhales the smoke through his nose and mouth; this is to act as a purge, expelling the poison from the body and thus curing the disease.

They also have a plant which the Brazilians call "petum" and the Spaniards "tapaco." After carefully drying its leaves, they put them in the bowl of a pipe. They light the pipe, and, holding its other end in their mouths, they inhale the smoke so deeply that it comes out through their mouths and noses; by this means they often cure infections. Venereal disease is common among them, and they have several natural remedies for it.

(Reprinted with permission from Clements Library, University of Michigan.)

did not.[13] MWM's reductionist approach limited the spectrum of relevant issues it considered for Navajo patients. In contrast, Navajo TIM integrated a Navajo belief system about illness that dealt with alternative modalities relevant to a Navajo's concept of illness, which was significant for the eventual healing of Navajo patients.

There are other case studies that show how TIM positively influences the treatment of depression, stroke and aphasia, and arthritic pain when used in conjunction with western allopathic medicine.[14–16]

Negative Implications

What are the negative impacts of TIM on Indian health outcomes? I am unaware of any documented conse-

quences in the medical literature but can draw from extensive personal clinical observations and experience. Potential for TIM complications include physiologic complications and herbal drug complications.

Physiologic complications from fasting, sweating, or herbal drug use during various TIM ceremonies, such as the sweat lodge, Sun Dance, and Yuwipi or peyote ceremonies, can lead to dehydration, progressing to metabolic fluid and electrolyte imbalance. Although there are numerous factors to consider here, these potential complications would be more likely in the chronically ill (i.e., those with diabetes, end-stage renal disease, coronary artery disease, and hypertension). Patients on western medications, such as lithium or diuretics, might be at risk for dehydration if a ceremonial practice potentiated the action of their western medication.

Another enormous area of potential complications is the use of herbal medicine by many tribal TIM healers. More than 200 indigenous herbs used by one or more Indian tribes in the past have been official in the *Pharmacopoeia of the United States of America*, and the historic Indian uses of these drugs corresponded to those approved in the *Dispensary of the United States*.[17] For example, I served as a consultant for an Indian patient being treated for fever and malaise with tea from the red willow tree (containing salicylic acid) dispensed by a local healer that resulted in gastritis and dyspepsia.[17] I have also seen the complication of hypoglycemia in a diabetic Indian patient who was simultaneously taking glyburide and a tea made from the root of devil's club (*Fatsia horrida*), which contains potent hypoglycemic substances.[18] The patient was using devil's club tea to treat depression and emotional problems due to family dysfunction under the direction of a local healer as part of a 6-month treatment ceremony. Both these examples had eventual positive outcomes, due primarily to the collaboration that occurred between the patients, their healers prescribing the ceremonial use of the two herbal drugs, and myself.

In addition to these examples, there is also the potential for a multitude of other complications that can result from an Indian patient's use of herbal medicine. It is important for current practitioners to be aware of which Indian patients are using TIM so that obscure complications can be prevented. Avoidance of complications will require collaborative strategies and communication between the Indian patient, the traditional healer, and the western allopathic practitioner.

Core Concepts of Traditional Indian Medicine

Spirituality can be defined as a belief system focusing on intangible elements that impart vitality and meaning to life's events.[19] Throughout history, people across cultures have found that spiritual beliefs can be an important component of maintaining well-being and promoting the healing process when recovering from disease or injury. Spirituality is expressed through formalized religions. Indians are no different from Christians, Jews, Muslims, Buddhists, or others who incorporate faith in the meaning of life's events. However, the degree to which different cultures link medical and spiritual practices varies enormously across cultures. Religion and medicine are inextricably linked for American Indians who adhere to traditional belief systems. Almost all traditional religious ceremonies among Indians are also healing ceremonies. To live in good health is to live in accordance with certain "lifeways" or belief systems that strive to maintain harmony between the inner self and the outer universe.[20] Illness results from negative mental, physical, or spiritual activity or from disruptions or imbalances in the environment (i.e., disharmony). Correction of the imbalances and the restoration of health usually involve a ceremony that may include rituals such as prayers, chants, singing, and the use of herbal substances or physical manipulations.

Within the broad scope of American Indian religion or TIM, each tribe has its own belief system, rituals, and practices, much as Christianity manifests through different churches and Buddhism through various sects. Indian spiritual and healing beliefs, as they relate to health, can be summarized in 10 basic core concepts that are common to most tribes, although no one tribe will adhere precisely to the same 10 nor perceive them in exactly the same way as described by Carol Locust.[21]

1. *American Indians believe in a Supreme Creator.* The Supreme Creator is spiritual and powerful but is not usually personified in human form. Rather, the Creator manifests through deities, guardians, or spirits specific to individual tribes—for example, the Hopi Kachina and Apache animal spirits. The ultimate spiritual goal is reunion with the Creator.

2. *Each person is a threefold being comprised of mind, body, and spirit.* The physical body is the house for the spirit, the "I am." Mind is awareness and the link between body and spirit, and the physical and spirit worlds.

3. *All physical things, living and nonliving, are part of the spirit world.* Everything in the world has life, spirit, and power, and everything is inter-related. Plants; animals; inanimate objects, such as rocks and mountains; wind; celestial objects; and water are part of the spirit world. In TIM, the essence of a plant is its power to heal human suffering through sacred ritual.

4. *The spirit existed before it came into a body and it will exist after the body dies.* Spirit is primary and immortal. Most tribes regard existence as circular and believe that after death, a person's spirit spends time in another reality and then returns to earth in another body. The ultimate goal is to be reunited with the Supreme Creator, although there is no "final judgment" as in western religious traditions. Thus, many Indians do not fear death, and medicine men and women do not specifically seek to prolong life but rather to help patients regain harmony and improve quality of life.

5. *Illness affects the mind and spirit as well as the body.* TIM is holistic in its approach and treats all three components. Every thought and action creates ripples in the being, and the consequences of what we do and think and how we act are inescapable. Anger, fighting, drugs, or not adjusting to a situation can bring disharmony in the body, mind, spirit, or all three. Healing rituals that incorporate herbal medicines, sweat lodges, meditations, and prayer and the use of ceremonial items, such as an eagle

feather, corn pollen, crystals, or other symbols of faith, and sacred power are intended for simultaneous healing of the body, mind, and spirit.

6. *Wellness is harmony in body, mind, and spirit.* Harmony derives not from who a person is or what happens to a person but how he or she responds to individual circumstances. Each person must control his or her attitudes despite impairments or obstacles; thus, the specific meaning of harmony and the path for achieving it will vary for each person.

7. *Unwellness is disharmony.* If one part of the being is out of harmony, then the whole being is out of harmony. For example, mental worry or guilt can lead to headaches, ulcers, and general malaise. Unwellness can be vague or specific. The source can be a family problem or friction at work. Staying in harmony does not guarantee freedom from problems but rather means nothing can cause the person to be out of harmony unless other spirit energy is involved. Indians believe that environmental influences of our fast-paced, industrialized urban society can lead to chronic stress and disharmony.

8. *Natural unwellness is caused by the violation of a sacred or tribal taboo.* One of two categories of disharmony is a natural unwellness, which is a violation of a sacred or tribal taboo that may be moral, religious, or cultural. For example, seeing or getting near certain animals that carry negative energy (snakes) or that have powerful spirit energy (wolf, bear, or eagle) can disrupt the normal energy pattern of the human body and cause illness. Sacred objects contain powerful energy and should be cared for in proper manner. Certain cultural practices, such as caring for the dead, harvesting or preparing certain foods, or observing natural cycles or phenomena, require strict adherence to proscribed practices. A careless person who breaks a taboo will be affected in some way.

9. *Unnatural wellness is caused by witchcraft.* "Witchcraft" is a western term that is imprecise but the closest equivalent to the Indian concept of an energy, especially mental energy, or a power that can be manipulated and used for evil purposes. A witch is a man or woman who uses energy to harm another person. Certain animals (which vary from tribe to tribe) can be seen as a personification of evil (though the animal itself is not considered evil). Indians may attribute sudden illness, accidents, catastrophes, or spirit harassment to witchcraft.

10. *Each of us is responsible for our own health.* Traditional Indian belief holds that we each choose to be who we are and what we are and that we should not rationalize problems by blaming them on physical limitations, conditions of birth, education, or government. Indians who engage in TIM and healing practices must join with the medicine man or woman as full and equal participants and take responsibility for bringing their lives back into balance. By contrast, western medicine tends to attribute illness to outside causes, such as viruses, bacteria, food, noise, stress, or biochemical and physiologic abnormalities, over which the person may feel little control.

The medicine man or woman is a catalyst to healing and spends as much time as needed to help restore harmony and health. Healing ceremonies and practices usually will include family members, who are considered integral to the healing process and are the patient's primary support system. Traditional healers hold an honored place within a tribe and may be chosen for this role by their tribe, by an older healer, by a tribal medical society, or as a result of a personal vision quest. Mastery of the TIM healing craft requires many years of training and disciplined spiritual practice. Tribes view the elders as "keepers" of this traditional knowledge and grant them authority over use of TIM and the training and certification of apprentice healers.

TIM is in part natural and empirical and in part supernatural and spiritual. In pre-Columbian times, healers used a broad range of techniques, including history taking, physical examination, and treatment modalities that included surgery, massage, fracture setting, wound dressing, and herbal medicine. These treatments were used in addition to any necessary ceremony to restore harmony and result in healing. In modern times, Indian healers use fewer hands-on techniques, such as surgery, but more spiritual ceremony coupled with herbal medicine.

Comparison of Traditional Indian Medicine and Modern Western Medicine

Currently, many American Indians in the United States and Canada use dual systems to treat their health problems. Comparing how TIM and MWM deal with health problems is helpful. The treatment of disease by MWM practitioners is based, for the most part, on the reductionist approach.[13] Good health is restored by the removal of obstacles that prevent the body from being well.[13] Although western medicine tends to honor the physician for removing the obstacle, the TIM concept of becoming well emphasizes the patient's own power to restore good health.[21] Traditional Indian practitioners do not do the healing; rather, they assist individuals in healing themselves. Healing under TIM is not the same as curing under MWM. Coronary heart disease may not be cured, but healing may occur in the TIM way by restoring the patient's physical, mental, and spiritual balance, resulting in a return to harmony. The purpose of TIM is to promote harmony for the patient, not necessarily to prolong life. See Table 6-1 for a comparison of the qualities of both systems. Although there are differences between how each health care system approaches an

Table 6-1. Comparison of Traditional Indian Medicine (TIM) with Modern Western Medicine (MWM)

TIM	MWM
Mind, body, spirit; holistic approach	Reductionist approach
Patient's tribal beliefs of health and illness used along with physical, social, and spiritual data to make diagnosis	Reductionist data—biochemical, physiologic, anatomic, laboratory data—used to make diagnosis (social and spiritual not emphasized)
Teaches (via healer) patient to heal self	M.D.s taught that they do the healing
Ceremonies teach the patient how to be well	Teaches patient to depend on the medical system and remain sick
Healing and harmony emphasized	Disease and curing emphasized
Honors the patient for restoring wellness	Honors the physician for curing
History, physical examination, and family assessment used along with treatment plan	History, physical examination, and laboratory data used for treatment plan
Herbal medicine from nature may be used	Pharmaceuticals may be used
Preventive medicine taught to patient and family	Preventive medicine taught to patient and family

Indian patient's health problem, they both have the goal of removing obstacles that are preventing good health or wellness for the patient. The IHS's task force on TIM has reported the importance and benefit of the two systems working together to care for Indian health problems.[5] By combining the strengths of both systems in approaching Indian health problems, the results are sure to benefit the patient more than either system used alone.

Strategies to Enhance Collaboration of Traditional Indian Medicine with Modern Western Medicine

To Indians, religion and medicine are closely intertwined and inseparable. Healing and worship are not distinguishable from one another in Indian ceremonies; for most tribes, there is no difference between religion and medicine.[21] Carl Hammerschlage has observed that health is "not only a physical state but also a spiritual one."[22] Literature worldwide addresses the importance of religious and spiritual factors in health care.[23, 24] Reduced incidence of certain diseases such as cancer, coronary heart disease, and dementia has been correlated with religious affiliation.[25–27] By combining the positive influence of spirituality on health in general for all religions and the data presented here for TIM, there is evidence to support a rationale for current practitioners who care for Indians to identify those patients who use both systems to treat their health problems. Indian patients who use both systems are probably closer to the ideal of holistic health care that is universally recommended. Clinical strategies that facilitate collaboration between the Indian patient, the patient's family, the healer, and the physician would probably be beneficial for the health care outcome of Indian patients.

Obtaining a SPIRITual history from Indian patients, proposed by Maugan[19] for other religions, is recommended by the author to identify Indian patients who use TIM. Maugan recommended using the mnemonic SPIRIT as a guide to identify essential components of a spiritual history.[19] Although Maugan's SPIRIT mnemonic will work for any religion, including TIM, there are some questions to add to the mnemonic that will enhance obtaining key information from Indian patients. See Table 6-2 for a sample of questions making the Maugan mnemonic SPIRIT relevant for American Indians.

Before obtaining a SPIRITual history from Indian patients, several issues should be carefully weighed by the practitioner. Asking questions about an Indian's spirituality (or any other patient's for that matter) is best done when there is long-term continuity of care and a physician-patient relationship established. Acute emergent care settings are not the best time or place to perform this history. The history should be sought in newly established physician-patient care relationships only with caution, if at all, particularly if the physician is non-Indian. The practitioner should also have a strong background and training in cross-cultural and medical anthropologic care as designated by several authors in the medical literature.[28–32] This should also include special cross-cultural awareness strategies for American Indians emphasized by the Native American Research and Training Center at the University of Arizona.[33–35] The SPIRITual history can be taken in one sitting or in sequences over time as a practitioner takes a social or lifestyle history. Finally, some Indian patients have concerns about discussing TIM and healers with their physicians because of a fear of being judged as irrational. Because of these concerns, health care providers should initiate these discussions in a nonjudgmental manner.

Table 6-2. Sample Questions for the American SPIRITual History to Identify
Indians Using Traditional Indian Medicine (TIM)

Spiritual belief system	What is your spiritual belief system?
	Do you culturally identify with a tribe?
	Do you follow or ascribe to the traditional beliefs of your tribe?
	Do you know your tribe's creation story?
	Do you believe in the TIM of your tribe?
Personal spirituality	Describe the beliefs and practices of your spiritual system that you personally accept.
	What does your spirituality mean to you?
	Do you participate in the spiritual ceremonies of your tribe?
	Do you know the purpose of your tribal ceremonies?
	Do you know where your tribe's sacred places are?
Integration with spiritual community	Do you belong to an Indian spiritual or religious group such as Shaker church, Native American church, or tribal-specific religion?
	What is your position or role?
	Is it a source of support?
	Could this group help in dealing with health problems?
	Who are the traditional healers or herbalists that may help you with health problems?
	Would you like me as your physician to collaborate with your healer(s) in regard to your health?
Ritualized practices and restrictions	Do you participate in the spiritual ceremonies of your tribe (e.g., sweat lodge, smudging, shaking tent, blessing way, peyote)?
	Which ceremonies used vary by tribe and geographic location?
	Do you use herbal remedies recommended by your tribal healer? If so, how often?
	Are you allowed to share the herbal medicine you use?
	Are you using both TIM and modern western medicine (MWM) to treat your health problems?
	If you become hospitalized, are there ceremonies to be performed in this setting (e.g., birthing, illness specific)?
	Do you speak your tribal language?
	Are you knowledgeable of your tribe's native medicines?
Implications for medical care	What aspects of your spirituality would you like me to keep in mind as I care for you?
	Do you wish me to collaborate with your TIM healer as you make your decisions about your health care?
	Is it important to you that I am aware of the TIM practices and herbs you use?
	Do you want a MWM perspective in the TIM practices and herbs you use (to acknowledge a positive outcome or to prevent side effects or potential harm with drug interactions)?
	Do you want me to participate, if asked, in TIM ceremonies used as a part of your health care?
Terminal events planning	As we plan for your health care near the end of your life, how does your faith impact your decisions?
	Are there particular aspects of western allopathic health care you wish to forgo because of your faith?
	Are there TIM ceremonies that may be required near the end of your life in which my role may be to facilitate these occurring in a hospital, nursing home, or long-term care facility? (Be aware that discussing terminal events with certain tribes—e.g., Navajo—should only be done, if at all, with special technique.)

Source: Adapted from TA Maugan. The spiritual history. Arch Fam Med 1996;5:11–16.

Primary care practitioners caring for Indians should adopt new roles and responsibilities for fostering and nurturing traditional health practices in the western health care system for American Indians. Some of these roles include advocating for Indian patients in matters relating to health care that includes traditional practices and traditional healers, and acknowledging and respecting the fact that TIM practices and spiritual needs are crucial to the health and wellness of American Indian communities. Physicians should provide a means to ensure delivery of traditional health practices for Indian patients. Western physicians should also ensure and advocate for cooperation with traditional practitioners. Western medicine should make a commitment to develop a cooperative spirit to create opportunities in which traditional healers can work side by side as peers in the care of Indian patients.

Conclusion

TIM is being increasingly used by American Indians in the United States. Reported rates for urban Indian use are 38–74%, and estimates for reservation Indians are 70–90%. Indians are using dual health care systems to care for their health problems, and there is evidence of positive health outcomes when TIM is used. Although there is the potential for complications, if there is collaboration between the Indian patient, the traditional healer, and the western physician, these can be minimized or eliminated.

References

1. Eisenberg DM, Kessler RC, Foster C, et al. Unconventional medicine in the United States: prevalence, costs and patterns of use. N Engl J Med 1993;328:246–252.
2. Guyette S. Selected characteristics of American Indian substance abusers. Intl J Addictions 1982;17:1001–1014.
3. Fuchs M, Bashshur R. Uses of traditional medicine among urban Native Americans. Medical Care 1975;13:915–927.
4. Marebella AM, Harris MC, Diehr S, Ignace G. The uses of Native American healers among Native American patients in an urban Native American health center. Arch Fam Med 1998;7:182–185.
5. Indian Health Service. A Roundtable Conference on the Traditional Cultural Advocacy Program. Indian Health Service, U.S. Department of Health and Human Services, November 1993.
6. Young TK. The Health of Native Americans: Towards a Bicultural Epidemiology. New York: Oxford University Press, 1994;213.
7. Stull DD. Victims of modernization: accident rates and Papago adjustments. Human Organization 1972;31:227–240.
8. Levy JE, Kunitz SJ. Indian reservations and social pathologies. SW J Cult Anthropol 1971;27:97–128.
9. Levy JE, Kunitz SJ. A suicide prevention program for Hopi youth. Soc Sci Med 1987;25:931–940.
10. Ferguson F. Navajo drinking: some tentative hypotheses. Human Organization 1968;27:159–167.
11. Ferguson F. Stake theory as an explanatory device in Navajo alcoholism treatment response. Human Organization 1976;35:65–78.
12. Slagle AL, Orlando JW. The Indian Shaker Church and Alcoholics Anonymous: revitalistic curing arts. Human Organization 1986;45:310–319.
13. Couleham J. Navajo Indian medicine: implications for healing. J Fam Pract 1980;10:55–61.
14. Thompson J, McKay S, Roundhead D, et al. Depression in a Native Canadian in NW Ontario: Sadness, grief or spiritual illness. Canada's Mental Health 1988;2:5–8.
15. Hufflinger KW, Tanner D. The peyote way: implications for cultural care theory. J Transcultural Nursing 1994;5:5–11.
16. Morse J, Young D, Swartz L. Cree Indian healing practices and western health care: a comparative analysis. Soc Sci Med 1991;32:1361–1366.
17. Vogel V. American Indian Medicine. Oklahoma City: University of Oklahoma Press, 1988;392–393.
18. Large RC, Brocklesby HN. A hypoglycemic substance from the roots of the devil's club (*Fatsia harrida*). Can Med Assoc J 1938;30:32–35.
19. Maugan TA. The spiritual history. Arch Fam Med 1996;5:11–16.
20. Avery C. Native American medicine: Traditional healing. JAMA 1991;265:2271–2273.
21. Locust CS. American Indian concepts concerning health and unwellness. Monograph Series, Native American Research and Training Center, University of Arizona, 1985;2–19.
22. Hammerschlage C. The spirit of healing in groups. Monograph from a modified text of the presidential address delivered to the Arizona group of Psychotherapy Society in Oracle, Arizona, Phoenix Indian Medical Center, April 1985;2.
23. Schreiber K. Religion in the physician/patient relationship. JAMA 1991;266:3062–3066.
24. McKee DD, Chappel JN. Spirituality and medical practice. J Fam Pract 1992;35:201, 205–208.
25. Lyon J, Garden K, Gress RE. Cancer incidence in Mormons and non-Mormons in Utah, United States, 1971–1985. Cancer Causes Control 1994;5:149–156.
26. Goldbourtm U, Yarri S, Makalie JH. Factors predictive of long-term coronary heart disease mortality among 10,059 male Israeli civil servants and municipal employees: a 23-year mortality follow-up in the Israeli ischemic heart disease study. Cardiology 1993;82:100–121.
27. Glein P, Beeson WL, Fraser GE. The incidence of dementia and intake of animal products: preliminary findings from the Adventist health study. Neuro-Epidemiology 1993;12:28–36.
28. Kleinman A, Eisenberg L, Good B. Culture, illness and care: clinical lessons from anthropologic and cross-cultural research Ann Intl Med 1978;88:251–258.
29. Galazka SS, Eckert KJ. Clinically applied anthropol-

ogy: concepts for the family physician. J Fam Pract 1986;22:159–165.

30. Eckert JK, Galazka SS. An anthropologic approach to community diagnosis in family practice. Fam Med 1986;18:274–277.

31. Borkan JM, Neher JO. A developmental model of ethnosensitivity in family practice training. Fam Med 1991;23:212–217.

32. Berlin EA, Fowkes WC. A teaching framework for cross-cultural health care. West J Med 1983;139:934–938.

33. Jackson E. Communicating with Native American Patients (video). Native American Research and Training Center, University of Arizona, 1992.

34. Evaneshko V. Culture's Impact on Health Care (video). Native American Research and Training Center, University of Arizona, 1992.

35. Brislin R. Understanding Cultural Diversity: The Challenge of Providing Care to Native Americans (video). National Institute on Deafness and Communication Disorders, University of Arizona, 1994.

Chapter 7
Environmental Health Issues

Thomas E. Crow

Most American Indians (AIs) and Alaska Natives (ANs) live in environments typified by severe climatic conditions; rough, often treacherous geography; extreme isolation; infestations of disease-carrying insects and rodents; inadequate housing; unsanitary methods of sewage and garbage disposal; and unsafe water supplies. Such harsh environments, coupled with decades of economic deprivation and compounded by the lack of basic environmental essentials in many homes (such as running water and toilet facilities), historically have contributed significantly to the exceptionally high incidence of disease, injury, and early death among AIs and ANs.

Developing solutions to the many environmental concerns affecting AIs and ANs requires the maintenance of close partnerships between the Indian Health Service (IHS) and the more than 500 tribes served by the IHS. IHS and tribal environmental health staffs provide services to AIs and ANs through a network of approximately 150 field programs, approximately 60% of which are directly managed by the tribes under either Title I or Title III of Public Law (P.L.) 93-638, the Indian Self Determination and Educational Assistance Act. These IHS and tribal environmental health programs are staffed at the area, district, and service unit levels by sanitarians, engineers, environmental health technicians, engineering aides, injury prevention specialists, and institutional environmental health specialists.

The years of potential life lost (YPLL) for AIs and ANs in 1991–1993 of 81.1 per 1,000 population was less than half of that of 1972–1974 (188.3 per 1,000 population). However, the YPLL for AIs and ANs is still 1.5 times the U.S. all races rate (54.1 per 1,000), and 1.7 times the white rate (47.7 per 1,000).[1] This chapter discusses those environmental factors that contribute to this disparity and presents an agenda for action that may be followed by clinical care providers in addressing the problem.

Injuries—Intentional and Unintentional

The age-adjusted injury death rate for AIs and ANs dropped from 188.0 per 100,000 in 1972–1987 to 83.4 in 1992. However, the rate is still nearly triple the U.S. all races rate of 29.4 for 1992.[1] Injuries account for 46% of the total YPLL among AIs and ANs, and every year more than 1,500 AIs and ANs die and more than 10,000 are injured seriously enough to be hospitalized. The IHS conservatively estimates an annual acute medical care cost for injury treatment of $100 million. More than one-fourth of the entire IHS Catastrophic Emergency Fund is spent for the medical care of injured AIs and ANs.[2] The primary contributors to the problem of injury-related mortality are summarized in Table 7-1.

The single most important factor in successfully addressing the problem of injury-related morbidity and mortality is to recognize that injuries are not "accidents." Injuries are predictable events that may be prevented by applying the same principles of public health epidemiology that are applied in addressing chronic and infectious diseases. Since 1987, the injury-related mortality rate among AIs and ANs has been successfully reduced by 55% through the efforts of IHS and tribal staffs, who have applied the epidemiologic approach to injury prevention to implement a variety of community-based environmental interventions. This successful effort hinges on the building of an effective local injury-prevention infrastructure to adequately address community injury problems. An effective community injury-prevention infrastructure encompasses the following components, which are modeled on the Institute of Medicine report.[3]

Assessment

The assessment component includes

- A trained professional staff capable of assessing local injury problems and identifying possible inter-

Table 7-1. Leading Causes of Death: American Indians and Alaska Natives, 1992

Cause of Death	Age-Adjusted AI/AN Mortality Rate Per 100,000 Population	Age-Adjusted U.S. All Races Mortality Rate Per 100,000 Population
Motor vehicle crash	32.0	15.4
Suicide	16.2	11.1
Homicide	14.6	10.5
Drowning	4.1	1.6
Residential fire	2.5	1.4

AI = American Indian; AN = Alaska Native.
Source: Adapted from Indian Health Service. Trends in Indian Health, 1996. Washington, DC: U.S. Department of Health and Human Services, Indian Health Service, Office of Planning, Evaluation, and Legislation, Division of Program Statistics, 1997; and Centers of Disease Control and Prevention. National Vital Statistics. Atlanta: National Center for Health Statistics, Centers for Disease Control and Prevention, 1996.

vention measures. The IHS currently coordinates a state of the art injury-prevention training program that provides IHS and tribal staffs with the ability to apply the principles of epidemiology and public health practice in addressing local injury problems and advocating for the support of those programs.

- A comprehensive injury surveillance and data management system that permits practitioners to effectively characterize local injury problems.

Policy

The policy component includes

- An effective advocate capable of communicating the need for injury-prevention policy to local governments. In the area of injury prevention, it is not always enough to simply know what must be done: There are frequently issues that demand well-trained, articulate champions at the local, regional, and national levels.
- Community partnerships and broad-based coalitions comprising key individuals and community stakeholders.
- Multiple intervention strategies that include both environmental and behavioral modifications.

Assurance

The assurance component includes

- A formalized system for conducting evaluation and assurance activities.

- Adequate staffing to ensure access to required services.

A few prominent injury-prevention success stories are cited here as an example of what can be accomplished when broad-based community coalitions apply sound public health principles to recognized community problems.

After studying more than 150 cases of severe injuries on the White Mountain Apache Indian Reservation, injury prevention staff identified two previously unrecognized injury problems: motor vehicle crashes with animals and nighttime pedestrian collisions. A coalition of concerned agencies and individuals developed an action plan to correct identified deficiencies in the cluster area, which entailed illuminating a 1.1-mile strip of roadway. In the years since completion of the project, no deaths or severe injuries have occurred in the target area.

An injury profile established for the community of Browning, Montana, indicated a cluster of 59 severe trauma cases (including 13 fatalities) over a 7-year period resulting from motor vehicle crashes and collisions with pedestrians walking between two local taverns. Most of the injuries occurred while pedestrians were crossing the highway. Others involved drivers who collided when entering or exiting the parking lots. With joint cooperation between the IHS, Browning citizens, the local electric utility, and the Montana Highway Department, overhead street lights were installed along the highway between the taverns and concrete curbing was installed in the parking lots to create controlled entry and exit points. Since the project was implemented in October 1988, injury and fatality incidents have been totally eliminated at the cluster site. Total cost of the project was approximately $6,500, with the Highway Department covering ongoing street-light electrical costs at $600 per year.

The first surveys of seatbelt use conducted within the Navajo Nation in the early 1980s showed that less than 5% of drivers and passengers used seat belts. In 1988, the Navajo Nation Tribal Council modified its motor vehicle safety code to require the use of safety belts and infant car seats for all motor vehicle occupants. After an extensive public information campaign sponsored by the Department of Highway Safety, IHS, and other interested parties, the tribal law enforcement officers began to strictly enforce the new tribal law. By December 1990, seatbelt usage had climbed to 50%. In 1992, the seatbelt usage rate had climbed to almost 70%. During the same period, 1987–1992, hospitalizations as a result of injuries sustained in motor vehicle collisions decreased by more than 25%, and hospitalizations for all causes decreased by 6%, resulting in an estimated savings in patient-care costs of approximately $2 million annually.

The important thing to note with regard to these interventions is the fact that they were able to achieve significant results over a short period through the application of relatively simple environmental modifications. Situations are frequently encountered in the practice of public health, such as the problem of unintentional injuries or domestic violence, that cause people to shrug their shoulders and attribute events to fate or the whim of human behavior. What these successful projects effectively demonstrate is that community action coupled with sound public health principles can make a real difference.

Water and Wastewater

During the years from 1900 to 1955, several major surveys were conducted for the purpose of assessing the health of AIs and ANs.[4] All of these surveys cited the lack of adequate water supplies and waste disposal facilities as major contributing factors to the high rates of infectious diseases experienced by AIs and ANs. The Indian Sanitation Facilities Act (P.L. 86-121) was signed into law on July 31, 1959, authorizing the IHS to provide essential water and wastewater facilities to AI and AN homes and communities. With the completion of all projects approved for funding through fiscal year 1995, approximately 200,000 AI and AN homes will have been provided with sanitation facilities since the program's inception in fiscal year 1960. As with other IHS activities, sanitation facilities projects are carried out cooperatively with the people who are to be served by the completed facilities. Projects are initiated only after receipt of a tribal request expressing a willingness on the part of the tribe to participate in carrying out the project and to execute a tribal agreement to assume ownership responsibilities for completed facilities. Experience shows that 60–70% of the actual construction work in these projects is performed by Indian tribes or tribal firms.

The impact of improved community sanitation brought about by the provision of sanitary water and wastewater disposal facilities has been demonstrated by significant reductions in morbidity and mortality rates. Infant mortality rates among AI and AN children have been reduced from 22.2 deaths per 1,000 live births in 1972–1974 to 8.8 in 1991–1993, a decrease of 60%. The U.S. all races and white populations' rates for 1992 were 8.5 and 6.9, respec-

tively.[1] The age-adjusted gastrointestinal disease death rate for AIs and ANs has decreased 76% since 1972–1974, when the rate was 6.2 deaths per 100,000 population. In 1991–1993, the AI/AN rate of 1.5 deaths per 100,000 population was only slightly higher that the 1992 U.S. all races rate of 1.3.[1] Although many factors have undoubtedly contributed to this dramatic improvement, such as improved nutrition and improved access to prenatal and other primary health care, the importance of improved water and wastewater facilities cannot be underestimated.

Although significant progress has been achieved since the program's inception in fiscal year 1960, much work remains to be done. At the end of fiscal year 1995, IHS and tribal environmental health staffs identified a continuing unmet need for funds of approximately $630 million for sanitary facilities,[5] as indicated in Table 7-2.

Solid Waste

The Indian Lands Open Dumps Cleanup Act of 1994 (P.L. 103-399) identified congressional concerns that solid waste, open-dump sites located on AI and AN lands threatened the health and safety of residents of those lands and adjacent areas.[6] The act mandated that the IHS conduct a study and inventory of open dumps on Indian lands and develop a 10-year plan to address solid waste deficiencies and identify the level of funding necessary to bring these sites in compliance with applicable provisions of the Resource Conservation and Recovery Act. In conformance with that mandate, IHS and tribal environmental health personnel completed the inventory, which indicated that there are approximately 730 open dumps meeting the criteria established in P.L. 103-399 located on AI and AN lands, of which approximately 600 are designated as "actively used" and are still receiving waste.[6] The IHS has estimated a need for approximately $154 million to provide for initial cleanup of those sites and to provide long-term solid waste collection and disposal services to 135,000 AI and AN homes currently served by the open dumps. In the absence of congressional funding to specifically address these sites, the IHS will continue to address the solid waste needs of AI and AN homes and

Table 7-2. Sanitation Facilities Deficiency Summary (Fiscal Year 1996)*

Water		Sewer		Solid Waste		Operation and Maintenance	
Housing Units	Costs (thousands)	Housing Units	Costs (thousands)	Housing Units	Costs (thousands)	Housing Units	Costs (thousands)
104,551	$306,308	70,511	$203,272	134,545	$112,745	44,247	$7,226

*Total need = $629,552,559.
Source: Adapted from Indian Health Service. Trends in Indian Health, 1996. Washington, DC: U.S. Department of Health and Human Services, Office of Planning, Evaluation, and Legislation, Division of Program Statistics, 1997.

communities in accordance with the policies, procedures, and funding priorities established for implementing P.L. 86-121.[5] Priority for funding under this plan is determined in large part by the health impact of the proposed project and the priority that is assigned to the project by the local tribal government.[6]

Hantavirus

During the spring and summer of 1993, an outbreak of acute respiratory illness associated with a previously unrecognized Hantavirus was reported in the southwestern United States.[7] Because of the disproportionate percentage of Native Americans contracting this disease (72% of the first 17 patients meeting the case definition) and the high fatality rate (76% of the first 17 patients), the IHS responded aggressively with colleagues in the Centers for Disease Control and Prevention (CDC), the Navajo Nation Division of Health, and state health departments in Arizona, Colorado, and New Mexico to determine the cause of the disease and to reduce risks among AI and AN people. A case-control study was initiated that identified the primary reservoir as the deer mouse (*Peromyscus maniculatus*), although serologic evidence of infection was also found in pinon mice (*Peromyscus truei*), brush mice (*Peromyscus boylii*), and western chipmunks (*Tamias* spp.).[7] Cases were epidemiologically associated with the following situations:

- Planting or harvesting field crops
- Occupying previously vacant cabins or other dwellings
- Cleaning barns and other outbuildings
- Disturbing rodent-infested areas while hiking or camping
- Inhabiting dwellings with indoor rodent populations
- Residing in or visiting areas in which the rodent population has shown an increase in density

In controlling outbreaks of Hantavirus-associated respiratory distress syndrome, eradication of the reservoir hosts is neither feasible nor desirable.[7] Control measures should consist of eliminating rodent infestation in and around the home by eliminating food sources and rodent harbor areas. The IHS and CDC have published detailed control measures,[7, 8] which are summarized as follows:

- Eliminate rodents and reduce the availability of food sources and nesting sites used by rodents inside the home. Before rodent elimination work is begun, ventilate closed buildings or areas inside buildings by opening doors and windows for at least 30 minutes. Use an exhaust fan or cross ventilation if possible.
- Prevent rodents from entering the home by covering all openings into the home that have a diameter of at least 0.25 in.

- Reduce rodent shelter and food sources within 100 ft of the home.
- Clean up rodent contaminated areas in a manner that limits the potential for aerosolization of dirt or dust from all potentially contaminated surfaces and household goods.

Special precautions are indicated for individuals who will be engaged in cleaning homes or buildings that are the sites of confirmed Hantavirus infection or heavy rodent infestations.[5] Persons conducting activities in these areas should contact the responsible local, state, or federal public health agency for guidance.

Hazardous Materials

Hazardous materials incidents that affect AI and AN communities typically occur as a result of the transportation of hazardous materials across tribal lands via highway or railway systems, although some hazardous materials releases have occurred from reservation-based industry. Tribal communities in close proximity with urban areas are also at risk to hazardous materials releases that are the result of illegal dumping by off-reservation polluters. IHS field staff work in collaboration with tribal staff to implement the provisions of Title III of the Superfund Amendments Reauthorization Act regarding emergency planning and community right-to-know. Tribal groups typically work with local emergency-response agencies to respond to incidents involving hazardous materials, although some tribes do maintain a limited emergency-response capability. Most tribes have formal local emergency planning committees in place, of which IHS and tribal environmental health staff are key members. The area office of environmental health and engineering maintains the responsibility for providing program support and technical assistance to local IHS and tribal staff in the area of hazardous materials management.

The IHS has entered into an interagency agreement with the Agency for Toxic Substances and Disease Registry (ATSDR) to provide mutual support in handling hazardous materials. The ATSDR provides IHS and tribal staff with training in hazardous materials management and the community risk assessment process, and the IHS assists the ATSDR in performing field surveys of sites on or adjacent to Indian lands for which the ATSDR has been petitioned to perform a risk assessment.

Lead

The 1992 amendments of the Indian Health Care Improvement Act (P.L. 94-437) mandate that the IHS reduce the prevalence of blood lead levels exceeding 15 µg/dl among AI and AN children ages 6 months to 5 years and eliminate the incidence of blood lead levels exceeding 25 µg/dl. The IHS has entered into a collaborative relationship with the CDC to identify the baseline blood lead levels of AI and AN children. Blood lead samples are taken by IHS clinical providers and submitted to state testing laboratories that are funded through CDC blood lead–prevention program grants. IHS and tribal environmental health staffs follow up with an environmental evaluation of the home of any individual with a blood sample that exceeds 10 µg/dl. Although the preliminary data are incomplete at the time of this writing, data observed in blood lead screening of approximately 5,000 children to date are summarized in Table 7-3.

As the data indicate, blood lead poisoning among AI and AN children appears to be limited to situations involving the home environment of specific children. Instances involving elevated blood lead levels among children in a community as a result of mining activities have been observed[9, 10] and have been addressed through the collaborative efforts of tribal governments, state departments of health, the IHS, and other federal agencies such as the Environmental Protection Agency and the ATSDR.

Institutional Environmental Health

IHS and tribal environmental health staffs perform institutional environmental health surveys of community facilities that serve the most vulnerable segments of tribal communities: the very young and the elderly. Approximately 25% of all ambulatory medical visits for AI and AN children ages 5 to 14 years are for respiratory diseases and infectious and parasitic diseases.[1] In an effort to control the transmission of infectious organisms and parasites among young children, the IHS has entered into an interagency agreement with the Head Start Bureau of the Administration for Children and Families (ACF) that ensures that tribally operated Head Start facilities comply with standard environmental health guidelines. The IHS worked in collaboration with the ACF and tribal Head Start programs to develop a national environmental health standard that is applied to all tribal Head Start facilities that receive funding from the ACF. IHS and tribal environmental health staff conduct compliance surveys, and the ACF works with the tribal contractors to bring deficiencies into compliance.

Although the gastrointestinal disease mortality rate among AIs and ANs has decreased by 76% since 1973,[1] foodborne illness continues to be a serious national concern that affects an estimated 24–81 million people annually.[11] Foodborne illness may be especially devastating for elderly members of the community, who bear a disproportionate share of the 10,000 annual deaths related to foodborne illness.[11] To address this situation,

Table 7-3. Blood Lead Levels Observed in AI/AN Children, Ages 6 Months to 5 Years; 1994–1996 (N = 4,984)

0–9 µg/dl (%)	10–14 µg/dl (%)	15–19 µg/dl (%)	>19 µg/dl (%)	Total
4,733 (95)	176 (3.5)	40 (0.8)	35 (0.7)	4,984 (100)

AI = American Indian; AN = Alaska Native.
Source: Adapted from reports submitted to the Indian Health Service from Centers for Disease Control and Prevention-funded state lead poisoning prevention programs 1992–1996.

the IHS has entered into an interagency agreement with the Administration on Aging to ensure that nutrition programs that provide meals to elderly members of the community are operated in compliance with the most recent version of the U.S. Food and Drug Administration food code. This program operates within a framework similar to that described for the Head Start program.

Agenda for Action

Primary care providers play a key role in promoting preventive health programs in AI and AN communities. Throughout history, AIs and ANs have viewed healers with deep respect and admiration. Because of the regard with which they are held in the community, IHS primary care providers are afforded a unique opportunity to serve as an important voice to communicate the health needs of AIs and ANs. The following agenda for action is offered as an example of how IHS primary care providers can use their unique position to promote environmental health issues within the community.

Provide Environmental Health Staff with Timely and Complete Referrals

It should go without saying that, for field-based follow-up to be effective, field staff must be provided with relevant information in as timely a manner as possible. Furthermore, IHS and tribal environmental health personnel use data provided by the clinical provider to conduct epidemiologic assessments of community risk factors. This is especially critical with regard to the injury surveillance database discussed earlier, under Injuries—Intentional and Unintentional. To accurately identify those factors that are significant contributors to the community injury problem, it is vital that the external cause of injury portion of the ambulatory patient care form be completed as completely and accurately as possible.

Take Advantage of Teachable Moments

Clinical providers share a unique relationship with their patients that is not enjoyed by other members of the health care team. Providers should maintain a close relationship with environmental health professionals to maintain an awareness of important community environmental health issues to be communicated to their patients. It is not always practical or desirable to discuss such matters at the time of the patient's initial presentation in the clinic. However, follow-up visits and other patient-provider encounters provide a unique opportunity to discuss how a given incident might have occurred and what the patient could have done to prevent the incident.

Become a Community Voice

As stated, healers enjoy a unique status within AI and AN communities. Providers should step outside the confines of the clinic and get to know the members of the community as individuals, rather than simply as patients, and establish the provider's credibility as a public health professional. Once credibility has been established, the provider's position can be used as a basis for speaking out in the community to encourage community and tribal leaders to practice healthy lifestyles and adopt public policies that will enhance the quality of life within the community.

Publish Research

During the course of a provider's clinical duties, he or she will be presented with the opportunity to observe and report on a wide range of epidemiologic phenomena. The provider should consider publishing his or her observations in an appropriate professional forum, such as the *IHS Primary Care Provider,* a journal for health professionals working with AIs and ANs, or a professional journal (after appropriate tribal consultation and approval). Publication of the provider's work will not only provide important information to clinical colleagues in the IHS, it could also prove to be a useful tool in raising the awareness of others with regard to the unique health challenges that confront AIs and ANs.

Summary

Although a tremendous amount of progress has been realized in improving the health status of AIs and ANs, much work remains to be done. Despite a 13% reduction in the rate of unintentional injury deaths since 1989, AIs and ANs still die from injuries at rates that are almost triple the U.S. all races rate.[1] Despite significant improvements in community water and wastewater facilities that have played an important role in reducing the gastroenteric mortality rate by 76% since 1973, approximately 12% of AI and AN homes and communities still lack adequate sanitation facilities.[5] A true team effort that combines the skills of primary care providers, community health professionals, and AI and AN tribal and community leaders is essential if the IHS is to achieve its goal of improving the health status of AIs and ANs to the highest possible level.

References

1. Indian Health Service. Trends in Indian Health, 1996. Washington DC: U.S. Department of Health and Human Services, Indian Health Service, Office of Planning, Evaluation, and Legislation, Division of Program Statistics, 1997.
2. Indian Health Service. Injury Prevention Program Five Year Plan: Immunizing Against the Injury Epidemic. Washington, DC: U.S. Department of Health and Human Services, Indian Health Service, Office of Environmental Health and Engineering, 1992.
3. Institute of Medicine, Committee for the Study of the Future of Public Health. The Future of Public Health. Washington, DC: National Academy Press, 1988;140–142.
4. Indian Health Service. The American Indian and Alaska Native: Their Environment, Health and the Environmental Health Program—A Historical Perspective: 1955–1985.Washington, DC: U.S. Department of Health and Human Services, Indian Health Service, Division of Environmental Health, 1985.
5. Indian Health Service. Fiscal Year 1998 Justifications of Budget Estimates to the Office of Management and Budget. Washington, DC: U.S. Department of Health and Human Services, Indian Health Service, 1997;110–139.
6. Indian Health Service. First Annual Report: Open Dumps on Indian Lands—Indian Lands Open Dump Cleanup Act. Public Law 103-399. Washington, DC: U.S. Department of Health and Human Services, Indian Health Service, Office of Environmental Health and Engineering, 1997;3–8.
7. Centers for Disease Control and Prevention. Hantavirus infection—southwestern United States: interim recommendations for risk reduction. MMWR Morb Mortal Wkly Rep 1993;42(RR-11):1–12.
8. Indian Health Service. Handbook of Environmental Health (1994). Washington, DC: U.S. Department of Health and Human Services, Indian Health Service, Division of Environmental Health, 1994;236–239.
9. Jones, et al. Blood lead screening in the San Carlos service unit. IHS Primary Care Provider 1993;(December):202–207.
10. Environmental Protection Agency. Tar Creek Superfund Site: Summary of Removal Response Activities. Washington, DC: Environmental Protection Agency, September 1995.
11. Food and Drug Administration. Food Code: 1995 Recommendations of the United States Public Health Service Food and Drug Administration (1995). Pub # PB95-265492CEH. Springfield, VA: National Technical Information Service, 1995.

Part II
Infectious Diseases

Chapter 8
Gastroenteritis

Raymond Reid

Gastroenteritis, known more commonly as *diarrhea*, is generally defined as the frequent passing of loose or watery stool. It is an ailment of people of all ages worldwide. Certain populations experience this ailment more frequently than others, such as residents of underdeveloped countries and people who live in homes with poor sanitation and who practice poor hygiene. It is also well known that infants have much higher rates of enteric infections than older children and adults.

Diarrheal illnesses in adults, for the most part, are mild, brief, and primarily considered an inconvenience. In infants and young children, even mild diarrhea can progress rapidly to a life-threatening situation if appropriate therapy is not instituted quickly.

This chapter discusses the problem of gastroenteritis in Indian populations, especially in infants and young children, and diagnosis and treatment are considered.

Epidemiology

Around the world, it is estimated that diarrhea and its complications are responsible for one death every 6 seconds.[1] Most of these deaths occur in developing countries. Factors associated with increased rates of diarrhea include lack of sanitary water supplies and waste disposal, improper food handling, and decreased attention to personal hygiene. Some of these factors reflect the socioeconomic and political status of the population and the logistical difficulties in making the required improvements. In the United States, a developed country, it is estimated that 400–500 deaths due to diarrhea occur each year.

Because of its high prevalence, many Indian parents have long considered diarrhea an illness that every child gets, like colds and chickenpox. Diarrhea in a child attracts little attention. Often, however, the potential for milder forms of the illness to develop into a serious or life-threatening illness is realized too late.

The incidence of a number of infectious diseases is known to be higher among American Indians than among the general U.S. population. With the increased availability of medical care facilities on reservations and the improvements in sanitation and home conditions, many of the formerly high rates of infectious diseases have decreased. Among tribes whose members once had strong faith in the practice of traditional medicine, increasing numbers of people have developed greater acceptance of modern medicine to provide cure.

In Indian populations, bacterial and viral agents are responsible for most cases of diarrhea. Lactose intolerance in infants is a significant additional cause of diarrhea. Other etiologies, such as endocrinopathies, anatomic defects, or diarrhea resulting from other ongoing chronic diseases, occur far less frequently.

Only since the early 1980s have high rates of diarrheal illnesses declined among Indians of all ages. During the years 1972–1977, gastroenteritis, with incidence rates of 5,060–8,015 per 100,000 population, was the "second leading notifiable disease," and bacillary dysentery (255–595 per 100,000) was "ranked between 8 and 12 (1970–1978) among the leading notifiable diseases."[2] Not included among gastroenteritis in this report were amebiasis (1.5–3.0 per 100,000), botulism, bacterial "food poisoning," and salmonellosis (13.4–36.3 per 100,000); but each of these separately listed diseases was responsible for significant numbers of diarrheal illness. Between 1970 and 1978, approximately half of the new cases of diarrhea occurred in children 4 years of age and younger. For this same period, no information could be found to determine the numbers or rates of deaths among Indians due to diarrhea. During the years 1991–1993, however, diarrhea was no longer among the top 10 causes of deaths in Indian children 4 years of age and younger.[3]

Current data prevent the determination of the number of clinic visits and hospitalizations for diarrhea among

Indian patients. In the latest year for which data are available, fiscal year 1994, the broad category of infectious and parasitic diseases was among the top six causes for hospitalization of children age 4 years and younger.[3] Similarly, infectious and parasitic diseases were among the top five causes for clinic visits in this age group. This broad category is not further broken down to indicate more precisely the extent to which enteric infections were responsible for hospitalizations and clinic visits.

The most recent extensive studies to determine the epidemiology of diarrhea in an Indian population were performed on the White Mountain Apache Reservation in east central Arizona during the 5-year period 1981–1985.[4, 5] The population of the tribe was approximately 10,000, with half the population younger than 15 years of age and approximately 20% younger than 5 years old. The applicability of data and information derived from these studies to other Indian tribes or groups is not known because similar extensive studies have never been performed in other tribal groups. However, it is thought that the findings in Apaches are similar to other tribal groups.

One study performed from 1981 to 1983 involved a cohort of 112 children, who were followed from birth until age 3 years.[5] Weekly home visits were made, at which information was collected on the occurrence of diarrhea since the last visit. If diarrhea had occurred, stool specimens were obtained for the identification of the etiologic agent. The data collected and analyzed indicated a diarrhea prevalence of 2.8% (2.552 days of diarrhea per 90,374 total days of observation). Additional analyses revealed a median of four episodes of diarrhea per child per year and a maximum of 15 episodes per year. Peak attack rates of diarrhea occurred in 4- to 12-month-old infants (an average of 6.4 episodes per year). Attack rates were slightly higher in male infants than in female infants.

Although hospitalizations for diarrhea occurred throughout the year, most occurred during the summer and fall months, and bacterial agents were primarily responsible for causing disease. Diarrhea caused by viruses was most prevalent during the early winter months.

Other studies were conducted among patients who visited clinics or were hospitalized because of enteric infections. During the 5-year period 1981–1985, 488 patients of all ages were hospitalized.[4] Of these, 377 (77.3%) were younger than 12 months old, and 64 (13.1%) were 12–23 months of age. Among 488 infants younger than 24 months of age, 107 were hospitalized once, 80 were hospitalized two times, and 23 were hospitalized three times. Also during this period, 535 children younger than 5 years old were seen for diarrhea in outpatient clinics. Of these, 368 children (68.8%) were younger than 12 months old, and another 133 (24.9%) were 12–23 months old. Almost all hospitalized infants younger than

24 months old exhibited various degrees of dehydration caused by excessive body fluid loss via the stool. These data demonstrate the clear predominance of diarrhea among infants compared to individuals in other age groups in this tribe.

Laboratory analyses of stool specimens of patients in all age groups revealed that rotavirus was responsible for most cases (24%). Bacterial agents causing disease included enterotoxigenic *Escherichia coli* (14%) and *Clostridium difficile* (9.2%). Significant numbers of cases of diarrhea were also caused by *Shigella* (5.6%), *Campylobacter* (3.1%), and adenovirus (5.4%). A separate study also found enterotoxic *Bacteroides fragilis* to be significantly associated with diarrhea, especially in children.[6]

These findings with respect to the age with the highest prevalence of enteric infections, etiologic agent, and seasonality are strikingly similar to patterns found in many less developed countries of the world. Studies conducted throughout the world have shown that rotavirus accounts for approximately 40% of all diarrheal illnesses in most populations, especially in infants younger than 1 year of age.[1, 7, 8] It is estimated that by the age of 3 years, each person has had at least one episode of rotaviral diarrhea,[9] thus demonstrating the high prevalence worldwide of rotavirus diarrhea. Additionally, in infant populations throughout the world, including the Apache population, *Shigella* and enterotoxic *E. coli* infections are more common during the second and third years of life.

Further information collected in the studies among Apache patients with diarrhea, regardless of etiologic agent, showed that 58–79% had respiratory symptoms. Studies conducted in this and in another population have suggested that the rotavirus was spread via respiratory secretions.[10, 11] Other findings accompanying diarrhea in hospitalized patients were fever, vomiting (60–70%), blood in the stool (<5%), six to eight stools per 24 hours before admission, 4–5 days of diarrhea before admission, and a 5- to 6-day hospital stay.[4]

Sporadic outbreaks or small epidemics of diarrheal illness caused by specific infectious agents have occurred among various tribes; some have been reported in the medical literature, but many others go unreported, except perhaps by the local media. For example, outbreaks of diarrhea caused by *Salmonella*[12] have been attributed to the lack of proper preparation or refrigeration of foods served at large gatherings. Outbreaks of *Shigella* infection are usually localized to small communities or small areas but cause large numbers of patients to flood reservation clinics and hospitals.

In the fall of 1981, while studies were being conducted among White Mountain Apaches to determine the epidemiology of diarrheal diseases, an outbreak of rotavirus diarrhea occurred in this population of approximately 10,000.[10] During the 3 weeks of the outbreak, 342 new cases of diarrhea occurred suddenly in patients who came from scattered locations on the reservation. Of the 289 patients of all ages who sought medical attention, stools from 233 patients were tested in the laboratory, and 169 (73%) were positive for the rotavirus antigen. Of all age groups, infants 3–5 months old had the highest percentage (67%) of rotavirus-positive stools. Of the 169 patients whose stools tested positive for the rotavirus antigen, hospitalization was required only for infants younger than 12 months of age. Infants younger than 3 months of age comprised the greatest number (134, 47%) of those requiring hospitalization. Forty-four (33%) of these infants had accompanying respiratory infections, which suggest that the rapid spread of this disease throughout the reservation occurred via respiratory secretions.

Sparse information is available about other outbreaks of infectious diarrhea among Indians. Thus, the frequency with which these have occurred among tribes cannot be precisely determined.

Diagnosis

Although the diagnosis of diarrhea might seem simple, easy diagnosis is often complicated by other concurrent symptoms and signs. Certainly, the frequent occurrence of loose or watery stools is pathognomonic of this illness. Diarrhea also occurs at several levels of severity.

A good history of the illness should include the duration of diarrhea before the clinic visit or hospitalization, the number of diarrheal stools passed during the previous 24 hours, the consistency of the stool (pasty to outright watery), the presence of fever and vomiting, symptoms of dehydration, appetite, whether the patient is lactose intolerant, types of home therapy used, other concurrent illnesses, and all medications being taken. Besides performing the standard physical examination, the physician should assess the patient's composure, mental status, and degree of dehydration as determined by examining the fontanelle, the lips and tongue, skin turgor, and weight change as well as noting whether the eyes are sunken.

No standard method exists for assigning a level of severity of a diarrheal illness. Labeling the illness as mild, moderate, or severe is often a subjective judgment based on the experience of the individual physician. However, the degree of severity can be assigned by considering the findings made during the physical examination. One recommended method in infants[13] that combines these findings is as follows: Mild diarrhea is determined by 5–6% dehydration, watery stools, increased thirst, or slightly dry mucous membranes. Moderate diarrhea exists with 7–9% dehydration, loss of skin turgor, sunken eyes, very dry mucous membranes, and depressed anterior fontanelle. Severe illness exists with more than 9% dehydration; the patient exhibits all

the signs of moderate dehydration along with a rapid weak pulse, cold extremities, and coma.

Laboratory analyses of blood specimens should include determining any electrolyte imbalances, the white cell count, and hematocrit. Stool should be examined for its consistency (pasty to watery) and for the presence of blood, mucus, and parasites. Stool can be cultured for bacterial agents and assessed for antigens of viral agents using appropriate enzyme-linked immunosorbent assay tests.

Lactase deficiency, a significant cause of diarrhea and abdominal pain, is known to have a high prevalence in certain populations, such as those of Asian origin, blacks, and American Indians. Whole cow's milk and many infant formulas contain lactose (milk sugar), which requires the lactase enzyme for digestion. Many young parents, especially, are not familiar with this condition and often confuse diarrhea caused by lactose intolerance with diarrhea caused by infectious agents. Thus, in determining the probable cause of diarrhea in an infant, lactose intolerance must be considered to avoid the institution of therapies that are more appropriate for infectious causes of diarrhea.

Treatment

Appropriate treatment depends on (1) obtaining a careful history of the diarrheal episode, (2) performing a good physical examination, (3) obtaining the necessary blood specimens for laboratory analyses, and (4) examination of stool. Various degrees of dehydration are present in almost all patients with diarrhea because varying amounts of body water have been lost with the diarrheal stool. Rehydrating the infant patient is the prime consideration of treatment.

Oral rehydration therapy (ORT) has increasingly become the mainstay for correcting dehydration caused by diarrhea, regardless of etiology. Before the use of ORT, patients with dehydration were rehydrated using solutions given intravenously. The simplicity and effectiveness of rehydrating patients by mouth using an appropriate oral rehydration solution (ORS) was first recognized in developing countries, which often lacked the necessary trained personnel, equipment, and supplies for intravenous therapy.[13] ORS is a mixture of specific concentrations of water, electrolytes (sodium, potassium, chloride, and bicarbonate), and glucose. It is used to replace water and electrolytes lost from the body because of diarrhea. The attractiveness of the use of ORS is that many mothers, given simple instructions and minimal supervision, can administer the solution to their infants to correct dehydration. This obviates the need for intravenous equipment and paraphernalia and frees the nurse to perform other pressing tasks. Also, infants are more receptive to ORS given by the mother than by others unfamiliar to them. Bonding between the mother and infant is continued and is enhanced, especially when the mother holds the infant while giving ORS.

Although many infants with diarrhea who show no sign of dehydration or are minimally dehydrated can be treated as outpatients using ORS, other infants with mild diarrhea or worse require hospitalization. Normally, ORS can fully rehydrate infants with mild or moderate dehydration within 4 hours. The recommended amount to be given hospitalized infants who are mildly dehydrated is 60 ml/kg; moderately dehydrated infants should receive 80 ml/kg of ORS. If dehydration persists after 4 hours, ORS can continue to be administered at these amounts until rehydration has been achieved. In infants who are severely dehydrated, rehydration should begin immediately with intravenous administration of Ringer's lactate or similar solutions at a rate of 40 ml/kg per hour. When pulse, blood pressure, and state of awareness have returned to normal, the child can then be given ORS to correct any remaining dehydration.

The maintenance phase of ORT in hospitalized patients begins when the infant has been adequately rehydrated, in most cases, after 4 hours. Maintenance consists of the continued administration of ORS in amounts to replace the water lost in the stool on a 1 to 1 basis. Lactose-free formula can also be given at a rate of 150 ml/kg/24 hours. Frequent reassessment of the child's vital signs and status should also be performed to ensure that the child remains adequately rehydrated and is progressing satisfactorily toward recovery. With this treatment regimen, most infants recover from their diarrheal illness.

Any abnormal electrolyte values noted on laboratory analyses of serum specimens can usually be corrected by the ORS without supplemental administration of medicines normally used to correct abnormal electrolyte values. Also, treatment for other concurrent illnesses, such as otitis media or lower respiratory infection, can be instituted at any time without interrupting ORT.

Infants seen in clinic who are minimally dehydrated or who show no signs of dehydration can be treated as outpatients using ORS. The recommended outpatient treatment consists of alternating the administration of ORS at a rate of 75 ml/kg/24 hours with the feeding of lactose-free formula. Mothers experienced with the use of ORS can purchase these solutions in supermarkets and drugstores.

In-house policies for antibiotic treatment of diarrhea caused by bacterial agents differ among clinics and hospitals on different reservations. For many cases of mild infection that require no hospitalization, no antibiotics are administered because the diseases in these cases are usually self-limiting, and antibiotic-resistant strains, particularly of *Shigella,* exist in many scattered locations. Severe cases of diarrhea caused by bacterial agents are generally treated with antibiotics, however, depending on the agent isolated from the stool.

Summary

Despite dramatic declines in the rates of enteric infections since the mid-1980s, these diseases continue to exist, and the rates are higher among American Indians (especially infants) than in the general U.S. population. Deaths secondary to diarrhea and its complications are extremely rare in Indian populations. Bacterial and viral agents are responsible for most cases of diarrhea. It is estimated that approximately half of cases are due to rotavirus, which is thought to be transmitted from person to person via respiratory secretions. The patterns of enteric infections among American Indians are strikingly similar to patterns found in many underdeveloped countries of the world.

ORT is a recently developed, simple mode of therapy now widely used to safely and effectively correct dehydration caused by diarrhea. The development of ORS and its proved efficacy are rooted in an Indian reservation, but its beneficial effects have been realized in populations throughout the rest of the United States and the world. Despite past efforts, which have contributed significantly to lowering formerly high rates of disease, much remains to be done by all sectors of the Indian population, including government, educational programs, and health programs, but mainly by individuals, to reduce even more these high rates among Indians.

References

1. Salata RA. Preventive Pediatrics and Epidemiology. In Behrman RE, Kleigman RM, Nelson WE, Vaughn VC III (eds), Textbook of Pediatrics (14th ed). Philadelphia: Saunders, 1992;158.

2. Indian Health Service. Illness among Indians and Alaska Natives, 1970–1978. DHEW Publication No. (HSA) 79-12040:4,11. Washington, DC: U.S. Department of Health, Education, and Welfare, Public Health Service, Health Services Administration, Indian Health Service, Division of Resource Coordination, Office of Program Statistics, 1979.

3. Indian Health Service. Trends in Indian Health, 1996. Washington, DC: U.S. Department of Health and Human Services, Indian Health Service, Office of Planning, Evaluation, and Legislation, Division of Program Statistics, 1997.

4. Sack RB, Santosham M, Reid R, et al. Diarrhoeal diseases in the White Mountain Apaches: clinical studies. J Diarrhoeal Dis Res 1995;13:12–17.

5. Santosham M, Sack RB, Reid R, et al. Diarrhoeal diseases in the White Mountain Apaches: epidemiologic studies. J Diarrhoeal Dis Res 1995;13:18–28.

6. Sack RB, Myers LL, Almeido-Hill J, et al. Enterotoxigenic *Bacteroides fragilis*: epidemiologic studies of its role as a human diarrhoeal pathogen. J Diarrhoeal Dis Res 1992;10:4–9.

7. Kleigman RM, Plotkin SA. Infectious Diseases:

Rotavirus. Preventive Pediatrics and Epidemiology. In Behrman RE, Kleigman RM, Nelson WE, Vaughn VC III (eds), Textbook of Pediatrics (14th ed). Philadelphia: Saunders, 1992;831.

8. Pickering LK, Cleary TG. Approach to Patients with Gastrointestinal Tract Infections and Food Poisoning. In Feigin RD, Cherry JD (eds), Textbook of Pediatric Infectious Diseases (3rd ed, vol 1). Philadelphia: Saunders, 1992;574.

9. Greenberg HB. Viral Gastroenteritis. In Wilson JD, Braunwald E, Isselbacher KJ, et al. (eds), Harrison's Principles of Internal Medicine (12th ed, vol 1). New York: McGraw-Hill, 1991;716.

10. Santosham M, Yolken RH, Wyatt RG, et al. Epidemiology of rotavirus diarrhea in a prospectively monitored American Indian population. J Infect Dis 1985;152: 778–783.

11. Santosham M, Yolken RH, Quiroz E, et al. Detection of rotavirus in respiratory secretions of children with pneumonia. J Pediatr 1983;103:583–585.

12. Horwitz MA, Pollard RA, Merson MH, Martin MS. A large outbreak of food-borne salmonellosis on the Navajo nation Indian reservation: epidemiology and secondary transmission. Am J Public Health 1971;67: 1071–1076.

13. Santosham M, Brown KH, Sack RB. Oral rehydration therapy and dietary therapy for acute childhood diarrhea. Pediatr Rev 1987;8:273–278.

Chapter 9
Otitis Media

Diana C. Hu

Otitis media (OM) and middle ear diseases are not illnesses unique to Native Americans, but they occur with greater frequency and cause more long-term morbidity in the Native American population throughout North America than in the rest of the U.S. population. The epidemiology and natural history also differ from the general population. This chapter reviews historic studies that describe the increased prevalence of middle ear disease in various Native American and Alaska Native groups, presents the current standards of diagnosis and treatment of middle ear disease, and explores areas of future endeavor to decrease OM in this population.

Definitions

OM has an array of presentations that represent a continuum in the time course of ear disease.

1. *Acute suppurative OM (AOM)*. This is usually the initial presentation of middle ear disease in children. It is associated clinically with ear pain or irritability, with or without fever or ear drainage. Physical examination with pneumatic otoscopy shows a reddened and thickened tympanic membrane (TM) or a TM with an effusion and injection. Decreased mobility of the TM is noted.
2. *Perforation*. Perforation of the TM may be found in two forms: (1) associated with an AOM with purulent drainage present, often with spontaneous resolution after treatment with antimicrobial agents, and (2) dry perforation associated with chronic OM and often associated with conductive hearing loss. This perforation is not likely to heal spontaneously, despite antimicrobial treatment.
3. *Serous OM (SOM)*. This condition is now also called *OM with effusion* (OME) and consists of nonpurulent fluid visible behind the TM on pneumatic otoscopy without accompanying signs or symptoms of acute infection. Mobility of the TM may be decreased or normal

with insufflation. Retraction of the TM may be seen. Duration of the effusion may be temporary after an episode of AOM or may be more chronic—that is, persisting for longer than 3 months.
4. *Chronic OM*. Chronic OM is usually described in three subsets:

1. Chronic OM with effusion is middle ear effusion persisting for longer than 3 months.
2. Chronic suppurative OM is purulent middle ear effusion associated with otorrhea for more than 6 weeks.
3. Chronic OM with perforation is a dry perforation with scarring of the TM and a low rate of spontaneous healing of the perforation.

All the above chronic OM manifestations may have an associated conductive hearing loss.

Epidemiology

Middle ear infection is one of the most common childhood infections in Native and non-Native populations. Although AOM affects both Native Americans and non-Natives with equally high incidence, it is the complications of acute and chronic OM that mark the difference between these two populations. In examining rates of acute infection alone, studies in the 1980s found that 17% of U.S. children had three or more episodes of OM in a 6-month period.[1] Teele and Klein[2] found that more than two-thirds of Boston-area children younger than 3 years of age had at least one episode of AOM, and more than one-third had three or more episodes in the first 3 years of life. Historically, the prevalence of AOM in the Native American population has equaled or exceeded that of the North American population. Studies of Alaska natives in the 1960s showed that 58% of Eskimo children had at least one episode of acute otorrhea in the first year of life.[3] This markedly underestimated the incidence of AOM because recall of otorrhea was used as the definition of an episode of AOM, which selects only the small subset of all AOM that presents with perforation. In a survey of four Southwestern tribes in the late 1970s, more than 1,000 children were followed: 60% had an attack of AOM during the first year of life and 47% had two or more episodes of AOM by age 2 years.[4] Data taken from the Navajo population (a reservation-based population of almost 200,000) in 1990 showed that 40% of all children younger than age 4 years had at least one new episode of OM during the 12-month period surveyed.[5]

Uncomplicated AOM remains a significant health problem for the Native American population, but the distinction between Native American-Alaska Native populations and non-Native populations is most evident when looking at complications of OM, specifically the rates of chronic perforation and hearing loss. The literature quotes widely divergent rates for chronic OM in the Native American population, ranging from 15 to 60 times that in the non-Native population. In the mid-1970s, OM and its long-term complications were estimated to be 15 times more prevalent in Native Americans than in whites.[6] During the 1970s and 1980s, the prevalence of chronic suppurative OM and perforation in other non-Native American populations was as low as 0.5% in school children in Pittsburgh and Sweden[7] but with rates averaging approximately 2% in other non-Native populations. In contrast, Brody et al.[7] in 1965 described a population surrounding Bethel, Alaska, where more than 1,000 children were surveyed. Thirty-one percent of the respondents had had at least one episode of draining ear in the first 3 years of life. Severe hearing loss occurred in 1–13% of the population of children studied (all available children were tested regardless of history of ear disease), but of those with severe loss, 86% had a history of a draining ear, implying a role of perforation in development of hearing loss. In the 10-year follow-up study of Eskimo children in 1973, Kaplan et al. found that 76% of 489 Eskimo children had a history of chronic OM, with 41% having chronic perforation.[3] Sixteen percent of the children had a 26-dB hearing loss, and 9% of all examined children had suppurative otorrhea at the time of examination.

Descriptions of chronic OM in Southwestern Indians were given by Zonis in 1968[8] and in Navajos by Jaffe in 1969.[9] They found that Navajo and Apache children had a higher-than-normal prevalence of chronic OM with perforation (4.2% and 8%, respectively, which was 2–5 times the rate in the general population at a comparable time). Zonis also noted that the non-Athabascan tribes of the Southwest did not have significantly higher rates of chronic OM than did the Athabascan tribes of the Southwest.

Rates of chronic OM clearly have changed in the 30 years since these observations. A 16-year comparison study of OM in an Apache population showed no change in the overall prevalence of middle ear disease but a significant decrease in the number of examined patients with evidence of chronic ear disease (especially perforation), with a decrease from 7.7% to 3.3% of examined ears.[10] A study by Gregg et al.[11] comparing ear disease in 1963–1965 and 1982 in two early–school-age South Dakota populations found a history of ear disease or hearing loss in more than 25% of the surveyed Native American children. Native American and non-Native children were included, and the numbers of Native Americans in the second sample were small, but the prevalence of ear disease showed no decrease during the almost 20-year interval. However, physical examination findings showed less evidence of chronic ear disease (retraction, scarring, perforation) in the more recently surveyed group. In prevalence data on other populations in 12 developing countries during a similar time period (1980s), Berman found rates of perforation varying from 0.4% to 5.7%.[12] Access to medical care and antimicrobial therapy appears to have affected the sequelae of OM, but there remains a suggestion of more chronic ear disease in Native American children.

Causal Associations

Many studies have looked at the role of socioeconomic status and poor housing conditions on the rates of OM in Native Americans. There has been no clear consensus on the impact of environmental factors on rates of OM for different tribal groups. A study published in 1973 by Johonnott[13] noted a significant difference in the prevalence of chronic OM in urban versus rural Alaska Native children: Urban Anchorage had a 4.4% prevalence, whereas rural Alaska had an 18.3% prevalence. A comprehensive study of a subset of Navajos, Hopis, San Carlos Apaches, and Colorado River Indian patients included home visitation as well as self-assessment questionnaires. The study showed no consistent, statistically significant relationship between many environmental factors (i.e., crowding, number of rooms in house, water supply, sewage disposal, heating, cooling, electricity, distance to health care facility, mother's education) and the development of AOM.[14] Studies in the Alaska Natives looking at the role of urban versus rural environment in the development of chronic OM also had conflicting results.

Other indigenous peoples, such as Australian aborigines and Melanesian islanders, were studied in the 1970s and were also found to have a high prevalence of perforation. Almost 12% of ears studied had perforation, and so these populations were thought to be very similar to the Native American populations in epidemiology of middle ear disease. These populations are also of low socioeconomic status and have had variable access to medical care. Berman's study of varying rates of OM and complications in developing countries found that access to medical care and changes in socioeconomic status were significant determinants in lowering the rates of chronic OM and complications.[12] Data on rates of chronic OM in the 1990s are not available. As societal and economic changes occur in the tribes studied, it will be important to see if rates of complication fall.

Familial and genetic issues have been raised as a predisposing factor for acquisition of OM. Early work (in the 1960s) found higher rates of chronic otitis for Athabascan tribes than for other Southwestern tribes. In the 1980s, Shaw et al.[14] reviewed data from Phoenix-area Indian Health Service providers. They found continued higher attack rates of acute suppurative OM in the Apache and Navajo children than in the Colorado River and Hopi children.[14] However, a 1985 study by Todd and Feldman[15] examined the impact of "allergic airway disease" (asthma or allergic rhinitis) on recurrent OM. They found that the patterns of recurrent OM in San Carlos Apache and Colorado River Indians were the same, 55% of the children having had at least two separate episodes of OM before 2 years of age.[15]

The most-studied Southwestern Native American population is the White Mountain Apache tribe on the Whiteriver Apache reservation, in whom multiple longitudinal studies on OM have been done. In 1977, Spivey and Hirschorn[16] compared the risk of pneumonia, diarrheal illness, and AOM in Apache children adopted by non-Native American middle class families to that of their non-Apache adoptive siblings and other Apache children still residing on the Whiteriver Apache reservation. The adopted Apache children continued to have an incidence of OM similar to the reservation Apache children, and the rates of pneumonia and diarrheal illness decreased, but they were still higher than in non-Apache adoptive siblings. The authors concluded there may be an inherent "genetic" predisposition to OM. A family study in the White Mountain Apache tribe showed no statistically significant difference between chronic OM prevalence in children with first-degree relatives with ear disease than in those without, but there was a suggestion of familial concurrence.[17]

Two studies looked at the role of facial structure as a possible predisposing cause for AOM and chronic OM in Athabascan tribes. In Athabascan tribes, a high incidence of facial clefting has been noted; it is similar to rates in Asian populations. The association of high rates of OM with cleft lip and palate is well established in all ethnic groups. The Athabascan tribes also have a high incidence of bifid or cleft uvula. The hypothesis was that bifid uvula could be a *forme fruste* of facial clefting that predisposes to OM. Despite an established prevalence of cleft uvula in 20% of San Carlos and White Mountain Apaches (compared to 1–3% in mixed-ethnic or primarily white groups

in Denver and Washington, DC), however, no association between clefting and increased risk of chronic OM was noted in Apaches.[18, 19]

Eustachian tube function in Native Americans may play a role in increased rates of OM. In the White Mountain Apaches, Berry and associates[20] studied eustachian tube function in young children and adults with chronic perforation and showed a functional difference from white populations with traumatic and chronic perforations. Differences in the eustachian tube function were hypothesized to predispose to recurrent AOM as well as perforation.

In addition to structural and familial risk factors, increased risk of bacterial infection has also been hypothesized as a cause of increased AOM. Historically, the Apache, Navajo, and Alaska Native tribes have had an increased incidence of invasive pneumococcal and *Haemophilus influenzae* disease before immunization for these pathogens. Researchers have studied the immune processing of these bacteria by Native Americans. Although no specific immune deficiency or processing defect has been found in the Athabascan tribes, it is postulated that causes other than environment account for the increased incidence of bacterial disease. It is known that Apaches and Navajos have a lower immunologic response than white children to specific types of *H. influenzae* type b (Hib) conjugate vaccines as well as to wild-type Hib disease.[21] Given that pneumococcus and untypable *H. influenzae* are the primary pathogens in almost 60% of cases of AOM in the general population, it may be that processing of these pathogens or environmental factors that predispose to these infections (or both) increases the risk of AOM in the Native American Athabascan population.

Diagnosis and Treatment

Because of discussions about increasing antimicrobial resistance in pneumococcus and other bacteria and about the role that outpatient antibiotics play in development of resistance, the criteria for the diagnosis of OM have been reviewed extensively in the pediatric literature. In the general population, 42% of all ambulatory antimicrobial prescriptions are attributed to the diagnosis of OM.[22] Application of stringent diagnostic criteria and the more judicious use of antimicrobials for treatment of AOM, with resultant reduction of antimicrobial use, are part of a changing standard of practice that has evolved throughout the 1990s in response to the evolution of antimicrobial resistance. The Centers for Disease Control and Prevention (CDC), with the American Academy of Pediatrics and American Academy of Family Practice, have published guidelines addressing diagnosis and treatment of middle ear disease and other common ambulatory care infections in pediatrics.[23] A review of current guidelines follows.

Acute Otitis Media

Use of pneumatic otoscopy remains the standard for diagnosis, and the presence of middle ear effusion *with* signs or symptoms of acute local or systemic illness (i.e., specific signs, such as otalgia or otorrhea, or nonspecific signs, such as fever) are necessary for the diagnosis of AOM. Use of other diagnostic methods, such as tympanometry and acoustic reflectometry, have been suggested, but these are not readily available to the general primary care practitioner. Even with these criteria, there is evidence in the literature and from clinical experience that more than 80% of AOM resolves spontaneously without antimicrobial treatment. Because of this, the standard in some European countries is to not initiate antibiotics on the first presentation with uncomplicated AOM (no otorrhea or recent previous AOM) but to schedule a return visit in 48 hours and treat only those who have persistent symptoms. However, studies show it is not possible on clinical examination to distinguish those patients with uncomplicated AOM who will spontaneously improve without treatment from those that will not; therefore, the standard in the United States has been to initiate therapy on presentation. The new guidelines do not suggest delay in therapy but, rather, more stringent initial examination and 5-day antimicrobial treatment courses for uncomplicated AOM in children older than 2 years of age. Abbreviated antimicrobial coarses (<10 days) in children younger than 2 years of age have been associated with higher recurrence rates than standard 10-day therapy, although younger infants have a higher recurrence rate than older children even when 10-day therapy is used. Although no specific bacteriologic studies have been done in Native Americans, the bacterial pathogens causing AOM in childhood in the Native American population are presumed to be the same as in the general population, with a predominance of pneumococcus and untypable *H. influenzae* and a minority of *Moraxella catarrhalis*.

Otitis Media with Effusion

AOM must be distinguished from OME, which is the presence of a middle ear effusion without coincident signs or symptoms associated with AOM. Recommendations of no antimicrobial treatment for OME of less than 3 months duration differ from past recommendations. Past myringotomy studies of OME have shown that bacteria are present in the effusion fluid, which led to guidelines in the 1970s for antimicrobial treatment of all chronic effusions. Although meta-analysis of subsequent data does establish that such treatment improves short-term resolution of the effusion, the cure rate above placebo is small enough that seven children would need to be treated for one to clearly benefit.[23] The natural cure rate of OME is quite high: More than 90% of OME after AOM clears spontaneously within 3 months with no treatment. The collaborative report in 1994 on practice guidelines for the treatment of OME in young children endorsed either no treatment or antimicrobial treatment.[24] The desire to reduce use of ambulatory antimicrobials, the accompanying increased risk of colonization by resistant bacteria, and the marginal benefit with treatment has now led the CDC to recommend no treatment. Data has been generated to show that antihistamine and decongestant use are not effective in the treatment of OME.

Chronic Otitis Media with Effusion

In the child with chronic OME lasting more than 3 months with hearing loss, a more aggressive approach is warranted. The Agency for Health Care Policy Research guidelines suggest either antimicrobial therapy or myringotomy and tympanostomy tube placement for these patients.[24] The use of steroids and antimicrobials to treat chronic OME has been suggested as an alternative to tympanostomy tube placement, but this recommendation has not been included in the 1994 collaborative panel report.[1]

Suppurative Otitis Media with Perforation

The diagnosis of AOM with perforation is made with visualization of discharge clearly originating from the middle ear space. The microbiology of the acute perforation is the same as with AOM without perforation, but in the setting of chronic suppurative OM with perforation, colonization with *Staphylococcus aureus, Pseudomonas*, and some fungi can complicate treatment.

Antimicrobial Treatment

In the Native American-Alaska Native patient, the same treatment regimens are currently recommended as for the general population. In 1997, the issue of increased antimicrobial resistance, especially for pneumococcus, has had more impact on *whether* to treat (and perhaps how long to treat) than *what* to treat with. Amoxicillin is still considered the first-line medication. Trimethoprim-sulfamethoxazole (TMP-SMX) is used for the penicillin-allergic patient or as second-line treatment for recurrent AOM. The efficacy, cost, and side effects of amoxicillin have led to its continued use as first-line treatment, even in light of the rising penicillin resistance of pneumococcus, the beta-lactamase production of untypable *H. influenzae* and *M. catarrhalis*, and the high spontaneous resolution rate of AOM. A wide array of oral cephalosporins (e.g., cefixime, loracarbef, cefuroxime axetil, cefprozil, cefpodoxime), macrolide combinations (e.g., erythromycin/sulfisoxazole [Pediazole], azithromycin, clarithromycin) and amoxicillin-clavulanic acid (Augmentin) are usually third- or fourth-line oral treatment of persistent or recurrent AOM.

Green and Rothrock[25] postulated a role for injectable ceftriaxone in the treatment of AOM in a study showing that single-dose ceftriaxone, 50 mg/kg given intramuscularly, yielded resolution rates similar to amoxicillin therapy. The role of ceftriaxone therapy in the treatment of isolated, uncomplicated AOM is unclear. Given the frequent use of intramuscular ceftriaxone for empiric treatment of the febrile infant with either no source for the fever or as initial therapy for presumed serious bacterial infection, many children with coincident AOM receive ceftriaxone therapy. However, concerns about overuse of antimicrobials and increasing resistance of pneumococcus to cephalosporins as well as penicillins should prompt practitioners to try to limit the use of broad-spectrum agents to treat infections that can be treated with narrower-spectrum agents.

Certain special cases of AOM may require different therapeutic selections. In the neonate, the higher likelihood of gram-negative enteric infection as a cause of AOM has led to suggestions for myringotomy and culture before initiation of antimicrobials and use of parenteral antibiotics. On culture, however, the most common causative agents remain the same as those for older children. The presence of bullae on the TM on pneumatic otoscopy is associated with *Mycoplasma pneumoniae* infection, but, more commonly, pneumococcal infection causes bullae formation. In this instance, many practitioners opt for a macrolide-containing preparation to cover any possibility of *Mycoplasma* infection as well as pneumococcal infection, but amoxicillin is usually adequate in most cases.

Chronic OM with perforation carries the risk of infection with *Staphylococcus* or *Pseudomonas*. Some practitioners advocate the use of topical gentamicin in the external ear if the otorrhea suggests *Pseudomonas* (i.e., green chronic discharge). However, use of 2% acetic acid solution (Domeboro drops) varies the pH of the canal enough to suppress *Pseudomonas* growth without use of topical antimicrobials; the patient often resists because of stinging. Use of oral antibiotics (as opposed to topical agents alone) is recommended for treatment of OM with perforation and otorrhea. This same principle applies to children with tympanostomy tubes and otorrhea.

The child with recurrent OM presents a special problem to the practitioner. First, the question of whether the infection is *recurrent* or *persistent* must be answered. Persistent infection is defined as pneumatic otoscopic findings consistent with AOM and symptoms within 2 weeks of AOM or during therapy for AOM. A change in antimicrobial therapy to a beta-lactamase–resistant preparation, under the supposition that the persistent symptoms may be due to resistant bacteria, is the standard course. Many practitioners think that recurrent otitis can be treated with repeated courses of amoxicillin, as opposed to second- or third-line agents, if the duration between episodes of AOM exceeds 30 days.

The child with multiple recurrences of AOM (the "high-risk" or "otitis-prone" child) is the subject of controversy about treatment. Many practitioners advocate the use of antimicrobial prophylaxis for the child who has three episodes in 6 months or four episodes in 1 year.[23] Multiple studies have been done with multiple agents (erythromycin, amoxicillin, TMP-SMX, or sulfisoxazole), all showing efficacy in decreasing the recurrence rate. However, other studies have noted that the risk of colonization with drug-resistant pneumococci increases greatly with proximity to a short course of oral antibiotics and also with use of amoxicillin prophylaxis for OM. This has led to discussions of the risk-benefit ratio of the use of prophylactic antibiotics to prevent recurrences. The CDC report stresses that selecting the patient most likely to benefit from prophylaxis is most important (i.e., the child younger than 2 years of age, those in out-of-home child care, and Native Americans) rather than using antimicrobial prophylaxis for all patients with recurrent AOM. They also note that poor compliance with the daily regimen greatly decreases the efficacy of the prophylaxis because continuous daily therapy is more successful than intermittent therapy in all studies. Because of this, once-daily prophylactic therapy with sulfisoxazole or amoxicillin for less than 6 months is recommended. Surgical intervention with tympanostomy tubes for failures is another option if antimicrobial prophylaxis fails.

Surgical Intervention

Surgical interventions for OM and its sequelae depend on the age of the patient, degree of hearing loss, and language function in the young patient. The use of tympanostomy tubes for SOM with hearing loss in the 20- to 25-dB range in the speech frequencies is an indication for tube placement. Language delay in the young child with recurrent AOM or persistent OME at a time when language acquisition is critical may benefit from otolaryngologic evaluation and surgical intervention. The timing of tympanoplasty for the child with chronic dry perforation of the TM is more variable. Many surgeons prefer to wait until the child is of school age (out of the otitis-prone age) and able to follow simple postoperative care instructions before embarking on a tympanoplasty. Mastoiditis, especially that necessitating surgical intervention, is extremely rare in the Native American population: In the 1990s, the prevalence was less than 1% of pediatric patients.

Future Work

It is still unknown why Native American populations are more predisposed to OM and its sequelae. As Native American populations become more assimilated and socioeconomic changes occur on reservations, it will be important to follow disease trends to determine the genetic versus environmental contributions to disease acquisition. Development of pneumococcal conjugate vaccines for use in infancy, similar to the conjugate Hib vaccines developed in the 1980s, may have great impact on the incidence of AOM during the otitis-prone period (younger than 2 years of age). Standards for early identification of the child who is otitis prone, intervention by primary care providers, access to and appropriate referral to otolaryngology, and developmental follow-up should be established for the high-risk Native American population.

Summary

OM remains a problem for both Native American and non-Native populations. Although historic data show an increased predisposition to chronic OM in Native Americans, more recent epidemiologic studies are lacking to see if complications have decreased with increased access to care, increased use of antimicrobials, improvements in socioeconomic conditions, and changes in bacterial epidemiology. Data on the spontaneous resolution rates of AOM and OME, as well as increasing concern about antimicrobial resistance in bacteria and overuse of antimicrobials, should lead to more stringent application of diagnostic criteria for the child with middle ear effusion to determine the need for and type of intervention.

Acknowledgments

The author thanks Drs. Steve Holve, Steve Moul, Jane Oski, and Paul Moller for their review of and advice on the preparation of this manuscript.

References

1. Berman S. Otitis media in children. N Engl J Med 1995;332:1560–1565.
2. Teele DW, Klein JO, Rosener BA. Epidemiology of otitis media in children. Ann Otol Rhinol Laryngol 1980;89(Suppl 68):5–6.
3. Kaplan GJ, Fleshman JK, Bender TR, et al. Long term effects of otitis media: a ten-year cohort study of Alaskan Eskimo children. Pediatrics 1973;52:577–585.
4. Goodwin MH Jr, Shaw JR, Feldman CM. Distribution of otitis media among four Indian populations in Arizona. Public Health Rep 1980;95:589–594.
5. IHS Headquarters, West Data Center. The Navajo Health Status Report 1996. (draft).
6. Weit RJ. Patterns of ear disease in the Southwestern American Indian. Arch Otolaryngol 1979;105:381–385.
7. Brody JA, Overfield T, McAlister R. Draining ears and deafness among Alaska Eskimos. Arch Otolaryngol 1965;81:29–33.
8. Zonis RD. Chronic otitis media in the southwestern American Indian. Arch Otolaryngol 1968;88:361–365.
9. Jaffe BF. The incidence of ear disease in the Navajo Indians. Laryngoscope 1969;79:2126–2134.
10. Todd NW Jr, Bowman CA. Otitis media at Canyon Day, Ariz. A 16 year follow-up in Apache Indians. Arch Otolaryngol 1985;111:606–608.
11. Gregg JB, Roberts KM, Colleran MJ. Ear disease and hearing loss, Pierre, South Dakota, 1962–1982. S D J Med 1983;10:9–17.
12. Berman S. Otitis media in developing countries. Pediatrics 1995;96:126–131.
13. Johonnott SC. Differences in chronic otitis media between rural and urban Eskimo children. Clin Pediatr 1973;12:415–419.
14. Shaw JR, Todd NW, Goodwin MH Jr, Feldman CM. Observations on the relation of environmental and behavioral factors to the occurrence of otitis media among Indian children. Public Health Rep 1981;96:342–349.
15. Todd NW, Feldman CM. Allergic airway disease and otitis media in children. Int J Pediatr Otorhinolaryngol 1985;10:27–35
16. Spivey GH, Hirschorn N. Migrant study of adopted Apache children. Johns Hopkins Medical Journal 1977;140:43–46.
17. Todd NW. Familial predisposition for otitis media in Apache Indians at Canyon Day, Arizona. Genet Epidemiol 1987;4:25–31.
18. Todd NW, Fischler RS. Bifid uvula and otitis media in Apache Indians. Cleft Palate J 1986;23:318–320.
19. Fischler RS, Todd NW, Feldman C. Lack of association of cleft uvula with otitis media in Apache Indian children. Am J Dis Children 1987;141:866–867.
20. Beery QC, Doyle WJ, Cantekin EI, Weit RJ. Eustachian tube function in an American Indian population. Ann Otol Rhinol Laryngol 1980;89:28–33.
21. Santosham M, et al. Prevention of *Haemophilus influenzae* type b infections in Apache and Navajo children. J Infect Dis 1992;165(Suppl 1):144–151.
22. Nelson WL, Kennedy DL, Lao CS, Kuritsky JN. Outpatient systemic anti-infective use by children in the United States, 1977–1986. Pediatr Infect Dis 1988;7:505–509.
23. Dowel SF (ed). Principles of judicious use of antimicrobial agents for pediatric upper respiratory infections. Pediatrics 1988;101(Suppl):163–184.
24. Stool SE, Berg AO, Berman S, et al. Otitis Media with Effusion in Young Children. Clinical Practice Guideline. AHPCR Publication No. 94-0622. Washington, DC: Agency for Health Care Policy and Research 1994.
25. Green SM, Rothrock SG. Single dose intramuscular ceftriaxone for acute otitis media in children. Pediatrics 1993;91:23–30.

Chapter 10
Bacterial Meningitis

George Brenneman

Bacterial meningitis among American Indian (AI) and Alaska Native (AN) infants and children before 1990 occurred with an impressive frequency that few other populations in the nation experienced. Professionals providing health care services to AI and AN patients documented high rates of invasive bacterial diseases (e.g., meningitis, septicemia, pneumonia, and septic arthritis) due to *Haemophilus influenzae* (Hi). Most of these were serotype b (Hib), when serotyping was performed and recorded, or one of a number of serotypes of *Streptococcal pneumoniae* (Spn).

High mortality rates and devastating sequelae associated with bacterial meningitis were common emotionally wrenching experiences for Indian Health Service (IHS) health care workers, AI and AN communities, and families. Thus, emergence of technology that promised safe and effective vaccines against Hib was very welcome and prompted systematic epidemiologic studies of invasive Hib disease among several AI and AN communities in the 1980s.

After clinical trials, which began in the mid-1980s, effective Hib vaccines became available in 1991 and were used widely in AI and AN communities. Based on published[1, 2] and unsystematic clinical observations from several IHS areas, invasive Hib diseases, especially meningitis, among AI and AN infants have significantly decreased since 1991. Physicians serving AI and AN children now seldom face the need to care for an infant with bacterial meningitis. This decline in Hib meningitis cases most likely will be followed by a welcome decline in AI and AN infant mortality due to meningitis.

The success in reducing a serious infectious disease among AI and AN children is a remarkable achievement. Many laboratory, clinical, and research professionals and indigenous outreach workers are entitled to much credit for this achievement. Greatest credit, however, goes to AI and AN infants, their families, and their communities, who willingly participated in many studies that defined the epidemiology of bacterial meningitis and that tested the safety, immunogenicity, and efficacy of new Hib vaccines.

Epidemiologic Studies

Incidence

Clinical observations and published retrospective health record reviews clearly indicated excessive rates of bacterial meningitis,[3] especially Hi meningitis, among AI and AN infants and young children. (At the time data were collected, many IHS hospital laboratories could not determine Hi serotypes. In the clinical setting, clinicians assumed that an invasive Hi infection was most likely Hib.) Review of health records from 1957 to 1964 in a Yupik Eskimo population in Alaska found that an annual average of 1 in 74 Eskimo infants experienced purulent meningitis and 1 in 200 infants died from the disease.[4] Later review in the same Alaska region (July 1971 to June 1974) showed an annual incidence of Hi meningitis of 474 per 100,000 children younger than 5 years of age.[5] A third report based on retrospective data from 1971 to 1977 from the same region in Alaska revealed a bacterial meningitis rate of 84.4 cases per 100,000 population, which was more than 10 times that of other U.S. populations. Hi accounted for 68% of these cases (409 per 100,000 children younger than 5 years of age).[6] Table 10-1 highlights data from these retrospective studies and shows clearly that the dominant cause of meningitis among AI and AN patients was Hi and that most meningitis occurred in the first year of life.

Early documentation of high rates of meningitis among AI and AN children and the promise of effective Hib vaccines led investigators to work on clarifying the epidemiology of Hi meningitis and other invasive Hi diseases among children in several AI and AN communities.

Table 10-1. Retrospective Health Record Surveillance: Meningitis Data from Selected American Indian and Alaska Native Populations

Region	Dates	Age	Etiology	Total Cases	Annual Rate (per 100,000)	Total Deaths	Mortality Rate
Southwestern	1957–1964	Infants	?	43	1,342	16	?
Alaska		1–4 yrs	?	9	?	2	?
	1971–1974	Infants	Hi 72%	32	63	?	?
		<5 yrs	?	?	474	?	?
	1971–1977	<5 yrs	Hi 68%	?	409	?	?
Navajo	1968–1973	Infants	69% Hi	136	?	?	12%
			26% Spn		?	?	24%
			5% Nm		?	?	?
		1–4 yrs	64% Hi	42	?	?	?
			12% Spn				
			7% Nm		?	?	?
			17% other				
Arizona	1978–1983	Infants	82% Hi	76	Overall Hib 136	5	8%
(other than			15% Spn			2	17%
Navajo)			3% Nm			1	50%
		1–4 yrs	58% Hi	26			
			8% Spn			0	0
			4% Nm				
			30% other				

Hi = *Haemophilus influenzae*; Spn = *Streptococcus pneumoniae*; Nm = *Neisseria meningitidis;* Hib = *Haemophilus influenzae* serotype b.

In a study on the Apache reservation, retrospective review of hospital records from January 1973 to December 1981 and prospective surveillance from October 1981 to January 1983 revealed an overall Hi meningitis incidence rate of 254 per 100,000 in Apache children younger than 5 years of age. Yearly incidence during this study of Hi meningitis among Apache infants was 500 to 2,917 cases per 100,000 and, among children younger than 5 years, 108 to 692 cases per 100,000. These high rates are eight times the incidence in the general U.S. population.[7] A prospective laboratory-based surveillance from January 1980 to December 1982 among AN (Eskimo-Aleut and Indian) children younger than 5 years of age revealed similar high rates of invasive Hib disease. For Eskimo children younger than 5 years of age, the rate of invasive Hib disease was found to be 705 per 100,000 and 401 per 100,000 in AI children. In this same period, non-Native children experienced a rate of 129 cases per 100,000. Among Eskimo children, Hib meningitis accounted for approximately 40% of cases, whereas 60% of cases among AIs were meningitis.[8]

Early Disease

An important characteristic of Hi meningitis among AI and AN children when compared with the general population is the younger age of highest incidence. Among

Navajo children, 81% of meningitis in children younger than 5 years of age occurred in infants younger than 1 year of age. Sixty-four percent of cases clustered between 4 and 8 months of age. The median age for Hib meningitis in AN children was 11.5 months.[7]

Chronic Disease and Sequelae

General literature reporting long-term follow-up in children who experienced meningitis, Hi meningitis in particular, reveals very high rates of serious sequelae due to central nervous system (CNS) damage.[9, 10] Chronic sequelae among AI children also have been reported. Review of Navajo children who had meningitis (68% due to Hi and 22% due to Spn) 3.6–15.0 years earlier, revealed significantly lower mean IQ scores when compared with their siblings. Of the 29% of the children in this study cohort with severe neurologic sequelae, 24% were found to be mentally retarded, 5% had hearing loss, 7% had cerebral palsy, and 12% had seizures.[11]

Genetic Predisposition

Excessive rates of invasive Hib meningitis and other invasive Hib diseases and high recurrent Hib disease[12] raised the question of possible impaired immune responses to bacterial infections in AI and AN children. In one study,

Figure 10-1. Postneonatal mortality from 1986 to 1993 resulting from meningitis and septicemia.

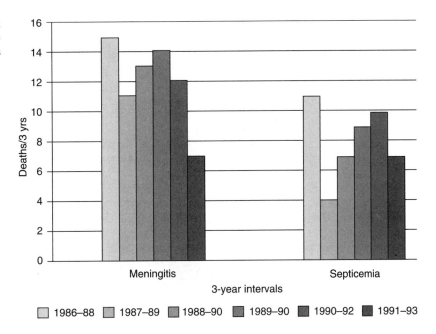

immunoglobulin G (IgG), IgM, and IgA responses after Hib capsular polysaccharide vaccination in 24-month-old apache children were 10 times lower than in white children of a similar age.[13] Responses to tetanus toxoid and diphtheria toxoid, however, were only two times lower.[13] In genetic studies done between 1971 and 1982 among 103 Alaska Eskimo children who had invasive Hib disease (mostly meningitis) and among matched controls, some genetic factors appeared to contribute to susceptibility to invasive Hib disease.[14] These studies among Alaska Eskimo children also revealed a positive association between the presence of a polymorphic genetic variant of uridine monophosphate kinase-3 and invasive Hib disease and a tendency toward a younger age at onset of illness.[15, 16]

Trends

Mortality

The story of meningitis among AI and AN children parallels events in development, testing, and public health use of effective Hib vaccines. The story is dramatic, interesting, and most gratifying. Meningitis and septicemia were among the five or six leading causes of AI and AN postneonatal infant mortality before 1990, but available data suggest declining death certificate diagnoses of postneonatal meningitis, as shown in Figure 10-1.[17] These data from IHS no longer include meningitis or septicemia among the five leading causes of AI and AN postneonatal infant mortality.

Morbidity

Dramatic decrease in number of diagnosed cases of Hib meningitis, the single most important cause of bacterial meningitis in infants and children younger than 5 years of age, clearly reflects the success of effective Hib vaccines and Hib immunization programs for AI and AN children beginning in early 1991. Figure 10-2 shows this decline of Hib meningitis among Navajo children younger than 5 years of age, which occurred after implementation of a reservation-wide Hib vaccination program in 1991. Information from other high-risk AI and AN populations reveal similar remarkable reductions in meningitis as well as other invasive Hib diseases.[1]

Primary Prevention

Various Vaccines

Licensure of the first Hib vaccine in 1984 was based on efficacy data from a national vaccine efficacy trial in Finland.[18] This vaccine was purified capsular polysaccharide, known as *polymer (of) ribose phosphate* (PRP). As seen with other polysaccharide immunogens, PRP was not immunogenic or effective in infants and was not recommended for children younger than 15–18 months of age. Because most invasive Hib diseases occurred in children younger than 2 years of age (in AI and AN children, younger than 1 year of age) and because postlicensure studies suggested weak efficacy,[19] PRP vaccine did not receive general enthusiastic reception.

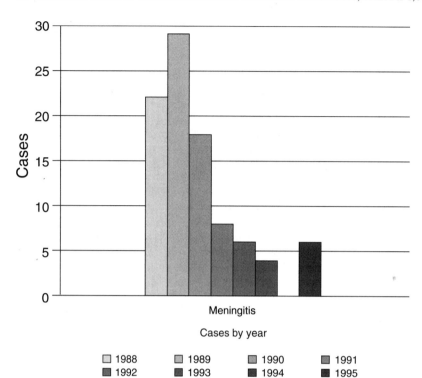

Figure 10-2. *Haemophilus influenzae* serotype b meningitis in Navajo children younger than 5 years of age from 1988 to 1995. There were no cases in 1994.

Cases by year

☐ 1988   ☐ 1989   ■ 1990   ■ 1991
■ 1992   ■ 1993   ■ 1994   ■ 1995

When a T-cell–independent polysaccharide immunogen (e.g., PRP) is bonded covalently (conjugated) with a highly immunogenic protein T-cell–dependent immunogen, T-cell–dependent characteristics transfer to the polysaccharide part of the conjugate. This knowledge was applied in development of conjugate Hib vaccines, and research and development by pharmaceutical companies produced four different conjugate vaccines (Table 10-2).

After phase I and II clinical testing in adults, these conjugate vaccines underwent evaluation when given to infants. Initial studies demonstrated promising immunogenicity in infants in a primary series of two to three injections at 2-month intervals at 2–6 months of age. Anamnestic responses followed booster doses at 12–18 months of age. Successful safety and immunogenicity studies of these conjugate vaccines led to efficacy trials. Eventually, three highly effective conjugate Hib vaccines (PRP-OMP, PRP-T,

HbOC) were approved by the U.S. Food and Drug Administration (FDA) for routine immunization of infants.

Immunogenicity

Except for PRP-D, conjugate Hib vaccines have demonstrated excellent immunogenicity in infants after a primary series given at 2, 4, and 6 months of age (PRP-T and HbOC) or at 2 and 4 months of age (PRP-OMP).[20, 21]

Two important observations on immunogenicity are relevant to primary prevention of Hib meningitis among AI and AN infants. Studies among AI and AN infants[22–24] and non-AI infants[25] receiving PRP-OMP demonstrated robust anti-PRP response after the initial vaccination at 2 months of age, in contrast to more sluggish responses after PRP-T or HbOC. Given that invasive Hib disease, especially Hib meningitis, occurs in early infancy

Table 10-2. Conjugate Vaccines: Polymer (of) Ribose Phosphate (PRP)

Trade Name	Company	Abbreviation	Carrier Protein
PedvaxHIB	Merck & Co, Inc., West Point, PA	PRP-OMP	Outer membrane protein of *Neisseria meningitidis*
ActHIB	Pasteur Merieux (Connaught Laboratories, Inc.), Swiftwater, PA	PRP-T	Tetanus toxoid
OmniHIB	SmithKline Beecham, Inc., Pittsburgh, PA	PRP-T	Tetanus toxoid
ProHIBit	Connaught Laboratories, Inc.	PRP-D	Diphtheria toxoid
HibTITER	Lederle-Praxis Biologicals, Pearl River, NY	HbOC	Nontoxic mutant diphtheria toxin

among AI and AN infants, PRP-OMP offers theoretical protective advantage during vulnerable early months of life.

The second observation is that conjugate Hib vaccines are interchangeable.[26] Also, higher sustained anti-PRP levels were induced when an initial PRP-OMP primary dose at 2 months of age was followed by either PRP-T or HbOC to complete the primary Hib immunization series.[27, 28] Navajo infants who received PRP-OMP as the primary immunizing series demonstrated more robust booster responses to HbOC than to PRP-OMP.[29] Based on these studies, some public health professionals in the IHS recommend a mixed vaccine primary series to give AI and AN infants the advantage of quicker and more sustained protection against invasive Hib disease.

Efficacy

Much credit for reduction of bacterial meningitis among AI and AN children, as well as among all American children, goes to many AI and AN infants, families, and communities. Recognizing the danger posed by Hib meningitis to their health, thousands of AI and AN families in a number of communities willingly participated in efficacy trials in the mid- to late 1980s.

In an important study[30] from July 1988 to August 1990, 4,161 Navajo and Hopi infants and their families participated in a double-blinded, placebo-controlled efficacy trial of PRP-OMP. The results of this trial were very gratifying and led to FDA approval of PRP-OMP, which was marketed as PedvaxHIB by Merck & Co., Inc. (West Point, PA). After the efficacy trial, Merck provided vaccine for all infants on the Navajo reservation, and soon the rates of Hib meningitis and other invasive Hib diseases began to decline.

Before the safety and efficacy of the conjugate Hib vaccines were established, the possible value of passive immunization with hyperimmune globulin, bacterial polysaccharide immune globulin (BPIG), was considered and studied.[31] When given to Apache infants, BPIG significantly reduced the incidence of invasive Hib and Spn diseases. Because it was known that young AI and AN infants were at increased risk of invasive Hib disease before active vaccines induced protective levels of antibody, combined active-passive immunization was an attractive prevention strategy.[32, 33] Public health use of active-passive Hib immunization in a high-risk AN population from July 1989 to December 1992 was followed by dramatic decline in Hib meningitis and other invasive Hib diseases.[1] Although active-passive immunization against invasive Hib extends protection into younger infancy before active vaccines alone induce protective antibody levels, public health use of passive vaccine diminishes when high community immunization levels confer herd immunity and reduce Hib pharyngeal carriage rates.

With respect to passive immunization against invasive Hib disease, studies among AN populations show significant protection against invasive Hib diseases in breast-fed infants compared to infants who were not breast-fed.[34] Before active Hib vaccines were available, maternal immunization with Hib capsular polysaccharide was considered a possible prevention strategy.[35] An important study completed in 1997 in Sacaton, Arizona, in which women of childbearing age receive Hib conjugate and Spn polysaccharide vaccines and are followed with their infants if and when pregnancy occurs, may demonstrate protective levels (up to 2 months of age) of placentally transferred anti-Hib and anti-Spn to their infants (personal communication, Mathuram Santosham, M.D., M.P.H., Center for American Indian and Alaska Native Health, Johns Hopkins School of Hygiene and Public Health, Baltimore, MD).

Hope in the Future

The excess burden of bacterial meningitis among AI and AN children is responding to effective primary prevention efforts with active Hib conjugate vaccines. As a result, Hi meningitis among AI and AN infants is relatively rare and is usually due to one of the other six Hi serotypes (type a, c, d, e, or f) or to inadequate immunization.

The primary cause of bacterial meningitis now is Spn. Among some AI and AN populations, high rates of invasive Spn disease have been reported. From 1980 to 1986, the annual Spn bacteremia rate among AN children younger than 2 years of age was 1,195 per 100,000 population.[36] The need for an effective Spn vaccine is urgent because 3.8–16.9% of Spn isolates among AN children have demonstrated relative penicillin resistance.[37] In studies on the White Mountain Apache Reservation, invasive Spn incidence rates for children between 1 and 2 years of age were 156 and 2,396 per 100,000, respectively.[38]

It is hoped that these excess rates also will fall under a successful primary prevention strategy similar to the Hib strategy discussed under Morbidity. The same technology applied in development of Hib conjugate vaccines is being applied to Spn. Because invasive Spn disease can be due to one of many serotypes (as many as 80 have been identified), conjugate vaccine development is more complex. However, surveillance in several AI and AN communities shows that 80–85% of invasive Spn disease among children younger than age 2 years is due to one of seven serotypes (personal communication, Mathuram Santosham, M.D., M.P.H., and Alan Parkinson, Ph.D., Arctic Investigations Laboratory, Centers for Disease Control and Prevention, Anchorage, AK). Conjugate vaccines with these seven most commonly implicated serotypes have been developed using the same protein carriers that were linked to PRP. These vaccines have undergone safety and immunogenicity testing and are ready for efficacy trials. In the near future, another cause of bacterial meningitis among AI and AN infants and children may become a rare event.

Table 10-3. Most Common Bacterial Agents Causing Meningitis

Age Group	Likely Organism	Antibiotic Choice
Younger than 3 mos	Streptococcus agalactiae Escherichia coli Listeria monocytogenes	Ampicillin and broad-spectrum cephalosporin
3 mos–18 yrs	Streptococcus pneumoniae Haemophilus influenzae Neisseria meningitidis	Broad-spectrum cephalosporin

Source: Adapted from VJ Quagliarello, MW Scheld. Treatment of bacterial meningitis. N Engl J Med 1997;336:711.

Clinical Management

An infant or child presenting with bacterial meningitis is a major clinical challenge. Prompt and accurate diagnosis followed by optimal treatment generally leads to a satisfactory outcome. However, bacterial meningitis is a life-threatening infection and can cause serious, disabling neurologic sequelae or death.

Early symptoms and signs of bacterial meningitis may appear to be those of routine benign illness, seen many times every day in the examining room. Since the advent of effective Hib vaccines, physicians in AI communities who several years ago diagnosed and treated bacterial meningitis regularly now rarely see an infant or child with bacterial meningitis.

The need for vigilance remains high. Hib meningitis among AI and AN infants and children continues to occur in spite of generally high community Hib immunization levels and is usually attributed to individual vaccine failure or a lapsed immunization schedule. Most Hi meningitis cases are now due to non–type b serotypes (e.g., serotypes a, c, d, e, or f). But other bacterial organisms, most often Streptococcus pneumoniae and Neisseria meningitidis, have emerged as dominant causes after the decline of Hib meningitis.

Clinical presentation, symptoms, and signs of bacterial meningitis in AI and AN infants and children are similar to those described in children generally. Response to recommended treatment for meningitis is identical to the expected responses for all other children. Thus, the clinician who decides on the management of an AI or AN infant or child with bacterial meningitis and his or her contacts provides optimal care by following current treatment and management recommendations published in respected journals and textbooks.[39, 40–42]

Bacterial Causes

The most likely bacterial agents causing meningitis in infants and children vary with age group, as shown in Table 10-3.

It should be noted that, before the advent of Hib vaccines, Hi meningitis occurred in AI and AN infants at an earlier age than in white infants. Although the use of Hib vaccines has changed the epidemiology of meningitis, clinicians should be aware that the age categories listed in Table 10-3 may have shifted to earlier ages.

Other less common organisms should always be remembered (e.g., Salmonella, staphylococci).

Symptoms and Signs

Symptoms and signs of bacterial meningitis are identical to those observed and documented in the general population. Variation by age is important to remember.

Diagnosis

Diagnosis of bacterial meningitis is made on evidence of bacteria or bacterial products in the cerebrospinal fluid (CSF). Definite bacteriologic diagnosis must be based on bacterial culture from the CSF or on Gram's stain evidence of bacteria in the CSF, but presumptive diagnoses can be made when compatible symptoms and signs are accompanied by finding bacteria in a culture of the blood or bacterial antigens in the CSF.

It is very important to avoid delay in making the diagnosis of bacterial meningitis. Delay in diagnosis is the most common reason for delay in treatment, which may result in irreversible CNS damage. Studies suggest that delay in treatment by a few hours may significantly increase risk of permanent auditory nerve or other CNS damage. Thus, the clinician should weigh the potential additional risks of delaying initiation of antibiotic therapy before doing certain diagnostic procedures.

Treatment

Table 10-4 lists current antibiotics that are usually effective against the specific organisms most frequently implicated in bacterial meningitis.[39]

Final choice of antibiotic should be based on local antibiotic resistance patterns and culture and susceptibility testing. In most clinical situations, however, it is necessary for the clinician to begin antibiotic therapy on empiric evidence while awaiting culture results. It may be necessary to continue a full course of empiric treatment in case an organism is not isolated, but adjustments may have to be made based on clinical response.

One review[40] presented important considerations about diagnostic procedures and starting antibiotics in an infant or child with suspected bacterial meningitis.

The need to perform cranial computerized tomography (CT) imaging before doing a lumbar puncture should

Table 10-4. Antibiotics and Doses for Bacterial Meningitis

Organism	Antibiotic	Dose/24 hrs (mg/kg)	Administration		Duration (days)
			Frequency		
Escherichia coli	Cefotaxime	100	Every 12 hrs <7 days old; every 8–6 hrs >7 days old		21
	Ceftriaxone*	100	Every 12 hrs		21
	Aminoglycoside	Standard dose	—		5
Streptococcus agalactiae	Ampicillin	150	Every 12 hrs <7 days old; every 8–6 hrs >7 days old		14
	Gentamicin	5	Every 12 hrs <7 days old; every 8 hrs >7 days old		5
Listeria monocytogenes	Ampicillin	150	Every 12 hrs <7 days old; every 8–6 hrs >7 days old		14
	Gentamicin	5	Every 12 hrs <7 days old; every 8 hrs >7 days old		14
Haemophilus influenzae	Cefotaxime	200	Every 8 hrs		7–10
	Ceftriaxone	100	Every 12 hrs		7–10
Neisseria meningitidis	Penicillin G	150	Every 5 hrs		5–7
	Cefotaxime	200	Every 8 hrs		5–7
	Ceftriaxone	100	Every 12 hrs		5–7
Streptococcus pneumoniae	Penicillin G	150	Every 4 hrs		10–21
	Cefotaxime	200	Every 8 hrs		10–21
	Ceftriaxone	100	Every 12 hrs		10–21

*Ceftriaxone should not be administered to jaundiced newborns.
Source: Adapted from AL Smith. Bacterial meningitis. Pediatr Rev 1993;14:16.

not delay empiric antibiotic treatment. Patients with suspected meningitis and with clear indication for CT imaging (e.g., coma, papilledema, focal signs) who may be some distance from the necessary technology or who cannot receive a lumbar puncture for other reasons should be given antibiotics empirically before transport to an appropriate referral center. If a lumbar puncture is not done before starting antibiotics, a blood culture should be obtained. Table 10-3 presents guidelines for the empiric use of antibiotics in children suspected of meningitis by age group and by most likely organism.

Although there is considerable discussion about the use of dexamethasone as adjunctive treatment in meningitis, it is generally recommended that children older than 2 months receive dexamethasone. It is more clearly beneficial in meningitis due to Hi and should be administered before the first antibiotic dose.

Regarding prophylactic treatment of children exposed to meningitis: Meningitis due to Hi or *N. meningitidis* should be considered contagious. Household and day care contacts should receive appropriate rifampin prophylaxis. Details on the administration of rifampin prophylaxis are clearly discussed in the 1997 *Red Book*.[41] Generally, it is advisable for clinicians involved with a case of contagious meningitis to consult a state epidemiologist for current recommendations.

Follow-up

Close follow-up of infants and children who have had meningitis is an essential part of meningitis care. It helps to ensure early detection of complicating sequelae and increases the opportunity for the family to ask questions.

References

1. Singleton RJ, Davidson NM, Desmet IJ, et al. Decline of *Haemophilus influenzae* type b in a region of high risk: impact of passive and active immunization. Pediatr Infect Dis J 1994;13:362–367.
2. Harrison LH, Tajkowski C, Croll J, et al. Post-licensure effectiveness of the *Haemophilus influenzae* type b polysaccharide–*Neisseria meningitidis* outer-membrane protein complex conjugate vaccine among Navajo children. J Pediatr 1994;125:571–576.
3. Feldman RA, Koehler RE, Fraser DW. Race-specific differences in bacterial meningitis deaths in the United States, 1962–1968. Am J Public Health 1976;66:392–396.
4. Fortuine R. Acute purulent meningitis in Alaska Natives: epidemiology, diagnosis and prognosis. Can Med Assoc J 1966;94:19–22.
5. Gilsdorf JR. Bacterial meningitis in southwestern Alaska. Am J Epidemiol 1977;106:388–391.

6. Ward JI, Margolis HS, Lum MK, et al. *Haemophilus influenzae* disease in Alaskan Eskimos: characteristics of a population with an unusual incidence of invasive disease. Lancet 1981;1:1281–1286.

7. Losonsky GA, Santosham M, Sehgal VM, et al. *Haemophilus influenzae* disease in the White Mountain Apaches: molecular epidemiology of a high risk population. Pediatr Infect Dis J 1984;3:539–547.

8. Ward JI, Lum MKW, Hall DB, et al. Invasive *Haemophilus influenzae* type b disease in Alaska: background epidemiology for a vaccine efficacy trial. J Infect Dis 1986;153:17–26.

9. Sproles ET, Azerrad J, Williamson C, Merrill RE. Meningitis due to *Haemophilus influenzae*: long-term sequelae. J Pediatr 1969;75:782–788.

10. Sell SHW, Merrill RE, Doyne EO, Zinsky EP. Long term sequelae of *Haemophilus influenzae* meningitis. Pediatrics 1972;49:206–209.

11. D'Angio CT, Froehlke RG, Plank GA, et al. Long-term outcome of *Haemophilus influenzae* meningitis in Navajo Indian children. Arch Pediatr Adolesc Med 1995;149:1001–1008.

12. Brenneman G, Silimperi D, Ward JI. Recurrent invasive *Haemophilus influenzae* type b disease in Alaskan Natives. Pediatr Infect Dis J 1987;6:388–392.

13. Siber GR, Santosham M, Priehs CM, et al. Impaired antibody response to *Haemophilus influenzae* b polysaccharide and low IgG2 and IgG4 concentrations in Apache children. N Engl J Med 1990;323:1387–1392.

14. Petersen GM, Silimperi DR, Rotter JI, et al. Genetic factors in *Haemophilus influenzae* type b disease susceptibility and antibody acquisition. J Pediatr 1987;110:228–233.

15. Petersen GM, Silimperi DR, Scott EM, et al. Uridine monophosphate kinase 3: a genetic marker for susceptibility to *Haemophilus influenzae* type b disease. Lancet 1985;2:417–419.

16. Petersen GM, Silimperi DR, Scott EM, et al. Uridine monophosphate kinase and susceptibility to invasive *Haemophilus influenzae* type b disease. Adv Exp Med Biol 1986;195[Pt A]:137–142.

17. Indian Health Service. Trends in Indian Health (Yearly Series 1987 to 1996). Washington, DC: U.S. Department of Health and Human Services, Indian Health Service, Office of Planning, Evaluation, and Legislation, Division of Program Statistics.

18. Peltola H, Kayhty H, Sivonen A, Makela PH. *Haemophilus influenzae* type b capsular polysaccharide vaccine in children: a double-blind field study of 100,000 vaccines 3 months to 5 years of age in Finland. Pediatrics 1977;60:730.

19. Harrison LH, Broome CV, Hightower AW. *Haemophilus influenzae* type b polysaccharide vaccine: an efficacy study. Pediatrics 1989;84:255–261.

20. Weinberg GA, Einhorn MS, Lenoir AA, et al. Immunologic priming to capsular polysaccharide in infants immunized with *Haemophilus influenzae* type b polysaccharide–*Neisseria meningitidis* outer membrane protein conjugate vaccine. J Pediatr 1987;111:22.

21. Decker MD, Edwards KM, Bradley R, et al. Comparative trial in infants of four conjugate *Haemophilus influenzae* type b vaccines. J Pediatr 1992;120:184–189.

22. Santosham M, Hill J, Wolff M, et al. Safety and immunogenicity of *Haemophilus influenzae* type b conjugate vaccine in a high risk American Indian population. Pediatr Infect Dis J 1991;10:113–117.

23. Santosham M, Riven B, Wolff M, et al. Prevention of *Haemophilus influenzae* type b infections in Apache and Navajo children. J Infect Dis 1992;165:S144–S154.

24. Bulkow LR, Wainwright RB, Letson GW, et al. Comparative immunogenicity of four *Haemophilus influenzae* type b conjugate vaccines in Alaska Native infants. Pediatr Infect Dis J 1993;12:484–492.

25. Granoff DM, Anderson EL, Osterholm MT, et al. Differences in the immunogenicity of three *Haemophilus influenzae* type b conjugate vaccines in infants. J Pediatr 1992;121:187–194.

26. Anderson EL, Decker MD, Englund JA, et al. Interchangeability of conjugated *Haemophilus influenzae* type b vaccines in infants. JAMA 1995;15:849–853.

27. Greenberg DP, Lieberman JM, Marcy SM, et al. Enhanced antibody responses in infants given different sequences of heterogeneous *Haemophilus influenzae* type b conjugate vaccines. J Pediatr 1995;126:206–211.

28. Bewley KM, Schwab JG, Ballanco GA, et al. Interchangeability of *Haemophilus influenzae* type b vaccines in the primary series: evaluation of a two-dose mixed regimen. Pediatrics 1996;98:898–904.

29. Reid R, Santosham M, Croll J, et al. Antibody response of Navajo children primed with PRP-OMP vaccine to booster doses of PRP-OMP vs. HbOC vaccine. Pediatr Infect Dis J 1993;12:812–815.

30. Santosham M, Wolff M, Reid R, et al. The efficacy in Navajo infants of a conjugate vaccine consisting of *Haemophilus influenzae* type b polysaccharide and *Neisseria meningitidis* outer-membrane protein complex. N Engl J Med 1991;324:1767–1772.

31. Santosham M, Reid R, Ambrosino DM, et al. Prevention of *Haemophilus influenzae* type b infections in high-risk infants treated with bacterial polysaccharide immune globulin. N Engl J Med 1987;317:923–929.

32. Santosham M, Reid R, Letson GW, et al. Passive immunization for infection with *Haemophilus influenzae* type b. Pediatrics 1990;85:662–666.

33. Letson GW, Santosham M, Reid R, et al. Comparison of active and combined passive/active immunization of Navajo children against *Haemophilus influenzae* type b. Pediatr Infect Dis J 1988;7:747–752.

34. Lum MK, Ward JI, Bender TR, et al. Protective influence of breast feeding on the risk of developing invasive *H. influenzae* type b disease [Abstract]. Pediatr Res 1982;16[Pt 2]:151.

35. Insel RA. Maternal immunization to prevent neonatal infections [Editorial]. N Engl J Med 1988;319:1219–1220.

36. Davidson M, Schraer CD, Parkinson AJ, et al. Pneumococcal disease in an Alaska Native population, 1980 through 1986. JAMA 1989;261:715–718.

37. Parkinson AJ, Davidson M, Fitzgerald MA, et al.

Serotype distribution and antimicrobial resistance patterns of invasive isolates of *Streptococcus pneumoniae*: Alaska 1986–1990. J Infect Dis 1994;170:461–464.

38. Cortese MM, Wolff M, Almeido-Hill J, et al. High incidence rates of invasive pneumococcal disease in the White Mountain Apache population. Arch Intern Med 1992;152:2277–2282.

39. Smith AL. Bacterial meningitis. Pediatr Rev 1993;14: 11–18.

40. Quagliarello VJ, Scheld MW. Treatment of bacterial meningitis. N Engl J Med 1997;336:708–714.

41. American Academy of Pediatrics Committee on Infectious Diseases. 1997 Red Book: Report of the Committee on Infectious Diseases (24th ed). Elk Grove Village, IL: American Academy of Pediatrics, 1997.

42. Berman S. Meningitis. In Berman S (ed), Pediatric Decision Making (3rd ed). St. Louis: Mosby–Year Book, 1996.

Chapter 11
Plague

Larry D. Crook and Bruce Tempest

Of all the diseases that a physician may be called on to treat while working with Native Americans, plague is the one that creates the greatest emotional response. This is no doubt related to the history of plague and to the fact that in the fourteenth century a pandemic of plague, referred to as the *Black Death*, killed approximately one-third of the population of Europe. The current pandemic of plague, beginning in the middle of the nineteenth century, has killed an estimated 13 million people.

Plague is a bacterial disease whose epidemiology and pathophysiology have been well described. The causative organism, *Yersinia pestis*, was named after its discoverer, Alexander Yersin. Yersin was a physician working at the Pasteur Institute in Paris when an epidemic of plague broke out in southern China and Hong Kong. He went to Hong Kong in June 1894 and injected material aspirated from buboes of plague patients into guinea pigs, thereby obtaining isolates of the organism. He also isolated the organism from dead rats found in the city, thus proving the connection between the disease and rats.[1] In Yersin's time, there was no effective treatment for plague, but excellent antiplague drugs are available today. Untreated bubonic plague has a 50–60% mortality rate, and untreated pneumonic plague is virtually 100% fatal. With modern treatment, however, the mortality rates should be less than 10%.

Epidemiology

Plague is primarily a disease of animals, and humans are infected only accidentally. Urban plague is a disease of rats and their fleas; it was the form of plague responsible for the epidemics in the Middle Ages. Rural plague is primarily a disease of small rodents, especially prairie dogs, ground squirrels, and rock squirrels, in the western United States. Rural plague is endemic in the rodent population and their fleas in the western United States, and all plague cases there are related to the intrusion of

humans into the animal cycle. Because such intrusions are most likely to occur in the warmer months, most cases of plague occur from May to September. Winter cases do occur, however, and are often related to the handling of infected animal tissues, especially those of rabbits.[2–4]

The most common risk factors for acquiring plague in the southwestern United States are living, hunting, or working in a rural area; a dog or cat in the home; a suitable habitat for rodents near the home; and fleas in or near the home.[5]

Pathogenesis

Plague is an acute febrile illness caused by the bacterium *Y. pestis*, a gram-negative bacillus. The organism has a distinct safety-pin appearance when it is stained with Giemsa's or Wright's stain, due to uptake of the dye at both ends of the bacillus.

The bacteria are introduced into a human most commonly by the bite of an infected flea. The fleas normally feed on small rodents, and when a flea ingests a blood meal from an animal infected with plague, the bacteria multiply in the foregut of the flea. Eventually, the plug of bacteria in the flea becomes large enough to obstruct the foregut; when the flea attempts to take a blood meal it regurgitates the blood, along with many bacteria, back onto the skin and the bite wound it has just created. An infected flea starves to death, but before it dies it may bite and infect many animals or people.

Y. pestis may also gain access to a human when he or she handles the carcass or the tissues of an animal infected with plague and bacteria pass through breaks in the skin to the lymphatic system.

A third, rare method of acquiring the bacterium is through direct inhalation from an animal or human with pneumonic plague. This leads directly to primary pneumonic plague. This form of plague has occurred in recent years as a result of exposure to domestic cats infected with pneumonic plague. Human-to-human spread of plague has not occurred in the United States in since 1925.

Clinical Presentation

After a flea bite, the usual incubation period is 5–7 days. Patients with plague present with an acute febrile illness. A history of a flea bite is often not obtained. A classic presentation of bubonic plague is easily recognized by the characteristic bubo. This enlarged, swollen, and exquisitely tender node, or group of nodes, drains the area of the site of the flea bite or the point of direct inoculation. The skin overlying the bubo is erythematous and shiny. The bubo is firm and not fluctuant early in the course of the disease, and there is often edema of the surrounding tissue. This presentation has been mistaken for other conditions, such as forms of lymphadenitis (particularly streptococcal or staphylococcal lymphadenitis), incarcerated hernia, and localized musculoskeletal injuries.

In septicemic plague, a bubo either does not develop or is so small or located in such a position as to be unrecognized. Septicemic plague may present as a viral syndrome, an upper respiratory syndrome, gastroenteritis, or as a number of other nonspecific syndromes. Vomiting and diarrhea are common. In both bubonic and septicemic plague, bacteremia is common, and the signs and symptoms of gram-negative sepsis, including shock, disseminated intravascular coagulation, and adult respiratory distress syndrome, may develop. In addition, the bacteria may spread to other organ systems, including the lung, central nervous system, and joints, via the bloodstream.

Various dermatologic manifestations of plague have been described, including pustules, vesicles, eschars, and papules. Purpura has also been described, and ecthyma gangrenosum and gangrene of the digits may also occur.[6]

Pulmonary involvement is either secondary to a bacteremia in bubonic or septicemic plague, or it is primary—that is, acquired by the inhalation of *Y. pestis* coughed up by a person or animal with pneumonic plague. The bacterium is not aerosolized, and face-to-face contact is necessary for spread. Plague pneumonia is most often bilateral and necrotizing, and pleural effusions are frequently detected. Gram-negative rods are usually seen in the sputum and pleural fluid, and the organism can be cultured from these specimens. Pneumonic plague is characterized by a very rapid course, and primary (inhalation) pneumonic plague is usually fatal if appropriate treatment is not begun on the first day of disease.[7]

Diagnosis

Culture of *Y. pestis* remains the most reliable method of diagnosis. The organism can be grown on routine laboratory media, and cultures of all relevant body fluids,

including blood, joint fluid, sputum, pleural fluid, and cerebrospinal fluid, should be obtained. Some authorities recommend obtaining several blood cultures over a period of 1 hour. The bubo should be aspirated, but usually no fluid can be obtained. In this case, a small amount of sterile saline should be injected into the bubo and quickly aspirated. This fluid should be gram-stained, cultured, and sent to a reference laboratory for fluorescent antibody testing. The fluorescent antibody test is both specific and sensitive, but a positive test only establishes a presumptive diagnosis of plague, and a negative test should never persuade the physician not to treat for plague.

Serum antibody titers can be measured at reference laboratories and can be helpful in diagnosing plague in retrospect. Titers should be obtained acutely and again at 6 weeks.

Treatment

Because of its long record of clinical efficacy, streptomycin is the drug of choice for treating plague. The usual dose with normal renal function is 15 mg/kg intramuscularly (IM) every 12 hours. Chloramphenicol and tetracycline have also been used extensively and are acceptable alternative drugs of choice. Chloramphenicol is especially useful when shock precludes reliable absorption of IM streptomycin and when infection involves hard-to-penetrate spaces, such as the cerebrospinal fluid, joint fluid, or eye. The usual initial dose is 25 mg/kg intravenously every 6 hours, which should be reduced by half once a clinical response has occurred. Tetracycline is useful as oral therapy to finish a 10- to 14-day course of treatment after the patient has responded to parenteral treatment.

Gentamicin has been used in the United States in recent years due to the unavailability of streptomycin. It appears to be effective, and it is acceptable in the treatment of a patient who is only suspected of having plague. Once the diagnosis is established, however, one of the drugs of choice should be used.

None of the beta-lactam antibiotics, including the newest penicillins and cephalosporins, have any proven efficacy in treating plague. They should not be used for this purpose. The resistance of *Y. pestis* to these drugs points out the high risk of relying on a beta-lactam for treating a case of lymphadenitis or undifferentiated sepsis in areas where plague is endemic. There are few clinical data in humans about other classes of antibiotics, such as the quinolones, and they should not be used to treat plague.

There is data to support the use of some sulfa drugs to treat plague, including sulfamethoxazole (used in Septra and Bactrim), but it is a second-line drug whose use is restricted to preventive treatment in children who cannot take tetracycline. It is not approved by the U.S. Food and Drug Administration for the treatment of plague.

Doxycycline has also been used in place of tetracycline, and it seems to be effective, but again there is not enough clinical data to recommend its use as a drug of choice.

Fatal cases of plague are often related to the failure of the physician to consider the disease in the differential diagnosis when the patient is first seen, and especially to the failure to begin a drug effective against plague.[8]

Prevention

Whenever a case of plague is suspected or diagnosed, it is imperative that the public health authorities be notified, and by law the state health department must be notified. All contacts of the patient should be identified.

Contacts of a case of plague that is not pneumonic should be observed carefully for 7 days. If a fever occurs, they should be treated as presumed cases of plague with a first-line drug. Contacts of a case of pneumonic plague who did not have face-to-face contact with the patient should be similarly observed and treated if they develop a fever.

Contacts of a case of pneumonic plague who have had face-to-face contact within 6 ft of the patient should be treated immediately as a presumed case of plague. *Y. pestis* is not aerosolized. It is spread in droplets, which quickly fall to the floor and cannot be propelled more than 6 ft by a cough. This important point should be made known to prevent misinformation and panic among the public and particularly the hospital staff.

A vaccine is available to protect against plague, but its use is recommended only for field workers who may be distant from treatment facilities and for researchers who may have regular exposure to *Y. pestis*.

Summary Points

- Plague is an acute febrile illness caused by a gram-negative bacterium.
- Plague is a disease of rodents and their fleas; humans are only accidentally involved in the natural cycles of plague.
- Plague generally presents either with a bubo (bubonic plague) or without a bubo (septicemic plague).
- Pneumonic plague is either secondary to hematogenous spread or due to inhalation of the organism (primary pneumonic plague).
- Diagnosis is made by standard bacteriologic methods of Gram's stain smear and culture, and by fluorescent antibody staining at reference laboratories.
- The drugs of choice are streptomycin, chloramphenicol, and tetracycline. Gentamicin may be used initially to cover the possibility of plague.

References

1. Gross L. How the plague bacillus and its transmission through fleas were discovered: reminiscences from my years at the Pasteur Institute. Proc Natl Acad Sci U S A 1995;92:7609–7611.
2. Reed WP, Palmer DL, Williams RC Jr, Kisch AL. Bubonic plague in the southwestern United States: a review of recent experience. Medicine (Baltimore) 1970;49:465–486.
3. Poland JD, Barnes AM. Plague. In Steele JF (ed), CRC Handbook Series in Zoonoses, Section A: Bacterial, Rickettsial, and Mycotic Diseases. Boca Raton, FL: CRC Press, 1979;1:515–559.
4. Barnes AM, Quan TJ, Beard ML, Maupin GO. Plague in American Indians, 1956–1987. MMWR Morb Mortal Wkly Rep 1988;37(SS-3):11–16.
5. Von Reyn CF, Weber NS, Tempest B, et al. Epidemiological and clinical features of an outbreak of bubonic plague in New Mexico. J Infect Dis 1977;136:489–494.
6. Welty TK, Grabman J, Kompare E, et al. Nineteen cases of plague in Arizona: a spectrum including ecthyma gangrenosum due to plague and plague in pregnancy. West J Med 1985;142:641–646.
7. Butler T. Yersinia infections: centennial of the discovery of the plague bacillus. Clin Infect Dis 1994;19:655–663.
8. Crook LD, Tempest B. Plague; a clinical review of 27 cases. Arch Intern Med 1992;152:1253–1256.

Chapter 12
Tuberculosis

Jeffrey M. Sippel and Anthony A. Marfin

Although *Mycobacterium tuberculosis* infection may have been endemic in pre-Columbian American Indians, the creation of Indian reservations after the Civil War created living conditions that increased the prevalence of tuberculosis among Native American (American Indian and Alaska Native) communities.[1] Today, these living conditions persist, and new promoters of tuberculosis have emerged: diabetes mellitus (DM) and end-stage renal disease (ESRD), along with alcoholism and homelessness among many urban-dwelling Native Americans.

Tuberculosis results from infection with *M. tuberculosis*, an aerobic acid-fast bacillus.[2] Infection most commonly occurs after inhalation of droplet nuclei generated by persons with pulmonary tuberculosis from coughing, sneezing, or talking. Because active cough is the most efficient mechanism for aerosolizing particles, patients with infiltrates or cavitary disease on chest radiograph or positive sputum smears are considered highly infectious. Persons with tuberculosis that does not involve the lungs or upper airways are generally considered noninfectious, but exceptions exist.

Tuberculosis infection involves the lungs in almost 90% of reported cases, although it can cause disease in virtually every organ system. Extrapulmonary tuberculosis is found more commonly in children younger than age 5 years, the elderly, and minorities, including Native Americans. Extrapulmonary disease occurs when there is contiguous spread of organisms into the pleural, pericardial, or peritoneal space or when organisms spread hematogenously from the lungs to lymph nodes, bone tissue, meninges, or other distant sites.

Mortality from tuberculosis was 60% until effective chemotherapy became available in 1946. In the United States, cure rates exceed 97% in most clinical settings. For this reason, tuberculosis is frequently thought of as a historic illness, yet it is still the leading cause of death worldwide. It is also a significant source of morbidity among Native Americans.

Epidemiology

Since the 1950s, tuberculosis incidence has dropped dramatically among all racial and ethnic groups in the United States, but it remains disproportionately high among Native Americans.[3] In 1955, the annual rate of tuberculosis among Native Americans exceeded 700 cases per 100,000; this decreased to 19 cases per 100,000 by 1990. Since then, tuberculosis incidence has only modestly decreased and still remains more than five times the rate in non-Hispanic whites.[4] In some states with large Native American populations, tuberculosis incidence is even greater. Alaska (annual rate 60.8 per 100,000), Arizona (32.9 per 100,000), New Mexico (25.3 per 100,000), Oklahoma (17.4 per 100,000), and California (17.3 per 100,000) account for nearly two-thirds of Native American tuberculosis cases.[5]

Morbidity and mortality attributable to tuberculosis are also disproportionately greater among Native Americans. In New Mexico, Native Americans are four times more likely to have tuberculous meningitis than the general population; they account for one-third of reported cases and make up less than 10% of the population. Similarly, although only 18% of U.S. tuberculosis cases have extrapulmonary manifestations, nearly three-fourths of these cases occur in minorities.[6] Although it is generally considered a treatable illness with high cure rates, tuberculosis causes 1% of the deaths among certain Native American groups, which is 35 times the all-race mortality rate from tuberculosis in the United States.

Tuberculosis is primarily a disease of reactivation among Native Americans. Native Americans older than age 65 years have the highest age-specific rate of tuberculosis among U.S.–born people (59 per 100,000). Such high rates most likely result from failure to prevent reactivation among at-risk members of this population. Persons at increased risk are those with positive tuberculin skin tests and comorbid illnesses, such as DM and ESRD. Reactivation among these persons, failure to identify and treat persons with active pulmonary tuberculosis, household crowding, and other coexisting socioeconomic factors promote ongoing transmission of tuberculosis.

The absolute number of Native American adults at increased risk for developing tuberculosis may be quite large. It is estimated that half of American Indians between the ages of 45 and 74 years living in Arizona, Oklahoma, North Dakota, and South Dakota have DM, and more than 50% have a history of tuberculosis or a positive tuberculin skin test. Because adults with positive tuberculin skin tests and DM may be up to five times more likely to reactivate than those without diabetes, the Indian Health Service adopted recommendations specifying tuberculosis-control activities and practice guidelines for Native Americans to reduce the morbidity attributable to tuberculosis.[7, 8] Special emphasis has been placed on identifying persons with DM or ESRD and a positive tuberculin skin test and encouraging preventive therapy.

Reactivation of old tuberculosis among elderly Native Americans contrasts with trends in the United States, where rapid progression of newly acquired infections has been increasing. The increase occurs especially among children younger than 15 years old, persons with HIV infection, the homeless, and recent immigrants from developing countries with high endemic rates of tuberculosis.[9] The influence that these new patterns of tuberculosis may have on Native Americans is unknown but do not appear to contribute significantly to the overall tuberculosis rate at this time.

Clinical Presentation

Exposure to an infectious case leads to aspiration of viable organisms and subsequent tuberculous infection in approximately 30% of those exposed. Of those who become infected, 5–7% will develop active tuberculosis within 1 year. After 1 year, an additional 5% will develop active tuberculosis sometime during their lifetime. The rest of the infected individuals are said to have inactive tuberculosis. This represents a significant proportion of Native American adults (see Preventive Therapy). Among HIV-infected persons, there is a 10% per-year risk of developing active tuberculosis.

Eighty percent of active tuberculosis in the United States involves only the lungs. Up to 5% of patients have both pulmonary and extrapulmonary sites of disease, and 15% present with extrapulmonary disease only. Cough is the most common symptom of pulmonary tuberculosis. A nonproductive cough frequently progresses to a productive cough over weeks to months. Dyspnea is unusual unless there is widespread parenchymal involvement. Hemoptysis can also accompany widespread lung disease, but it also results from bronchiectasis as a residual of healed tuberculosis. Pleuritic chest pain may be present if there is either subpleural parenchymal involvement or pleural effusion. Nonspecific symptoms of fever, weight loss, and night sweats are frequently present with more advanced disease. Physical findings associated with pulmonary tuberculosis are nonspecific. Rales, bronchial breath sounds, or egophony may be heard over the involved area if consolidation is present. Dullness to percussion and diminished breath sounds at the lung base may be noticeable if pleural effusion is present. Extrapulmonary manifestations of tuberculosis include lymphatic (30%), pleural (23%), genitourinary (12%), bone and joint (10%), miliary (7%), and meningeal (5%) involvement.

Diagnosis

Because symptoms and physical findings are nonspecific, diagnosis of active tuberculosis requires a high degree of clinical suspicion plus the use of ancillary tests, including chest radiographs, sputum analysis, and sputum cultures. Skin testing with purified protein derivative (PPD) may also be useful, although 20% of individuals with active tuberculosis have a negative skin test at initial evaluation. Skin testing is more often used in screening for inactive disease among high-risk populations.

Chest Radiograph

Pulmonary tuberculosis almost always has abnormalities detectable on chest radiograph. Although the findings are not specific for tuberculosis, they can provide a presumptive diagnosis in the correct clinical setting, especially in high-risk patients. Tuberculosis occurring from progression of recent infection often appears as a mid- or lower-lung zone infiltrate, and may have associated ipsilateral hilar adenopathy. Hilar and mediastinal adenopathy are particularly common in infected children. Pleural effusion can also be present with recent infection, and it frequently occurs in the absence of parenchymal infiltrate. Tuberculosis occurring from reactivation of remote infection usually causes upper-lobe changes. Cavitation and fibrotic scarring are common, as is volume loss with retraction of the ipsilateral hilum upward. Apical and posterior segments of the upper lobes and the superior segment of the lower lobes are most frequently involved. Isolated upper lobe anterior segment disease is rare.

Sputum Analysis

Analysis of expectorated sputum provides the first direct evidence of infection with *M. tuberculosis*. Collection and analysis of three early-morning samples reveals organisms in up to 70% of culture-positive cases. The most commonly used procedure for microscopic sputum examination is the modified acid-fast stain, or Ziehl-Neelsen technique. Stain sensitivity can be increased if the specimen is centrifuged and enzymatically digested before staining. At least 10^4 bacilli/ml must be present to be detected by light microscopy. Other methods of sputum analysis, including polymerase chain reaction and DNA or RNA amplification techniques, have been developed, but they are expensive and not widely available. These tests may be most useful in cases of presumed smear-negative pulmonary disease, but they have not yet been accepted as a diagnostic tool.

Mycobacterial Cultures

Definitive identification of mycobacterial species and susceptibility testing require organism culture. Two solid media are commonly used: Löwenstein-Jensen (egg-based) and Middlebrook-Cohn (agar-based) media. Although isolates may grow more rapidly on agar-based media, egg-based media are generally regarded as the reference standard and may yield more positive cultures per inoculum. BACTEC (Becton Dickson and Co., Franklin Lakes, NJ) liquid culture media that incorporate radiometric identification systems are now widely used in clinical laboratories. Liberation of radiolabeled CO_2 by growth of mycobacteria provides increased sensitivity and rapid detection within 9–16 days.

Skin Testing

If a combination of risk factors, symptoms, and chest radiograph support a diagnosis of active tuberculosis, neither a positive nor a negative tuberculin skin test should preclude completion of the full diagnostic evaluation. Although tuberculin skin testing is the standard method for identifying infected persons,[10] it cannot differentiate between active and inactive disease. There is a false-negative rate of 20% for tuberculin skin testing in the face of active pulmonary tuberculosis.

Intradermal PPD skin testing for delayed-type hypersensitivity, also called the *Mantoux procedure*, is the most widely used tuberculin skin test and is more specific than multiple-puncture devices. Although three concentrations of PPD antigens are available, it is generally most appropriate to begin testing with intermediate-strength (5-TU) preparation. Forty-eight to 72 hours after intradermal injection of 0.1 ml of 5-TU PPD antigen, the induration around the injection site should be measured by palpation and recorded in millimeters, not simply as "positive" or "negative." Erythema without induration does not indicate infection and should not be measured as part of the reaction.

Previously, an induration of 10 mm or more was considered evidence of infection with *M. tuberculosis*. Since 1990, however, both the Centers for Disease Control and Prevention (CDC) and the American Thoracic Society have endorsed revised criteria in an attempt to decrease the number of false-negative tests in high-risk individuals and decrease the number of false-positive tests in low-risk individuals.

Other host factors may influence the likelihood of false-negative or false-positive skin tests. In active tuberculosis, the tuberculin reaction is falsely negative in approximately 20% of cases at initial evaluation. Anergy states are also associated with false-negative skin tests; these are most commonly seen with increasing age (older than 70 years), hypoalbuminemia (<2 g/dl), malignancy, immunosuppressive drugs, or systemic infection (particularly viral infections, including infectious mononucleosis, mumps, influenza, and human immunodeficiency virus [HIV]). Control antigens may be helpful in some instances but are of uncertain usefulness and not universally recommended.[10] False-positive tests rarely occur due to errors in test administration and are often seen in individuals from tropical regions with high prevalence of naturally occurring nontuberculous mycobacterial infections or in those with recent bacille Calmette-Guérin vaccination. Neither of these conditions should preclude use of PPD skin testing if clinically indicated. Nontuberculous mycobacterial infection is rarely a problem among Native Americans, except for those from the southeastern United States.

The probability that a skin test reaction is truly from *M. tuberculosis* infection increases with any one of the following factors:

1. As the size of the reaction increases
2. When the patient is a contact of a person with known tuberculosis
3. When a family history of tuberculosis exists
4. When the patient's community has a high prevalence of tuberculosis

Differential Diagnosis

The constellation of exposure history or previous infection, other risk factors, symptoms, radiographic findings, and sputum analysis often leads to a presumptive diagnosis of active tuberculosis. However, other illnesses may have similar findings. Cavitary lung disease detected on chest radiograph is frequently seen with bronchogenic carcinoma, *Aspergillus* or other fungal infections, pyogenic bacterial infection with *S. aureus*, *Klebsiella pneumoniae*, or anaerobic organisms, and rarely with nocardiosis or Wegener's granulomatosis. Acid-fast organisms on sputum analysis are seen with infections from nontuberculous mycobacterial species, *Nocardia*, and some *Legionella* species. Cultures can differentiate between species of mycobacteria. Causes of false-negative and false-positive skin tests are mentioned in the previous section.

Treatment

Chemotherapy for active tuberculosis has undergone important changes during the 1990s. Previously, therapy consisted of daily medication with two effective agents, given for 18–24 months. However, these lengthy treatment courses were associated with significant risks of drug side effects and noncompliance. The emergence of drug-resistant tuberculosis has further complicated treatment of tuberculosis. Newer studies have documented the efficacy and safety of much shorter courses of chemotherapy. Cornerstones to the newer regimens are the use of four medications until drug susceptibilities are known, and using directly observed therapy (DOT) two to three times per week. Relapse rates are less than 3% in most populations with susceptible organisms.

Because antibiotic susceptibility testing takes many weeks, initial therapy for active disease is always empiric. Empiric regimens should take into account history of prior treatment, the regional likelihood of drug-resistant organisms, and HIV status. Table 12-1 shows a four-drug regimen: isoniazid (INH), rifampin (RIF), pyrazinamide (PZA), and either ethambutol or streptomycin. A three-drug regimen with INH, RIF, and PZA should be used only if there are no risk factors for drug-resistant tuberculosis and community rates of INH resistance are less than 4%. DOT is recommended for all individuals, regardless of the provider's perception of patient reliability.

The importance of compliance with antituberculous therapy should not be underestimated: Noncompliance is the most important cause of drug therapy failure throughout the world, and it contributes significantly to the development of drug-resistant tuberculosis. Only 55% of persons with active tuberculosis in New York City completed self-administered therapy in 1990. Given low completion rates of self-administered programs, rising prevalence of drug-resistant tuberculosis, and the inability to identify patients at high risk for noncompliance, the American Thoracic Society and the CDC endorse DOT as the standard of care for all patients.[11] Using incentives and enablers, facilitating access to health and social services, and addressing unique cultural and linguistic backgrounds of patients is particularly important among minority populations, including Native Americans.

Along with prompt institution of multiple-drug chemotherapy, the ongoing risk of transmission of tuberculosis must be minimized. Until the patient is considered noninfectious, he or she should be prohibited from entering environments where previously unexposed people are present or to wear a mask if contact is unavoidable. Two weeks of effective chemotherapy is often considered sufficient time to render a patient noninfectious. After an average of 16 days of multiple-drug therapy, cough is reduced by 65%, and there is a 99% reduction in organisms recoverable from sputum, from 10^6 to 10^4 organisms. However, each case must be individually assessed. Patients with cavitary disease, persistently high sputum counts, or prolonged cough may remain infectious much longer. After beginning antibiotics, surveillance of sputum for staining and culture is recommended at 2 weeks, 4 weeks, and then monthly until negative.

Preventive Therapy

A PPD-positive person with no evidence of active disease is considered to have clinically inactive tuberculosis infection. Preventive therapy given to patients with inactive tuberculosis significantly reduces the likelihood of

Table 12-1. Initial Empiric Treatment of Tuberculosis in Human Immunodeficiency Virus-Negative Adult Patients*

Regimen 1	First 8 Wks of Therapy	Next 16 Wks (two times or three times wkly, DOT)

	INH 300 mg/day
	RIF 600 mg/day
	PZA 15–30 mg/kg/d, 2 g maximum
	EMB 15 mg/kg/day or SM 20–30 mg/kg/day,
	   1 g maximum
		INH 15 mg/kg (900 mg maximum each dose)
		RIF 10 mg/kg (600 mg maximum each dose)
		If sensitivities not known or if organism is resistant
		   to INH or RIF, then continue: EMB (25 mg/kg
		   if three times wkly, 50 mg/kg if two times wkly)
		   or SM 25–30 mg/kg (1.5 g maximum each dose)

Regimen 2	**First 2 Wks of Therapy**	**Next 22 Wks (two times wkly, DOT)**

	INH, RIF, PZA, and either EMB or SM taken
	   daily, dosed as above
		INH, RIF, PZA, and EMB or SM dosed as above
		Can stop PZA at 8 wks and can stop EMB or SM
		   when susceptibilities known

*Other effective drug treatment regimens are available in published Centers for Disease Control and Prevention guidelines.[14]
DOT = directly observed therapy; INH = isoniazid; RIF = rifampin; PZA = pyrazinamide; EMB = ethambutol; SM = streptomycin.

subsequent disease reactivation. Without preventive therapy, a PPD-positive person has a lifetime risk of approximately 10% for reactivation. Factors that increase an individual's lifetime risk for reactivation include fibrotic lesions on chest radiograph, inadequate treatment for tuberculosis in the past, corticosteroid therapy, and silicosis. HIV-infected individuals have a 10% per-year rate of reactivation. The most important risk factors for reactivation among Native Americans are DM and ESRD (Table 12-2). Providers serving Native American populations should consider preventive therapy for the following persons, in order of priority:

Group 1: Recent skin test converters (from negative to positive within the past 2 years), regardless of age

Group 2: "Positive" skin test of uncertain duration in patients with DM or ESRD, regardless of age

Group 3: "Positive" skin test of uncertain duration in patients younger than 35 years old, even in the absence of risk factors

Group 4: "Positive" skin test of uncertain duration in patients older than 35 years old, even in the absence of risk factors

Because DM and ESRD affect a large proportion of many Native American populations, the greatest reductions in the incidence of tuberculosis may be made by identifying and treating persons in group 2.[7, 8] Persons of any age with medical conditions associated with reactivation (specifically DM and ESRD) should be consistently encouraged to complete preventive therapy. The CDC has reviewed other groups that may benefit from preventive therapy.[10, 12]

Because the first 2 years after skin-test conversion is the period of greatest risk for developing active disease, anyone known to have converted, regardless of age (group 1), should be strongly encouraged to complete preventive therapy. Because younger persons have a slightly greater cumulative risk of disease reactivation and less risk of preventive drug side effects, persons in group 3 should also be encouraged to complete preventive therapy. Older persons without medical conditions (group 4) are generally not offered preventive therapy because the risk of disease is low and the risk of preventive drug side effects are greater. In some settings, they may be offered preventive therapy, but this should be done only on a case-by-case basis, after a person with significant experience with tuberculosis has performed a rigorous risk assessment.

INH is the drug of choice for preventive therapy and is given in a dose of 10 mg/kg daily, with a maximum dose of 300 mg. Twelve months of INH is highly effective and reduces the likelihood of reactivation by 93%.[13] However, 6–9 months of INH may provide a more favorable risk-benefit ratio in some cases. The estimated incidence of INH-associated hepatitis in persons younger than 20 years old is 0%; in those age 20–34 years, it is 0.3%; for 35 to 49 year olds, 1.2%; 50–64 years of age, 2.3%; and for persons older than age 64 years, 0.8%. Risk for hepatitis increases with concomitant alcohol consumption. Elevations of liver enzymes occur in 10–20% of patients taking INH. Preventive therapy should be stopped if liver enzymes exceed five times the normal laboratory values in an asymptomatic individual.

Conclusions

The incidence of tuberculosis among Native Americans is five times greater than that of non-Hispanic whites in the United States and is responsible for disproportionately elevated morbidity and mortality. Because tuberculosis is largely a disease of reactivation among Native Americans, identification of individuals at risk for tuberculosis and offering preventive therapy, where appropriate, can favorably modify outcomes. Particular attention should be paid to individuals at increased risk for reactivation, including those with DM and ESRD. Although skin testing is an excellent method for screening individuals for the presence of infection with *M. tuberculosis*, it does not differentiate between active and inactive disease. For this reason, the diagnosis of active tuberculosis requires a high degree of clinical suspicion and a thorough evaluation, including chest radiograph, sputum smear analysis,

Table 12-2. Clinical Interpretation of Intermediate Strength Purified Protein Derivative Skin Testing

Size of Skin Reaction (mm)	Considered Positive when Associated with These Factors:
5	Persons at high risk for *Mycobacterium tuberculosis* infection, including close contacts with infected patients, those with chest radiograph findings consistent with prior infection (old, healed tuberculosis), and those with human immunodeficiency virus
10	Persons at increased risk for *M. tuberculosis* infection, including foreign-born individuals from Asia, Africa, or Latin America; other minorities; intravenous drug users; medically underserved low-income groups; residents of long-term care facilities; and individuals with significant comorbid illnesses such as diabetes mellitus or end-stage renal disease
15	Persons with no identifiable risk factors

and sputum culture. Treatment regimens using multiple antibiotics have cure rates exceeding 97% in most circumstances, provided that DOT is used.

Acknowledgments

The authors would like to thank Dr. Tom Welty (recently retired from the Indian Health Service) and Dr. Mary Ann Ware (Multnomah County Health Department, Oregon) for their many contributions to the completion of this chapter.

References

1. Stead WW, Eisenach KD, Cave MD. When did *Mycobacterium tuberculosis* infection first occur in the New World? Am J Respir Crit Care Med 1995;151: 1267–1268.
2. Hopewell PC, Bloom BR. Tuberculosis and Other Mycobacterial Diseases. In Murray JF, Nadel JA (eds), Textbook of Respiratory Medicine (2nd ed). Philadelphia: Saunders, 1994:1094–1160.
3. Rhoades ER. The major respiratory diseases of American Indians. Am Rev Respir Dis 1990;141:595–600.
4. Centers for Disease Control and Prevention. Reported Tuberculosis in the United States 1995. Atlanta: Centers for Disease Control and Prevention, 1996.
5. Sugarman J, Chase E, Johannes P, Helgerson SD. Tuberculosis among American Indians and Alaska Natives, 1985–1990. IHS Primary Care Provider 1991; 16:186–190.
6. The NHLBI Working Group. Respiratory diseases disproportionately affecting minorities. Chest 1995;108: 1380–1392. [Published erratum appears in Chest 1996;109:295.]
7. Welty TK, Helgerson SD, Tempest B, et al. Control of tuberculosis among American Indians and Alaska Natives. IHS Primary Care Provider 1989;14:53–54.
8. Welty TK, Follas R. IHS standards of care for tuberculosis: INH preventive therapy. IHS Primary Care Provider 1989;14:54–58.
9. Cantwell MF, Snider DE, Cauthern GM, Onorato IM. Epidemiology of tuberculosis in the United States, 1985 through 1992. JAMA 1994;272:535–539.
10. Advisory Council for the Elimination of Tuberculosis. Screening for tuberculosis and tuberculosis infection in high-risk populations: recommendations of the Advisory Council for the Elimination of Tuberculosis. MMWR Morb Mortal Wkly Rep 1995;44[RR-11]: 18–34.
11. Bayer R, Wilkinson D. Directly observed therapy for tuberculosis: history of an idea. Lancet 1995;345: 1545–1548.
12. Centers for Disease Control and Prevention. Core Curriculum on Tuberculosis: What the Clinician Should Know. Atlanta: DHHS, PHS, CDC, 1994.
13. IUAT Committee on Prophylaxis. Efficacy of various durations of isoniazid preventive therapy for tuberculosis: five years of follow-up in the IUAT trial. Bull World Health Organ 1982;60:555–564.
14. Centers for Disease Control and Prevention. Treating Tuberculosis. A Clinical Guide. Atlanta: Centers for Disease Control and Prevention, 1994.

Chapter 13
Human Immunodeficiency Virus Infection

Jonathan Vilasier Iralu

The care of the Native American patient with human immunodeficiency virus (HIV) infection presents a special challenge to physicians and other providers in Indian country. Native American patients with acquired immunodeficiency syndrome (AIDS) differ from patients in the general population in their approach to illness and wellness. Poverty and the rural location of Indian reservations make HIV care especially challenging. This chapter focuses on the basic management of HIV infection and the recognition and treatment of four complications of AIDS.

Epidemiology

In 1992, the seroprevalence of HIV among American Indians (AIs) and Alaska Natives (ANs) was 0.3 of 1,000 women receiving prenatal care and 4.5 of 1,000 men seeking care in sexually transmitted disease (STD) clinics at 58 Indian Health Service facilities (40 rural, six urban, 12 mixed). The rate of HIV seroprevalence among AI women in the western states was found to be four to eight times higher than the rates in childbearing women for all races.[1]

The first case of AIDS in an AI or AN was reported to the Centers for Disease Control and Prevention (CDC) in 1982. Since then, 1,554 cases have been reported to the CDC, representing 0.3% of total U.S. cases for all races. The first half of 1996 marked a turning point in AIDS mortality in the United States. For the first time since the beginning of the epidemic, the death rate in the general population fell (by 13%) compared with the preceding 6-month period. The mortality rate among AIs showed a much more dramatic decline (32%) over the same time period. It has been postulated that this decline in mortality reflects the use of new, highly potent combination antiretroviral drugs and increased use of prophylactic agents for prevention of opportunistic infections.[2]

Primary Care

This section explains the basic approach of the primary care provider to the patient with newly diagnosed HIV infection. The initial workup and a rational approach to antiretroviral therapy in Indian patients are discussed. A warning is in order. State-of-the-art HIV primary care changes every single day. The recommendations below (especially for antiretroviral therapy) are likely to change at least in part soon after publication. Please consult current editions of newsletters and Web sites listed in the bibliography for the most up-to-date guidelines.

History and Physical Examination

History should focus on risk factors for HIV acquisition and possible exposures to other pathogens that may become relevant as immune function declines. It is crucial to use discretion in discussing high-risk behaviors, such as substance abuse and sexual activity, which might be culturally sensitive issues. Patients should be questioned about travel history, history of tuberculosis exposure, STD history, use of alcohol and other drugs, and pet ownership. The clinician should look for signs and symptoms of depression and anxiety, which often accompany news of a diagnosis of HIV infection. It is also helpful to determine a patient's attitudes toward religion and traditional healing and to encourage participation in these activities early on if desired.

The physical examination should be thorough. A careful skin examination is critical to look for malignancies, such as Kaposi's sarcoma, and for infections, such as cryptococcosis, bacillary angiomatosis, and herpes zoster. The fundi of the HIV-positive patient should be examined for cytomegalovirus at the first visit and *at every subsequent* visit. A complete dental examination looking for Kaposi's sarcoma, thrush, gingivitis, and hairy leuko-

Table 13-1. Primary Care Screening

Test	Frequency	Comments
CD4 count	Every 3–4 mos	Use same laboratory
HIV viral load	Every 3–4 mos	Use same method and laboratory
RPR/VDRL	Every yr	LP if positive
PPD	Once	12 mos isoniazid if positive
HBsAb, HBsAg, HCV Ab	Once	HBV vaccinate if unprotected
Cytomegalovirus Ab	Once	Test if low risk only
Toxoplasma Ab	Once	Prophylaxis if CD4 <100
CBC, chemistry panel	Every 3 mos	—
Chest x-ray	Once	If symptomatic or PPD is positive
Pap smear	Every 6 mos for 2 yrs, then annually	Every 6 mos if positive

RPR = rapid plasma reagin (test); LP = lumbar puncture; HBV = hepatitis B virus; HBsAb = hepatitis B surface antibody; HBsAg = hepatitis B surface antigen; HCV = hepatitis C virus antibody; PPD = purified protein derivative; HIV = human immunodeficiency virus; Ab = antibody; CBC = complete blood count.
Source: Adapted from J Bartlett. Update on HIV management. Hopkins HIV Report 1997;9:3–4.

plakia should likewise be performed at every visit. All lymph node groups and the liver and spleen should be palpated for signs of pathology. A screening rectal examination and testicular examination should be performed, given the increased risk of tumors at these two sites. Finally, a complete neurologic examination is warranted at every visit.

Laboratory Testing, Screening, and Vaccinations

All patients newly diagnosed should have a baseline CD4 count and viral load determination. Additional commonly ordered tests are listed in Table 13-1.

Table 13-2. When to Start Therapy

Clinical Category	CD4 Count and HIV RNA	Recommendation
Symptomatic (AIDS, thrush, fever)	Any value	Treat
Asymptomatic	CD4 <500/μl or HIV RNA >10,000 (bDNA)	Recommend treatment
Asymptomatic	CD4 >500/μl and HIV RNA <10,000 (bDNA)	Consider observation alone

AIDS = acquired immunodeficiency syndrome; HIV = human immunodeficiency virus.
Source: Adapted from Feinberg MB, Carpenter C, Fauci AS, et al. Guidelines for the use of antiretroviral agents in HIV-infected adults and adolescents. Ann Intern Med 1998;128:1086.

Antiretroviral Therapy

Recent advances in antiretroviral therapy have revolutionized the care of the HIV-positive patient. In the late 1980s and early 1990s, monotherapy with zidovudine (AZT) was the treatment of choice for HIV. In the fall of 1995, the AIDS Clinical Trials Group Study 175 clearly demonstrated the advantage of double therapy with two nucleoside drugs over traditional AZT monotherapy in decreasing HIV viral loads and decreasing progression and mortality. The year 1997 saw an explosion in the use of triple-drug combination therapy in American patients. It has become possible to lower the amount of HIV in a patient's blood below the lower limits of detectability and to see subsequent improvement in patients' health status. My patients' progress during 1997 on triple-drug therapy, including weight gain, recovery from chronic opportunistic infections, and living longer, has been nothing short of astounding.

Not long ago, the U.S. Department of Health and Human Services convened the Panel on Clinical Practice for Treatment of HIV Infection. Recommendations for treatment were made based on CD4 count and viral load (Table 13-2). (The Infectious Diseases Society of America [ISDA] has published very similar guidelines.[3])

Therapy should also be considered for the patient with acute HIV infection. This is usually administered for up to 12 months.

The initial regimen for treating HIV infection in patients who need treatment should include three drugs. Monotherapy with AZT is contraindicated. The staged approach of starting two nucleoside agents and adding a protease inhibitor later when patients fail to respond is no longer recommended. Recommended combinations are listed. Indinavir is featured because it is by far the least expensive protease inhibitor with a tolerable side-effect profile.

Table 13-3. Antiretroviral Drugs

Drug	Dose	Side Effects
AZT (zidovudine)	200 mg PO tid	Cytopenias, headache, gastrointestinal upset, confusion, myositis, steatosis, macrocytosis
3TC (lamivudine)	150 mg PO bid	Headache, diarrhea, fatigue, leukopenia
ddI (didanosine)	200 mg PO bid, if ≥60 kg 150 mg PO bid, if <60 kg	Neuropathy (25%), pancreatitis (10%), diarrhea, hyperuricemia
ddC (zalcitabine)	0.75 mg PO tid	Neuropathy (30%), pancreatitis (1%), oral ulcers, cardiomyopathy
d4T (stavudine)	40 mg PO bid	Neuropathy, elevated LFTs, agitation, macrocytosis
Indinavir	800 mg PO tid	Nephrolithiasis (4%), elevated indirect bilirubin
Nelfinavir	750 mg PO tid	Diarrhea
Nevirapine	200 mg PO bid	Rash

LFTs = liver function tests; PO = orally.

AZT, lamivudine (3TC), indinavir
AZT, didanosine (ddI), indinavir
AZT, zalcitabine (ddC), indinavir
3TC, stavudine (d4T), indinavir
ddI, d4T, indinavir

The 3TC-containing regimens may be especially prone to induce drug resistance, a negative characteristic. The recommended drugs, dosages, and side effects are listed in Table 13-3.

The ultimate goal of triple-drug therapy is an undetectable viral load. Drug therapy failure can be defined as follows:

1. Failure to achieve a 0.50 to 0.75 log reduction in viral load at 1 month or a 10-fold reduction at 2 months
2. Failure to achieve an undetectable viral load at 4–6 months
3. Return to a detectable viral load (>500/ml) after previous undetectability
4. Threefold increase in viral load from a nadir value
5. Persistently falling CD4 count
6. Clinical deterioration (new AIDS-defining illness)

If treatment fails or if the patient develops toxicity with the original drugs, it is time to change therapy. As a rule, one should never add a new drug to a failing regimen without changing at least two of the original drugs. Recommendations for modifying therapy are covered in detail in the U.S. Department of Health and Human Services guidelines.

If drugs are being changed simply because of toxicity and there has been no adverse change in the viral load, it is not necessary to change more than two drugs. The combinations of AZT-d4T, ddC-ddI, ddC-d4T, and ddC-3TC should never be used because of lack of proved efficacy.

Prevention of Opportunistic Infections

The prevention of opportunistic infections has played a major role in prolonging life in persons infected with HIV. Following are the current recommendations from the U.S. Public Health Service (USPHS) for prophylactic therapy (Table 13-4).

Treatment with trimethoprim-sulfamethoxazole offers coverage for pneumocystosis and toxoplasmosis. Oral desensitization therapy can be performed if a history of non–life-threatening allergy to this drug is obtained. The pneumococcal vaccine is the principal vaccine recommended by the USPHS and IDSA for patients with HIV infection. *Haemophilus influenzae* vaccines are not indicated in adults. Live vaccines, such as polio, yellow fever, and varicella, are contraindicated in HIV-positive patients.

Clinical Syndromes

Four major clinical syndromes are likely to be seen by the practitioner in Indian country in patients with AIDS. This section provides a framework for the diagnosis and management of these syndromes.

Undifferentiated Fever

Undifferentiated fever is one of the most important clinical syndromes seen in patients with AIDS.

The causes of fever in patients with advanced HIV disease are protean and include drug allergy (especially sulfa), infections, and malignancy. The important pathogens and neoplasms to consider in the differential diagnosis are as follows:

Mycobacterium avium bacteremia
Miliary *Mycobacterium tuberculosis* infection
Pneumocystosis, disseminated
Cryptococcosis
Coccidioidomycosis
Histoplasmosis
Bartonellosis

Table 13-4. Opportunistic Infection Prophylaxis*

Organism	Indication	First Choice	Second Choice
Pneumocystis carinii	CD4<200; unexplained fever; thrush	TMP-SMX 1 DS/day	TMP-SMX 1 DS three times/wk or dapsone 100 mg/day or pentamidine nebulizer 300 mg/mo
Toxoplasma gondii	CD4<100 and positive *Toxoplasma* IgG	TMP-SMX 1 DS/day	TMP-SMX 1 DS three times/wk or dapsone 50 mg/day + pyrimethamine 50 mg/wk + folinic acid 25 mg/wk
Mycobacterium avium	CD4<50	Azithromycin 1,000–1,200 mg/wk or Clarithromycin 500 mg PO bid	Rifabutin 300 mg/day
Streptococcus pneumoniae	All patients	Pneumovax 0.5 ml IM q6yrs	—

TMP-SMX = trimethoprim-sulfamethoxazole; PO = orally; IM = intramuscular; DS = double strength.
*Prophylaxis is not recommended for *Haemophilus influenzae*, cytomegalovirus, *Cryptococcus neoformans*, *Histoplasma capsulatum*, *Coccidioides immitis*, and varicella zoster.
Source: Adapted from USPHS/IDSA Prevention of Opportunistic Infections Working Group. USPHS/IDSA guidelines for the prevention of opportunistic infections in persons infected with human immunodeficiency virus: a summary. Ann Intern Med 1996;124:349–368.

Cytomegalovirus viremia
Non-Hodgkin's lymphoma

The approach to the patient with undifferentiated fever should begin with a noninvasive evaluation followed by more invasive testing. The physical examination is key, with special attention paid to the dilated funduscopic examination, the skin, lymph nodes, and liver and spleen. The following tests should then be considered:

1. Routine chemistries, complete blood count (CBC), urinalysis, chest x-ray (CXR), and blood cultures
2. Lysis centrifugation blood culture (available via many state laboratories)
3. Purified protein derivative skin test
4. Lumbar puncture for cell counts, chemistries, acid-fast and fungal cultures, cryptococcus antigen, *Coccidioides* complement fixation (if there is a history of travel), and *Toxoplasma* antibody
5. Sputum induction for *Pneumocystis carinii* (if any pulmonary findings are present)

The lysis centrifugation culture is of critical importance because several of the pathogens listed can be detected by this method. Cytomegalovirus cultures and serology are of little value. The lumbar puncture is useful because cryptococcosis can present with no headache. A computed tomography (CT) scan is traditionally performed before the lumbar puncture to rule out mass lesions.

If the diagnosis remains elusive, the more invasive stage of the evaluation should follow up on findings from the physical examination and routine laboratory findings. Skin lesions and abnormal lymph nodes should be biopsied. If there are no clues from the physical examination or routine tests, two tests are of key importance: the bone marrow biopsy and the abdominal CT scan. Nuclear medicine scans are usually of extremely low yield. A liver biopsy should be obtained as a last resort because other, less risky tests often yield the diagnosis. Endoscopic biopsies are helpful if there are any gastrointestinal complaints to make the diagnosis of cytomegalovirus enteritis and lymphoma.

Pulmonary Infiltrates

Pulmonary infections are a common manifestation of AIDS. The differential diagnosis of pulmonary infiltrates in AIDS is immense.

The approach to pulmonary infiltrates in the patient with AIDS is based on the stage of HIV infection. Patients with early HIV infection (CD4 count above 200) are at greatest risk for recurrent bacterial pneumonias and for tuberculosis. Patients with CD4 counts less than 200 are more likely to have infection with one of the opportunistic organisms such as *Pneumocystis, Coccidioides, Histoplasma, Toxoplasma,* or *M. avium* complex.

The workup of the patient with pulmonary infiltrates begins with the routine CXR. Patients with focal areas of consolidation are more likely to have bacterial pneumonia or tuberculosis, and patients with diffuse interstitial infiltrates are more likely to have one of the fungal or parasitic pathogens listed. The next stage of the evaluation is sputum induction using nebulized, hypertonic saline. Sputum should be sent immediately for *Pneumocystis* immunofluorescence, acid-fast smear and culture, and fungal culture. If a diagnosis is not forthcoming and the patient is deteriorating, it would be reasonable to proceed with bronchoscopy or fine-needle aspiration of the infected lobe. Open-lung biopsy is performed only as a last resort.

Treatment should focus on the specific etiologic agent once a diagnosis is made. While waiting for a diagnosis, empiric therapy should be started. In the patient with a very high CD4 count (above 500), it is reasonable to treat for routine bacterial pathogens, such as pneumococcus, and atypical bacteria, such as *Mycoplasma*, with the combination of a third-generation cephalosporin and a macrolide antibiotic (erythromycin). Patients with a CD4 count less than 500 are at risk for infection with *Pneumocystis* and should be covered for this infection empirically. A combination of a third-generation cephalosporin and trimethoprim-sulfamethoxazole would be reasonable in this setting. If the diagnosis is not confirmed but the patient improves with trimethoprim-sulfamethoxazole therapy, a full 3-week course to cover *Pneumocystis* is warranted.

Diarrhea

Diarrhea is a common cause of morbidity and mortality of patients with advanced HIV disease, affecting up to 50% of patients. The differential diagnosis is broad.

The initial history should dwell on chronicity, whether there is fever, bleeding, or tenesmus; medications given; and travel history. The physical examination is focused on the fundi, the presence or absence of lymphadenopathy and hepatosplenomegaly, and the stool guaiac. The initial basic laboratory workup should include the following:

1. CBC, electrolytes, BUN, creatinine, liver function tests
2. Routine stool culture
3. *Clostridium difficile* toxin assay
4. Stool for ova and parasites
5. Stool for trichrome stain (microsporidiosis)
6. Stool for modified acid-fast bacillus stain (cryptosporidiosis and cyclosporiasis)

If these initial screening tests are not revealing, invasive workup with upper and lower endoscopy is indicated.

Discussion of the treatment of all possible causes of diarrhea is beyond the scope of this chapter. Some general points should be made. First, acute diarrhea, particularly in rural reservation sites, is often caused by *Shigella* or *Salmonella* and warrants empiric therapy with ciprofloxacin while awaiting cultures. Second, some pathogens, such as cytomegalovirus, can be present on culture of a tissue biopsy of the gut without being the etiology of diarrhea. It is crucial to document invasive disease (such as cytomegalic inclusiona in enterocytes) before attributing the diagnosis to a single pathogen. Third, as in opportunistic infection at other sites in AIDS, multiple pathogens are the rule rather than the exception. Finally, some conditions have a particularly poor response to therapy, most notably cryptosporidiosis. The clinician and the patient are often faced with the difficult ethical decision of whether prolonged therapy with total parenteral nutrition is justified.

Headache

The neurologic manifestations of AIDS are protean, and detailed discussion is beyond the scope of this chapter. Rapid diagnosis of headache in AIDS is of critical importance because some of the opportunistic illnesses in AIDS are treatable and possibly 100% reversible.

The history and review of systems in AIDS patients with headache are usually nonspecific. In cryptococcal meningitis (*Cryptococcus* being an important fungal pathogen), the majority of patients complain of headache and malaise. Only 22% complain of stiff neck.[5] Similarly, in toxoplasmosis, fever is seen in only 7%, whereas focal neurologic findings are seen in 73%.[6] The routine physical examination in both conditions is usually normal unless the disease is advanced and focal findings have developed.

The initial laboratory workup includes a neuroimaging study followed by a lumbar puncture if there is no evidence for increased intracranial pressure. Brain magnetic resonance imaging is superior to CT for detecting mass lesions, but CT is less expensive and provides a rapid screening test for increased intracranial pressure. The lumbar puncture in cryptococcal meningitis is often deceptively benign, with only 21% of patients in one study showing white cell counts more than 20 per µl and only 55% showing protein more than 45 mg/dl.[7] A lumbar puncture is probably not necessary if the patient has a positive serum *Toxoplasma* serology, with multiple typical ring-enhancing lesions on CT in the basal ganglia and gray-white matter junction.

Cryptococcal meningitis is traditionally treated with amphotericin B at a dose of 0.6–0.7 mg/kg per day for a minimum of 2 weeks. It is mandatory to follow this up with lifelong suppressive oral fluconazole therapy because otherwise, the majority of patients will relapse. Toxoplasmosis can be treated empirically without brain biopsy with pyrimethamine plus either sulfadiazine or clindamycin in the patient with multiple ring-enhancing lesions and a positive anti-*Toxoplasma* antibody. Patients with an atypical imaging study or those with negative serologies are candidates for immediate brain biopsy. Patients who fail empiric anti-*Toxoplasma* therapy after 10–14 days should also be biopsied.

Conclusion

This chapter focuses on the initial clinical approach to patients with AIDS and the evaluation and treatment of four common complications of AIDS. The subject matter changes rapidly. The reader is urged to review the newsletters and Web sites listed below for the most up-to-date recommendations.

Summary Points

- HIV infection is a significant cause of disease in Native Americans.
- Measurement of the viral load has become a critical measure of prognosis in AIDS.
- Zidovudine monotherapy is no longer acceptable as treatment for HIV.
- Triple-drug therapy with two nucleoside reverse transcriptase inhibitors and a protease inhibitor are now the treatment of choice for HIV.
- The evaluation and early management of fever, pneumonia, diarrhea, and headache can easily be performed even at remote reservation health centers. Concise recommendations are provided in this chapter.

Useful Resources

Books

Bartlett J. Medical Management of HIV Infection. Baltimore: Port City Press, 1997.
Kazanjian P. Ambulatory Care of the HIV Infected Patient. Ann Arbor, MI: University of Michigan Press, 1996.

Newsletters

Hopkins HIV Report
Johns Hopkins University AIDS Service
1830 East Monument St, 4th Floor
Baltimore, MD 21205

AIDS Clinical Care
1440 Main Street
Waltham, MA 02154-1600

Web Sites

Johns Hopkins University AIDS Service:
 http://www.hopkins-aids.edu
University of San Francisco AIDS Program:
 http://hivinsite.ucsf.edu

References

1. Conway GA, Ambrose TJ, Chase E, et al. HIV infection in American Indians and Alaska Natives: surveys in the Indian Health Service. J Acquir Immune Defic Syndr 1992;5:803–809.
2. Centers for Disease Control and Prevention. Update: trends in AIDS incidence, deaths and prevalence—United States, 1996. MMWR Morb Mortal Wkly Rep 1997;46:165–173.
3. Carpenter CJ. Antiretroviral therapy for HIV infection in 1997, updated recommendations of the Infectious Disease Society-USA panel. JAMA 1997;277:1962–1969.
4. Feinberg MB, Carpenter C, Fauci AS, et al. Guidelines for the use of antiretroviral agents in HIV-infected adults and adolescents. Ann Intern Med 1998;128:1079–1100
5. Chuck SL, Sande MA. Infections with Cryptococcus neoformans in the acquired immunodeficiency syndrome. N Engl J Med 1989;321:794–799.
6. McArthur JC. Neurologic manifestations of AIDS. Medicine 1987;66:407–436.

Chapter 14
Hepatitis

Theresa Cullen

Each year, hepatitis and its sequelae cause serious morbidity and mortality among American Indian (AI) and Alaska Native (AN) populations. The three common viruses, hepatitis A, B, and C, account for more than 100,000 cases of acute hepatitis each year in the United States. In AI and AN communities, the incidence of hepatitis A is more than 10 times that of the general population.[1] The increased incidence in this population is reflected by cyclic epidemics and an increase in the occurrence of fulminant hepatitis A with subsequent mortality. Moreover, urban AI and AN populations have a higher incidence of hepatitis A than do rural AIs and ANs (151 per 100,000 vs. 106 per 100,000).[1]

Chronic hepatitis, particularly as a result of hepatitis B, affects more than 1 million Americans a year. AN communities have high rates of this disease; in these communities, hepatitis B is the major risk factor for developing hepatocellular carcinoma. The increased risk of developing hepatocellular carcinoma in AN men is 3.7 times higher than in white men in the United States.[2] Once again, urban AIs and ANs have a higher incidence of this disease than do rural AIs and ANs (47 per 100,000 vs. 25 per 100,000).

Hepatitis C is a silent epidemic, infecting an estimated 4 million Americans.[3] It is the major cause for posttransfusion hepatitis, primarily in patients older than 55 years old. It is the most common cause of nonalcoholic liver disease in the United States. AI and AN incidence is currently unknown for this chronic disease.

Chronic liver disease and cirrhosis are the second leading causes of death for AI and AN populations between 25 and 44 years of age. AI and AN have an age-adjusted alcoholism death rate 5.6 times the U.S. all-races rate.[4] These data reflect an increased risk of alcoholic hepatitis and its cirrhotic sequelae. Clearly, alcohol and its hepatic sequelae continue to account for significant morbidity and mortality in AI and AN communities.

However, most communities are capable of preventing most cases of hepatitis. Appropriate immunizations, hand washing, adequate sanitation and housing, safer sex, and decreased alcohol use can result in a significant impact on the incidence of these diseases.

Hepatitis A

It is 3 A.M. on September 1 in the emergency room of a small rural reservation hospital. You are a board-eligible family practitioner who finished your residency in June. A 4-year-old child, complaining of stomach pain and vomiting, is brought in by her mother. The mother reports that she has watched the child's fluid intake closely, but the child has seemed listless for the past few days. No one else is ill at home. The child attends one of the day-care centers in the community. The child has a low-grade temperature and mild, nonfocal abdominal pain. You realize that this is the third child with similar complaints that you have seen within the past few days. The other children all looked well and were sent home with viral gastroenteritis treatment guidelines. Now, however, you wonder if there is a pattern, and you decide to order laboratory tests. The child's aspartate aminotransferase (AST) and alanine aminotransferase (ALT) levels are in the 1,000 range, with a minimally elevated bilirubin. Clearly, your patient has hepatitis; given the presenting situation, it is most likely hepatitis A.

Pathology

The hepatitis A virus (HAV) is an RNA virus (picornavirus) that causes only this disease. Pathologically, typical lesions of hepatitis A consist of panlobular infiltration with mononuclear cells, variable degrees of cholestasis, and hepatic cell necrosis. Despite this serious pathology, there is no chronic hepatitis due to hepatitis A.

Transmission and Incidence

Formerly called *infectious hepatitis*, hepatitis A is transmitted almost exclusively by the fecal-oral route, usually from person to person or by ingestion of infected food or water. Parenteral transmission has been documented but is very rare. AIs and ANs have the highest reported incidence of hepatitis A (121.2 cases per 1,000, compared to the U.S. total of 10.3 per 1,000 in 1994),[5, 6] with periodic epidemics in unimmunized communities. Communities with high rates of infection are usually characterized by poor housing, overcrowding, and lack of sanitation. These three factors are intimately connected. Families who live in homes with no running water or outdoor privies may find it difficult to initiate safe hand washing.

Clinical Course and Diagnosis

Incubation period for HAV infections is usually 2–6 weeks, with an average incubation period of 1 month. Clinical presentation can be variable. Constitutional signs can include anorexia, nausea and vomiting, myalgias, headache, pharyngitis, low-grade temperatures, and fatigue. Dark-colored urine and clay-colored stools may precede noticeable jaundice. Jaundice is usually detected clinically by icteric sclera. Children younger than the age of 2 years are rarely symptomatic, and most adults exhibit minimal, if any, signs of disease.

As a result, in endemic areas of HAV infection, clinicians must maintain a high index of suspicion about this disease. The presenting clinical picture can be very vague, especially with young patients. Early in epidemic situations, many cases can be missed or attributed to other viral infections, such as gastroenteritis.

If you suspect an acute case of hepatitis A, laboratory evaluation can be helpful. Liver function test elevation usually precedes symptoms. ALT is usually greater than AST. Occasionally, bilirubin can be markedly elevated and may continue to rise even though liver enzymes decrease. Jaundice does not usually appear until the bilirubin exceeds 2.5. Most laboratory abnormalities resolve within 6 months after acute infection.

Hepatitis serology is diagnostic, with positive serology for immunoglobulin M (IgM) antibody to HAV (anti-HAV) indicating a recent infection. Ninety-nine percent of people have an elevation in IgM anti-HAV at the onset of symptoms. IgG anti-HAV usually appears 2–6 months after infection. However, total antibody to HAV (IgM and IgG anti-HAV) determines immunity and is usually present 2–6 months after infection.

The clinical course of HAV is usually unremarkable in children. Occasionally, children must be admitted for secondary complications, primarily dehydration. Adults who contract HAV can develop more serious complications, including liver failure. This is an extremely rare complication, however, occurring primarily in patients with underlying liver disease. Signs of hepatic failure include hypoglycemia, change in mental status, prolonged prothrombin time, and serum bilirubin levels above 10.

Therapy

There is no specific treatment for acute HAV infections. A low-fat, high-carbohydrate diet can be recommended. Alcohol and other hepatotoxic drugs should be avoided. As noted, hospitalization may be required for hypoglycemia or dehydration. Clinic and hospital staff must be reminded about the need for proper prevention, including adequate hand washing.

Prevention

During acute infections or epidemics, spread of the disease usually occurs before the infected individual seeks medical care. In acute infections, close household contacts and day care contacts should be offered immunoglobulin. This antibody preparation confers protection on the recipient through passive transfer of antibody. Immunoglobulin does *not* result in a false-positive IgM, so patients can be diagnosed even after receiving this postexposure prophylaxis.

The most significant advances in prevention have occurred with the introduction of the HAV vaccine, which is available free for AI and AN populations through Vaccines for Children programs. This inactive vaccine is available as a two-dose series (some older vaccine has a three-dose program). In epidemic situations among AI and AN communities, vaccination of 70–80% of children stops the epidemic.[4–10] Due to the proved efficacy of this vaccine and the known high incidence of HAV in AI and AN communities, the Centers for Disease Control and Prevention recommends routine vaccination for young AI and AN children (age 2 years or older) and catch-up vaccination for older children.[6] Vaccination is also recommended for patients with chronic liver disease, patients with clotting disorders, homosexual males, travelers to certain countries, illegal-drug users and, occasionally, health care workers and food handlers. The current vaccine is not licensed for children younger than the age of 2 years.

Epidemics

Tribal health workers, community health representatives, environmental health workers, and public health nurses function as the eyes and ears in the community. Providers must pay close attention to their concerns and to any changes in the pattern of patient complaints in high-risk areas. Epidemic situations may not be recognized initially, especially if more than one health center provides care to the population, or if there are new health care providers. On reservations, however, public health nursing has historically tracked epidemics and can help predict the next cycle. This cycle usually occurs every 5–10 years in communities with high rates of disease and HAV seroprevalence rates of 30–40% in children by the age of 5 years.[6]

As soon as an outbreak is suspected, the appropriate local, state, and national agencies should be notified. Traditionally, county and state health departments are very helpful in responding to epidemic situations. In addition, the Indian Health Service has epidemiologic help available for these situations.

It is critical to involve other concerned on-reservation groups early, including schools, restaurants, day care centers, and environmental health groups. Remember: Timing is critical. The earlier you recognize an epidemic, the more likely you are to halt the spread quickly. Some on-reservation facilities have developed early-intervention teams to address epidemic settings. Even if your facility does not have an early-intervention team, environmental health policies should dictate reporting procedures. In epidemic situations, leave nothing to chance, because chance will win.

Hepatitis B

In the small community in Alaska where you work, your next patient, a quiet man in his 40s, has come in complaining of fatigue of several months' duration. He has worked in an off-reservation town for the last 10 years, has made few visits to the clinic, and has no known chronic medical problems.

On further discussion, he reveals other concerns, including itching and some abdominal pain. He had a cholecystectomy a "long time ago," during which he received some blood due to some unknown complication. He denies any fever, weight loss, nausea, vomiting, or other constitutional complaints. He does not drink alcohol or smoke tobacco. His examination is unremarkable, but his blood work reveals minimally elevated liver function tests. Hepatitis serology is positive for hepatitis B surface antigen (HBsAg).

Pathology

The hepatitis B virus (HBV) is a double-stranded DNA virus that is a major cause of acute and chronic hepatitis. Chronic infection with HBV can result in hepatocellular carcinoma. The incidence of this carcinoma is increased in ANs.

Transmission and Incidence

HBV is transmitted primarily through blood or sexual contact. Vertical transmission from mother to child occurs in approximately 50% of mothers who have chronic HBV infection. In Alaska, transmission of HBV occurs primarily from carrier children to uninfected children. This transmission route has resulted in increased cases among many villages in Alaska, with approximately 8–13% of ANs developing hepatitis B surface seropositivity.[3]

Clinical Course and Diagnosis

There is a high risk for infant infection due to maternal transmission. Most of these cases are asymptomatic but have a high risk of developing chronic hepatitis. In children, most cases are also asymptomatic, and chronic HAV infection also develops in up to 50% of cases. Adults usually exhibit clinical signs during acute infection, including icteric symptoms. As with HAV, however, there is a broad spectrum of clinical severity, with a small percentage of acutely infected adults developing fulminant hepatitis. Chronic hepatitis usually develops in less than 5% of adults.

Hepatitis serology is diagnostic, and it includes three HBV-associated viral antigens or corresponding antibodies (HBsAg and core antigens c and e [HBcAg, HBeAg]). HBsAg is found in both acute infection and chronic HBV infection. HBsAg disappears during convalescence, when antibody develops. The persistence of HBsAg for more than 12 weeks is a predictor of chronic infection; the presence of HBsAg for 6 months or longer indicates chronic infection. All prenatal and high-risk patients should be screened for HBsAg.

HBcAg is not easily measured, but antibody to HBcAg is clinically available. IgM anti-HBc detects recent infection, and IgG anti-HBc persists for years after acute infection. These tests offer little help in a primary care setting for diagnosing and treating this disease.

HBeAg develops within 6 weeks of infection and disappears after the peak of infection, with the development of antibody. Persistence of HBeAg means ongoing viral replication: Patients are infectious during this stage. Hepatocellular carcinoma develops more frequently in patients who develop anti-HBe and persistent HBsAg.

Therapy

Most therapy is supportive but is also aimed at detecting chronic infection. If cirrhosis develops, the 5-year survival rate can be as low as 55%. Interferon has been approved for treatment of chronic hepatitis B, but treatment has not been shown to prevent the development of hepatocellular carcinoma. Additional new agents, including antiviral medications, are also available for treatment of the chronically infected patient.

In certain high-risk communities, including ANs, alpha-fetoprotein testing should be offered every 6 months to patients with chronic hepatitis B. This testing can help identify patients in the early, resectable stages of hepatocellular carcinoma. This early identification has led to decreased 1-year mortality rates for this cancer.[3]

Prevention

The hepatitis B vaccine is effective in preventing HBV disease. The hepatitis B vaccine program in certain areas of Alaska has resulted in a significant decrease in symptomatic hepatitis B infection (from rates of 100–220 per 100,000 down to 1–20 per 100,000 over a 5- to 10-year period). It is available free through the Vaccines for Children program for AIs and ANs. All children should be routinely immunized with this vaccine. In addition, high-risk adult groups should be offered this vaccine, including health care workers, patients with high-risk sexual behavior, and dialysis patients. The hepatitis B series consists of three shots, given at birth, 1 month, and 6 months. At this time, the need for booster doses is unclear, especially in children immunized before 1 year of age.

After high-risk exposure, hepatitis B immunoglobulin should be given, preferably within 24 hours. This should be combined with the first of three vaccine doses. If the patient has been previously immunized, test for HBsAb. If this result is negative, repeat a vaccine booster dose.

Hepatitis C

Your dialysis patient complains of feeling poorly. She has been your patient for the last 5 years and has been on dialysis for the past 8 years. During this time, she has rarely voiced any complaints, but today is clearly different. Her oldest daughter has accompanied her to the clinic; wanting to make sure that her mother tells you how she feels. Your patient is unable to clarify for you what is wrong, but she knows that somehow she is not well. Her last chemistries from dialysis show minimally elevated liver function tests. Further serology, done over the next few weeks, confirms a diagnosis of hepatitis C.

Pathology

The hepatitis C virus (HCV) is an RNA virus that is less infectious than HBV. It is responsible for most of the cases of what was formerly known as non-A, non-B hepatitis. HCV was only recently identified (1989), and testing for anti-HCV in clinics and blood donors became available in 1990.

Transmission and Incidence

HCV is transmitted by infected blood, either by transfusion or intravenous drug use; sexual transmission occurs at a very low rate. Hepatitis C is also a major factor in dialysis patients. It accounts for up to 75% of acute hepatitis cases in hemodialysis patients. However, risk factors are not identifiable in more than 40% of cases. Approximately 1% of the U.S. population is chronically infected with HCV. Acute hepatitis C develops into a chronic infection in most infections (up to 90%).

Clinical Course and Diagnosis

Most cases of acute hepatitis C are clinically mild. The virus has an incubation period of 2–20 weeks, with only 25% of patients manifesting clinical jaundice. Eighty-five percent of infections go on to become chronic. This chronic condition is also subclinical, although most patients show mild to moderate hepatitis on biopsy. Neither symptoms nor degree of ALT elevation correlate with the severity of the disease on biopsy.

Cirrhosis develops in up to 25% of patients followed over several years; after 20 years, cirrhosis may develop in up to 50% of patients. Liver failure and other complications of cirrhosis reflect the insidious and indolent nature of this disease: These complications usually do not develop for years after infection. Age at time of diagnosis, duration of infection, and degree of histologic damage at biopsy correlate with progression of liver disease. Alcohol intake and infection with HBV may also affect the progression of this disease. Hepatitis C is the leading reason for orthotic liver transplant at many centers.

Diagnosis is based on serologic tests, but some of these tests may not have the sensitivity desired. IgM and IgG antibodies develop slowly and may not be detectable in some infections. Early diagnosis may be helpful because patients respond to acute treatment better during the acute phase than when the disease is already chronic.

Diagnosis of chronic hepatitis C is based on immunoassays that look for anti–hepatitis C surface antibodies. A positive enzyme-linked immunosorbent assay (ELISA) detects chronic hepatitis C. Chronic infection is confirmed by use of recombinant immunoblot assay testing (RIBA). Both ELISA and RIBA testing can show HCV within 3 months of exposure. If both the ELISA and RIBA are positive, referral to gastroenterology is indicated for evaluation and possible liver biopsy.

Hepatitis C may also be implicated in the development of hepatocellular carcinoma. However, there is currently no known pathogenic mechanism for this association. It is speculated that the chronic HCV infection, by causing chronic hepatocyte damage, increases the risk of hepatocellular carcinoma.

Therapy

Acute therapy is supportive, as for HAV and HBV. If serologic tests are consistent with hepatitis C, consider referral to a gastroentemologist The treatment options for hepatitis C are changing rapidly, and a consultant can work with primary care physicians to manage these patients appropriately. Currently, interferon is effective in approximately 20–40% of selected patients; patients who receive interferon can be followed by primary care providers. Important side effects include depression, fatigue, headaches, and an influenzalike response. Adjunct therapy includes alcohol restriction: Patients with chronic hepatitis C should limit their intake to no more than 10 g of alcohol (one glass of wine, one beer) once a week.

Prevention

Modification of risk factors through changes in transfusion screening protocols has resulted in decreased transmission of this disease. Universal precautions can also result in decreased transmission in health care workers. Vaccine development for HCV is ongoing.

References

1. Grossman DC, Kreiger JW, Sugarman JR, Forqera RA. Health status of urban American Indians and Alaska Natives. A population based study. JAMA 1994;271: 845–850.
2. Wainwright RB. The US Arctic Investigations Program: infectious disease prevention and control research in Alaska. Lancet 1996;347:517–520.
3. Wainwright RB, Bulkow LR, Parkinson AJ, et al. Protection provided by hepatitis B vaccine in a Yupik Eskimo population: results of a 10 year study. J Infect Dis 1997;175:674–677.
4. Welty TK, Darling K, Dys S, et al. Guidelines for prevention and control of hepatitis A in American Indian and Alaska Native communities. S D J Med 1996;49: 317–322.
5. McMahon BJ, Beller M, Williams J, et al. A program to control an outbreak of hepatitis A in Alaska by using an inactivated hepatitis A vaccine. Arch Pediatr Adolesc Med 1996;150:733–739.
6. Centers for Disease Control and Prevention. Prevention of hepatitis A through active or passive immunization. MMWR Morb Mortal Wkly Rep 1996;45[No. RR-15]:1–30.
7. Indian Health Service. Trends in Indian Health, 1996. Washington, DC: U.S. Department of Health and Human Services, Office of Planning, Evaluation, and Legislation, Division of Program Statistics,1997.
8. Sjorgen MH. Serological diagnosis of viral hepatitis. Gastroenterol Clin North Am 1994;23: 457–477.
9. Hoofnagle JH, Biscegli AM. The treatment of chronic viral hepatitis. N Engl J Med 1997;335:347–356.
10. Sharara AI, Hunt CM, Hamilton JD. Hepatitis C. Ann Intern Med 1996;125:658–668.

Chapter 15
Hydatid Disease

Bruce Tempest and Joseph F. Wilson

Hydatid disease *sensu lato* causes serious health problems on all continents of the world. In some regions, it ranks among the most important of public health issues. For example, in the Turkana district of Kenya, the prevalence of this infection was 200 per 100,000, and, in western China, Chai reported 26,065 surgical cases in recent years from just six provinces.[1] In North America, hydatid disease is relatively uncommon. It occurs primarily in local populations in which the parasite is hyperendemic and among immigrants from countries where the disease is highly endemic (mostly sheep- and cattle-raising countries). However, these diseases occur disproportionately among Native Americans.

Among four species of tapeworm of the genus *Echinococcus* that are pathogenic to humans, two are of clinical importance in North America: *E. granulosus* and *E. multilocularis*.[2]

A second form of CE is caused by a northern or non-synanthropic biotype of *E. granulosus*. That cestode occurs naturally wherever a predator-prey relationship exists between wolves and large members of the deer family, usually moose and caribou.[5] Dogs may replace wolves as final host if they have access to cysts. This disease, also called the *sylvatic form*, is clinically benign. It tends to be self-limiting, with treatment usually required only in the management of "complicated" cysts (i.e., cysts that have ruptured or become secondarily infected). Although indigenous to most regions of Alaska and much of northern Canada, this hydatid disease occurs largely in small villages of the interior where a subsistence lifestyle is practiced, with only 2% of cases found in whites. It is believed that the European biotype evolved from this form when humans first began to domesticate animals.

Cystic Echinococcosis

Cystic echinococcosis (CE), also called *cystic hydatid disease* (CHD), results from infection by *E. granulosus* and is characterized by the development of fluid-filled cysts, seen most commonly in the liver or lungs. There are two biotypes of *E. granulosus*, with distinct life cycles and symptoms, and requiring dissimilar management.[3]

The classic form of CE is caused by the European biotype of *E. granulosus*. This is the disease generally described in textbooks and in the extensive worldwide literature on hydatid disease. It is sometimes called the *pastoral form* because it is perpetuated by a cycle in synanthropic hosts (i.e., in domestic animals closely associated with people). A high percentage of locally acquired infections of this type in North America occur among Indians in western sheep-raising communities, such as the Navajo tribes in Arizona.[4]

Alveolar Hydatid Disease

Alveolar hydatid disease (AHD) is caused by *E. multilocularis*, the most pathogenic of all cestodes. This is a small fox tapeworm that is indigenous to the circumpolar tundra. It has a wide distribution across the northern latitudes of the Eurasian continent, where it creates major medical problems in Central Europe, Russia, China, and northern Japan. It is also present in foxes across much of the north-central United States and Canada, where it has now been found in 11 states and three provinces of Canada, and its range appears to be enlarging.[2] In North America, all but two of 44 known, active infections in humans have been among Yupik/Inupiat Eskimos from a small area in northwestern Alaska. Infection by this parasite results in an indolent but devastating, cancerlike disease that, if untreated, almost invariably progresses to a fatal outcome.[6]

Table 15-1. Clinical Features of Three Forms of Hydatid Disease

Disease	Cystic Echinococcosis, European Biotype	Cystic Echinococcosis, Northern Biotype	Alveolar Hydatid Disease
Adult tapeworm	European biotype of *E. granulosus*	Northern biotype of *E. granulosus*	*E. multilocularis*
Geographic distribution	Major livestock countries of the world: China, Mediterranean area, Argentina, and Australia	Tundra and boreal forest of the Holarctic: Russia, Alaska, and Canada	Across northern Eurasia and Central Europe: Russia, China, Japan, and northwest Alaska
Host:			
Definitive	Dog	Wolf	Fox
Intermediate	Sheep, cattle, pigs, and other ungulates	Moose and caribou	Voles, lemmings, and other rodents
Location:			
Lung	19%	57%	Metastatic lesions only
Liver	70%	43%	100% primary
Other sites	11%	0.30%	Lungs, bone, brain and mediastinum metastatic lesions only
Median age at diagnosis	23 yrs (pulmonary), 23 yrs (hepatic)	22 yrs (pulmonary), 65 yrs (hepatic)	55 yrs (all cases)
Pathophysiology:			
Size of cysts (cm)	7.2–15.0	3–4	Solid, cancerlike growth
Laminated membranes	Thick, white, opaque	Thin, translucent, fragile	N/A
Daughter cysts	Present in 30–50% of cases	Never reported	N/A
Symptoms at diagnosis	Common: 80–99%	Rare: 6–10%	85% historically, 35% recently
Spontaneous resolution	<1%	83% (30 of 36 cases)	40%
Prognosis	Many complications	Benign clinical course	High mortality and morbidity
Severe complications:			
Anaphylaxis	Common if cyst ruptures	Not reported	None
Dissemination	0–13% (a serious complication if cyst ruptures)	Not reported	None
Giant cysts (>10 cm)	Common	Rarely seen	N/A
Mortality	4–10%	0%	80% (untreated), 14% (treated)
Treatment	Aggressive	Very conservative	Aggressive: radical surgery and chemotherapy

N/A = not applicable.

Thus, three clinical disease entities are caused by two species of *Echinococcus*. Some of the important differences among these three diseases are presented in Table 15-1. Health providers for Native Americans require a working knowledge of these problems because in each case the disease occurs almost exclusively, or at least disproportionately, among Native Americans.

Life Cycle

Echinococcosis is perpetuated by a cycle involving a canine predator (final host, harboring the adult tapeworm) and a prey species (intermediate host, harboring the larval stage of the parasite) (Figure 15-1). Dogs (occasionally cats, in the case of *E. multilocularis*) serve as the important source

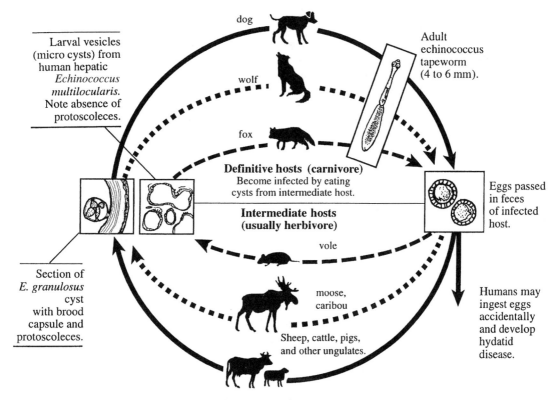

Larval vesicles (micro cysts) from human hepatic *Echinococcus multilocularis.* Note absence of protoscoleces.

Section of *E. granulosus* cyst with brood capsule and protoscoleces.

dog

wolf

fox

Adult echinococcus tapeworm (4 to 6 mm).

Definitive hosts (carnivore) Become infected by eating cysts from intermediate host.

Intermediate hosts (usually herbivore)

vole

moose, caribou

Sheep, cattle, pigs, and other ungulates.

Eggs passed in feces of infected host.

Humans may ingest eggs accidentally and develop hydatid disease.

Figure 15-1. Diagram illustrating the lifecycle of echinococcosis.

of infection for humans in each of the three diseases when they ingest rodents or the viscera of moose or sheep.

Clinical Presentation

Pathogenesis

Echinococcosis results when eggs are ingested through contact with feces of infected dogs. The egg releases the embryo (oncosphere) in the small intestine; the embryo then enters the portal bloodstream and passes to the liver, lung, or some other tissue, where it develops into the larval stage. In infections by *E. granulosus*, the larval stage has the form of a more or less spherical, fluid-filled cyst. The cyst is enclosed by a fibrous capsule of host origin, called the *ecto-cyst.* The endocyst consists of an external laminated membrane lined by a single-celled layer of germinal membrane. The germinal membrane gives rise to brood capsules, which in turn produce protoscoleces, each of which forms the scolex of the adult cestode of the next generation (Figure 15-1). When cysts degenerate or are poorly preserved, the brood capsules become detached, and the protoscoleces collect in dependent parts of the cyst; such material is often called *hydatid sand.* Germinal tissue, including that in

brood capsules and protoscoleces, can undergo proliferation and regeneration of new cysts if spilled into a body cavity, often resulting in disseminated disease. (The laminated membrane appears to be a nonliving mucopolysaccharide; it cannot proliferate and is inert. Germinal membrane from any structure can proliferate and form new cysts.)

When a canid (e.g., dog, wolf, or fox) ingests a cyst, the cyst is disrupted by the digestive process and the protoscoleces are released. Protoscoleces become scoleces when they attach to the mucosa. There they grow two or three segments to become mature, egg-producing tapeworms (4–6 mm long). About a month after the initial egg of *E. multilocularis* is ingested (45–50 days in the case of *E. granulosus*), new eggs appear in the animals' feces. The cycle then begins anew.

Symptomatology

European Synanthropic Form of Echinococcus Granulosus

Infection in humans by this biotype of *E. granulosus* is characterized by the presence of one or more cysts. Serious complications, such as dissemination of disease after rupture into a serosal cavity, the formation of giant cysts or hepatopulmonary fistulae, and other bizarre problems, commonly occur. The mortality rate may be 4–10%. The cysts in human infections are usually located in the liver (55–75%), with the lungs being the next most frequent site (10–30%). Other, less frequent sites (5–24%) include the brain, peritoneum, pancreas, spleen, kidney, heart, musculoskeletal tissue, subcutaneous fat, and breast.[7] These cysts have thick, opaque, whitish, laminated membranes (Figure 15-2A).

Northern Nonsynanthropic Form of Echinococcus Granulosus

Compared to the European form, these cysts are smaller (4 cm vs. 7–15 cm), the disease is more benign, and it is usually self-limiting. The laminated membranes of these cysts are thin, fragile, bluish, and translucent (Figure 15-2B). When a pulmonary cyst ruptures, the fluid and membranes are often coughed up, frequently without the patient's knowledge. The majority of "simple" (intact and not infected) pulmonary cysts (83%, 30 of 36 patients followed) "silently" disappears if left untreated (Figure 15-3). At the time of diagnosis, symptoms from pulmonary cysts are observed in only 6–10% of cases, usually as a result of complications after cyst rupture or secondary infection. Pain, hemoptysis, coughing up clear fluid, and fever are the most common symptoms. Bacterial infection of a ruptured pulmonary cyst may result in pneumonia or pulmonary abscess. Hepatic cysts seldom cause symptoms,[5] and symptoms are more common in children than in adults.[8]

Alveolar Hydatid Disease

AHD differs from CE in that the larval stage does not develop as a cyst. Rather, it develops into an irregular, solid, white to yellowish, cancerlike mass that is virtually always primary in the liver. It enlarges by proliferation and invasion of adjacent tissues (Figure 15-4). It may extend to regional lymph nodes or metastasize to distant organs. Growth of the lesion is slow, and therefore, the preclinical or prepatent period (the time between the initial infection and the onset of symptoms) may be up to 20–30 years.[6] Symptoms generally do not appear until an advanced stage is reached. At diagnosis, the larval cestode is not resectable in approximately 80% of patients. Pain (29%) or a palpable mass in the right upper quadrant (27%), hepatomegaly (24%), jaundice (12%), and neurologic findings secondary to brain metastases (7%) are the most common presenting symptoms.

Diagnosis

Serology

Serologic studies are important in confirming the diagnosis in uncertain cases, especially for AHD and the European form of CE.[9] Patients with intact simple cysts of the Northern biotype almost invariably (13 of 14 cases, or 93%) have negative serology, but this changes promptly to positive if the cyst ruptures.[3]

History

A history of contact with dogs that may have acquired the parasite is very important in establishing a diagnosis of echinococcosis. *A careful history is usually all that is required to differentiate the two forms of CE under consideration.* A history of contact with a dog from a sheep-raising farm in Arizona is quite different from contact with a dog from a remote village of Alaska, where there are wolves and where moose or caribou are hunted. The geographic distributions of the two biotypes of *E. granulosus* do not significantly overlap in North America.

Imaging Techniques

The diagnosis of hydatid disease often is the result of incidental x-ray or computed tomography (CT) studies for unrelated problems. Mass ultrasound screening for detection of AHD and the classic biotype of CE is another increasingly important technique used to diagnose echinococcosis in some hyperendemic regions (e.g., Saint Lawrence Island, Alaska; Turkana, Kenya). Ultrasonography is a useful modality in evaluating the extent and distribution of the cysts.

European Biotype

Plain radiographs are useful in evaluating pulmonary cysts of this biotype. In half of such patients (50%), a very well-defined, round cyst of uniform water density is present. In 20% of patients, the appearance is that of a lung abscess with a thick-walled cavity and an air-fluid level. Ultrasound and CT studies are highly sensitive and often specific for hydatid disease of the liver.[10]

Cyst rupture may be the first sign of hydatid disease, with resulting allergic, infective, or obstructive complications. Additionally, a change in the appearance of the radiographic image of the cyst may result from rupture. Rupture of the cyst may be of three types.[11] In a contained rupture, the endocyst collapses as fluid escapes into the potential space between it and the pericyst. On ultrasound and CT, an undulating membrane may be seen. With a communicating rupture, the cyst may rupture into the biliary or bronchial tree that the cyst eroded into. In the biliary tree, obstruction can result. In the lung, air may replace fluid. The classic "water-lily" and "crescent" signs are interesting and often diagnostic findings occasionally seen with both types of CE. With direct rupture, the cyst contents empty into the peritoneal or pleural space. Additionally, ultrasound may reveal a reduction in cyst size, which occurs in response to medical therapy and resultant death of the cyst.

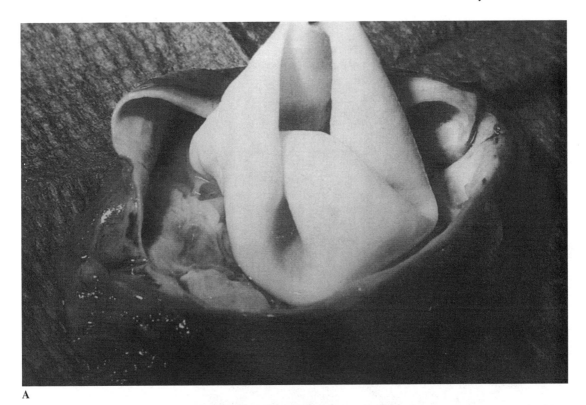

A

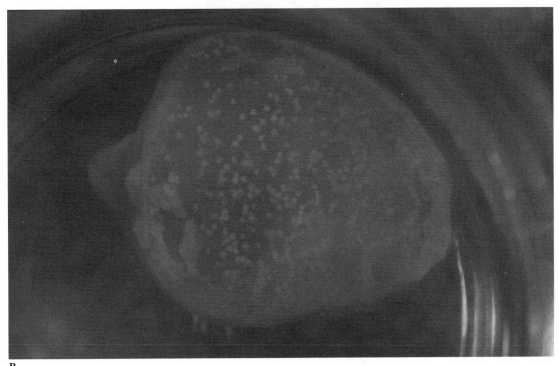

B

Figure 15-2. A. An *Echinococcus granulosus* cyst of the European biotype and its pericyst removed from the sartorius muscle. Note the thick, opaque, white laminated membrane held by forceps. (Reprinted with permission from Rask, MR. Primary muscular hydatidosis. Surgical Rounds 1979;June:63.) B. An *E. granulosus* cyst of the Northern biotype in a Petri dish. Note the thin, translucent laminated membranes with brood capsules clearly visible.

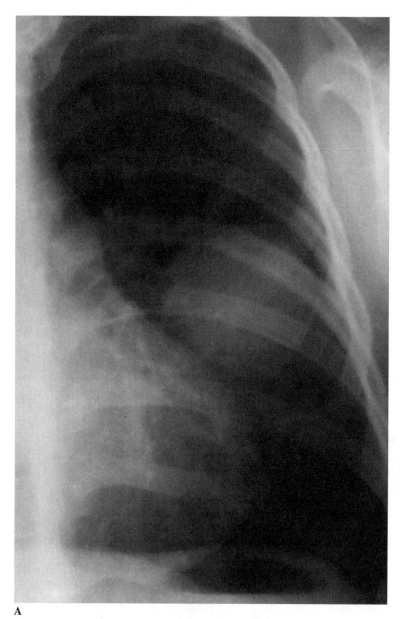

Figure 15-3. A. Date: 5/26/69. An anterior-posterior chest x-ray of an 8-year-old boy showing a 4.5 cm×5.0 cm, asymptomatic cyst of the Northern biotype in the left lower lung. Conservative, nonoperative management was elected. B. Date: 1/12/72. Follow-up chest x-ray of the same patient showing that the cyst had silently disappeared. The patient was unaware that the cyst had ruptured.

A

Northern Biotype

In Alaska and Canada, most cases of the Northern biotype of CE were diagnosed after x-ray screening for tuberculosis control.[5] The finding of one or more rounded, smooth-walled, cystic lesions 2–5 cm in diameter, if accompanied by an appropriate history, is generally diagnostic, especially in a young person (median age is 22 years). Daughter cysts, seen in approximately 30–50% of patients with the European biotype, have never been described in patients with the Northern form of disease.[1] The finding of daughter cysts strongly suggests that the parasite is of the European biotype.

Alveolar Hydatid Disease

Hepatomegaly or right upper quadrant pain or mass are common presenting symptoms. Areas of diffuse or mottled calcification in the liver on plain films may be the first sign of AHD, but the lesions are more clearly defined by CT. Areas of calcification are often in evidence, and in large lesions, central liquefaction may be apparent.[6]

Echinococcosis may also be diagnosed initially at exploratory laparotomy, laparoscopy, thoracotomy, or thoracoscopy. AHD of the liver presents as a white to yellowish, cancerlike mass. Metastases to regional lymph nodes or omentum and invasion of adjacent structures

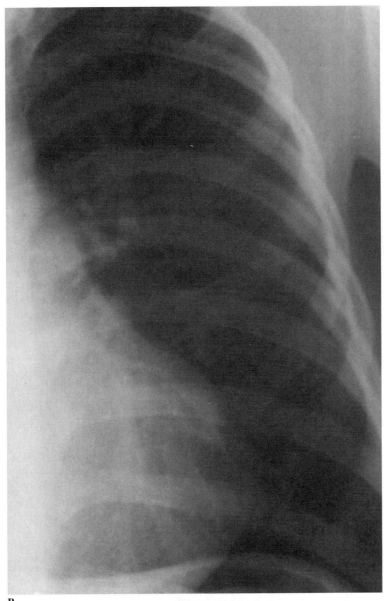

B

may be observed. Obstruction of the inferior vena cava may have been the reason for surgery.

Treatment

Hydatid disease has been recognized for a long time. Evidence of echinococcosis has been found in ancient Egyptian mummies and in the writings of Hippocrates (460–379 B.C.). Yet, until the late 1970s, there was no useful medical treatment. As a result, diagnosis and treatment were relegated to surgeons.

Surgical Aspects

The European biotype of CE remains largely a surgical problem.[12] However, this surgery is complex and carries a high morbidity and some mortality. Pulmonary cysts are generally treated quite conservatively by cystectomy, with an important objective being the preservation of pulmonary function.[12, 13] The management of hepatic cyst is more controversial. Many surgeons recommend radical resection, including the excision of the pericyst (pericystectomy),[14–16] but others favor a more conservative evacuation of only the endocyst (cystectomy).[12, 17] The

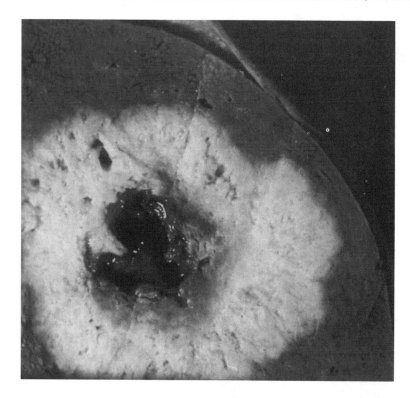

Figure 15-4. A typical hepatic lesion of alveolar hydatid disease. A few microcysts and a zone of central necrosis with cavitation are visible. Such cavities may become very large (25 cm in diameter in one case from Alaska).

appropriateness of injecting the cyst with a scolecide as part of the surgical procedure is being debated. It is not clear which scolecide is the safest. Formaldehyde and hypertonic saline should be avoided because of the risk of a fatal fibrosing cholangitis.[18] Silver nitrate (0.5%), hydrogen peroxide, and cetrimide (0.5% solution) are generally recommended.[19] Ultrasound-guided, percutaneous needle aspiration followed by injection of a scolecide, a technique called *PAIR* (*p*uncture, *a*spiration, *i*njection, and *r*easpiration), is increasingly being used as the primary means of treatment of hepatic cysts.[20] A report from Spain, however, indicates that nearly all scolecides can cause caustic sclerosing cholangitis.[21] The authors recommended that all injection of scolecides be abandoned and greater reliance be placed on pre- and postoperative chemotherapy. In addition, in a study of hepatic CE from Rome, the authors "are confident that surgical management must always be preceded and then followed by treatment with benzimidazole anthelminthics."[16]

The Northern biotype of CE usually does not require either medical or surgical therapy. Complications after infection or rupture of cysts, such as pulmonary abscess or pneumothorax, may need surgical intervention, but this is usually limited to chest-tube drainage.

In AHD, complete surgical resection of the primary hepatic lesion was, until recently, the only hope for cure. Resection often requires radical surgery, including trisegmentectomy. In Alaska, nine patients have undergone resection for cure, and each eventually had a good result.

The average postdiagnosis survival time is now 24 years, and four patients are still living (five died of unrelated causes).

It has been found that in some cases AHD lesions of the liver may undergo spontaneous resolution. Small, partially, or fully calcified hepatic lesions, even in the presence of positive serologic and histologic studies, may in fact be inactive, "burned-out" lesions, requiring no treatment other than follow-up.[22] There have been 29 such inactive cases diagnosed in Alaska; thus, 41% of all identified cases (29 of 71 cases) have taken this self-limiting course.

Medical Treatment

Mebendazole was first described as having an effect on the larval stage of echinococcus by Heath and Chevis in 1974.[23] Since that time, there has been worldwide interest in the role of the benzimidazole compounds in the treatment of hydatid disease. Numerous clinical trials with mebendazole have been reported, with both controversial and favorable results.[24] More recently, albendazole has been evaluated in the treatment of the European biotype of CE and AHD. Uses have included inoperable patients; before surgery; prophylactically after surgery; and perioperatively for urgent surgery.[25] A controlled, prospective trial has also been reported with albendazole involving treatment times of 1 and 3 months.[26] Very favorable results were reported. Clinical side effects with both mebendazole and albendazole have included neutropenia,

Figure 15-5. Cases of active alveolar hydatid disease among Alaska Natives from 1947 to 1996.

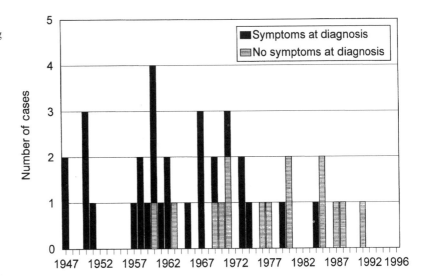

abnormalities of liver function tests, and, rarely, renal dysfunction, and they are sometimes quite severe. Liver function abnormalities do not appear to be related to the duration of treatment; therefore, *appropriate monitoring is required throughout therapy.* In the management of resectable AHD, albendazole is recommended (400–600 mg bid orally given with meals) both preoperatively and postoperatively for 2 years or more. The experience in Alaska suggests that chemotherapy is parasiticidal, at least in some cases, and should be considered as an alternative to surgery in poor-risk patients.[27] In patients who are not candidates for surgery, a longer course of uninterrupted, high-dose albendazole may be beneficial.

Prevention

Hydatid disease has been recognized as ideally suited for preventive programs. This is especially true for the European biotype of *E. granulosus* because the animals involved in the cycle are all domestic. This synanthropic cycle can be effectively interrupted by preventing dogs' access to the discarded viscera of sheep and other ungulates. Some preventive programs have been highly successful, with eradication of the parasite from the region (e.g., Iceland). Yet most programs have been unable to eliminate the parasite. In both cycles that commonly occur in Alaska, wild animals are involved. The eradication of the parasite in those cycles is not practical. Human infections can be expected to occur in these regions indefinitely into the future.

Discussion

In general, echinococcosis is a preventable disease. When it occurs in a community, it serves as an indicator that educational or other preventive programs are needed. It is difficult to assess the individual contributions of various factors that may lead to a reduction in the risk of hydatid disease. This is especially true for AHD because of its long prepatent period and the indolent growth of the lesion. Nevertheless, a review of a 50-year, multidisciplinary approach to a difficult health problem in a remote community in Alaska suggests that a favorable effect is being achieved. The combined effects of education, early-detection screening efforts by ultrasound and serosurveys, dog control and deworming programs, and important progress in chemotherapy are evident in Figure 15-5 and Table 15-2. Decreasing annual rates of infection, size of lesions, and frequency of symptoms at the time of diagnosis are observed. Survival time has doubled from 1972 through 1996.

Health providers can take the following important measures to prevent echinococcosis:

1. In sheep- or cattle-raising communities, the prevailing animal husbandry techniques should be reviewed with the local authorities. The need to properly dispose of the viscera of slaughtered animals must be recognized. All new cases of the European form of CE must be reported to the appropriate public health officials, in the same way that a new tuberculin conversion or active case of tuberculosis requires reporting, with a prompt search for the source of infection by a team of experts. A new infection of CE demonstrates that the cycle is being perpetuated in the area and calls for the establishment of an effective detection and prevention program. Public health officials must be notified, the offending dogs must be identified and treated, unrestrained dogs must be eliminated, and all dogs of the area must be treated approximately every 6 weeks with praziquantel. A well-executed program should eliminate the parasite from the area.

Table 15-2. Statistics on Active Cases of Alveolar Hydatid Disease*

	First 25 Yrs (1947–1971)	Second 25 Yrs (1972–1996)	p Value	1987–1996
Number of cases	28	14	?	3
Number/yr	1.1	0.56	?	0.30
Annual rate/100,000	2.61	0.75	<.001	0.33
Number of lesions	(10)	(11)	?	(3)
Mean size of lesions	13.0 cm	6.5 cm	.032	2.2 cm
Symptoms on admission	22 (79%)	5 (36%)	.006	0 (0%)
Annual rate of symptomatic disease/100,000	2.05	0.27	<.001	0.0
Mean survival time	12.4 yrs	24.2 yrs	.267	?

*The same results are statistically significant if the first 10 years of study (1947–1956) are omitted and the remaining period is divided into two 20-year periods.

2. Although the Northern biotype of *E. granulosus* cannot be eliminated from its natural hosts, the incidence of CE can be reduced through education. In endemic areas, those in the community who hunt should know that the lungs of moose and caribou should be destroyed or frozen so that dogs cannot feed on them.[28] It should be clearly understood that people cannot acquire the disease through contact with or by eating these game animals. Even when cysts are found in the lungs, there is no reason not to fully use this valuable food source.

3. Communities at great risk of infection by *E. multilocularis* should have well-established, ongoing programs for early detection of disease and an effective dog control and treatment program.[29] A community's degree of risk can be determined by field analysis of an adequate sample (100–200) of the local rodents (voles and lemmings) trapped in and around villages or other inhabited areas, looking for *E. multilocularis* lesions in the liver. If no hepatic lesions are found in them, the risk factor is relatively low.

The nature of the cycle of the parasite should be an ongoing part of the local school curriculum. In high-risk areas, individuals not included by an organized preventive program should be taught to treat their dogs and cats monthly with praziquantel.

Summary

Three disease entities (the European biotype of CE, the Northern biotype of CE, and AHD), caused by two species of the small, canine tapeworm, genus *Echinococcus*, have different symptoms, different clinical presentations, and require quite different treatment. They should be recognized as distinct clinical problems. In North America, two of these diseases (the Northern biotype of CE and AHD) occur almost exclusively among Native Americans, and in the third (the European biotype of CE),

Native Americans are infected disproportionately to the population at large. There have been significant advances in the diagnosis, treatment, and prevention of these clinical problems, making it important that health providers working with Native Americans have knowledge of the biology, diagnosis, and treatment of each of these zoonoses.

The majority of Native Americans lives in areas where at least one of these diseases is endemic. When unusual cystic lesions of the lung or liver are encountered, it is important to remember CE in the diagnosis, or if a firm, solid, cancerlike, hepatic mass is found on physical examination, at surgery, or on imaging studies, AHD as well as cancer must be considered in the differential diagnosis.

Acknowledgments

The authors wish to thank Dr. Robert L. Rausch, University of Washington School of Medicine, and Dr. Randall J. Basaraba, Veterinary Diagnostic Laboratory, Kansas State University, for reading the manuscript; and Lesa Bulkow, Centers for Disease Control and Prevention, Anchorage, Alaska, for statistical analysis and preparation of graphs.

References

1. Anderson FL, Chai J, Liu F. Surgical Treatment of Cystic Echinococcosis. In Anderson FL, et al. (eds), Compendium on Cystic Echinococcosis. Provo, UT: Brigham Young University Press, 1993.
2. Wilson JF, Rausch RL, Wilson FR. Alveolar hydatid disease, review of the surgical experience in 42 cases of active disease among Alaskan Eskimos. Ann Surg 1995;221:315–323.
3. Pinch LW, Wilson JF. Non-surgical management of cystic hydatid disease in Alaska. Ann Surg 1973;178:45–48.
4. Schantz PM. Echinococcosis in American Indians living in Arizona and New Mexico. Am J Epidemiol 1977;106:370–379.

5. Wilson JF, Diddams AC, Rausch RL. Cystic hydatid disease. A review of 101 autochthonous cases of *Echinococcus granulosus* infection. Am Rev Respir Dis 1968;98:1–15.

6. Wilson JF, Rausch RL. Alveolar hydatid disease: a review of clinical features of 33 indigenous cases of *Echinococcus multilocularis* infections in Alaskan Eskimos. Am J Trop Med Hyg 1980;29:1340–1355.

7. Jerry M, Benzarti M, Garrouche A, Abdelaziz H. Hydatid disease of the lungs. Am Rev Respir Dis 1992; 146:185–189.

8. Wilson JF, Rausch RL. Experience with 59 children with cystic echinococcosis of the Northern biotype from Alaska and Canada. Unpublished manuscript.

9. Gottstein B, Schantz PM, Wilson JF. Serologic screening for *Echinococcus multilocularis* infections with ELISA. Lancet 1985;1:1097–1098.

10. Gharbi HA, Hassine W, Brauner MW, et al. Ultrasound examination of the hydatid liver. Radiology 1981;139: 459–463.

11. Lowall DB, McCorkoll SJ. Rupture of echinococcus cysts: diagnosis, classification, and clinical implications. AJR Am J Roentgenol 1986;146:391–394.

12. Morris DL, Richards KS. Hydatid Disease. Current Medical and Surgical Management. Oxford, England: Butterworth–Heinemann, 1992;57–75.

13. Mutaf O, Arikan A, Yazici M, et al. Pulmonary hydatidosis in children. Eur J Pediatr Surg 1994;4:70–73.

14. Pawlowski ZS. Critical Points in the Clinical Management of Cystic Echinococcosis: A Revised Review. In Anderson FL, Ouhelli H, Kachani M (eds), Compendium on Cystic Echinococcosis in Africa and in Middle Eastern Countries with Special Reference to Morocco. Provo, UT: Brigham Young University Press, 1997:119–135.

15. Aeberhard P, Fuhrimann R, Strahm P, et al. Surgical treatment of hydatid disease of the liver: an experience from outside the endemic area. Hepatogastroenterology 1996;43:627–636.

16. Di Matteo G, Bove A, Chiarini S, et al. Hepatic echinococcus disease: our experience over 22 years. Hepatogastroenterology 1996;43:1562–1565.

17. Fenton-Lee D, Morris DL. The management of hydatid disease of the liver: part 1. Trop Doct 1996;26:173–176.

18. Belghiti J, Benhamoic JP, Houry S. Caustic sclerosing cholangitis. A complication of the surgical treatment of hydatid disease of the liver. Arch Surg 1986;121: 1162–1165.

19. Schaefer JW, Yousuf Khan M. Echinococcosis (hydatid disease): lesson from experience with 59 patients. Rev Inf Dis 1991;13:243–247.

20. Salama H, Adbel-Wahab MF, Strickland GT. Diagnosis and treatment of hepatic cysts with the aid of echo-guided percutaneous cyst puncture. Clin Infect Dis 1995;21:1372–1376.

21. Castellano G, Moreno-Sanchez D, Gutierrez J, et al. Caustic sclerosing cholangitis: report of four cases and cumulative review of the literature. Hepatogastroenterology 1994;41:458–470.

22. Rausch RL, Wilson JF, Schantz PM, McMahon BJ. Spontaneous death of *Echinococcus multilocularis*: cases diagnosed serologically (by EM2 ELISA) and clinical significance. Am J Trop Med Hyg 1987;36: 576–585.

23. Heath DD, Chevis RAF. Mebendazole and hydatid cysts [Letter]. Lancet 1974;2:218–219.

24. Wilson JF, Rausch RL. Mebendazole and alveolar hydatid disease. Ann Trop Med Parasitol 1982;76: 165–173.

25. Horton RJ. Chemotherapy of echinococcosis infection in man with albendazole. Trans R Soc Trop Med Hyg 1989;83:97–102.

26. Gil-Grande LA, Rodriguez-Caabeiro F, Prieo JG, et al. Randomised controlled trial of efficacy of albendazole in intra-abdominal hydatid disease. Lancet 1993;342: 1269–1272.

27. Wilson JF, Rausch RL, McMahon BJ, et al. Parasiticidal effect of chemotherapy in alveolar hydatid disease: review of experience with mebendazole and albendazole in Alaska Eskimos. Clin Infect Dis 1992;15: 234–249.

28. Wilson JF. An unusual Alaskan disease. Alaska: Magazine of Life on the Last Frontier 1971;Oct:2–3.

29. Rausch RL, Wilson JF, Schantz PM. A programme to reduce the risk of infection by *E. multilocularis*: the use of praziquantel to control the cestode in a village in the hyperendemic region of Alaska. Ann Trop Med Parasitol 1991;84:239–250.

Chapter 16
Hantavirus Pulmonary Syndrome

Bruce Tempest and Larry D. Crook

In May 1993, we identified five previously healthy young Native Americans (Navajo) who died of rapidly progressive respiratory failure after a brief nonspecific prodrome. An intensive investigation followed, which involved the Indian Health Service, the New Mexico Department of Health, the Centers for Disease Control and Prevention, and the University of New Mexico School of Medicine. Within 3 weeks, a previously unrecognized hantavirus was identified as the causative agent transmitted to humans from infected deer mice.[1] Although hantaviruses had been earlier identified and associated with rodents in the western hemisphere, no human disease had been associated with these viruses. On the other hand, in much of Eurasia and Scandinavia, several hantaviruses are associated with acute renal failure accompanied by hemorrhagic manifestations (hemorrhagic fever with renal syndrome [HFRS]). Cardiopulmonary dysfunction with the rapid progression of respiratory failure and shock differentiates hantavirus pulmonary syndrome (HPS) from HFRS. Native Americans were the initial focus when the newly recognized disease first received attention. Because of the Indian Health Service's involvement, the majority of the patients initially identified with HPS were Native Americans. HPS is now recognized to be widely dispersed in the western hemisphere, although Native Americans are overrepresented, constituting 23.8% of the U.S. total.

Clinical Findings

Because of the nonspecificity of the initial presentation, a carefully taken history is critically important. Before the abrupt onset of respiratory failure, patients have prodromal symptoms for 2 days to 2 weeks (median 4 days) (Table 16-1). The prodrome consists of symptoms of fever and myalgia in all patients. The myalgia is quite striking in most patients and usually is the symptom causing the most distress. Headache is frequent, as are gastrointestinal symptoms. The latter consist of combinations of nausea, vomiting, abdominal pain, and diarrhea. Although cough and shortness of breath are frequently listed as symptoms, it has been our experience that they occur later in the prodrome, usually just before the acute onset of respiratory failure. In other words, if a patient has the onset of cough and dyspnea at the same time as the other prodromal symptoms noted, it is not likely that HPS is the cause of the patient's illness. In addition, coryza, nasal congestion, and sore throat are not part of the prodrome. Although the HPS prodrome has often been described as "flulike," several clinical points differentiate it from culture-confirmed influenza. Patients with influenza more commonly have a history of sore throat, nasal symptoms, cough at the outset, and findings of an injected throat. As the patient with HPS progresses to respiratory failure, the cough is productive of copious, nonpurulent secretions.

Unless the patient with HPS is already in respiratory failure, the most common physical findings are tachycardia, tachypnea, and fever. In general, these patients look much sicker than their symptoms and physical findings would suggest. There are no hemorrhagic manifestations, such as petechiae.

The most important laboratory findings include thrombocytopenia and a left-shift neutrophilic leukocytosis with myelocytes (often seen), both of which usually progress during the prodrome. In addition, large immunoblastic lymphocytes are seen in the peripheral smear and are most helpful in establishing a presumptive diagnosis. The other laboratory abnormalities are less helpful and include mildly increased lactate dehydrogenase, aminotransferase, and alanine aminotransferase. The coagulation parameters are mildly abnormal. Renal function tests are normal. With the onset of respiratory failure, the Pao_2-Fio_2 ratio is low in all patients needing oxygen, with the majority of patients having a value less than 100.

Table 16-1. Symptoms in 17 Patients
with Hantavirus Infection

Symptom	No. of Patients (%)
Fever	17 (100)
Myalgia	17 (100)
Headache	12 (71)
Cough	12 (71)
Nausea or vomiting	12 (71)
Chills	11 (65)
Malaise	10 (59)
Diarrhea	10 (59)
Shortness of breath	9 (53)
Dizziness or light-headedness	7 (41)
Arthralgia	5 (29)
Back pain	5 (29)
Abdominal pain	4 (24)
Chest pain	3 (18)
Sweats	3 (18)
Dysuria or frequent urination	3 (18)
Rhinorrhea or nasal congestion	2 (12)
Sore throat	2 (12)

Source: Reprinted with permission from JS Duchin, FT
Koster, Peters CJ, et al. Hantavirus pulmonary syndrome: a
clinical description of 17 patients with a newly recognized disease. N Engl J Med 1994;330:949–955. Copyright 1994 Massachusetts Medical Society. All rights reserved.

The chest radiograph of patients with respiratory failure changes rapidly, faster than the changes in patients
with adult respiratory distress syndrome (ARDS).[2] HPS
produces a radiographic pattern of noncardiogenic pulmonary edema. The heart size is normal. The radiographic findings are characterized by prominent
interstitial edema with progression to air-space disease in
the majority of patients. Interstitial edema is manifest by
Kerley's B lines, hilar indistinctness, or peribronchial
cuffing and is present in all patients with respiratory failure. Alveolar flooding subsequently develops in the
majority of those with interstitial edema. Pleural effusion
is also common. HPS differs from ARDS by the lack of a
peripheral distribution of initial air-space disease and the
prominence of interstitial edema early in the disease.
Manifestations of interstitial edema, such as Kerley's B
lines or peribronchial cuffing, are seen in fewer than 10%
of patients with ARDS. The radiographic changes of HPS
have been compared to those of patients with bacteremic
pneumococcal pneumonia.[3] Lobar infiltration was
strongly associated with pneumococcal pneumonia,
whereas bilateral alveolar or interstitial disease was present or developed in HPS.

Patients with the most rapid evolution of hypoxemia
and radiographic progression are the ones most likely to
progress to cardiac dysfunction and death in cardiogenic

shock with electromechanical dissociation. Hemodynamic monitoring demonstrates low initial pulmonary
artery occlusion pressures.[4] In patients progressing to
shock, there is a drop in the cardiac index and an increase
in the systemic vascular resistance. These findings are the
opposite of the expected findings in septicemic or viremic
shock. Decreased oxygen delivery is reflected in rising
lactate levels. Lactate concentrations of 4 mmol/liter or
less correlate with mortality. If patients survive the cardiopulmonary dysfunction, their recovery is rapid and
without sequelae.

Pathology

Pathologic abnormalities at autopsy are largely limited to
the lungs. Pleural effusions and edematous, airless lungs
were found in all autopsied patients. Histologically, septal
and alveolar edema is present with only moderate interstitial infiltrate by mononuclear cells. The kidneys are
grossly and histologically normal. Except for gastric
mucosal hemorrhage in a minority of patients, evidence
of hemorrhage is absent. In contrast to the severe cardiac
dysfunction before death, there are no gross or microscopic changes in the myocardium.

Immunohistochemical staining of autopsy specimens
from HPS patients demonstrates widespread distribution of
hantaviral nucleocapsid antigens in the endothelial cells of
all organs examined, although the concentration was greatest in the lung.[5] It is not clear why only the lung demonstrates the major pathologic findings. The universal
presence of immunoglobulin G (IgG) and IgM antibodies
to the virus at the onset of HPS suggests that the pulmonary
manifestations occur late in the course of the infection.
Analyses of fluid suctioned from the trachea in patients with
fatal disease is notable for the lack of cells and for a fluid
protein to serum protein ratio more than 80%. Noncardiac
edema fluid has a ratio of protein content to serum protein
of 60% or greater. The mechanism proposed to explain the
clinical and laboratory findings is as follows. The virus is
widely distributed in endothelial cells after infection. Antibodies develop, and the immune system is activated.[6] In the
lung, a vascular leak develops, resulting in the lung being
flooded with fluid having the properties of serum. This
results in impairment of gas exchange. The mechanism of
the cardiac dysfunction is unclear, but the lack of histologic
changes suggests no direct myocardial injury.

Treatment

Treatment is supportive. These patients are typically young
and without pre-existing disease; management of the cardiopulmonary abnormalities in an intensive care setting
seems to favorably affect the outcome.[7] Because of the
rapid progression of the cardiorespiratory dysfunction, it is

critical to make a presumptive diagnosis on the basis of history and simple laboratory findings and to move the patient to an intensive care setting. Actual diagnosis of HPS is done serologically, with the most rapid results usually obtained by consulting the state health laboratory.

Oxygen is required with half or more of patients needing mechanical ventilation, frequently with high levels of positive end-expiratory pressure. Pulmonary artery catheterization and hemodynamic monitoring facilitates fluid replacement in the face of worsening pulmonary edema. The progression of left ventricular function can be monitored by echocardiography. If cardiac dysfunction progresses, inotropic agents, such as dobutamine, dopamine, and norepinephrine, are preferred over continued fluid boluses. Ribavirin intravenously has been used in an open labeled trial with no clear benefit. This is in contrast to its usefulness in HFRS, which, having a more prolonged course, allows time for the drug to demonstrate efficacy. Platelet transfusions are not needed for treating the thrombocytopenia.

The prodrome of HPS and subsequent pulmonary edema and respiratory failure can be similar to disease caused by other infectious agents. We have seen disease initially suspected to be HPS caused by gram-positive organisms (e.g., primary pneumococcal bacteremia or multilobar bacteremic pneumonia), gram-negative organisms (e.g., septicemic plague), spirochetes (e.g., relapsing fever), and the other viruses (e.g., primary influenza A pneumonia). Other infectious agents might also mimic HPS, at least superficially. Consequently, it is important to maintain universal precautions and respiratory isolation. For the same reason, antibiotics appropriate for sepsis should be included in treatment.

Hantaviruses

Hantavirus nucleotide sequences detected in patient tissue specimens by reverse transcriptase polymerase chain reaction initially confirmed the previously unrecognized hantavirus. Later designated *sin nombre virus* (SNV), it is the cause of HPS. Identical sequences were also identified in deer mice, *Peromyscus maniculatus*, trapped in case households. The wide range of the deer mouse includes most of the continental United States and much of Canada and Mexico. Subsequently, HPS occurred outside the range of the deer mouse. Black Creek Canal virus, identified in a Florida case, and Bayou virus, identified from a patient with HPS in Louisiana, represent additional pathogenic hantaviruses separate from SNV.[8] The preferred host rodents for these new strains of hantavirus are the cotton rat and rice rat, respectively. It is of interest that both of the patients just mentioned had azotemia in addition to respiratory failure. HPS has also been identified in Canada, Brazil, Uruguay, and Argentina. The genetic diversity of SNV suggests that this virus is neither newly emergent nor newly virulent. Indeed, frozen tissue from rodents captured in 1983 demonstrate SNV-like sequences. The dates for human cases of HPS diagnosed retrospectively continue to be pushed back: 1959 for a case diagnosed serologically and 1978 for a case identified by immunohistochemistry of the virus in autopsy tissue.

The outbreak in 1993 would appear to be due to a change in human-rodent equilibrium. Biologists in New Mexico, monitoring small-mammal populations, noted a 10-fold increase in deer mouse populations over previous years. This appeared to follow a wet winter, which resulted in increased vegetation and abundant food for rodents. Rodent trapping at a household where a case of HPS originated was compared to trapping results at a nearby household and at households 24 km or more away. More small rodents were trapped at the case household than at the near or far control households. The seroprevalence of hantavirus antibodies in *Peromyscus* animals did not differ significantly between the three types of households.

Epidemiology

Asymptomatic, chronically infected rodents serve as reservoirs for hantaviruses. Typically, up to one-third of deer mice are infected. Transmission to humans appears to result from inhalation of aerosols of rodent urine and feces, which can occur when dried material contaminated with rodent excreta is disturbed. Arthropod vectors are not known to have a role in transmitting hantaviruses to humans. Nearly all patients with HPS are from rural areas. In urban areas, the deer mouse is displaced by the house mouse. A case-control study to evaluate risk factors for HPS found an association between cases and peridomestic cleaning and agricultural activities.[9] These results are consistent with patient histories of opening and cleaning storage areas or previously unoccupied buildings.

All this would suggest that eliminating rodents from the human environment should be a central issue in preventing HPS.[10] Eradicating the reservoir rodents is not feasible. Hantaviruses have lipid envelopes that are susceptible to most disinfectants, including dilute bleach (hypochlorite solution), 70% ethyl alcohol, detergents, and most household disinfectants. General precautions for those in affected areas follow:

1. Eliminate rodents inside the home with spring-loaded traps and rodenticides.
2. Reduce the availability of food sources in the home.
3. Prevent rodents from entering the home with appropriate barriers.
4. Reduce rodent shelter and food sources around the home.

When eliminating rodents from previously closed buildings, open the doors and windows to ventilate before beginning work. To empty traps, wear gloves, put the carcasses in plastic bags containing enough disinfectant to wet the carcasses, and bury or burn them. Workers who handle or are frequently exposed to rodents should be informed of the symptoms of HPS and be given detailed instructions on preventing exposure. They should also be given appropriate equipment, including respirators, gloves, and disinfectants. Those engaging in outdoor activities should avoid rodent burrows and not use rodent-infested cabins until they are appropriately cleaned.

As of May 1997, 4 years after the initial recognition of HPS, there had been 160 cases of HPS. The age distribution was from 11 to 69 years, with a mean of 36 years. In the United States, cases have been reported in 26 states, mostly west of the Mississippi. The mortality rate has been 47.5%. There have been very few clinically mild cases of HPS.

In an effort to evaluate the frequency of subclinical disease, serologic studies have been done of a number of populations. These included people who work with rodents, medical personnel who cared for patients with HPS, household contacts of cases, and patients whose symptoms suggested the HPS prodrome and who were evaluated in facilities serving the area where the 1993 outbreak first occurred.[11] None of these groups had serologic evidence of infection by SNV. This suggests that in the initial outbreak, there was no person-to-person spread. In an HPS outbreak in Argentina that was associated with another hantavirus (Andes), however, there has been strong epidemiologic evidence for person-to-person spread.[12]

Summary Points

- The diagnosis of HPS is suspected on the basis of history and a limited number of laboratory tests. Confirmation of hantavirus infection requires testing at state laboratories and is time consuming.
- If HPS is suspected, expeditious transfer to a facility with intensive care capabilities is indicated and should not be delayed to await confirmatory testing.

- Anticipate rapid cardiopulmonary decompensation. Treatment consists of cardiopulmonary support in an intensive care unit.

References

1. Duchin JS, Koster F, Peters CJ, et al. Hantavirus pulmonary syndrome: clinical description of seventeen patients with a newly recognized disease. N Engl J Med 1994;330:949–955.
2. Ketai LH, Williamson MR, Telepak RJ, et al. Hantavirus pulmonary syndrome (HPS): radiographic findings in 16 patients. Radiology 1994;191:665–668.
3. Moolenaar RL, Dalton C, Lipman HB, et al. Clinical features that differentiate hantavirus pulmonary syndrome from three other acute respiratory illnesses. Clin Infect Dis 1995;21:643–649.
4. Hallin GW, Simpson SQ, Crowell RE, et al. Cardiopulmonary manifestations of hantavirus pulmonary syndrome. Crit Care Med 1996;24:252–258.
5. Nolte KB, Feddersen RM, Foucar K, et al. Hantavirus pulmonary syndrome in the United States: a pathological description of a disease caused by a new agent. Hum Pathol 1995;26:110–120.
6. Zaki SR, Greer PW, Coffield LM, et al. Hantavirus pulmonary syndrome: pathogenesis of an emerging infectious disease. Am J Pathol 1995;146:552–579.
7. Levy H, Simpson SQ. Hantavirus pulmonary syndrome. Am J Respir Crit Care Med 1994;149:1710–1713.
8. Khan AS, Ksiazek TG, Peters CJ. Hantavirus pulmonary syndrome. Lancet 1996;347:739–741.
9. Zeitz PS, Butler JC, Cheek JE, et al. A case control study of hantavirus pulmonary syndrome during an outbreak in the southwestern United States. J Infect Dis 1995;171:864–870.
10. Centers for Disease Control and Prevention. Hantavirus infection: southwestern United States: interim recommendations for risk reduction. MMWR Morb Mortal Wkly Rep 1993;42:RR-11.
11. Vitek CR, Breiman RF, Ksiazek TG, et al. Evidence against person-to-person transmission of hantavirus to health care workers. Clin Infect Dis 1996;22:824–826.
12. Wells R, Estani SS, Yadon ZE, et al. An unusual hantavirus outbreak in southern Argentina: person-to-person transmission? Emerg Inf Dis 1997;3:1–4.

Chapter 17
Infectious Skin Disorders

Ann Andonyan and Norman Levine

Infectious skin disorders are common among all peoples and cultures. Native Americans who live in close quarters and with limited resources are at increased risk of contracting cutaneous infections. In this chapter, we present a practical guide to the Native American patient with a suspected infection involving the skin. Six common skin infections in Native Americans are discussed: candidiasis, dermatophytosis, pediculosis capitis, pyoderma, scabies, and verruca.

Candidiasis

Etiology and Epidemiology

Candida albicans, the organism responsible for most candidal infections, colonizes the esophagus, skin, oral cavity, and vagina.[1] Circumstances that favor candidiasis include obesity, diabetes mellitus, warm and moist environments, and chronically macerated skin.[1]

Clinical Presentation

Patients with oral candidal infections (thrush) present with white plaques overlying a red mucosa. When the plaques are dislodged from the mucosal surface, there is underlying erosion with punctate bleeding points.[1]

Affected skin is pruritic, red, and scaly and is patterned into poorly marginated plaques with satellite papules and pustules (Figure 17-1). The favored sites of involvement include intertriginous areas, such as the inframammary, interdigital, intergluteal, and groin areas. In men, the scrotum is often beefy red and edematous; in women, the vulva is similarly inflamed. Sites of occlusion, such as occurs under a diaper, also favor *Candida* overgrowth.

Diagnostic Evaluation

Confirmation is made either by a microscopic evaluation or with a culture for *Candida*.[1] A microscopic examination is done by scraping the scaly border of a lesion or examining the contents of a pustule with a drop of 10% KOH. A positive scraping shows budding yeast forms or branching pseudohyphae, which look like empty tubes without septations.[1]

Differential Diagnosis

- *Atopic or irritant diaper dermatitis*: As candidiasis, the skin is red and scaly, but it lacks satellite papules and pustules and does not favor intertriginous areas.
- *Erythrasma:* This bacterial infection presents as scaly plaques in intertriginous sites, but the plaques are reddish brown, do not have satellite papules and pustules, and display a coral red fluorescence under Wood's light.
- *Intertrigo*: This noninfectious inflammation of the intertriginous skin has red and sometimes scaly plaques that may be difficult to differentiate from candidiasis. The absence of satellite lesions and a negative KOH examination and culture are often necessary to rule out an infectious process.
- *Tinea cruris*: Dermatophyte infections of the groin in men present with red, scaly plaques; however, the scrotum is spared and satellite papules and pustules are not present.
- *Folliculitis*: Inflammatory or bacterial involvement of hair follicles gives red papules and pustules that may resemble those of candidiasis. The lack of interfollicular involvement distinguishes it from candidiasis.

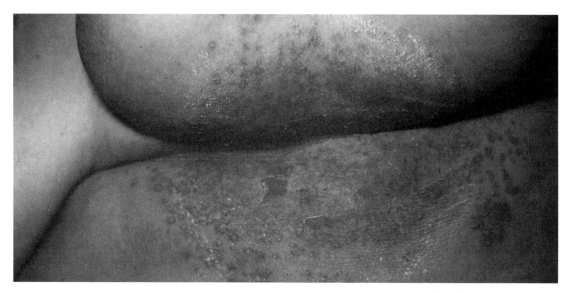

Figure 17-1. Candidiasis of the inframammary fold with scaly plaques and satellite papules.

Treatment

In uncomplicated oral candidiasis, treatment with clotri-mazole troches (10 mg) sucked on five times daily for 14 days is usually curative. In patients whose compliance may be problematic, another option is oral fluconazole as a single 150-mg dose.

Cutaneous candidiasis is usually responsive to one of the topical imidazole antifungal agents, such as clotrima-zole, econazole, or miconazole, applied twice daily for 14–21 days.[1] Avoid imidazole-corticosteroid combination preparations because the corticosteroid is often too potent for the intertriginous location being treated and could pro-duce cutaneous atrophy. Recurrence of *Candida* infec-tions can be minimized by emphasizing good hygiene, which includes the use of drying powders, frequent cleansing, and weight loss.

Dermatophytosis

Etiology and Epidemiology

A dermatophyte is a fungus that infects keratinized skin and hair. *Trichophyton rubrum* is the organism commonly responsible for infections of the body (tinea corporis), feet (tinea pedis), and groin (tinea cruris). *Trichophyton tonsurans* is the most common cause of fungal scalp infections (tinea capitis). These infections occur most often in warm, moist environments, and they may spread through direct contact.[2]

Clinical Presentation

Tinea capitis caused by *T. tonsurans* presents with patchy scalp alopecia, with broken hairs that give the appearance of black dots (Figure 17-2). With other organisms, such as *Microsporum Canis* there is more of an inflammatory response, consisting of red, scaly, edematous plaques.

Tinea corporis and tinea cruris present with red, scaly, sharply marginated, and often annular (ringlike) plaques. In men, when the groin is involved, the medial thighs are the site of the lesions; the scrotum is spared.

Tinea pedis presents with scaling, red, sometimes pru-ritic plaques between the toes extending onto the sides and bottoms of the feet in a moccasinlike distribution (Figure 17-3). It may also present with vesicles, bullae, and collarettes on the instep.

Diagnostic Evaluation

To confirm a clinical suspicion of a tinea infection, a KOH preparation or fungal culture can be done, as with candidiasis. One looks for hyphae, which appear as branching filaments with indentations (septations), giv-ing the appearance of boxcars lined up in a row.

Differential Diagnosis

- *Discoid lupus erythematosus (DLE)*: The lesions of scalp DLE show alopecia and scale, but there is also hyper- and hypopigmentation and evidence of cuta-neous atrophy.

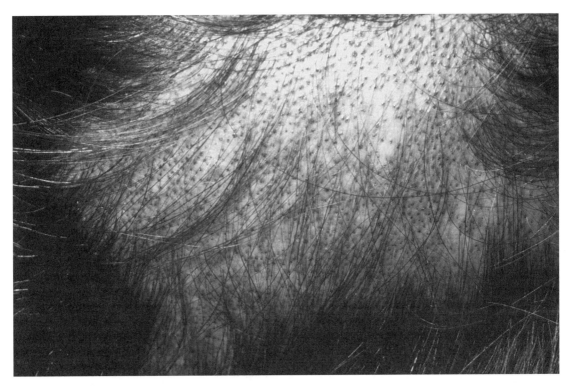

Figure 17-2. Tinea capitis with alopecia and "black dots," which are broken hairs.

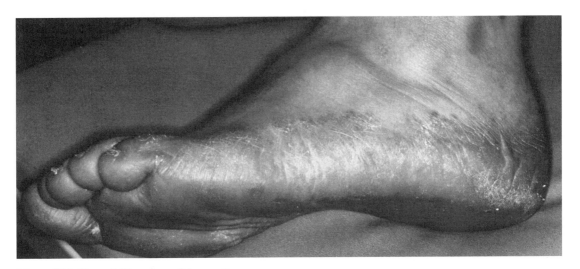

Figure 17-3. Moccasinlike pattern of tinea pedis.

- *Pityriasis rosea*: Red, scaly plaques on the trunk and proximal extremities resemble those of tinea corporis, but the lesions are oval rather than round and often line up in a Christmas-tree pattern along cleavage lines in the skin. A negative KOH examination confirms the absence of fungal elements.

- *Dyshidrotic eczema*: In dyshidrotic eczema of the feet, vesicles on the instep are similar to those seen in vesicular tinea pedis. Involvement of the fingers is a clue that the patient has dyshidrotic eczema. A KOH examination of the roof of a vesicle is often needed to distinguish the two entities.

- *Erythrasma*: As tinea pedis, there are interdigital, red, scaly plaques of the feet. A negative KOH examination and positive coral red fluorescence differentiate it from a fungal infection.
- *Psoriasis*: Psoriasis of the scalp and trunk may resemble tinea capitis and tinea pedis in that both have well-demarcated, scaly, red plaques. The scale in psoriasis is thick and white, there is little or no alopecia, and lesions are often found over elbows and knees, which rarely have fungal infections.
- *Seborrheic dermatitis*: Scale and erythema are present in the scalp, but alopecia is uncommon, and the lesions are usually not as well demarcated, as in tinea capitis.
- *Secondary syphilis*: The lesions of secondary syphilis are scaly and red but not annular. A negative KOH examination may be necessary to rule out fungal skin infection.
- *Trichotillomania*: Habitual hair pulling can produce a patchy alopecia similar to "black-dot ringworm." It differs in that the length of the broken hairs varies and is seldom flush with the scalp, as seen in *T. tonsurans* infection.

Treatment

Treatment for dermatophyte infections should not begin until there is laboratory evidence that an infection is present because these infections so closely mimic other processes.

The treatment of choice for tinea pedis and tinea cruris is a topical imidazole cream, such as clotrimazole or miconazole, applied twice daily for 3 weeks in tinea cruris and for 1 month in tinea pedis. Tolnaftate should be used only if one of the imidazoles is not available. Nystatin is ineffective in dermatophyte infections.

Tinea capitis must be treated by an oral medication; topical therapy alone is not useful. Ultramicronized griseofulvin is given for 6 weeks at a dose of 10 mg/kg daily for children and 500 mg twice daily for adults. The newer antifungal agents, terbinafine and itraconazole, may also be effective, but there is far less experience with these agents.

Systemic therapy is usually needed for tinea corporis and recalcitrant tinea pedis and tinea cruris. The most effective treatments are oral itraconazole or terbinafine. For tinea corporis and tinea cruris, the adult dose of itraconazole is 200 mg per day for 1 week, and the adult dose of terbinafine is 250 mg per day for 2 weeks. For tinea pedis, the itraconazole dose is 400 mg per day for 1 week or 250 mg terbinafine per day for 2 weeks. Should terbinafine and itraconazole not be available, oral griseofulvin is the next line of therapy, and is used at a dose of 10 mg/kg per day (for children) and 500 mg twice daily (for adults) for 2–4 weeks.

Pediculosis Capitis (Head Lice)

Etiology and Epidemiology

Pediculosis capitis, caused by *Pediculus humanus capitis*, affects children more than adults, girls more than boys; it commonly occurs as epidemics in schools.[3] The infestation propagates by direct head-to-head contact with an infected person. The risk factors for spread of the infection include overcrowding, poor hygiene, and shared towels, brushes, hats, or combs.[3]

Clinical Presentation

Patients present with pruritus of the scalp, especially of the occipital region. A louse may be barely visible as a minute brown moving object. There may also be small red papules at the site of bites. Eggs (nits) are found attached to the hair shaft near the scalp (Figure 17-4).

Diagnostic Evaluation

Definitive diagnosis is made by performing a wet-mount examination under low-power magnification to visualize the lice or nits on the hair shaft.

Differential Diagnosis

- *Hair casts*: Hair casts are the outer coverings of the hair shaft. Like nits, these are white; unlike nits, they move freely on the hair shaft.
- *Dandruff (seborrheic dermatitis)*: The scale of seborrheic dermatitis can be mistaken for pediculosis. The scale is often a greasy yellow-brown, however, occurs along the anterior and lateral hairline, and does not move spontaneously, as a live organism (head lice has been called "walking dandruff").
- *Impetigo*: Superficial bacterial scalp infections can produce pruritic, red, crusted papules in the scalp. These do not attach themselves to the hair shaft, however.

Treatment

Pediculosis of the scalp is treated with permethrin (Nix) 1% rinse or gamma benzene hexachloride (lindane) shampoo. The medications are applied for 10 minutes and then rinsed. Nits are removed with a fine-toothed comb or with a dilute solution of acetic acid used as a rinse.* All household members and close contacts should be examined for lice. In addition, clothes, towels, linens, and combs used at the time of treatment should be washed.

---

*Avoid the use of permethrin in children younger than 2 months old and lindone in children younger than 2 years old. Use both medications with caution in pregnant women.

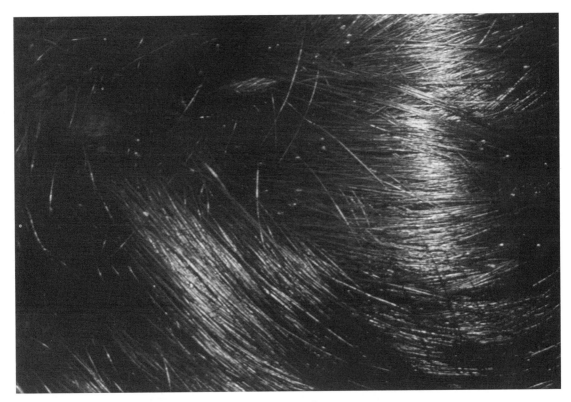

Figure 17-4. Head lice with numerous nits attached to the hair shafts.

Pyoderma

Etiology and Epidemiology

Pyoderma is a bacterial infection of the skin and soft tissues, usually caused by *Staphylococcus aureus* or *Streptococcus pyogenes* (group A beta-hemolytic streptococcus).[4] Impetigo is an infection of the superficial epidermis.[5] The bullous form is due to *S. aureus*, whereas nonbullous impetigo is often due to a combination of *S. aureus* and *S. pyogenes*.[6] Impetigo is the most common skin infection in children and is contagious via direct person-to-person contact and fomites that have been in contact with infected skin.[7]

Ecthyma is a deeper infection, through the epidermis and into the superficial dermis, producing a shallow ulcer. Erysipelas is an infection of the dermis, and cellulitis involves the deep dermis and subcutaneous fat.[5]

A skin break provides an opportunity for entry of the infective organisms, which often colonize the surface of the skin. Risk factors seen in Native Americans include hot and humid environments, poor hygiene, inadequate sanitation, inadequate water supply, and crowded living conditions.[4]

A potentially serious sequela of streptococcal impetigo is acute poststreptococcal glomerulonephritis.

This rarely occurs in the general population with impetigo, but Native American populations have an increased incidence of this complication.[8]

Clinical Presentation

Impetigo presents as a single, 2- to 4-mm erythematous macule that quickly evolves into a vesicle or pustule that erodes, producing a honey-colored exudative crust[7] (Figure 17-5). Lesions spread onto adjacent skin and coalesce into crusted plaques. The bullous variant of impetigo begins as superficial bullae that quickly rupture, leaving a round or oval, crusted erosion with a collarette of scale.

Ecthyma begins as a vesicle or pustule arising from an erythematous base, which evolves into larger crusted papules and plaques.

Erysipelas often presents on the face or extremity as a warm, tender, sharply marginated, erythematous plaque with raised borders that spreads to adjacent skin. There are usually fever, chills, lymphadenopathy, and leukocytosis.[4] Cellulitis is similar in presentation, but, unlike erysipelas, it is a poorly marginated, rapidly spreading, warm, tender, indurated, erythematous plaque (Figure 17-6). It is accompanied by chills, fever, malaise, ascending lymphangitic streaking, and regional lymphadenopathy.

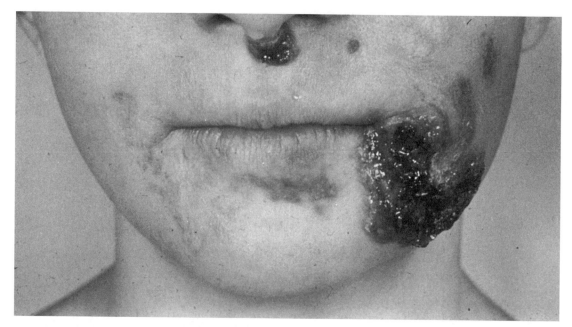

Figure 17-5. Impetigo of the face with crusted plaques.

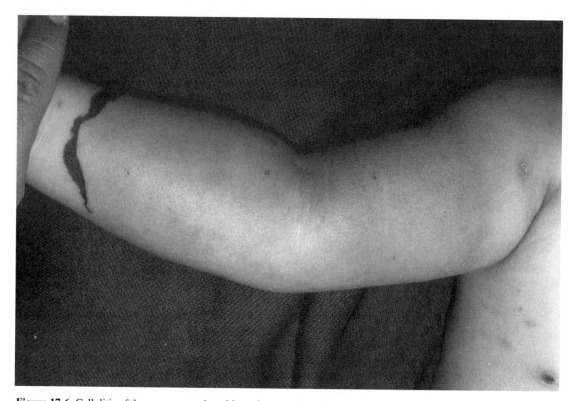

Figure 17-6. Cellulitis of the upper extremity with erythema and marked edema.

Diagnostic Evaluation

Fresh, exudative lesions can be gram-stained or cultured for gram-positive bacteria. A skin biopsy can also be stained for organisms.

Differential Diagnosis

- *Candidiasis*: *Candida* infections produce pustules and, occasionally, crusted plaques. The scaly red plaques of candidiasis are different from the lesions of impetigo.
- *Contact dermatitis*: Acute contact dermatitis may resemble impetigo with crusted red plaques. Both conditions may be linear, but contact dermatitis usually has more geometric shapes, which approximate the configuration of the contactant.
- *Herpes simplex virus infection*: As pyoderma, there are vesicles that rupture and form crusted plaques. A culture is often needed to differentiate the two entities. However, impetigo will culture bacteria. Herpes simplex may be identified by a Wright's stained smear, which shows multinucleated giant cells.
- *Stasis dermatitis*: It is often difficult to differentiate the warm, red lesions on the distal lower extremity involved in stasis dermatitis from cellulitis. In fact, cellulitis may supervene over chronic dermatitis. Cellulitis should be suspected when constitutional signs and symptoms accompany the eruption. When in doubt, one should treat for cellulitis.

Treatment

The treatment of choice for impetigo, ecthyma, or mild erysipelas is oral dicloxacillin, in a dose of 12–25 mg/kg per day four doses daily (in children) and 250–500 mg four times daily (in adults) for 10–14 days. Another first-line alternative is cephalexin given in a dose of 250–500 mg four times daily for 10 days in adults.* In penicillin-allergic patients, erythromycin is an alternative, at a dose of 30–50 mg/kg per day in divided doses four times daily for children and 250–500 mg four times per day for 10 days in adults.[6]

In severe erysipelas or cellulitis, intravenous nafcillin is indicated: Give 500 mg every 6 hours in adults and 150 mg/kg per day divided into four doses in children.[4] In penicillin-allergic patients, vancomycin 6.5–8.0 mg/kg should be administered intravenously every 6 hours. These are given until 2–3 days after signs of acute illness have passed, at which time, treatment is switched to oral dicloxacillin, cephalexin, or erythromycin for 7–10 days.

---

*In children, the dose of cephalexin is 25–50 mg/kg per day divided into four doses daily.

Scabies

Etiology and Epidemiology

The parasite for scabies, *Sarcoptes scabiei*, affects any age, race, or socioeconomic class, but it is very common among many Native American tribes, where it occurs in mini-epidemics. The infection is transmitted by direct contact with an infected person and only rarely through fomites, such as towels, linen, and clothing.[9] Close living conditions predispose whole households to this infestation, but individual sensitivity to the mite dictates the degree of clinical involvement.

Clinical Presentation

Scabies presents with severe pruritus, which is often worse at bedtime. The infected person develops poorly defined, red papules; nodules; and vesiculopustules, which may become excoriated and lichenified (skin thickening) after vigorous scratching. Burrows containing the mite appear in finger web spaces as thin, wavy, gray-white lines with a vesicle and a punctate black spot.

In older children and adults, the infection is limited to the skin below the neck, but in those younger than 2 years of age, the entire body, including the face, may be affected with vesicular and pustular lesions.[9, 10] In a child, likely sites of involvement include the palms, soles, scalp, face, and postauricular fold. In older children and adults, the web spaces (Figure 17-7), volar wrists, belt line, areola in females, penis and scrotum in males, axilla, and intertriginous areas are the most common sites of involvement.

Diagnostic Evaluation

A definitive diagnosis of scabies is made by taking a skin scraping from a burrow or a scaly papule and identifying a mite, eggs, or excrement under a low-power microscope. A negative scraping does not rule out the diagnosis because most lesions represent a hypersensitivity response rather than a site of infestation.

Differential Diagnosis

- *Atopic dermatitis*: The lesions of atopic dermatitis are pruritic, crusted, and scaly papules, but the face is usually involved, the genitals are spared, and there is more lichenification and few, if any, inflammatory papules.
- *Dermatitis herpetiformis*: As scabies, there are vesicular, intensely pruritic, and crusted papules. The vesicles are bilateral, symmetric, and clustered, however, without burrows.
- *Insect bites*: Multiple insect bites may mimic a scabies infestation because the lesions are red and intensely itchy. The papules seldom involve the genitalia, however, do not have burrows, and resolve spontaneously.

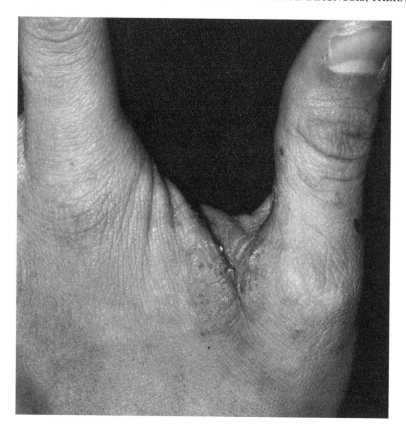

Figure 17-7. Scabies with burrows of the finger web spaces.

Treatment

For patients older than 2 months of age, permethrin 5% cream is the treatment of choice. It should be applied overnight. The treatment is repeated after 7 days in case of incomplete initial application or reinfection. Use permethrin with caution in pregnant women.

Lindane 1% lotion is also effective against scabies but cannot be used in pregnant patients or in children younger than the age of 2 years. Like permethrin, lindane is applied overnight and reapplied in 7 days. All clothing and bed linens used on the night of treatment should be washed the next morning. There is no need to cleanse clothing not worn within 24 hours of being treated. One need not scrub the house, carpets, and so forth.

Follow-up evaluation should be made at 2 and 4 weeks after treatment to evaluate for any new or persistent lesions and to watch for possible secondary bacterial infection.[9]

Verruca (Warts)

Etiology and Epidemiology

Verruca, or warts, are classified by location and morphology. They include verruca vulgaris (common wart),

verruca plantaris (plantar wart), and verruca plana (flat wart). Warts occur most commonly during the first three decades of life and are spread through direct person-to-person contact and autoinoculation.[11]

Clinical Presentation

Warts may occur on any skin surface but are most common on the hands, plantar aspects of the feet, and in the genital area. They are usually asymptomatic unless traumatized.

Warts are typically discrete, skin-colored, rough-surfaced (verrucous) papules (Figure 17-8). On the feet (plantar warts), the normal skin lines are obliterated. Warts may appear around the nail (periungual warts), where they present as less well-demarcated verrucous papules that may extend under the nail plate. When warts are pared, punctate hemorrhages are noted, which represent thrombosed capillaries that are traumatized by the paring process.[12]

Diagnostic Evaluation

Clinical inspection is usually sufficient to diagnose most warts. In questionable lesions, a diagnostic skin biopsy shows characteristic changes.

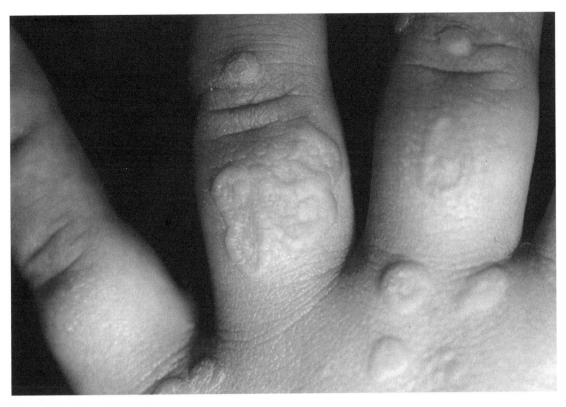

Figure 17-8. Warts of the hand.

Differential Diagnosis

- *Callus*: Plantar calluses may resemble plantar warts in that both are hyperkeratotic papules. Calluses differ in that they have intact skin lines over the surface and lack punctate bleeding points when pared.
- *Compound nevus (mole)*: Compound nevi have a verrucous surface but are fleshier in consistency than most warts and are brown rather than flesh-colored.
- *Seborrheic keratosis*: A seborrheic keratosis may present as a verrucous papule indistinguishable from a wart. It differs in that it occurs mostly in older people, is usually multiple, occurs on the trunk rather than on the distal extremities, and is often pigmented.
- *Skin tags*: Like flat warts, skin tags are small skin-colored papules, but they are pedunculated and fleshier and usually occur on the neck and in the axilla, unusual sites for warts.

Treatment

Asymptomatic, nonproblematic warts do not need to be treated because 67% of warts spontaneously resolve in 2 years without therapy.[11] For warts that require treatment, there are dozens of potential treatment modalities, but there is no treatment of choice.

Persistent or symptomatic lesions can be treated with cryotherapy with liquid nitrogen. This is accomplished by applying liquid nitrogen to the wart, with either a spray canister or a cotton swab, such that a 1- to 3-mm white "freeze" border surrounds the wart.[13] This should remain for 5–30 seconds, depending on the size of the wart. This regimen is repeated every 2–3 weeks until the wart resolves. The patient should be informed that postinflammatory hypopigmentation, very visible in darker Native American skin, is a possibility.

Salicylic acid, applied as a 10–16% solution, 40% patch, 15–20% gum, or 1% cream, is a safe and reasonably effective modality. The verruca is soaked in warm water for 5 minutes and then pared or filed with an emery board; salicylic acid treatment is applied once a day until the wart resolves. If a patch is used, it should be changed every 48 hours. Months of treatment are often needed to clear the lesions.

Electrodesiccation and curettage of problem warts has the advantage of physically removing the lesion in one sitting. Scarring is almost ensured with this procedure and, as with all wart therapies, there is a risk of recurrence.

Special care must be exercised in treating plantar warts because painful scars after overaggressive therapy can feel like having a permanent stone in one's shoe. Asymptomatic plantar warts do not need treatment.

Conclusion

Several health and environmental factors contribute to a high incidence of skin infections in Native Americans. To modify these risk factors and decrease the risk of infection, diet modification, exercise, good hygiene, adequate sanitation, and an ample water supply should be implemented.

Summary Points

- Cutaneous candidiasis presents with scaly, red plaques with satellite papules and pustules.
- Before starting treatment of dermatophytosis (tinea infections), confirmation with diagnostic examination is strongly recommended.
- Treatment of pediculosis capitis includes permethrin or lindane rinses. Close contacts should be examined for infestation.
- Oral dicloxacillin, cephalexin, or erythromycin are the treatments of choice for impetigo, ecthyma, and mild erysipelas. Severe erysipelas and cellulitis are treated with intravenous nafcillin or vancomycin.
- Intractable pruritus with multiple inflammatory papules is highly suggestive of scabies. Microscopic examination of the contents of a skin burrow confirms the diagnosis.
- Most warts resolve in 2 years without therapeutic intervention. There are dozens of treatments for warts, but there is no treatment of choice.

References

1. Fotos P, Lilly J. Clinical management of oral and perioral candidosis. Dermatol Clin 1996;14:273–280.
2. Wargon O. Tinea of the skin, hair and nails. Med J Aust 1996;164:552–556.
3. Janniger C, Kuflik A. Pediculosis capitis. Cutis 1993;51:407–408.
4. Carroll J. Common bacterial pyodermas: taking aim against the most likely pathogens. Postgrad Med 1996;100:311–322.
5. Feingold D. Staphylococcal and streptococcal pyodermas. Semin Dermatol 1993;12:331–335.
6. Shriner D, Schwartz R, Janniger C. Impetigo. Cutis 1995;56:30–32.
7. Darmstadt G, Lane A. Impetigo: an overview. Pediatr Dermatol 1994;11:293–303.
8. Nicolle L, Postl B, Urias B, et al. Group A streptococcal pharyngeal carriage, pharyngitis, and impetigo in two northern Canadian native communities. Clin Invest Med 1990;13:99–106.
9. Peterson C, Eichenfield L. Scabies. Pediatr Ann 1996;25:97–100.
10. Pruksachatkunakorn C, Duarte A, Schachner L. Scabies: how to find and stop the itch. Postgrad Med 1992;91:263–269.
11. O'Brien J. Common skin problems of infancy, childhood, and adolescence. Primary Care 1995;22:99–115.
12. Moghaddas N. Periungual verrucae: diagnosis and treatment. Clin Podiatr Med Surg 1995;12:189–199.
13. Landow K. Nongenital warts: When is treatment warranted? Postgrad Med 1996;99:245–249.

Chapter 18
Sexually Transmitted Disease

Deborah L. Goldsmith

The diagnosis, treatment, and prevention of sexually transmitted diseases (STDs) have always been hampered by reluctance to address sexual health issues openly and by the higher prevalence of STDs in poor and underserved populations. In many American Indian cultures, concerns related to cultural inappropriateness and privacy on the part of the patient and the provider hinder the ability to fully elucidate the sexual history.[1] These concerns may impair the ability to deal effectively with STDs. These issues are compounded by the fact that there are numerous "tribal groupings in the United States, each with its own language, religion, folkways, mores, and patterns of interpersonal relationships."[2] Outreach programs should be specialized to individual tribes to bring patients in for timely treatment and prevent spread of these contagious diseases in a community.

Epidemiology

The epidemiology of STDs in the Native American population is as varied as the tribes themselves. Some studies have revealed that Alaska Native women, who often live in rural areas, have high rates of gonorrhea, chlamydia, and human papillomavirus (HPV).[3] Many studies have shown high rates of particular STDs in certain Native American populations.[1, 4, 5] However, methods of record keeping make it hard to obtain good nationwide epidemiologic data because many public health rosters group Native Americans in the "Other" ethnic groups category.

Nonetheless, Toomey et al.[6] performed an excellent epidemiologic study documenting high rates of gonorrhea and syphilis in American Indian populations in states with large numbers of Native American residents. The average Native American gonorrhea rate over the 1984–1988 period was 501 per 100,000, which was more than twice the rate among non–Native Americans in the states studied. The findings for syphilis rates were very similar. Other studies have shown evidence of *Chlamydia trachomatis* infection in up to 30% of screened women.[1, 5] This finding is particularly disturbing because women often are asymptomatic, and infection can lead to sterility and perinatal transmission.

Multiple socioeconomic and cultural factors likely contribute to the risk of STDs in the Native American population. When looking at minority groups, Rice et al.[7] found that "sexual behaviors leading to exposure to gonorrhea include early onset of sexual intercourse, large numbers of casual partners, and particularly selection of partners who are themselves members of high-risk core groups." Other behaviors identified to increase transmission of gonorrhea include "failure to recognize symptoms of gonorrhea, delay in seeking treatment after onset of symptoms, continued sexual activity after onset of symptoms, delay in notifying sexual partners of exposure to infection, nonuse of barrier prophylaxis, and noncompliance with therapy."[7] These behaviors may be influenced by substance abuse, low socioeconomic status, low levels of schooling, limited access to health care, or delayed use of available resources, which may be frequently encountered in the Native American population. Cultural perceptions of health and disease may also play a role.

Diagnosis and Treatment

Once a Native American patient presents for evaluation, the diagnosis and treatment of infection are no different from that of the non-Native patient. It is useful to divide the various STDs into ulcerative and nonulcerative diseases. This facilitates a reasonable diagnostic and treatment algorithm.

Ulcerative Lesions

The ulcerative STDs affecting the Native American population include syphilis, chancroid, and herpes simplex virus (HSV). Lymphogranuloma venereum also presents early with ulcerative lesions, but these are so seldom recognized by the patient that the disease is rarely ulcerative at the time of presentation for treatment.

The lesions of HSV generally present as small clusters of painful vesicles that later form shallow, painful ulcers. The primary episode of this recurrent disease may be accompanied by tender regional adenopathy and systemic symptoms of fever, headache, malaise, and, rarely, meningitis. Although presumptive diagnosis can often be made by history and physical appearance of the lesions, definitive diagnosis requires either a positive Tzanck smear or HSV culture from the base of the ulcer. Serology is generally not helpful in diagnosing acute disease. Acute primary outbreaks may be treated with acyclovir 200 mg orally (PO) five times a day for 7–10 days. The newer agents, valacyclovir and famciclovir may also be used but are more costly. Treatment of the primary outbreak may shorten the course until the painful lesions crust over and alleviate the systemic symptoms, but it does not prevent future recurrence.

Recurrent episodes tend to be less severe than the initial outbreak. If a patient begins antiviral treatment during the prodrome stage or the first 48 hours of the outbreak, there may be a decreased time to lesion healing. Treatment in the immunocompetent patient is not generally suggested due to the cost and limited benefit of therapy. Patients with frequent recurrence (six or more episodes per year) may receive daily suppressive therapy to decrease the number of outbreaks. The dosing regimen is variable, ranging from 200–400 mg of acyclovir PO bid to qid. The goal is to place the patient on the minimal inhibitory dose. It is reasonable to discontinue suppressive therapy after 1 year, reinitiating if the patient again had frequent recurrences. Although patients appear to be most infectious when they have active lesions, it is known that some shed virus even when no lesions are present. Barrier methods, such as condoms, are useful to prevent transmission of HSV.

Differentiating the ulcerations of chancroid from HSV and syphilis is difficult but vital. Definitive diagnosis by culture of the causative organism, *Haemophilus ducreyi*, is not feasible due to lack of commercially available culture medium and low sensitivity. A patient presenting with one or more painful genital ulcers with a history inconsistent with HSV is suspicious for chancroid. Tender inguinal adenopathy is seen in approximately one-third of chancroid patients; if it is suppurative, the diagnosis is virtually certain. The clinician should rule out syphilis either by dark-field microscopy of the ulcer exudate or negative nontreponemal serology at least 1 week after the appearance of the original ulceration. Although there are no repercussions from lack of treatment for HSV lesion incorrectly diagnosed as chancroid, the same cannot be said of syphilis. If syphilis cannot be ruled out, the patient should be treated for both chancroid and syphilis.

Recommended chancroid regimens include erythromycin 500 mg PO qid for 7 days, azithromycin 1 g PO as a single dose, or ceftriaxone 250 mg intramuscularly (IM) as a single dose. Although the former treatment is the most cost effective, the latter two regimens offer the advantage of single-dose, observed therapy. Patients should be reexamined in 1 week to document improvement of the lesions. If the patient has not had pain relief and significant ulcer healing in this time, alternative diagnoses must be considered.

A patient with a solitary, painless ulcer is most likely to have syphilis caused by the spirochete *Treponema pallidum*. This must be the working diagnosis until proved otherwise. Given the relatively high incidence in some minority communities and the repercussions of untreated disease, appropriate diagnosis of syphilis is a priority.

The definitive tests for early syphilis are either darkfield microscopy or direct fluorescent antibody tests to identify spirochetes from the base of the chancre. Many clinics do not have the necessary testing equipment; thus, serologic tests must be performed. Presumptive diagnosis can be made by the combination of a positive nontreponemal test, such as rapid plasma reagin or VDRL test, and a specific antitreponemal antibody test, such as microhemagglutinin-*T. pallidum* or fluorescent treponemal antibody absorbed. Up to 30% of patients with a primary chancre have initially negative serology, however, prompting repeat testing in several weeks if no alternative diagnosis is made. The treatment of choice for primary syphilis is parenteral penicillin, generally benzathine PCN G, 2.4 million units IM as a single dose. In the nonpregnant, penicillin-allergic patient, either doxycycline 100 mg PO bid or tetracycline 500 mg PO qid for 14 days may be used if the patient can be followed closely. Erythromycin at a dose of 500 mg PO qid is clearly less effective and requires strict compliance and diligent repeat testing. In the penicillin-allergic patient who is pregnant or suspected of noncompliance, penicillin desensitization should be followed by standard treatment, as outlined.

Patients who go untreated have resolution of the primary chancre. These patients may progress to secondary syphilis within 2–8 weeks. This stage is attributed to the widespread dissemination of the spirochete. The manifestations may be protean, but the skin is nearly always involved. Papular, macular, maculopapular, and pustular lesions may all be present. Systemic symptoms of fever, malaise, anorexia, arthralgias, and lymphadenopathy are frequent. Patients may also have mucous membrane, central nervous system, renal, and gastrointestinal manifestations. Diagnosis is made by indirect and direct treponemal tests, as noted. The treatment is the same as for primary syphilis, but many clinicians give a second dose of benzathine penicillin 1 week after the first treatment.[8]

Many more patients are diagnosed by screening serology than by direct observation of a primary chancre or signs of secondary syphilis. These asymptomatic patients have latent syphilis. Patients with known primary infection within the last year have early latent disease. Those in whom the duration of infection is unknown are considered to have late latent syphilis. All such patients should be evaluated for signs or symptoms of tertiary disease, such as aortitis, iritis, syphilitic gummas, or neurosyphilis. Any patient with evidence of the preceding conditions should undergo lumbar puncture to assess for neurosyphilis. If there is no evidence of neurosyphilis, patients with latent disease should be treated with benzathine penicillin G. Treatment of early latent disease is with 2.4 million units IM as a single dose. The dose for late latent syphilis is also 2.4 million units IM, but it should be repeated weekly, for a total of three doses.

Diagnosis and treatment of neurosyphilis and congenital syphilis are outside the scope of this book. The clinician faced with these problems should consult specialty texts in infectious diseases, Centers for Disease Control and Prevention guidelines, or an infectious disease specialist.

Another organism causing genital ulcers is lymphogranuloma venereum (LGV), which is caused by the serovars L1, L2, and L3 of *C. trachomatis*. The ulcers are painless, self-limited, and likely to go unnoticed by the patient. Most patients present later in their infection with painful, generally unilateral, inguinal adenopathy. If left untreated, this lymphadenopathy may become extensive and fluctuant, causing scarring. Both clinical presentation and positive LGV serology lead to the diagnosis. Treatment consists of doxycycline 100 mg PO bid for 21 days and aspiration of any fluctuant nodes. Erythromycin 500 mg PO qid for 21 days may be used in the pregnant or doxycycline-intolerant patient. If a diagnosis of chancroid is also considered, it is reasonable to choose the erythromycin regimen while awaiting the LGV serology, keeping in mind that the course of treatment for LGV is 21 rather than 7 days.

All the ulcerative genital diseases may increase the likelihood of human immunodeficiency virus (HIV) transmission. Syphilis and chancroid are clearly associated with increased HIV rates; all patients who present with these STDs should be counseled and offered HIV testing. This is particularly important because concomitant HIV infection may change the treatment recommendations for these STDs.

Nonulcerative Lesions

A nonulcerating STD that is becoming increasingly well known is HPV. HPV types 6 and 11 most often cause benign, though potentially disfiguring, exophytic anogenital warts. Other than the unusual case in which these grow large enough to block either the vaginal or urethral orifice, the effects of these growths are mainly cosmetic. Researchers suspect that these exophytic warts may more easily spread HPV than subclinical infection; therefore,

debulking and possible obliteration of these warts is reasonable. Various methods may be used, including cryotherapy, podophyllin, CO_2 laser, conventional surgery, electrocautery, and, most recently, imiquimod cream. Most of these methods require multiple applications over weeks to months to achieve resolution of the warts. However, the recurrence rate is quite high. Of more concern than these cosmetically disturbing warts is asymptomatic HPV infection with types 16, 18, 31, 33, or 35, which have been strongly associated with genital dysplasia and cervical or rectal carcinoma. There is a high incidence of these infections in certain Native American populations.[4, 9] There is no treatment for HPV infection *per se*. Patients need close clinical follow-up with special attention paid to timely cervical Papanicolaou (Pap) smears and consideration of anal Pap smears as well.

HIV and hepatitis B virus have significant morbidity and mortality associated with them. They are covered elsewhere and are not further discussed in this chapter. The remaining STDs to be considered are best grouped by clinical syndrome rather than specific pathogen. Of most import are urethritis, mucopurulent cervicitis (MPC), and pelvic inflammatory disease (PID).

Urethritis

Urethritis is usually diagnosed in men and for treatment purposes is classified as gonococcal or nongonococcal urethritis (NGU). Both cause dysuria and itching or burning of the urethra. Gonococcal disease generally produces a thick, purulent discharge that may range in color from white to a yellow-green. Classically, NGU causes a clear and thin or mucoid discharge; often there is no discharge at all. Differentiation between NGU and gonococcal disease *must not* be made on appearance of discharge, which can be misleading. Gram's stain of the urethral discharge is the initial diagnostic test, allowing for presumptive diagnosis and immediate treatment. The presence of more than five polymorphonuclear cells per high-power (100×) field is consistent with urethritis. If intracellular gram-negative diplococci are seen, treat the patient for gonorrhea (see treatment of MPC section) and chlamydia. If no gonococcal organisms are seen, the patient has a presumptive diagnosis of NGU and should be treated accordingly until results of gonorrhea and chlamydia cultures are available.

NGU has been associated with multiple pathogens. The most common is *C. trachomatis*, followed by *Ureaplasma urealyticum*. *Trichomonas vaginalis* occasionally causes NGU, as does HSV. There are many cases of NGU in which the etiology remains unknown. Other than obtaining chlamydia cultures, the diagnosis is not pursued further unless the patient has persistent symptoms despite multiple attempts at treatment. In this case, a wet mount of urethral discharge should be searched for *Trichomonas*, and urethroscopy should be considered. Doxycycline 100

Table 18-1. Treatment of Pelvic Inflammatory Disease

I. Outpatient treatment of pelvic inflammatory disease
   A. Ceftriaxone, 250 mg, IM, single dose **or** cefoxitin, 2 g, IM plus probenecid, 1 g, PO **plus** doxycycline, 100 mg, PO bid for 14 days
   B. Clindamycin, 450 mg, PO qid **or** metronidazole,[a] 500 mg, PO bid for 14 days **plus** ofloxacin, 400 mg, PO bid for 14 days
   C. Clindamycin, 600 mg, PO tid for 14 days **plus** ciprofloxacin, 250 mg, PO bid for 14 days
II. Inpatient treatment of pelvic inflammatory disease
   A. Cefoxitin, 2 g, IV q6h **or** cefotetan, 2 g, IV q 12 hrs **plus** doxycycline, 100 mg, IV or PO bid (This regimen should be continued at least 48 hrs; when patient improves, she may then continue doxycycline, 100 mg, PO bid to complete a 14-day course.)
   B. Clindamycin, 900 mg, IV q8h **plus** gentamicin loading dose of 2 mg/kg IV followed by 1.5 mg/kg q8h[b] (This regimen should be continued at least 48 hrs; when patient improves, she may then continue clindamycin at the dose of 450 mg PO qid or switch to doxycycline, 100 mg, PO bid to complete a 14-day course. If there is evidence or suspicion of *Chlamydia trachomatis*, the patient should be switched to the doxycycline regimen for the remainder of the 14-day course.)

[a]Patients should be advised to avoid alcohol consumption to avoid Antabuse-like reactions.
[b]Gentamicin dosing must be adjusted for renal function. Although usage of q12h or daily dosing is likely to be efficacious, there are no studies to support this.
Source: Adapted from Centers for Disease Control and Prevention. 1993 Sexually transmitted diseases treatment guidelines. MMWR Morb Mortal Wkly Rep 1993;42(suppl RR-14):47–83.

mg PO bid for 7 days is therapy of choice for NGU because it covers both *Chlamydia* and *Ureaplasma*. Erythromycin 500 mg PO qid for 7 days is an alternative regimen, as is azithromycin 1 g PO as a single dose. The azithromycin has the advantage of directly observed therapy in clinic, but it is more costly. On the rare occasion that *Trichomonas* is involved, metronidazole 2 g PO as a single dose or 250 mg PO tid for 7 days should be used.

Mucopurulent Cervicitis

Although women generally do not experience urethritis, they can get MPC from the same organisms. Women may be asymptomatic or have abnormal vaginal discharge or bleeding. On direct examination, yellow or green exudate is visible from the cervical os. Culture the exudate for both gonorrhea and chlamydia, although often neither organism can be isolated. Because many women are unlikely to return for treatment after culture results are back, it is prudent to treat at the initial visit. Unless the patient is from a community with a high prevalence of gonorrhea, it is reasonable to treat presumptively for chlamydia alone. As with NGU, the recommended regimen is doxycycline 100 mg PO bid, erythromycin 500 mg PO qid for 7 days, or azithromycin 1 g PO as a single dose. If the gonorrhea culture is positive, every effort must be made to contact and further treat the patient; therefore, patients who cannot be contacted or are likely to miss follow-up should also be treated presumptively for gonorrhea. The recommended regimens for gonococcal, MPC, or urethritis include ceftriaxone 125 mg IM, cefixime 400 mg PO, ciprofloxacin 500 mg PO, or ofloxacin 400 mg PO, all given as a single dose. Azithromycin given as a 2-g single dose provides adequate coverage for both gonorrhea and chlamydia, but there is a high incidence of gastrointestinal side effects, which prompts fears of the patient vomiting up the medicine and thereby receiving treatment for neither organism.

Pelvic Inflammatory Disease

When infection enters the upper female genital tract, it can cause a spectrum of disorders, such as endometritis, salpingitis, tubo-ovarian abscess, and peritonitis. These are known collectively as *PID*. There is a wide variation in signs and symptoms, with many women being asymptomatic or having very subtle findings. Minimum criteria for making the diagnosis of PID include lower abdominal pain and adnexal and cervical motion tenderness.[10] Additional, fairly routine criteria are often used to make a diagnosis of PID. These include temperature higher than 38.3°C, abnormal cervical or vaginal discharge, laboratory documentation of either gonococcal or chlamydial cervical infection, and elevation of the nonspecific tests of inflammation, such as the sedimentation rate or C-reactive protein. Strict adherence to these criteria increases the specificity of diagnosis at the cost of severely limiting sensitivity, thereby missing the diagnosis in women with fairly mild PID.

Treatment decisions may be difficult because there are many organisms, alone or in combination, which may cause PID, including *Neisseria gonorrhoeae*, *C. trachomatis*, anaerobes, gram-negative facultative bacteria, and streptococci (Table 18-1). Although cervical cultures for *N. gonorrhoeae* and *C. trachomatis* should always be performed, often no microbiological diagnosis is made, which forces the clinician to treat empirically. For the patient well enough for outpatient therapy, there are several reasonable options. All these require clinical follow-up in 72 hours with physical and microbiologic reexamination in 7–10 days to confirm cure. Those who cannot or will not comply with this follow-up should be considered for inpatient treatment.

Other parameters for hospitalization of a woman with PID include pregnancy, inability to differentiate from appendicitis or ectopic pregnancy, suspicion of pelvic abscess, adolescence, HIV or another serious underlying illness, severe nausea and vomiting, toxic appearance, or failure of outpatient therapy. Hospitalized patients should show substantial improvement within the first 72 hours of appropriate therapy. Those who do not improve may require further diagnostic workup and surgical evaluation.

Summary

All the infections discussed share the factor that they are readily communicable to sexual partners. Therefore, a vital part of treating any of these STDs is identification and treatment of all at-risk sexual partners. Cultural factors in the Native American population may further complicate this obligation because speaking about sexual partners may be considered improper[1]; this makes it difficult to contact people who have potentially become infected with an STD.

During a syphilis outbreak on an Indian reservation in Arizona, standard infection-control measures were found to be inadequate to control the outbreak.[11] This prompted a "novel approach to secondary disease prevention using 'cluster' interviewing techniques."[11] Patients with STDs were asked about sexual partners as usual but also were asked about "persons who might 'profit from serologic testing.'" In addition, persons identified by community health care workers as "close associates" of the case patient were identified. All three groups of at-risk people (i.e., sexual partners, those suspected by patient of needing testing, and "close associates") were then contacted and offered serologic syphilis testing and treatment. Only by using these unconventional methods were the health care workers able to stem the outbreak.[11]

Clearly, use of these nontraditional means of outbreak investigation may enable the health care giver to ensure the health of the community at large. Cultural and socioeconomic issues also affect risk factors[3]; therefore, better understanding of cultural risk factors will help community and public health officials formulate more tailored STD prevention plans for the Native American population. Correct diagnosis and treatment of STDs can help the health of an individual Native American patient, but providing an easily accessible, nonjudgmental environment for patients with possible STDs is essential for the health of the individual as well as the community at large.

References

1. Harrison HR, Boyce WT, Haffner WH, Crowley B, et al. The prevalence of genital *Chlamydia trachomatis* and mycoplasmal infections during pregnancy in an American Indian population. Sex Transm Dis 1983;10:184–186.
2. Bullough VL, Bullough B. Health Care for the Other Americans. New York: Appleton-Century-Crofts, 1982;109.
3. Davidson M, Schnitzer PG, Bulkow LR, Schloss ML, et al. The prevalence of cervical infection with human papillomaviruses and cervical dysplasia in Alaska Native women. J Infect Dis 1994;169:792–800.
4. Jolly AM, Orr PH, Hammond G, Young TK. Risk factors for infection in women undergoing testing for *Chlamydia trachomatis* and *Neisseria gonorrhoeae* in Manitoba, Canada. Sex Transm Dis 1995;22:289–295.
5. Cullen TA, Helgerson SD, LaRuffa T, Natividad B. *Chlamydia trachomatis* infection in Native American women in a southwestern tribe. J Fam Pract 1990;31:552–554.
6. Toomey KE, Oberschelp AG, Greenspan JR. Sexually transmitted diseases and Native Americans: trends in reported gonorrhea and syphilis morbidity, 1984–88. Public Health Rep 1989;104:566–572.
7. Rice RJ, Roberts PL, Handsfield HH, Holmes KK. Sociodemographic distribution of gonorrhea incidence: implications for prevention and behavioral research. Am J Public Health 1991;81:1252–1258.
8. Tramont EC. Treponema Pallidum (Syphilis). In GL Mandell, JE Bennett, R Dolin (eds), Principles and Practice of Infectious Diseases. New York: Churchill Livingstone, 1995:2117–2133.
9. Kenney JW. Ethnic differences in risk factors associated with genital human papillomavirus infections. J Adv Nurs 1996;23:1221–1227.
10. Centers for Disease Control and Prevention. 1993 sexually transmitted disease treatment guidelines. MMWR Morb Mortal Wkly Rep 1993;42[Suppl RR-14]:47–83.
11. Gerber AR, King LC, Dunleavy GJ, Novick LF. An outbreak of syphilis on an Indian reservation: descriptive epidemiology and disease-control measures. Am J Public Health 1989;79:83

Part III
Cardiovascular Disease

Chapter 19
Coronary Artery Disease and Hypertension

James M. Galloway and Joseph S. Alpert

Despite a marked decline in cardiovascular mortality in the general U.S. population, significant increases in coronary artery disease (CAD) and its manifestations have been seen in the Native American population. Cardiovascular disease has become the leading cause of death for Native Americans. This trend is associated with a dramatic increase in the frequency of cardiovascular risk factors, with disturbing implications for the future rates of coronary artery, cerebrovascular, and peripheral vascular disease among Indian people. The clinical diagnosis and initial management of CAD are discussed, and risk factors are reviewed briefly. The role of hypertension is discussed in greater depth.

Coronary Artery Disease

In the general U.S. population, the overall age-adjusted mortality from CAD has declined by more than 50% since 1968.[1] This appears to be substantially related to primary and secondary prevention activities involving lifestyle changes (e.g., regular exercise, diminishing tobacco use, and a diet lower in calories, animal fat, and saturated fat) with subsequent declining serum cholesterol levels. Improved therapies and greater public and physician awareness have resulted in better control of other modifiable risk factors, such as hypertension.

In the Native American population, the rates of CAD seemed to be relatively low in the past and remain lower on average than in the general U.S. population. Nevertheless, there is dramatic regional variation. The northern plains tribes, such as the Sioux, have a very high CAD incidence and mortality rate, and the southwestern tribes (e.g., the Pima) have a relatively low rate.[2] Table 19-1 shows the Strong Heart Study's findings on regional variation in CAD incidence relative to the strongest risk factor, diabetes.[3] The study compared Native Americans in Arizona (Pima, Maricopa, Papago), Oklahoma (Apache, Caddo, Comanche, Delaware, Fort Sill Apache, Kiowa, and Wichita), and the Dakotas (Oglala, Cheyenne River Sioux, Devil's Lake Sioux).

Moreover, the incidence, prevalence, and mortality of CAD seem to be increasing significantly in Native Americans generally.[4, 5] The reason for this apparent increase has not been fully elucidated but appears to be due largely to a cultural change from a traditional lifestyle to a more westernized lifestyle, with concomitant changes in levels of exercise, diet, weight, and associated diabetes.[4, 5]

In the 1940s, CAD rates appeared to be low among Indian people, and atherosclerosis was less common than in the white population. In fact, in more than 10,000 admissions to one Navajo hospital during 1949–1952, Gilbert[6] found no cases of acute myocardial infarction (AMI). Fulmer and Roberts[7] evaluated the adult population of a Navajo community (Many Farms) from 1956 to 1962 and found four new cases of ischemic heart disease, two each of AMI and angina, among 508 persons age 30 and older. The annualized attack rate for AMI was 0.7 per 1,000.[7] Sievers[8] reviewed 138 documented AMIs in patients from various southwestern tribes and calculated an annual attack rate of 1.0 per 1,000 for Navajo and Hopis older than age 40 years from 1957 through 1966. Because cigarette smoking, hypertension, and hypercholesterolemia were infrequent in southwestern Indians, it was thought that the low incidence of CAD was related to the relative lack of these risk factors.[8]

As predicted in 1986 by Coulehan et al.,[9] subsequent data suggested that the incidence rates for CAD were gradually beginning to increase. In the 1970s, when inpatient and population censuses were used, it was found that myocardial infarction among the Crow and northern Cheyenne Indians equaled or exceeded the rate for men and women in Framingham, Massachusetts.[10] This was the first study to report a high CAD rate among Native

Table 19-1. Regional Prevalence Rates for Coronary Heart Disease, Strong Heart Study, 1989–1992*

Region	Definite Myocardial Infarction			
	Nondiabetic Female	**Nondiabetic Male**	**Diabetic Female**	**Diabetic Male**
Arizona	0.4	0.5	0.3	1.5
Oklahoma	0.6	3.9	2.0	8.9
Dakotas	0.2	2.9	3.1	8.0
	Possible Coronary Heart Disease			
Arizona	16.1	9.8	20.9	18.0
Oklahoma	17.4	12.9	25.3	23.4
Dakotas	17.9	15.6	24.3	21.4

*Prevalence rates per 100 American Indians, ages 45–74 years, in each location.
Source: Adapted from BV Howard, ET Lee, LD Cowan, et al. Coronary heart disease prevalence and its relation to risk factors in American Indians. The Strong Heart Study. Am J Epidemiol 1995;142:254–268.

Americans. Data from the 1975–1978 period suggested that the AMI rate among southwestern Native Americans increased significantly (75 per 100,000 annually) from the 1957–1966 rate (35 per 100,000 annually).[11]

Reeves et al.[12] studied the mortality of chronic diseases among the Native American population in Wisconsin. They found that the mortality from CAD was significantly greater in both Native American men and women age 45–64 years than in whites of the same age. Mortality rates for those older than 65 years, however, were still lower than mortality rates for whites of similar ages.

The same pattern is found nationally, with heart disease becoming the leading cause of death for both sexes among American Indians (AIs) and Alaska Natives (ANs). In addition, the AI and AN heart disease mortality rates exceed the rates among U.S. whites and all races in all age groups ages 1–65 years (Table 19-2). Overall, 21.9% of all deaths in AIs and ANs are from diseases of the heart. Again, there was significant regional variation, with diseases of the heart responsible for 32.4% of the deaths in the Oklahoma area and only 15.4% in the Tucson area (although they were still the leading cause of death in that area as well).[13]

Acculturation into western society has brought with it an apparent decrease in physical activity, significant cultural disruption, and additional psychological stress. This change is thought to be related to the increased occurrence of myocardial infarction and CAD. In addition, as the traditional lifestyles of Native Americans change (with the accompanying changes in diet, activity, and weight), the prevalence of diabetes has developed to epidemic proportions in some Native American tribes, leading to a further increase in CAD through this major risk factor. The incidence of hypertension, dyslipidemia, and tobacco use is also increasing, thereby raising significant concerns about the future cardiovascular health of Native American people. In its Year 2000 Health Objectives for AIs and ANs, the Indian Health Service made the reduction of the death rate from CAD its number one objective.[14]

Table 19-2. American Indian and Alaska Native Cardiac Disease Mortality Rates per 100,000 Compared with U.S. White and All-Race Rates by Age

Age (yrs)	American Indian and Alaska Native	All Races (United States)	Whites (United States)
1–4	2.5	1.8	1.5
5–14	0.9	0.8	0.6
15–24	3.0	2.7	2.2
25–44	21.6	19.6	16.6
45–54*	127.0	114.6	103.6
55–64*	380.8	346.5	325.6
65+*	1,353.2	1,844.5	1,849.7

*Heart disease is the leading cause of death for age group.
Source: Adapted from Indian Health Service. Trends in Indian Health, 1996. Washington, DC: U.S. Department of Health and Human Services, Indian Health Service, Office of Planning, Evaluation, and Legislation, Division of Program Statistics, 1997.

Diagnosis and Therapy

The medical diagnosis and management of CAD among Native Americans is not significantly different from that in other populations. A classic history of exertional, substernal, nonpleuritic chest pressure with radiation to the arms, neck, or shoulders and associated with shortness of breath, nausea, or diaphoresis should prompt the same immediate response and initial interventions.

If the patient is not currently in pain and the chest discomfort is chronic and stable, a basic evaluation is made, including a physical examination (looking for, among other things, the presence of aortic stenosis or other valvular disease, hypertrophic cardiomyopathy, and congestive heart failure). An electrocardiogram (ECG), complete blood count, renal panel, chest x-ray (CXR), and arterial oxygen saturation should be performed. A functional evaluation may be needed to determine the presence and severity of CAD, including an exercise stress test, stress echocardiography, or radionuclide stress evaluation, as appropriate. An evaluation of left ventricular function should be entertained in patients with evidence of current or past congestive heart failure or a prior myocardial infarction, particularly because significant benefit in terms of quality of life and survival has been shown in patients with a reduced ejection fraction (45% or less) treated with an angiotensin-converting enzyme (ACE) inhibitor.[15–19] Chronic anti-ischemic medications should include aspirin, and, as needed, nitrates and beta-blockers. Long–acting calcium channel blockers are occasionally used.

On the other hand, if the patient presents with ongoing chest discomfort that may be secondary to CAD, immediate evaluation with an ECG and a physical examination is essential. Prompt administration of oxygen, sublingual nitroglycerin (unless the patient is significantly hypotensive or bradycardic), and aspirin, if appropriate, is important, along with placement of an intravenous line. If chest discomfort persists, consideration should be given to pain relief with intravenous morphine and aggressive intervention with thrombolytics (if AMI with 1 mm or more ST segment elevation in appropriate leads or a left bundle branch block is present), unless contraindicated. Heparin, beta-blockers, ACE inhibitors, and potentially a transfer for intensive care, acute catheterization, and subsequent mechanical intervention should be considered, if appropriate. The standard thrombolytic guidelines from the American Heart Association and the American College of Cardiology are clearly suitable for use in this patient population, although local factors may influence some aspects of this protocol. In most Native American health settings, streptokinase has become the thrombolytic agent of choice, primarily because of economic considerations and excellent efficacy.

The evaluation of chest pain of unclear etiology is somewhat more problematic, partly due to the vast differential for potential causes of chest pain. However, some basic guidelines are helpful in deciding who is at high risk and should therefore be admitted for observation and intervention as indicated.[20]

The most important aspect of chest pain evaluation is the history. A description of recent "ischemic-sounding" chest pain lasting more than 15 minutes should prompt an extended period of observation and repeat evaluations (including repeat ECGs) or admission to rule out unstable angina or AMI, even in the face of initially normal ECG and cardiac enzymes.

Ischemic chest pain at rest carries a relatively high short-term risk for death or infarction. Chest discomfort associated with deep T-wave inversions also carries a relatively high short-term risk. Patients with "ischemic-sounding" chest discomfort associated with the findings of congestive heart failure, hypotension, or a new murmur of mitral regurgitation are also at substantial risk.

For patients who do not meet the criteria for high risk after a careful history, physical examination, ECG, and standard laboratory evaluation, there may be a role for troponin T and I testing in the near future. These troponins are highly sensitive markers for myocardial necrosis occurring 3–12 hours before testing. Some studies have suggested that these may be reliable predictors of death and serious complications, especially if repeated in 6 hours.[21] However, confirmation of these results is necessary before full endorsement and widespread implementation can be advised.

Several caveats are relevant to the management of Native American patients with CAD:

- The majority of these patients have diabetes mellitus, and the manifestation of cardiac ischemia in diabetes is often atypical and even silent. Therefore, a high level of suspicion should be maintained in dealing with diabetic patients with any chest or epigastric discomfort.

- In general, in very rural settings without immediate access to hospitals with intensive care capabilities, the physician should use smaller, repeated doses of cardiovascular medications, such as beta-blockers, to avoid the potential adverse effects of high doses.

- In rural reservation settings, there are benefits to developing a working relationship with the traditional healers so that chest pain is quickly referred to the emergency room or clinic rather than after a long ceremony, in case acute thrombolytic therapy is needed. This working relationship has been successfully implemented on many reservations. After the evaluation, if no acute intervention is needed (or after the return of the patient if it is), the patient is referred back to the traditional healer for further care and follow-up. This may also allow for the development of a closer working relationship with the local traditional healers, to the benefit of patients who believe in both health systems.

Risk Factors

Until relatively recently, limited data were available on the classic cardiac risk factors in Native Americans. An early study by Coulehan et al.[9] revealed that diabetes was the major risk factor for AMI during the years 1976–1983 among the Navajo. A low incidence of cigarette smoking and lower levels of total serum cholesterol than in the corresponding white population were also noted. More recently, however, the Strong Heart Study group did a number of excellent studies on the role of classic coronary risk factors among 13 tribal groups of Native Americans in three separate geographic areas.[3, 5, 22] These studies showed that among several Native American tribes, the rates of definite myocardial infarction and definite CAD were higher in men than in women and that diabetes was the strongest independent risk factor. Besides age and sex, additional risk factors for CAD in Native Americans include hypertension, obesity, albuminuria, tobacco smoking, hyperinsulinemia, and low high-density lipoprotein (HDL) and high low-density lipoprotein (LDL) cholesterol.[3, 5]

The Navajo Health and Nutrition Survey[23] is the first population-based examination of CAD risk factors in the Navajo tribe. In addition to the risk factors found by the Strong Heart Study, this survey found that fasting hypertriglyceridemia and sedentary lifestyle were associated with CAD. Another study of risk factors among the Navajo revealed that hypertensive diabetics had a twofold increase in heart disease and a more than fivefold increase in cerebral and peripheral vascular disease over nonhypertensive diabetics.[24]

Diabetes

Although regional variations occur in the incidence and prevalence of diabetes among Native Americans, the overall rates have been rising by epidemic proportions since the 1970s. Current levels of diabetes are 70.9% for female Pima Indians ages 45–74 years and 64.7% for Pima men of the same age.[22] Among the Navajo, 17% of the men and 25% of the women between the ages of 20 and 91 years have diabetes.[23] These findings are 40% higher than any previous evaluation has demonstrated among the Navajo and four times higher than age-standardized U.S. estimates.[25]

Diabetes mellitus is a well-recognized risk factor for the development of atherosclerosis and cardiovascular disease. In fact, the most common complication of diabetes is atherosclerosis. Seventy-five to 80% percent of adult diabetics die from cardiovascular disease, as opposed to approximately 35% in the general U.S. population. In fact, the risk of cardiovascular disease in patients with diabetes is three to five times that of nondiabetics. (For a more detailed discussion of the role of diabetes among Native Americans, see Chapter 22.)

Dyslipidemia

Serum cholesterol levels in many Native American tribes also appear to be increasing. Some Native American tribes (e.g., the Pimas and the Papagos [Hohokam]) have had lower total serum cholesterol levels than those of the white population. In the tribal members evaluated by the Strong Heart study, however, levels of the cardioprotective HDL cholesterol were lower than in the general U.S. population.[22] The Cheyenne River Sioux have higher serum cholesterol levels than do the rest of the U.S. population.[26] Gillum et al.[27] studied 242 Chippewa Indians residing in an urban setting in Minnesota. They found serum cholesterol levels and other CAD risk factors that were similar to or greater than those observed in the general U.S. population. A study of the Zunis revealed values similar to those present in the surrounding white population (unpublished observations by RJ Goldberg, IS Ockene, and JS Alpert). Among the Navajo, serum concentrations of total cholesterol are similar to the general U.S. population, but serum triglycerides were elevated and HDL cholesterol concentrations were lower than expected for the general U.S. population, especially for Navajo women.[23] Similar findings were noted among the Pima.[28]

Although genetic factors may be the cause of variability in mean serum cholesterol values from tribe to tribe, differences in diet may also be an important determinant. Strong evidence favoring diet as the major determinant of serum cholesterol in Native Americans comes from observations made among the Tarahumara Indians of Mexico. This tribe eats a largely vegetarian diet that is very low in fat (12%) and cholesterol (72 mg/day). Mean serum cholesterol for members of this tribe is 136 mg/dl. When dietary fat and cholesterol were increased experimentally for only 5 weeks, serum total and LDL cholesterol levels dramatically rose in a fashion similar to that observed in a group of normocholesterolemic U.S. subjects. Thus, the low serum cholesterol values observed in the Tarahumaras seem to be, at least in large part, the result of their low-fat diet.[29]

With the dramatic changes in the diet (primarily changing from a high-carbohydrate diet to a high-fat diet) and lifestyle among Native Americans, as well as the increasing incidence of CAD and atherosclerosis in general, the normalization of serum lipid abnormalities in these individuals will likely become increasingly important. (For further detail on dyslipidemia and its therapy in Native Americans, see Chapter 21.)

Due to historically low levels of CAD in Native Americans, lipid evaluations have, in general, not been aggressively pursued in the past. In light of the epidemic of CAD and its risk factors in AIs and ANs, however, aggressive prevention efforts are essential. It is important to measure a fasting lipid profile (to include total and HDL cholesterol and triglycerides) in adult Native American patients 20 years of age and older, particularly those with other risk factors. If normal, this should be repeated at least every 5 years. In diabetics, the tests should be repeated annually. If levels are abnormal, intervention is indicated, with careful follow-up.

Tobacco

Tobacco use, once primarily a ceremonial adjunct, is similarly increasing within Native American communities. In the communities studied by the Strong Heart Study, 53.1% of men and 45.3% of the women interviewed from North and South Dakota currently smoked cigarettes. At the other end of the spectrum, 29.7% of male and 12.9% of female Pima Indians smoke cigarettes.[22] The use of tobacco among tribes appears to correlate crudely with the rates of CA. The frequency of tobacco smoking appears to be increasing.

Hypertension

Like diabetes, hypertension among AIs was relatively uncommon in the past, but it appears to be increasing simultaneously with obesity and other cardiovascular risk factors. Similarly, this increase in blood pressure among AIs appears to be related to marked changes in lifestyle and diet as a more westernized diet is adopted, with an overall increase in food availability and consumption. An associated increase in consumption of foods high in salt, fat, and cholesterol as well as a decrease in levels of activity and exercise also appear to contribute.[30]

Previous studies suggested that the microvascular as well as macrovascular complications of diabetes were relatively uncommon in Native Americans. Subsequent evaluations have shown that diabetes and hypertension eventually result in the same chronic disease manifestations in Indians as in other populations, with an increase in AMI[31] and renal failure.[32]

It is well recognized that people who are diagnosed with high blood pressure have up to three to four times the risk of developing CAD as opposed to those who do not have high blood pressure. Hypertension is closely related to obesity and glucose intolerance in studies of AI and non-AI populations. The additive risk of hypertension in AIs with non–insulin-dependent diabetes mellitus is remarkable, with a significant effect on overall and cardiovascular mortality as well as the development of proteinuria and renal failure, both of which are also associated with a higher mortality.[32, 33]

Sievers[34] published an excellent review of the prevalence of hypertension among AIs and ANs in 1977. In 1937, Salsbury[35] found only four cases of hypertension among 4,826 Navajos admitted to an Arizona hospital during a 5-year period, with a prevalence of 0.08%. In 1956, Darby et al.[36] reported the prevalence of hypertension to be 7.1% in one Navajo community (Ganado) and 4.2% in another (Pinon), with hypertension defined as a blood pressure higher than 140/90 mm Hg. Fulmer and Roberts[37] (study done at Many Farms between 1956 and 1962 and published in 1963) found that less than 5% (4.7%) of Navajo adults had hypertension.

In 1970, Alfred[38] reported that the blood pressure of migrant Navajo men was higher in an urban environment than while they were living on the reservation, which suggests that the stress of urban migration may contribute to the prevalence of hypertension.

Strotz and Shorr[39] (1973) found that 20% of Papago (Tohono O'odham) Indians age 15 years and older had hypertension with a blood pressure in excess of 160/95 mm Hg. The proportion of hypertension was about 43% for the diabetics but only 15% for nondiabetics. Broussard et al.[40] (1987) had similar findings: 37% of diabetic Native Americans treated at Indian Health Service facilities were hypertensive.

In 1979, Destefano et al.[41] reported that the prevalence of hypertension among Navajo Indians older than age 19 living on the reservation had risen to 17% (12% in men and 5% in women), with hypertension defined as a diastolic blood pressure above 90 mm Hg. They found a definite association between hypertension and the presence of obesity in both men and women and alcohol use in men. Others have suggested that the major causes of hypertension among Native Americans are related to obesity and high alcohol consumption.[4]

In 1986, Welty et al.[42] observed that Gila Bend Papago Indians age 25 years and older had an age-adjusted prevalence of hypertension of 19.5% for men and 24.7% for women (as defined by a blood pressure of 160/95 mm Hg or greater or taking antihypertensive medication). This was not significantly higher than the general U.S. rates.

In a 1991 survey of 704 Cree and Ojibwa Indians in Canada ages 20–64 years, Young[43] found that 27% had hypertension, as defined by a blood pressure higher than 140/90 mm Hg.

Some 23% of men and 14% of women from the Navajo Health and Nutrition Study[23] are hypertensive, as opposed to 16.6% in men and 19.7% in women evaluated in North and South Dakota by the Strong Heart Study. The rates of hypertension in the Pimas and the Oklahoma Indians were similar but substantially higher than those reported in either study (32.3% and 32.6%, respectively, in men and 30.4% and 32.0% in women).[22]

The impact of hypertension on the renal function of diabetic patients is of particular concern in this population. As described in Chapter 25, hypertension promotes a marked acceleration of the renal dysfunction associated with diabetes. The incidence of end-stage renal disease in some Native American populations (Pima and Zuni) is the highest in the world and more than 12 times that of the general U.S. population (unpublished data by A Narva, The IHS Kidney Disease Program). Therefore, aggressive hypertensive control with renal protective agents is essential. ACE inhibitors have been shown to significantly slow the relentless progression of renal dysfunction, including the associated proteinuria, even in normotensive individuals with proteinuria or moderate renal insufficiency.[44, 45]

Treatment

In general, without specific indications for individual antihypertensive agents and any specific contraindications, antihypertensive therapy should begin with the introduction of ACE inhibitors. They are recommended for their efficacy, relatively low cost, and low rates of adverse reactions and because of the high frequency of concomitant diabetes in this hypertensive population. ACE inhibitors have also been found to prolong survival in patients with moderate left ventricular systolic dysfunction or congestive heart failure. These agents are generally initiated at low doses with cautious upward titration. In patients with existing renal insufficiency or proteinuria, ACE inhibitors have been shown to delay progression of proteinuria and renal insufficiency.[44, 45] In this population with hypertension and renal insufficiency, the optimal goal blood pressure is generally approximately 125/75 mm Hg rather than higher. Primary contraindications include allergy or a history of significant adverse reaction to an ACE inhibitor, hyperkalemia, and significant renal insufficiency, generally manifested by a serum creatinine greater than 2.5–3.0.

In patients with a prior myocardial infarction, particularly if large, the use of beta-blockers for heart rate and blood pressure control has been shown to prolong survival. These agents can be combined with ACE inhibitors (generally at lower doses) for diabetic patients with renal dysfunction. The presence of type 2 diabetes does not contraindicate the use of beta-blockers, especially in patients with a history of AMI. The effects on serum glucose and lipid determinations are small, and the potential survival benefit may be substantial. Beta-blockers can be safely used in diabetics with careful monitoring of blood glucose and lipid status.

Low-dose loop diuretics are a cost-effective and generally well-tolerated alternative. Their adverse effect on a patient's lipid levels may limit their use, however, especially in those with CAD. Serum potassium levels must be monitored and supplemented where necessary.

Conclusion

Although CAD mortality is currently lower in AI and AN peoples than in the general U.S. population, there appears to be a steep upward trend in CAD incidence and, even more disturbing, in its risk factors. Diabetes mellitus is now at epidemic proportions in Native American communities and is the strongest risk factor for the development of CAD in this population.

Primary prevention of diabetes and CAD is essential and should be integrated into every outpatient and inpatient visit. Primary prevention should be the focus through measures to reduce risk factors, including obesity, diabetes, hypertension, smoking, and dyslipidemias. The prevention of CAD in known diabetics is important and should include close evaluation for other risk factors by aggressive screening and appropriate management, with a high suspicion of CAD (including atypical presentations). Daily aspirin administration of 160–325 mg for prevention of myocardial infarction is a high priority for individuals older than age 45 years. The prevention of recurrent events in patients with known CAD is essential, with even more aggressive risk factor modification, including the use of beta-blockers in addition to aspirin.

Treatment of CAD is not significantly different from that suggested for non-AIs but must be culturally specific and acceptable to this population to be optimally effective.

References

1. McGovern P, Pankow J, Shahar E, et al. Recent trends in acute coronary heart disease, mortality, morbidity, medical care and risk factors. N Engl J Med 1996;334: 884–890.
2. Welty TK, Coulehan JL. Cardiovascular disease among American Indians and Alaska natives. Diabetes Care 1993;16(Suppl 1):277–283.
3. Howard BV, Lee ET, Cowan LD, et al. Coronary heart disease prevalence and its relation to risk factors in American Indians, the Strong Heart Study. Am J Epidemiol 1995;142:254–268.
4. Alpert JS, Goldberg R, Ockene IS, Taylor P. Heart disease in Native Americans. Cardiology 1991;78:3–12.
5. Howard B, Go O, Lee E, et al. The rising tide of cardiovascular disease in American Indians: the Strong Heart Study (in press).
6. Gilbert J. Absence of coronary thrombosis in Navajo Indians. Calif Med 1955;82:114–115.
7. Fulmer HS, Roberts RW. Coronary heart disease among the Navajo Indians. Ann Intern Med 1963;59:740.
8. Sievers ML. Myocardial infarction among southwestern American Indians. Ann Intern Med 1967;67: 800–807.
9. Coulehan J, Lerner G, Helzlsouer K, et al. Acute myocardial infarction among Navajo Indians, 1976–83. Am J Public Health 1986;76:412–414.
10. Hrabovsky SL, Welty TK, Coulehan JL. Acute myocar-

dial infarction and sudden death in Sioux Indians. West J Med 1988;150:420–422.

11. Sievers ML, Fisher JR. Increasing rate of acute myocardial infarction in southwestern American Indians. Ariz Med 1979;36:739–742.

12. Reeves MJ, Remington PL, Nashold R, Pete J. Chronic disease mortality among Wisconsin Native Americans, 1984–1993. Wis Med J 1997;96:27–32.

13. Indian Health Service. Trends in Indian Health, 1996. Washington, DC: U.S. Department of Health and Human Services, Indian Health Service, Office of Planning, Evaluation, and Legislation, Division of Program Statistics, 1997.

14. Healthy People 2000 Midcourse Review and 1995 Revisions. Rockville, MD: U.S. Department of Health and Human Services, Public Health Services, 1995.

15. The CONSENSUS Trial Study Group. Effects of enalapril on mortality in severe congestive heart failure: results of the Cooperative North Scandinavian Enalapril Study. N Engl J Med 1987;316:1429–1435.

16. Cohn JN, Johnson G, Ziesche S, et al. A comparison of enalapril with hydralazine-isosorbide dinitrate in the treatment of chronic congestive heart failure. N Engl J Med 1991;325:303–310.

17. The SOLVD Investigators. Effect of enalapril on survival in patients with reduced left ventricular ejection fractions and congestive heart failure. N Engl J Med 1991;325:293–302.

18. The SOLVD Investigators. Effect of enalapril on the mortality and the development of heart failure in asymptomatic patients with reduced left ventricular ejection fractions. N Engl J Med 1992;327:685–691.

19. Pfiffer MA, Braunwald E, Maye L, et al. Effect of captopril on mortality and morbidity in patients with left ventricular dysfunction after myocardial infarction: results of the Survival and Ventricular Enlargement Trial. N Engl J Med 1992;327:669–677.

20. Hlatky MA. Evaluation of chest pain in the emergency department. N Engl J Med 1997;337:1648–1653.

21. Hamm C, Goldman B, Heeschen C, et al. Emergency room triage of patients with acute chest pain by means of rapid testing for cardiac troponin T or troponin I. N Engl J Med 1997;337:1648–1653.

22. Welty T, Lee E, Yeh J, et al. Cardiovascular disease risk factors among Native Americans. Am J Epidemiol 1995;142:269–287.

23. Mendlein J, Freedman D, Peter D, et al. Risk factors for coronary heart disease among Navajo Indians: findings from the Navajo Health and Nutrition Survey. J Nutr 1997;127:2099s–2105s.

24. Hoy W, Light A, Megill D. Cardiovascular disease in Navajo Indians with type 2 diabetes. Public Health Rep 1995;110:87–94.

25. Will J, Strauss K, Mendlein J, et al. Diabetes mellitus among Navajo Indians: findings from the Navajo Health and Nutrition Survey. J Nutr 1997;127(Suppl): 2106–2113.

26. Welty TK. Cholesterol levels among the Sioux. Indian Health Service Provider 1989;14:35.

27. Gillum RF, Gillum BS, Smith N. Cardiovascular risk factors among urban American Indians: blood pressure, serum lipids, smoking, diabetes, health knowledge and behavior. Am Heart J 1984;107:765–776.

28. Howard BV, Davis MP, Pettitt DJ, et al. Plasma and lipoprotein cholesterol and triglyceride concentrations in the Pima Indians: distributions differing from Caucasians. Circulation 1983;68:214–222.

29. Connor SL, Connor WE. The Importance of dietary cholesterol in coronary heart disease. Prev Med 1983;12:115.

30. Galloway JM. Hypertension in Native Americans: etiology, association and trends. The Federal Practitioner 1996;13:51–54.

31. Sugarman JR, Hickey M, Hall T, Gohdes D. The changing epidemiology of diabetes among Navajo Indians. West J Med 1990;153:140–145.

32. Lee ET, Lee VS, Lu M, et al. Incidence of renal failure in NIDDM: the Oklahoma Indian Diabetes Study. Diabetes 1994;43:572–579.

33. Nelson RG, Pettitt DJ, Carraher MJ, et al. Effect of proteinuria on mortality in NIDDM. Diabetes 1988;37: 1499–1504.

34. Sievers ML. Historical overview of hypertension among American Indians and Alaska Natives. Arizona Medicine 1977;34:607–610.

35. Salsbury CG. Disease incidence among Navajo. Southwest Med 1937;21:230–233.

36. Darby WJ, Salsbury CG, McGainity WJ, et al. A study of the dietary background and nutriture of the Navajo Indian. J Nutr 1956;60(Suppl):1–86.

37. Fulmer HS, Roberts RW. Coronary heart disease among the Navajo Indians. Ann Intern Med 1963;59:740.

38. Alfred BM. Blood pressure changes among male Navajo migrants to an urban environment. Can Rev Soc Anth 1970;7:189–200.

39. Strotz CR, Shorr GI. Hypertension in Papago Indians. Circulation 1973;48:1299–1303.

40. Broussard BA, Valway SE, Kaufman S, et al. Clinical hypertension and its interaction with diabetes among American Indians and Alaska Natives. Diabetes Care 1993;16(Suppl 1):292–296.

41. DeStefano F, Coulehan J, Wiant MK. Blood pressure survey on the Navajo Indian reservation. Am J Epidemiol 1979;109:335–345.

42. Welty TK, Freni-Titulaer L, Zack MM, et al. Effects of exposure to salty drinking water in an Arizona community: cardiovascular mortality, hypertension prevalence, and relationships between blood pressure and sodium intake. JAMA 1986;255:622–626.

43. Young TK. Prevalence and correlates of hypertension in a subarctic Indian population. Prev Med 1991;20:474–485.

44. Ravid M, Savin H, Jutrin I, et al. Long term stabilizing effect of angiotensin converting enzyme inhibition on plasma creatinine and on proteinuria in normotensive type 2 diabetic patients. Ann Intern Med 1993;118:577–581.

45. Ahmad J, Siddiqui MA, Ahmad H. Effective postponement of diabetic nephropathy with enalapril in normotensive type 2 diabetic patients with microalbuminuria. Diabetes Care 1997;20:1576–1581.

Chapter 20

Acute Rheumatic Fever, Rheumatic Heart Disease, and Valvular Heart Disease

Eric A. Brody

Acute rheumatic fever (ARF) and its sequela, rheumatic heart disease (RHD), continue to affect Native Americans more commonly than the general U.S. population. Between 1968 and 1977, age-adjusted mortality rates for chronic RHD in Native Americans were twice those of the non-Native population. More recently, data have suggested that mortality has decreased, only slightly exceeding that in the general U.S. population.[1] Attack rates of ARF have been favorably affected by improved public health measures and medical programs of surveillance and eradication.[2, 3] Nevertheless, ARF continues to be seen more commonly in lower socioeconomic groups and among certain ethnic groups, including Native Americans, blacks, Hawaiians, and Hispanics. Thus, patients continue to be at risk for significant cardiovascular morbidity and mortality from ARF and RHD, and an adequate understanding of the pathophysiology, natural history, and therapy of these entities is vital for practitioners caring for Native Americans.

Epidemiology and Pathogenesis

ARF follows only group A streptococcal infection of the upper respiratory tract and is not associated with streptococcal skin infections (impetigo). The incidence of streptococcal pharyngitis is equal in male and female patients, and its seasonal incidence parallels that of ARF. Streptococcal pharyngitis is generally, but not exclusively, a disease of school-age children, and epidemiologic studies in Native Americans suggest a similar peak incidence, with 53% of cases occurring between the ages of 5 and 14 years.[2] The incidence and prevalence of disease are variable in different countries. In developing countries, the incidence exceeds 100 per 100,000. In the United States, between 1935 and 1960, the incidence was 40–65 per 100,000 population. The incidence of streptococcal pharyngitis has significantly declined in recent years, with

current estimates at less than two cases per 100,000.[4] Epidemiologic data in Native Americans are limited but suggest rheumatic fever initial attack rates of 8–9 per 100,000 in 1974–1977, which, although higher than the rate for the general U.S. population, represents a decline in incidence.[2] The decline in incidence in the general U.S. population has been attributed to a number of possible factors, including antibiotic therapy for streptococcal pharyngitis, better housing conditions, decreased crowding in homes and schools, and improved access to medical care. Clearly, several of these factors are present in Native American populations as well and may account for the decreased incidence of ARF. Significantly, the resurgence of ARF in the United States in the mid-1980s occurred in geographically distinct regions of the country and amongst middle-class families with ample access to medical care, which suggests that other factors, such as a changing virulence of the infecting organism, may be playing a role.[4]

The evidence that group A streptococcal pharyngitis is the agent resulting in ARF is strong but indirect. As mentioned, the seasonal variation in streptococcal pharyngitis parallels that of ARF. Effective antibiotic therapy aimed at eradicating the organism virtually eliminates the possibility of ARF. Successful primary prevention and surveillance programs have been instituted in several Native American populations.[1, 5, 6] However, attempts to explain cardiac involvement as a result of direct infection have been unsuccessful. Host-related factors for susceptibility are suggested by the limited 3% incidence of ARF in patients with untreated streptococcal pharyngitis and up to 50% incidence in patients with a prior episode of ARF (thus the necessity for antibiotic prophylaxis aimed at secondary prevention).[4] The major factors suggesting heightened risk of ARF are the magnitude of the immune response to the streptococcal infection and persistence of the organism after the infection. These factors and others suggest that an abnormal immunologic response to the organism results in the rec-

Table 20-1. Guidelines for the Diagnosis of Initial Attacks of Rheumatic Fever (Jones Criteria, Updated 1992)

Major Manifestations	Minor Manifestations
Carditis	Clinical findings
Polyarthritis	Arthralgia
Chorea	Fever
Erythema marginatum	Laboratory findings
Subcutaneous nodules	Elevated acute-phase reactants
	Erythrocyte sedimentation rate
	C-reactive protein
	Prolonged P-R interval

Supporting Evidence of Antecedent Group A Streptococcal Infection

Positive throat culture or rapid streptococcal antigen test
Elevated or rising streptococcal antibody titer

Source: Reprinted with permission from AJ Dajani, E Ayoub, FZ Bierman, et al. Guidelines for the diagnosis of rheumatic fever: Jones criteria, updated 1992. JAMA 1992;268:2069. Copyright 1992, American Medical Association.

ognized clinical manifestations of ARF.[4] Although many theories have been proposed, the precise mechanisms through which group A streptococcal infection triggers the clinical manifestations of ARF remain unknown.

Diagnosis and Clinical Manifestations

The diagnosis of ARF is clinical but requires confirmatory laboratory studies as well. The Jones criteria, originally published in 1944, describe the features necessary for the diagnosis of ARF. These criteria have been revised and modified over the years to reflect the changing understanding of the illness. Confirmatory laboratory studies continue to evolve as well and remain a foundation of the diagnosis.[7]

The major criteria for the diagnosis of ARF include carditis, polyarthritis, chorea, erythema marginatum, and subcutaneous nodules (Table 20-1). Minor manifestations include arthralgias, fever, elevations of acute-phase reactants (erythrocyte sedimentation rate, C-reactive protein), and a prolonged PR interval. The presence of one major and two minor criteria or two major criteria alone make the diagnosis of ARF. Also required is supporting evidence of antecedent group A streptococcal infection through either positive throat culture, a rapid streptococcal antigen test, or an elevated or rising streptococcal antibody titer. It should be noted that the guidelines for diagnosis outlined in Table 20-1 are required for initial attacks of ARF.

Patients with prior episodes of ARF are at much higher risk for recurrences than the general population, and a greater index of suspicion must be held. Most patients with recurrent episodes do fulfill the Jones criteria, but in some cases, the diagnosis may be less clear. Because acute carditis may be difficult to diagnose in patients with prior episodes of ARF, a recurrence may be diagnosed in a patient with known RHD or a well-documented history of prior ARF by a single major criterion or several minor criteria. Even in recurrences, supporting evidence of recent group A streptococcal infection is necessary.[7]

The practitioner must also recall that a number of other illnesses may fulfill the Jones criteria and mimic ARF. The differential diagnosis includes infective endocarditis, serum sickness, connective tissue diseases, and rheumatoid arthritis. Clinical manifestations generally follow group A streptococcal pharyngitis after a latent period of approximately 3 weeks. In a substantial number of cases, pharyngitis may be mild or asymptomatic in patients who eventually develop ARF.[4]

Rheumatic carditis may affect the endocardium, pericardium, or myocardium to varying degrees. Carditis is almost always manifest clinically by a murmur of valvulitis. Carditis is generally thought to be among the most specific findings of ARF, occurring in at least 50–72% of patients.[4] Carditis, specifically valvulitis, should be suspected in patients without a history of valvular heart disease or known murmur who present most commonly with a new murmur of mitral regurgitation (MR) or aortic insufficiency (AI). Pulmonic and tricuspid valve involvement is rare.[4] The murmur of acute MR is high-pitched, blowing, and extends throughout systole; it is the hallmark of rheumatic valvulitis. It is best heard in the left lateral decubitus position at the apex and radiating to the axilla. Aortic insufficiency is less common than is MR. The diastolic murmur of AI is blowing in quality, decrescendo, and heard best at the left upper sternal border with the patient leaning forward.

Myocarditis is often manifest as tachycardia, and its absence makes the diagnosis of rheumatic carditis unlikely. Severe involvement may result in congestive heart failure with associated orthopnea, paroxysmal nocturnal dyspnea, or frank pulmonary edema. Pericarditis may manifest as characteristic pleuritic or positional chest pain with or without a pericardial friction rub and associated pericardial effusion. Pericarditis without valvular involvement is rare.[4, 6]

Migratory polyarthritis is the most frequently seen major manifestation of ARF, occurring in roughly 60% of cases. It is generally asymmetric, migratory, and involves the larger joints, including wrists, knees, ankles, and elbows. The arthritis is usually benign in that it causes no joint deformity. In untreated cases, the arthritis persists for 2–3 weeks. It responds rapidly to salicylate therapy, usually within 48 hours. The diagnosis of ARF should be considered doubtful if symptoms of arthritis persist despite adequate salicylate therapy.[4, 8]

Chorea or St. Vitus' dance is characterized by purposeless, involuntary, rapid movements of the head, trunk, or extremities and is often associated with muscle weakness. At times, chorea may be unilateral, and emotional lability may be noted. It is found in a minority of patients, approximately 20% of those with ARF. Chorea is generally a delayed manifestation of ARF, appearing 3 months or more after onset of the illness (in contrast to the 3-week latency of carditis and arthritis), and other manifestations may therefore not be present at the time of presentation. Thus, chorea may be the only manifestation of ARF and is sufficient to make the diagnosis.[4, 8]

Erythema marginatum is a unique rash appearing as nonpruritic macules with pale centers. The lesions vary greatly in size and may be rounded or serpiginous. They are found largely on the trunk and proximal extremities and generally not on the face. Erythema marginatum is an infrequent manifestation of ARF, seen in fewer than 5% of cases.[4, 8]

Subcutaneous nodules are firm and painless, approximately 0.5–2.0 cm. They are rare findings in ARF, seen in approximately 3% of cases. They are usually freely movable and found on the extensor surfaces of the elbows, knees, and wrists. They may also be found on the scalp of the occiput and over the spinous processes.[4, 8]

Laboratory diagnosis of ARF requires evidence of antecedent group A streptococcal infection. Positive throat cultures are found in a minority of patients at the time of presentation with ARF. However, serologic evidence is usually at a peak at the time of clinical presentation with ARF. Therefore, confirmatory evidence in the form of rising antistreptolysin O (ASO), deoxyribonuclease B (DNase B), or antistreptokinase titers should be sought. A positive rise is considered to be an increase of two or more dilutional increments between the acute-phase and convalescent-phase specimens, separated by 2–4 weeks.[7] The ASO titer is most widely used, and an antibody response is seen in 80% of patients with acute group A streptococcal pharyngitis. A single low-titer does not exclude ARF. If the clinical situation is highly suggestive, other serologic tests should be performed. An elevated titer for at least one serologic marker may be found in 95% of patients with ARF, except those presenting with chorea alone.[7]

Treatment of Acute Rheumatic Fever

Medical therapy of ARF has three primary goals: (1) eradication of the underlying group A streptococcal infection; (2) reduction of symptoms of associated inflammation, particularly arthritis; and (3) treatment of congestive heart failure, if present.

Primary prevention of ARF consists of identification of cases of streptococcal pharyngitis and prompt antibiotic treatment. Such therapy not only prevents episodes of ARF but also limits infectivity and the capacity to spread the disease. Penicillin remains the treatment of choice. Patients who are unlikely to be compliant with the required oral regimen of penicillin V (500 mg two to three times daily for 10 days) should be treated with a single intramuscular injection of benzathine penicillin G, 1.2 million units. For penicillin-allergic patients, erythromycin 250 mg qid for 10 days is an acceptable alternative. Dose adjustments in the pediatric population are necessary. Other effective regimens include newer macrolide antibiotics, such as azithromycin, which may be given as a 5-day course of therapy (500 mg on day 1, followed by 250 mg per day for days 2–5). Also, 10-day regimens of limited-spectrum, first-generation cephalosporins may be used.[4]

The arthritis of ARF is readily treated with salicylates, which generally provide prompt and dramatic relief of symptoms. Aspirin given in four to five divided doses to adults to provide a total dose of 100 mg/kg per day is recommended to achieve serum levels of 15–20 mg/dl; this should result in abatement of symptoms within 12–24 hours. In patients in whom the arthritis does not respond promptly, an alternative diagnosis should be entertained. It is strongly recommended, however, that neither salicylates nor steroids should be initiated until the diagnosis is clear. Withholding therapy poses no danger to the patient, and symptoms may be treated with other analgesics.[4]

Corticosteroids have a role primarily in the treatment of carditis, especially if complicated by evidence of congestive heart failure. Prednisone, given twice daily in doses of 2–4 mg/kg per day in adults, is recommended as the usual regimen, with a rapid taper over 2 weeks. If there is a clinical relapse, longer courses of therapy may be necessary. Salicylates and steroids are often given simultaneously, and this combination therapy is thought to be helpful in preventing reactivation of the illness.[4]

Essential to therapy of ARF is eradication of group A streptococcal infection. The organism may be cultured in only 11–25% of patients at the time of diagnosis of ARF. Nevertheless, all patients should receive treatment for the acute infection at the time of presentation with ARF with one of the regimens outlined in the preceding paragraphs.

Supportive care consists of bed rest for those with significant joint pain. Duration should be determined on an individual basis, depending on response to therapy. Hospital admission is recommended for all patients with evidence of carditis. If heart failure is noted, diuretics, oxygen therapy, and afterload reduction is reasonable, as is prompt evaluation by echocardiography. In these patients, cardiology consultation should be strongly considered and arrangements made for close follow-up.[4]

Secondary Prevention

Secondary prevention is vital in patients who have had prior episodes of ARF because the attack rate is signifi-

Table 20-2. Secondary Prevention of Rheumatic Fever

Agent	Dose	Mode
Benzathine penicillin G	1,200,000 units every 3–4 wks	IM
	OR	
Penicillin V	250 mg twice daily	PO
	OR	
Sulfadiazine	0.5 g once daily for patients ≤27 kg (60 lb); 1.0 g daily for patients >60 kg (60 lb)	PO
For patients allergic to both penicillin and sulfadiazine		
Erythromycin	250 mg twice daily	PO

IM = intramuscularly; PO = orally.
Source: Adapted from A Dajani, K Taubert, W Wilson, et al. Treatment of acute streptococcal pharyngitis and prevention of rheumatic fever: a statement for health professionals. Pediatrics 1995;96:758.

cantly higher in these patients. Recurrent infection need not be symptomatic for ARF to recur. Thus, the recommended approach to secondary prevention is continuous antibiotic prophylaxis in populations at risk. Patients with an increased risk of recurrence include caregivers of young children and adolescents, teachers, health care professionals, military recruits, and others in crowded housing situations. Economically challenged populations have been shown to be at higher risk as well. Patients with prior episodes of carditis are at greater risk of carditis recurrence, and subsequent episodes tend to increase in severity. The duration of continuous prophylaxis depends on the presence of cardiac involvement. Special consid-

eration should be given to lifelong prophylaxis in Native American populations with a history of rheumatic carditis, especially if the individual resides in an extended family setting.

Both oral and parenteral antibiotic regimens may be used for secondary prevention of ARF (Table 20-2). Parenteral prophylaxis should be considered the regimen of choice for patients who are at greatest risk, especially if compliance is in question. If compliance can be ensured, then oral therapy may be considered.[4]

Endocarditis Prophylaxis

All patients with a prior history of ARF and resultant valvular heart disease should be considered at increased risk for bacterial endocarditis. These patients are appropriate candidates for antibiotic prophylaxis before certain invasive dental and surgical procedures. The antibiotic regimens described for the prevention of ARF recurrence are inadequate in these settings, and additional therapy is mandatory. Patients with prosthetic heart valves are at particularly high risk.[9] Patients with prior ARF without evidence of carditis do not need prophylaxis.

The recommendations for the prevention of bacterial endocarditis have been updated.[9] Bacteremia may occur with daily activities, such as tooth brushing, but prophylaxis is recommended only for procedures commonly resulting in bacteremia with organisms associated with endocarditis (Table 20-3). Antibiotic regimens appropriate for bacterial endocarditis prophylaxis are listed in Table 20-4. High-risk patients are those with prosthetic heart valves, complex cyanotic congenital heart disease, and prior bacterial endocarditis. Considered at moderate risk are patients with most other congenital cardiac anomalies, hypertrophic cardiomyopathy, mitral valve prolapse with valvular regurgitation, thickened valve leaflets, or rheumatic valvular heart disease. A number of clinical entities are thought to present no greater risk than they do

Table 20-3. Procedures Requiring Endocarditis Prophylaxis

Respiratory tract
   Tonsillectomy or adenoidectomy
   Surgery involving the respiratory mucosa
   Bronchoscopy with a rigid bronchoscope
Gastrointestinal tract*
   Sclerotherapy for esophageal varices
   Esophageal stricture dilation
   Endoscopic retrograde cholangiography with biliary
      obstruction
   Biliary tract surgery
   Surgery involving the intestinal mucosa
Genitourinary tract
   Prostatic surgery
   Cystoscopy
   Urethral dilation

*Prophylaxis is recommended for high-risk patients; it is optional for medium-risk patients.
Source: Adapted from A Dajani, KA Taubertet, W Wilson, et al. Prevention of endocarditis, recommendations by the American Heart Association. JAMA 1997;277:1794–1801. Copyright 1997, American Medical Association.

Table 20-4. Prophylactic Regimens for Dental, Oral, Respiratory Tract, or Esophageal Procedures

Situation	Agent	Regimen[a]
Standard general prophylaxis	Amoxicillin	Adults: 2.0 g
		Children: 50 mg/kg PO 1 hr before procedure[a]
Unable to take oral medication	Ampicillin	Adults: 2.0 g IM or IV
		Children: 50 mg/kg IM or IV within 30 mins of procedure
Allergic to penicillin	Clindamycin	Adults: 600 mg
	Cephalexin[b] or cefadroxil[b]	Children: 20 mg/kg PO 1 hr before procedure
	Azithromycin or clarithromycin	Adults: 2.0 g
		Children: 50 mg/kg PO 1 hr before procedure
		Adults: 500 mg
		Children: 15 mg/kg PO 1 hr before procedure
Allergic to penicillin and unable to take oral medications	Clindamycin	Adults: 600 mg
		Children: 20 mg/kg IV within 30 mins of procedure
	Cefazolin	Adults: 1.0 g
		Children: 25 mg/kg IM or IV within 30 mins of procedure

[a]Total children's dose should not exceed adult dose for all situations referenced.
[b]Cephalosporins should not be used in individuals with immediate-type hypersensitivity reaction (urticaria, angioedema, or anaphylaxis) to penicillins.
IM = intramuscularly; IV = intravenously; PO = orally.
Source: Reprinted with permission from AS Dajani, KA Taubert, W Wilson, et al. Prevention of bacterial endocarditis. Recommendations by the American Heart Association. JAMA 1997;277:1798. Copyright 1997, American Medical Association.

for the general population and do not require prophylaxis for endocarditis (Table 20-5). These include isolated secundum atrial septal defect, prior aortocoronary bypass surgery, cardiac pacemakers and implantable defibrillators, mitral valve prolapse without valvular regurgitation, and innocent heart murmurs.[9]

Follow-up of Rheumatic Carditis and Valvular Heart Disease

History and physical examination should provide the basis of follow-up for patients with ARF and resultant valvular heart disease. Careful questioning about the patient's activity levels, exercise tolerance, and symptoms limiting these activities should be a routine feature of every follow-up visit. Symptoms suggestive of heart failure, including orthopnea, paroxysmal nocturnal dyspnea, chest pain and dyspnea on exertion, should be sought and attempts made to quantify their severity. Patients may report lower-extremity edema, fatigue, exercise intolerance, or palpitations. A careful cardiac physical examination is vital. Auscultation aimed not only at the detection of murmurs but an assessment of their severity is key, with special care taken to describe the murmur (i.e., intensity, location, duration, quality) to provide a basis of comparison for serial examinations. Assessment of jugular venous pressure, hepatojugular reflux, peripheral pulses, blood pressure, and lung auscultation and percus-

sion round out the complete cardiac physical assessment. A routine electrocardiogram (ECG) is appropriate because abnormalities of axis, chamber enlargement, and rhythm disturbances may reflect valvular disease progression in otherwise asymptomatic patients. Similarly, chest radiography may be useful in assessing cardiac chamber sizes, pulmonary vascular congestion, or pulmonary venous hypertension.

Patients presenting with ARF in the presence of a murmur, ECG abnormalities, or cardiac symptoms should be strongly considered for transthoracic echocardiography at the time of diagnosis. This study establishes the etiology of specific valvular abnormalities suspected on physical examination and provides baseline assessments of left ventricular function, cardiac chamber size, and lesion severity for longitudinal follow-up. Moderate to severe valvular lesions deserve close clinical follow-up. Repeat study should be considered in asymptomatic patients in 3–6 months, with prompt reassessment by echocardiography for any progression in symptoms or significant change in physical examination findings.

In the absence of ARF recurrence, repeat echocardiographic evaluation should follow published guidelines for valvular heart disease in general.[10] Routine reevaluation of asymptomatic patients with mild stenotic or regurgitant lesions is not indicated. Patients with mild to moderate valvular stenosis with stable symptoms may also be followed clinically, with reevaluation prompted only by symptom progression. It is reasonable to have yearly, rou-

Table 20-5. Procedures Not Requiring Endocarditis Prophylaxis

---

Respiratory tract
  Endotracheal intubation
  Bronchoscopy with flexible bronchoscope, with or
    without biopsy*
  Tympanostomy tube insertion
Gastrointestinal tract
  Transesophageal echocardiography*
  Endoscopy with or without gastrointestinal biopsy
Genitourinary tract
  Vaginal hysterectomy*
  Vaginal delivery*
  Cesarean section
In uninfected tissue
  Urethral catheterization
  Uterine dilation and curettage
  Therapeutic abortion
  Sterilization procedures
  Insertion or removal of intrauterine devices
Other
  Cardiac catheterization, including balloon angioplasty
  Implanted cardiac pacemakers, implanted defibrillators,
    and coronary stents
  Incision or biopsy of surgically scrubbed skin
  Circumcision

---

*Prophylaxis is optional for high-risk patients.
Source: Adapted from AS Dajani, KA Taubert, W Wilson, et al. Prevention of bacterial endocarditis. Recommendations by the American Heart Association. JAMA 1997;277:1794–1801. Copyright 1997, American Medical Association.

tine, scheduled echocardiographic reevaluations of moderate to severe stenotic lesions. These patients should also be strongly considered for regular clinical evaluation by a cardiologist for two reasons. First, the progression of symptoms is the indication for surgical intervention in these patients, and the symptom progression may be subtle. Second, a rare patient may develop severe stenosis with a relative paucity of symptoms and may require exercise treadmill testing to assess exercise tolerance. Exercise testing in this setting is higher risk than in the general population and should only be undertaken by practitioners skilled in both the interpretation of treadmill testing and the management of potential complications.

Regurgitant valvular lesions are often asymptomatic and may remain so even when severe. In this instance, changes in ventricular dimensions or systolic function may be the indication for surgical intervention. Such changes may occur in the absence of clinically apparent decreases in exercise tolerance or other symptoms and are indications of declining ventricular function. In this setting, valve replacement or repair may be recommended in asymptomatic patients to avoid irreversible ventricular

failure. Thus, moderate to severe lesions deserve yearly, scheduled echocardiographic study as well as clinical evaluation by a cardiologist. Echocardiographic evaluation is recommended for any progression in symptoms for patients with aortic regurgitation or MR. Such symptoms are generally an indication for surgical intervention, even when only moderate lesions are present.[11]

After valve replacement surgery, several important features deserve mention. Patients undergoing valve repair or replacement continue to be at increased risk for recurrence of ARF if they are in a high-risk profession or live with school-age children in an endemic population. Thus, continued monthly antibiotic prophylaxis against ARF may be appropriate. In addition, these patients are in the highest-risk group for endocarditis, and therefore, recommendations for antibiotic prophylaxis around the time of invasive procedures and dental work must be followed (Table 20-6).

Atrial fibrillation occurring in the setting of rheumatic valvular heart disease, specifically mitral valve disease, represents one of the highest-risk settings for embolic stroke. Such patients should be strongly considered for chronic warfarin therapy, with a goal international normalized ratio (INR) of 2.0–3.0. Patients having mechanical valvular prostheses require life-long anticoagulation therapy with warfarin; current recommendations suggest a goal INR of 2.5–3.5. Bioprosthetic valves do not require chronic anticoagulation in the absence of atrial fibrillation.

Summary Points

- Rheumatic fever and RHD continue to be a significant cause of morbidity and mortality in Native American populations, exceeding that in the general U.S. population.
- Antibiotic therapy is highly effective in both primary and secondary prevention of ARF.
- Strong consideration to lifelong rheumatic fever prophylaxis should be made in Native American populations, even for patients who have had valve replacement surgery.
- Endocarditis prophylaxis must be considered in all patients with known valvular heart disease undergoing invasive and dental procedures.
- Follow-up with a cardiologist should be considered in all patients with documented moderate to severe stenotic and regurgitant valvular lesions. Asymptomatic patients may progress to irreversible ventricular dysfunction in the absence of apparent symptoms.
- Anticoagulation should be used in selected patients with mitral valve disease and in those with atrial fibrillation. Close follow-up of the INR, no less often than once per month, is mandatory to ensure compliance and prevent potential morbidity and mortality.

Table 20-6. Prophylactic Regimens for Genitourinary and Gastrointestinal (Excluding Dental and Esophageal) Procedures

Situation	Agents[a]	Regimen[b]
High-risk patients	Ampicillin plus gentamicin	Adults: ampicillin 2.0 g IM or IV plus gentamicin 1.5 mg/kg (not to exceed 120 mg) within 30 mins of starting procedure; 6 hrs later, ampicillin 1 g IM or IV or amoxicillin 1 g PO Children: ampicillin 50 mg/kg IM or IV (not to exceed 2.0 g) plus gentamicin 1.5 mg/kg within 30 mins of starting the procedure; 6 hrs later, ampicillin 25 mg/kg IM or IV or amoxicillin 25 mg/kg orally
High-risk patients allergic to ampicillin or amoxicillin	Vancomycin plus gentamicin	Adults: vancomycin 1.0 g IV over 1–2 hrs plus gentamicin 1.5 mg/kg IV or IM (not to exceed 120 mg); complete injection or infusion within 30 mins of starting procedure Children: vancomycin 20 mg/kg IV over 1–2 hrs plus gentamicin 1.5 mg/kg IV or IM: complete injection/infusion within 30 mins of starting procedure
Moderate-risk patients	Amoxicillin or ampicillin	Adults: amoxicillin 2.0 g PO 1 hr before procedure or ampicillin 2.0 g IM/IV within 30 mins of starting procedure Children: amoxicillin 50 mg/kg PO 1 hr before procedure, or ampicillin 50 mg/kg IM or IV within 30 mins of starting procedure
Moderate-risk patients allergic to ampicillin or amoxicillin	Vancomycin	Adults: vancomycin 1.0 g IV over 1–2 hrs; complete infusion within 30 mins of starting procedure Children: vancomycin 20 mg/kg IV over 1–2 hrs; complete infusion within 30 mins of starting procedure

[a]Total children's dose should not exceed adult dose.
[b]No second dose of vancomycin or gentamicin is recommended.
IM = intramuscularly; IV = intravenously; PO = orally.
Source: Reprinted with permission from AS Dajani, KA Taubert, W Wilson, et al. Prevention of bacterial endocarditis. Recommendations by the American Heart Association. JAMA 1997;277:1799. Copyright 1997, American Medical Association.

References

1. Becker TM, Wiggins CL, Key CR, et al. Ethnic differences in mortality from acute rheumatic fever and chronic rheumatic heart disease in New Mexico, 1958–1982. West J Med 1989;150:46–50.
2. Coulehan J, Grant S, Reisinger K, et al. Acute rheumatic fever and rheumatic heart disease on the Navajo Reservation, 1962–77. Public Health Rep 1980;95:62–68.
3. Coulehan JL, Baacke G, Welty TK. Cost-benefit of a streptococcal surveillance program among Navajo Indians. Public Health Rep 1982;97:73–77.
4. Dajani AD. Rheumatic Fever. In Braunwald E (ed), Heart Disease. A Textbook of Cardiovascular Medicine. Philadelphia: Saunders, 1997;1769–1775.
5. Phibbs B, Taylor J, Zimmerman RA. A community-wide streptococcal control project. JAMA 1970;214:2018–2024.
6. Altha M, Enos E, Frank C, et al. How an American Indian tribe controlled the streptococcus. World Health Forum 1982;3:423–428.
7. Dajani AJ, Ayoub E, Bierman FZ. Guidelines for the diagnosis of rheumatic fever: Jones criteria, updated 1992. JAMA 1992;268:2069–2073.
8. Kaplan EL. Acute Rheumatic Fever. In Hurst JW, Schlant RC, Alexander RW (eds), The Heart. New York: McGraw-Hill, 1994;1451–1456.
9. Dajani AS, Taubert KA, Wilson W, et al. Prevention of bacterial endocarditis; recommendations by the American Heart Association. Circulation 1997;96:358–366.
10. Cheitlin MD, Alpert JA, Armstrong W, et al. ACC/AHA Guidelines for the clinical application of echocardiography. Circulation 1997;95:1686–1744.
11. Carabello B, Crawford F. Valvular heart disease. N Engl J Med 1997;337:32–41.

Chapter 21
Lipid Abnormalities

David C. Robbins, Wm. James Howard, and Barbara V. Howard

Cardiovascular disease (CVD) was rare among the ancestors of today's American Indians. The recent increase in coronary heart disease (CHD) in these populations, however, is undoubtedly a manifestation of the dietary and lifestyle changes of the past century. Smoking, diabetes, obesity, increases in dietary fat, and the transition to a sedentary lifestyle have played a role in raising the prevalence of atherosclerosis to epidemic proportions in many tribes.

Lipid abnormalities are potent risk factors for CVD. Most studies of lipid abnormalities have not traditionally focused on minority groups. In recent years, however, it has become evident that there are distinct ethnic differences in plasma lipoproteins. Genetic determinants and cultural and environmental influences unique to each ethnic group cause these differences.[1] Early reports showing healthy lipid profiles in American Indians led researchers to believe that these groups needed no further investigation in these areas. More recently, however, the skyrocketing incidence of atherosclerosis and diabetes in American Indians has led researchers to re-examine the associations among lipid alterations, diabetes mellitus, and CVD in these indigenous populations of the United States.

In 1988, the Strong Heart Study began to investigate CVD and its risk factors in geographically diverse groups of American Indians, to quantify the rates of disease, and to assess the importance of CVD risk factors.[2-4] The population for the clinical examination included American Indians ages 45–74 years examined between July 1989 and January 1992. They were resident members of the following tribes: the Pima, Maricopa, and Papago Indians of central Arizona, who live in the Gila River, Salt River, and Ak Chin Indian communities; the seven tribes of southwestern Oklahoma (Apache, Caddo, Comanche, Delaware, Fort Sill Apache, Kiowa, and Wichita); the Oglala and Cheyenne River Sioux in South Dakota; and the Spirit Lake Tribe in the Fort Totten area of North Dakota. Approximately 1,500 individuals from each center were included.

For the purposes of this review, we focus exclusively on lipid levels and lipid abnormalities in the American Indians in the Strong Heart Study populations. The link with CVD is amply covered in Chapter 19.

Lipid Levels and Prevalence of Dyslipidemia

Mean total cholesterol levels among the three centers of the Strong Heart Study were generally lower than those of age-matched adults from the general U.S. population, as was the prevalence of hypercholesterolemia (Figure 21-1).[5-7] Among the three centers, Arizona had mean total cholesterol concentrations more than 20 mg/dl lower than South and North Dakota, with Oklahoma having intermediate concentrations. Concentrations of 200 mg/dl or higher were found in 25% of Arizona versus 47% of South and North Dakota participants.[5] Patterns of mean low-density lipoprotein (LDL) cholesterol mirrored that of total cholesterol, although the differences between the lowest (Arizona) and highest (South and North Dakota) prevalence of elevated LDL cholesterol became more pronounced at higher LDL levels (Figure 21-2).[5] Approximately 25% of men and 10% of women had low high-density lipoprotein (HDL) (<35 mg/dl), and there was little difference between centers (Figure 21-3). Although mean concentrations of total triglycerides were higher among Arizona men, the proportions of men and women with elevated triglyceride concentrations were small and did not differ significantly among the centers (data not shown).[5]

Worsening Lipoprotein Profile in Diabetes

Dyslipidemia, or alterations in lipoprotein composition and metabolism, frequently accompanies non–insulin-

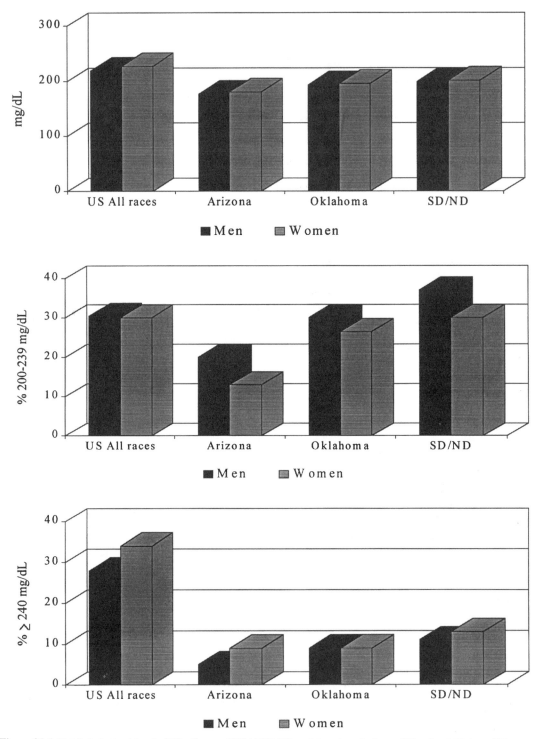

Figure 21-1. Total cholesterol levels: U.S. all races (NHANES III) and American Indians. (SD = South Dakota; ND = North Dakota.) (Adapted from TK Welty, ET Lee, J Yeh, et al. Cardiovascular disease risk factors among American Indians: the Strong Heart Study. Am J Epidemiol 1995;142:269–287; and DC Robbins, TK Welty, WY Wang, et al. Plasma lipids and lipoprotein concentrations among American Indians: comparison with the US population. Curr Opin Lipidol 1996;7:188–195.)

Figure 21-2. Low-density lipoprotein cholesterol in American Indians in three geographic areas. (SD = South Dakota; ND = North Dakota.) (Adapted from TK Welty, ET Lee, J Yeh, et al. Cardiovascular disease risk factors among American Indians: the Strong Heart Study. Am J Epidemiol 1995;142:269–287.)

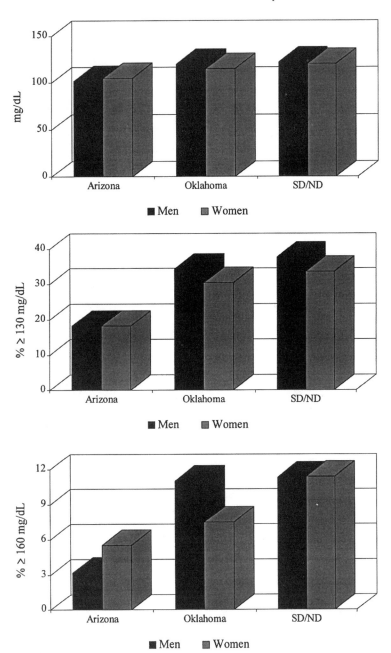

dependent (type 2) diabetes mellitus. Common alterations include increased very low-density lipoprotein (VLDL), LDL compositional changes, and decreased HDL with compositional changes. The insulin resistance syndrome that generally occurs in individuals with type 2 diabetes contributes to these lipoprotein abnormalities. The increase in triglycerides, decrease in HDL, and alterations in LDL composition in type 2 diabetes are thought to be responsible for stimulation of the atherosclerotic process.

Cholesterol is incorporated into several lipoprotein particles. LDL is the most cholesterol-rich and is best identified with deposition of lipids in vessel walls. LDL particles vary in size, and it appears that small LDL particles (the so-called *B phenotype*) are most closely associated with atherosclerosis. In addition, small LDL is phenotypically linked to hypertension, obesity, hypertriglyceridemia, and insulin resistance (syndrome X, or the insulin resistance syndrome).[8] Expression of the small LDL particle is influenced by genetics as well as

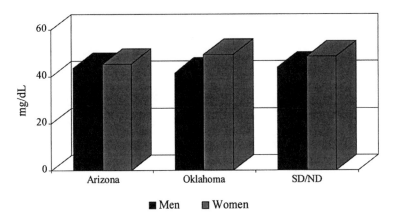

Figure 21-3. High-density lipoprotein cholesterol in American Indians in three geographic areas. (SD = South Dakota; ND = North Dakota.) Adapted from TK Welty, ET Lee, J Yeh, et al. Cardiovascular disease risk factors among American Indians: the Strong Heart Study. Am J Epidemiol 1995;142:269–287.)

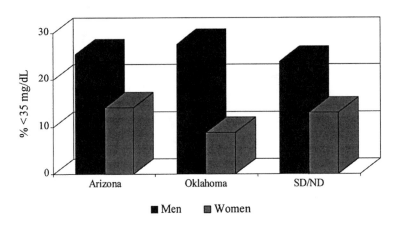

environment. American Indians in the Strong Heart Study showed a similar relationship between LDL and other aspects of the insulin resistance syndrome: Patients with small LDL particles were most likely to have other aspects of the insulin resistance syndrome, especially hypertriglyceridemia.

Another risk factor for atherosclerosis is the presence or absence of certain common variants in the structure of apolipoprotein E (apo E), a component of several lipid particles, including VLDL and HDL. There are three common types (phenotypes) of apo E. Some, such as E2, are associated with slight elevations in total cholesterol and early-onset Alzheimer's disease. Compared to whites, American Indians have a very low incidence of apo E2. Those with apo E4 had slightly higher levels of cholesterol.[9]

Lipoprotein (a) (lp[a]) levels among American Indians in the Strong Heart Study are generally low and do not correlate with CVD in a cross-sectional analysis. Lp(a) is a structurally heterogeneous protein bound to LDL-like particles.[10] Lp(a) levels are relatively independent of environmental factors, such as diet and diabetes, because the size and concentration of the protein seem to be determined primarily through inheritance. Those who express the larger phenotypes generally have the lowest levels of lp(a). Most epidemiologic studies demonstrate a direct correlation between lp(a) and prevalence of CHD. Conventional treatments for hyperlipidemia have relatively little impact on lp(a) levels.

Examination of lipid abnormalities in American Indians becomes more important as the prevalence of diabetes, especially type 2 diabetes, escalates dramatically in this segment of the population. In the three centers of the Strong Heart Study, the prevalence of diabetes ranges from 32% (South and North Dakota men) to 72% (Arizona women). These and similar data from other American Indian populations are disproportionate to those of the general U.S. population and stand in stark contrast to the low prevalence of diabetes in American Indians in the 1930s.

Roots of the Lipid Problem

Lifestyle changes are thought to be primarily responsible for the worsening lipoprotein profile in American Indians. These changes mainly encompass diet and level of physical activity. Since the 1980s, the link between dietary fat and prevalence of diabetes has been well established.[11–14] A comparison of the traditional Pima Indian diet of the eighteenth century with that of today shows a

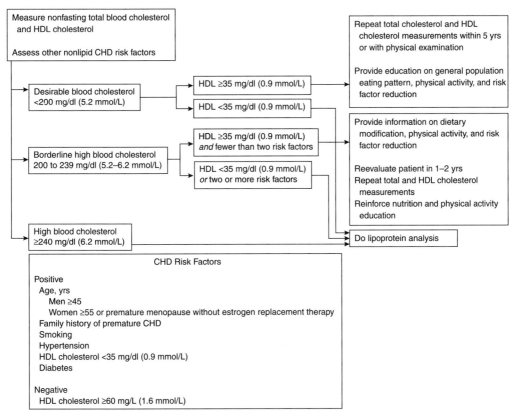

Figure 21-4. This algorithm summarizes the National Cholesterol Education Program guidelines for measurement of lipids and lipoproteins in adults. Note that the algorithm begins with a nonfasting blood sample. Further action is dictated by the levels of the total and high-density lipoprotein (HDL) cholesterol and associated risk factors for cardiovascular disease (CVD). The coronary heart disease (CHD) risk factors, both positive and negative, are summarized in the box at the bottom of the figure. Patients considered at risk for CVD should have a fasting lipoprotein analysis.

23–33% decrease in carbohydrates and a 27% increase in fat.[15] The increase in dietary fat was accompanied by an increase in the prevalence of obesity, a state that has consistently been associated with dyslipidemia.[16] Between 36% and 41% of American Indians in the Strong Heart Study are obese. These rates greatly exceed those for U.S. whites,[5] and they suggest a worsening lipoprotein profile because obesity has been identified as a risk factor for diabetes in this population.[17]

Dietary changes have been shown to induce potentially atherogenic changes in lipoprotein profiles in groups of Amerindian descent.[18] Two separate studies have examined the influence of diet on the lipoprotein profile of North American Indian populations: the Pima Indians of central Arizona[19] and the Tarahumara Indians of Mexico.[20] In both studies, subjects were fed their traditional low-fat, high-fiber diets and then high-fat modern diets. Results of this bolus of dietary fat representing the "contemporary" diet included a 24–31% increase in total cholesterol, a 17–31% increase in HDL cholesterol, and a 39% increase in LDL cholesterol.[19, 20] In the Mexican study, these changes were accompanied by an

18% increase in plasma triglycerides and a 7% mean increase in body weight after only 5 weeks on the high-fat diet.[20]

Intervention Strategies

The modified National Cholesterol Education Program (NCEP) guidelines are summarized in Figures 21-4 and 21-5.[21] The clinical approach to dyslipidemia is relatively straightforward and should be regularly integrated into the medical care of the adult. We suggest a stepwise approach that slightly modifies the 1993 NCEP guidelines. The approach begins with reliable accumulation of historic and laboratory data. Table 21-1 summarizes the historic risk factors on which the treatment algorithm is based, and Table 21-2 contains goals for serum lipoprotein and lipid concentrations. In addition, clinicians should be alert to multiple environmental and genetic causes of dyslipidemia, including medication (thiazides, steroids), alcoholism, obesity, pancreatitis, hypothyroidism, tobacco use, and familial dyslipidemias. Familial

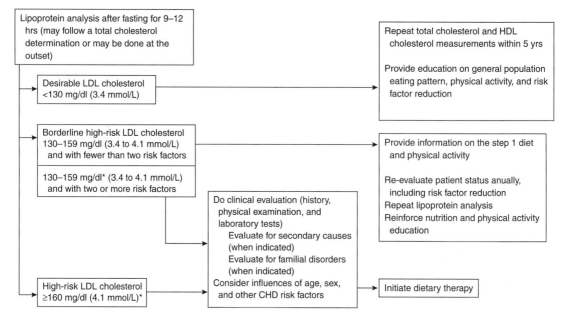

Figure 21-5. This algorithm summarizes the steps recommended by the National Cholesterol Education Program for patients requiring fasting lipoprotein analysis (measurement of total, high-density lipoprotein [HDL], and low-density lipoprotein [LDL] cholesterol and triglycerides). We consider these recommendations somewhat conservative, especially among populations with high rates of diabetes. When dietary therapy fails to produce desirable LDL cholesterol levels, appropriate drug therapy should be administered.
*On the basis of the average of two determinations. If the first two LDL cholesterol test results differ by more than 30 mg/dl (0.7 mmol/L), a third test result should be obtained within 1–8 weeks and the average value of the three tests used. (CHD = coronary heart disease.)

Table 21-1. Basis of Treatment for Dyslipidemia

Positive Risk Factors
   Age (yrs)
      Male ≥45
      Female ≥55 or premature menopause without estrogen replacement therapy
   Family history of premature CHD (definite myocardial infarction or sudden death before 55 yrs of age in father or other male first-degree relative, or before 65 yrs of age in mother or other female first-degree relative)
   Current cigarette smoking
   Hypertension (blood pressure ≥140/90 mm Hg, or taking antihypertensive medication)
   Low HDL cholesterol (<35 mg/dl or 0.9 mmol/L)
   Diabetes mellitus
Negative risk factors
   High HDL cholesterol (≥60 mg/dl or 1.6 mmol/L)

CHD = coronary heart disease; HDL = high-density lipoprotein.

dyslipidemias are characterized by the early appearance (before age 50 years) of CHD among close relatives.

The NCEP guidelines call for the measurement of fasting (12 hours since the last meal) concentrations of total and HDL cholesterol as the sole screening test. This allows lipid measurement in nonfasting patients but ignores the evolving importance of triglycerides in cardiovascular risk. The prevalence of hypertriglyceridemia is higher among overweight and diabetic patients, and the cost of adding triglycerides to the lipid panel is small. In addition, LDL cholesterol cannot be estimated without measuring triglycerides. Thus, we prefer to obtain fasting blood for the measurement of total cholesterol, triglycerides, HDL cholesterol, and calculation of LDL cholesterol.

The NCEP guidelines call for dietary and drug therapies based on the total number of risk factors carried by an individual, the presence of CHD, and the LDL cholesterol level. However, the clinical recognition of CHD is insensitive. Subclinical CHD is common, especially among populations at risk. Because we seek to treat as well as prevent heart disease, we tend to initiate dietary and drug therapy in patients with less conventional risk factors, such as hyper-triglyceridemia and obesity.[22] Consideration also is given to the presence of diabetes (fasting plasma glucose 126 mg/dl or greater) or even hyperglycemia (fasting blood sugars above 110 mg/dl). Furthermore, increasing attention is being given to the insulin resistance syndrome, a cluster of metabolic abnormalities that includes hypertension, central obesity, dyslipidemia (i.e., elevated triglycerides; low HDL; small, dense LDL particles; and increased residence time of VLDL and chylomicrons), varying degrees of hyperglycemia, and, occasionally in women, polycystic ovarian syndrome.[23, 24]

There is also controversy over the goal of treatment, especially among patients with diabetes. Cholesterol levels are classified as desirable, borderline, or high (see Table 21-2). Given the high prevalence of CHD among those with diabetes, it has been argued that the goal of treatment should be an LDL cholesterol level of 100 mg/dl or less, even *in the absence* of known CHD.[25] Most interventional studies designed to reduce CHD events have omitted diabetic patients from the analysis on the arguable assumption that their heart disease differs from that affecting nondiabetic participants. In our opinion, diabetic patients have accelerated atherosclerosis, which is fundamentally similar to that occurring in nondiabetic patients. The Scandinavian Simvastatin Survival Study demonstrated the importance of lowering lipids in diabetic patients.[26] Approximately 5% of the participants in the Scandinavian Simvastatin Survival Study were diabetic. During approximately 5 years of study, treatment with simvastatin lowered cholesterol in diabetic as much as in nondiabetic participants. More important, among the diabetic participants, the risk reduction for mortality and cardiac events was equal to or greater than that seen in non-

diabetic participants. The conventional guidelines for the initiation and goals of therapy are shown in Table 21-3.

Treatment always includes dietary changes. High-carbohydrate diets that are rich in both soluble and insoluble fiber (more than 25 g/day) and low in total and saturated fat (<30% of total daily calories as fat, with approximately equal amounts of polyunsaturated, monounsaturated, and saturated fats) can be expected to reduce total cholesterol by only 10–30%. In contrast to the American Heart Association step I diet, the traditional Pima diet contained 70–80% carbohydrate and only 12% fat.[15] Even short-term transition to the traditional diet results in rather dramatic improvements in glucose tolerance[27] and total and LDL cholesterol.[28] The reverse is also true, as illustrated by a marked worsening of cardiovascular risk factors, such as plasma LDL cholesterol (31%), and triglycerides (18%), when Mexican Tarahumara Indians switched to a higher-fat diet for only 5 weeks.

Table 21-2. Classification of Cholesterol Levels

Cholesterol Level	Initial Classification
Total Cholesterol	
<200 mg/dl (<5.2 mmol/L)	Desirable blood cholesterol
200–239 mg/dl (5.2–6.2 mmol/L)	Borderline high blood cholesterol
≥240 mg/dl (≥6.2 mmol/L)	High blood cholesterol
HDL Cholesterol	
<25 mg/dl (<0.9 mmol/L)	Low HDL cholesterol

HDL = high-density lipoprotein.

Table 21-3. Guidelines for Initiation and Goals of Therapy

Patient Category	Initiation Level	LDL Goal
Dietary Therapy		
Without CHD and with fewer than two risk factors	≥160 mg/dl (≥4.1 mmol/L)	<160 mg/dl (<4.1 mmol/L)
Without CHD and with two or more risk factors	≥130 mg/dl (≥3.4 mmol/L)	<130 mg/dl (<3.4 mmol/L)
With CHD	>100 mg/dl (>2.5 mmol/L)	≤100 mg/dl (≤2.6 mmol/L)
Drug Treatment		
Without CHD and with fewer than two risk factors	≥190 mg/dl (≥4.9 mmol/L)	<160 mg/dl (<4.1 mmol/L)
Without CHD and with two or more risk factors	≥160 mg/dl (≥4.1 mmol/L)	<130 mg/dl (<3.4 mmol/L)
With CHD	≥130 mg/dl (≥3.4 mmol/L)	≤100 mg/dl (≤2.6 mmol/L)

CHD = coronary heart disease; LDL = low-density lipoprotein.

In addition, a modest reduction in calories associated with weight loss quickly and often dramatically lowers triglycerides in obese patients with and without diabetes. Whenever tolerated, the therapy for dyslipidemia should also include recommendations for increased energy expenditure. Even modest increases in exercise are associated with beneficial changes in lipid profiles.[29–31] It should be emphasized that even a small (5%) drop in LDL cholesterol lowers the risk of CHD by approximately 10%.

Drug treatment is generally safe and should be instituted after an adequate attempt at reaching treatment goals with diet and exercise has failed. The NCEP guidelines suggest that attention be directed to secondary causes of hyperlipidemia, that blood lipoprotein measurements be repeated in 6–8 weeks, and that the treatment plan be re-evaluated after 3 months. Failure to achieve adequate risk reduction at this point indicates the need for drug treatment. The major drugs available are outlined in Table 21-4.

Treatment for Patients with Hypercholesterolemia and Normal Triglyceride Levels

The statin drugs are widely available and are cost-effective in appropriate patients. Niacin is probably a second-line agent, given its bothersome and potentially serious side effects. The dosage of the statin drug should be increased incrementally until LDL cholesterol level goals are obtained. Surveys of doctors' practices reflect a shocking disregard for compliance with NCEP guidelines, including titration of drugs to reach treatment guidelines. Occasional patients do not reach their goal even on maximum allowable doses. These patients should receive combination therapy, usually in the form of dietary fiber, oat bran, psyllium seed supplements, or bile

acid sequestrants. Colestipol is now available as a tablet, which improves its convenience. The bile-binding agents cause occasional constipation, which can be reduced by fiber supplements.

Treatment for Patients with Mixed Hyperlipidemia

Both cholesterol and triglycerides are elevated (above 200 mg/dl) in these patients, who frequently have secondary causes of dyslipidemia, especially diabetes and obesity, and obtain tangible benefits from weight loss and exercise. Metformin (Glucophage) may be the drug of choice in patients with type 2 diabetes and mixed hyperlipidemia because this hypoglycemic agent also lowers triglycerides and raises HDL cholesterol. Three drugs should be considered as primary therapy for this class of dyslipidemia: (1) a high-dose statin, (2) niacin, and (3) gemfibrozil. The Helsinki Heart Study demonstrated the usefulness of gemfibrozil on CVD rates, but overall mortality was unaffected.[32] Atorvastatin (Lipitor) is marketed as a highly potent statin drug having significantly more impact on triglyceride concentrations than do other members of the statin class. Its "unique" effects on triglycerides and HDL cholesterol are probably shared by other statins, however, especially when given to patients with high LDL cholesterol concentrations and triglycerides above 200 mg/dl, but in higher doses than currently recommended. Because atorvastatin has a longer half-life and its efficacy per milligram of drug administered is greater than that of other statins, a maximal dose results in greater LDL cholesterol and triglyceride reduction than that achieved with other statins. Patients with mixed hyperlipidemia who cannot be controlled on maximal doses of other statins should be given a trial of atorvastatin. Some patients require additional therapy even after

Table 21-4. Drugs Used to Treat Hyperlipidemia

Drug	Indications	Effects	Dosage	Side Effects
Niacin	↑ LDL-C ↑ TG	↓ LDL, ↓ TG, ↓ TC, ↑ HDL-C	1 g PO tid	Flushing, gastric upset, itching, tingling, skin rash, hypotension
Cholestyramine, colestipol	↑ LDL-C NOT for use in patients with ↑ TG	↓ LDL, ↓ TC, ↑ HDL-C, ↑ TG	8 g PO bid 10 g PO bid	↑ TG, binds certain drugs, vitamin K deficiency, constipation
Lovastatin, pravastatin, simvastatin,	↑ LDL-C	↓ LDL, ↓ TC, ↑ HDL-C, small ↓ TG	Up to 40 mg/day Up to 40 mg/day Up to 40 mg/day	Myositis, rhabdomyolysis, skin rash, LFT abnormalities
Atorvastatin	↑ LDL-C	↓ LDL, ↓ TC, ↑ HDL-C, ↓ TG	Up to 40 mg/day	Myositis, rhabdomyolysis, skin rash, LFT abnormalities
Gemfibrozil	↑ TG, combined hyperlipidemia	↓ TC, ↑ HDL-C, variable effect on TC	600 mg bid	Myopathy, hepatic damage, dyspepsia

LDL-C = low-density lipoprotein cholesterol; TG = triglycerides; TC = total cholesterol; HDL-C = high-density lipoprotein cholesterol; LFT = liver function test; PO = orally; ↓ = decreased; ↑ = increased.

an adequate trial on high-dose statin and diet. Combination therapy consisting of a statin plus niacin or gemfibrozil increases the risk of myositis, and it is best administered to very compliant patients by physicians who have experience with this combination.

Treatment for Patients with Elevated Triglycerides

Patients with triglyceride levels above 800 mg/dl are at risk for pancreatitis and should receive immediate attention for their lipid disorder. On the other hand, extreme hypertriglyceridemia may be a sign of or cause of pancreatitis. Thus, the workup should include tests for pancreatitis. Secondary causes of dyslipidemia are common among these patients, and they include obesity, diabetes, estrogen therapy, and excessive alcohol intake. Short periods (<1 week) of a very low-calorie diet or even starvation can dramatically lower triglyceride levels. Such therapies should be used with extreme caution in diabetic patients treated with insulin or sulfonylureas because the risk of hypoglycemia is high. Patients with a history of pancreatitis should be given gemfibrozil. Alternatives include niacin or the monounsaturated oil omega-3 fatty supplements (6–12 g/day), or both. Fish oil supplements, and especially niacin, raise plasma glucose. Niacin should therefore be used with caution, if at all, in people with diabetes.

Treatment for Patients with Low High-Density Lipoprotein Cholesterol

There are no prospective trials to indicate the benefits of specifically addressing patients with low HDL cholesterol, and treatment is speculative. No one would argue the wisdom of adhering to a "sensible" diet and engaging in regular aerobic exercise. Many lipid experts would treat this class of patients in the presence of CHD. Options are based, in part, on the other lipoprotein levels. The only drug therapies that significantly raise HDL are niacin (even in doses as low as 1 g/day), gemfibrozil (weekly), and possibly atorvastatin. The associated increase in HDL with niacin therapy is occasionally dramatic but usually small. It should be kept in mind that because of the relatively lower amounts of HDL cholesterol, small changes in the concentrations of HDL cholesterol translate into larger *percentage* changes. It is estimated that every 1% increment in HDL cholesterol lowers the risk of CHD by 2%. Thus, efforts aimed at raising HDL cholesterol levels may reduce the incidence of disease.

Treatment for Patients with Normal Lipoproteins and Established Coronary Heart Disease

Caution should be exercised in placing a patient in this category because lipid levels are known to be lower for several months after a coronary event. Lipoprotein profiles should be repeated several months after a myocar-

dial infarction. Many lipid experts would argue that such patients should be treated with a goal of lowering LDL cholesterol levels to at least 100 mg/dl. The usual prudent advice about lifestyle should be given. Estrogen replacement in early postmenopausal women should be considered, but with concern for patients who smoke or who have a history of abnormal thrombosis or hypertriglyceridemia. In addition, it is reasonable to seek less common causes of atherosclerosis, such as elevated levels of serum homocysteine or increased amounts of lp(a). In some patients, 1–2 mg per day of folate lowers homocysteine concentrations and may reduce the presumed injury to the vascular wall. Lp(a) levels are modestly lowered by niacin, estrogen (in women), and gemfibrozil, but the specific impact on cardiovascular risk is unknown.

Summary

There is a misconception about heart disease in American Indians. Many members of the medical profession continue to think that American Indians either are resistant to heart disease or are less likely to have it in the light of conventional risk factors. The Strong Heart Study and other surveys of American Indians show that American Indians, as do whites, experience atherosclerosis and that recognized risk factors, such as hypertension, diabetes, central obesity, and smoking, are taking their toll among the tribes. Although tribes vary in their rates of heart disease, both coronary and peripheral vascular diseases are common problems, and rates exceed that of the U.S. population in several tribes.

Clinicians treating American Indians should be aware of the risks facing this patient population. Strategies for prevention and treatment of atherosclerosis should focus on reducing the multiple risk factors by stressing weight loss, dietary changes, increased physical activity, and cessation of smoking and by the use of drugs for hypertension, diabetes, and hyperlipidemias. It is clear that aggressive treatment reduces the incidence of both primary and secondary events and may greatly improve the cardiovascular health of American Indians.

References

1. U.S. Department of Health and Human Services. Report of the Secretary's Task Force on Black and Minority Health (Vol 1). Washington, DC: U.S. Department of Health and Human Services, August 1985.
2. Lee ET, Welty TK, Fabsitz RR, et al. The Strong Heart Study: a study of cardiovascular disease in American Indians: design and methods. Am J Epidemiol 1990; 132:1141–1155.
3. Howard BV, Welty TK, Fabsitz RR, et al. Risk factors for coronary heart disease in diabetic and nondiabetic

Native Americans: the Strong Heart Study. Diabetes 1992;41:4–11.

4. Lee ET, Howard BV, Savage PJ, et al. Diabetes and impaired glucose tolerance in three American Indian populations aged 45–74 years. Diabetes Care 1995;18:599–610.

5. Welty TK, Lee ET, Yeh J, et al. Cardiovascular disease risk factors among American Indians: the Strong Heart Study. Am J Epidemiol 1995;142:269–287.

6. National Center for Health Statistics. Health, United States, 1993 (DHHS publication no. (PHS) 94-1232). Washington, DC: US Government Printing Office, 1994.

7. Johnson CL, Rifkind BM, Sempos CT, et al. Declining serum total cholesterol levels among US adults: the National Health and Nutrition Examination Surveys. JAMA 1993;269:3002–3008.

8. Gray RS, Robbins DC, Wang W, et al. Relation of LDL size to the insulin resistance syndrome and coronary heart disease in American Indians: the Strong Heart Study. Arterioscler Thromb Vasc Biol (in press).

9. Kataoka S, Robbins DC, Cowan LD, et al. Apolipoprotein E polymorphism in American Indians and its relation to plasma lipoproteins and diabetes. The Strong Heart Study. Arterioscler Thromb Vasc Biol 1996;16:918–925.

10. Scanu AM. Lipoprotein (a). A genetic risk factor for premature coronary heart disease. JAMA 1992;267:3326–3329.

11. Bennett PH, Knowler WC, Baird HR, et al. Diet and Development of Non–Insulin-Dependent Diabetes Mellitus: An Epidemiological Perspective. In Pozza G (ed), Diet, Diabetes and Atherosclerosis. New York: Raven, 1984:109–119.

12. Snowden DA. Animal produce consumption and mortality because of all-cause combined coronary heart disease, stroke, diabetes, and cancer in Seventh-Day Adventists. Am J Clin Nutr 1988;48:7399.

13. Marshall JA, Hamman RF. Dietary lipids and glucose tolerance. The San Luis Valley Diabetes Study. Ann N Y Acad Sci 1993;683:46–56.

14. Feskins EJM, Kromhout D. Epidemiologic studies on Eskimos and fish intake. Dietary lipids and insulin action. Ann N Y Acad Sci 1993;683:9–15.

15. Boyce VL, Swinburn BA. The traditional Pima Indian diet. Composition and adaptation for use in a dietary intervention study. Diabetes Care 1993;16:369–371.

16. Despres JP. Dyslipidaemia and obesity. Bailliere s Clin Endocrinol Metab 1994;8:629–660.

17. Knowler WC, Pettitt DJ, Saad MF, Bennett PH. Diabetes mellitus in the Pima Indians: incidence, risk factors, and pathogenesis. Diabetes Metab Rev 1990;6: 1–27.

18. Robbins DC, Welty TK, Wang WY, et al. Plasma lipids and lipoprotein concentrations among American Indians: comparison with the US population. Curr Opin Lipidol 1996;7:188–195.

19. Swinburn BA, Boyce VL, Bergmen RN, et al. Deteriora-

tion in carbohydrate metabolism and lipoprotein changes induced by modern, high-fat diet in Pima Indians and Caucasians. J Clin Endocrinol Metab 1991;73:156–165.

20. McMurry MP, Cerqueira MT, Connor SL, Connor WE. Changes in lipid and lipoprotein levels and body weight in Tarahumara Indians after consumption of an affluent diet. N Engl J Med 1991;325:1704–1708.

21. Summary of the Second Report of the National Cholesterol Education Program (NCEP) Expert Panel on Detection, Evaluation, and Treatment of High Blood Cholesterol in Adults (Adult Treatment Panel II). Expert Panel on Detection, Evaluation, and Treatment of High Blood Cholesterol in Adults. JAMA 1993;269: 3015.

22. Gates G. Dyslipidemias in diabetic patients. Is standard cholesterol treatment appropriate? Postgrad Med 1994;95:69–70.

23. Haffner SM. The insulin resistance syndrome revisited. Diabetes Care 1996;19:275–277.

24. Reaven GM. Pathophysiology of insulin resistance in human disease. Physiol Rev 1995;75:473–486.

25. Kannel WB, D'Agostino RB, Wilson PW, et al. Diabetes, fibrinogen, and risk of cardiovascular disease: the Framingham experience. Am Heart J 1990;120:672-676.

26. Pyorala K, Pederson TR, Kjekshus J, et al. Cholesterol lowering with simvastatin improves prognosis of diabetic patients with coronary heart disease. A subgroup analysis of the Scandinavian Simvastatin Survival Study. Diabetes Care 1997;20:614–620.

27. Swinburn BA, Boyce BL, Bergman RN, et al. Deterioration in carbohydrate metabolism and lipoprotein changes induced by modern, high fat diet in Pima Indians and Caucasians. J Clin Endocrinol Metab 1991;73: 156–165.

28. Howard BV, Abbott WG, Swinburn BA. Evaluation of metabolic effects of substitution of complex carbohydrates for saturated fat in individuals with obesity and NIDDM. Diabetes Care 1991;14:786–795.

29. Ronnemaa T, Marniemi J, Puukka P, Kuusi T. Effects of long-term physical exercise on serum lipids, lipoproteins and lipid metabolizing enzymes in type 2 (non-insulin dependent) diabetic patients. Diabetes Res 1988;7:79–84.

30. Lampman RM, Schteingart DE. Effects of exercise training on glucose control, lipid metabolism, and insulin sensitivity in hypertriglyceridemia and non-insulin dependent diabetes mellitus. Med Sci Sports Exerc 1991;23:703–712.

31. Bernard RJ, Inkeles SB. Diet and exercise in the treatment of NIDDM. The need for early emphasis. Diabetes Care 1994;17:1469–1472.

32. Frick MH, Elo O, Haapa K, et al. Helsinki Heart Study: primary-prevention trial with gemfibrozil in middle aged men with dyslipidemia. N Engl J Med 1987; 317:1237.

Part IV
Endocrine Disorders

Chapter 22

Type 2 Diabetes Mellitus: Epidemiology, Pathogenesis, Management, and Complications

Jonathan Krakoff and Charlton A. Wilson

Diabetes is the most common reason for visits to a physician for adult patients in the Indian Health Service. Excluding pregnancy, diabetes and its complications contribute to the most inpatient hospital days and are the fourth most common cause of death. Type 2 diabetes is a chronic disease epidemic among the Native American population, and large numbers of people in many tribes have diabetes. This chapter provides a practical approach to diabetes management and focuses primarily on type 2 diabetes because this is the sort found in the majority of Native Americans.

Epidemiology

Native Americans have the highest prevalence of diabetes of any minority group in the United States. The Strong Heart Study, a study to estimate cardiovascular disease rates among Native Americans in three separate geographic areas, found the prevalence of diabetes in Pimas of Arizona ages 45–74 years to be 65%. Data from Oklahoma and the Dakotas suggest prevalence rates of 38% and 33% for the same age group in each tribe.[1] Prevalence of diabetes in other groups may be lower but is rising. Diabetes was rarely diagnosed in Native Americans before the 1950s. Pima data suggest that since then, the diabetes rate has increased from 3.2% to their current figures.

Native Americans are diagnosed with type 2 diabetes at very young ages. In other settings, their ages would suggest that they have type 1 diabetes. Studies in Pimas suggest that even young people with diabetes lack the islet cell antibodies and other autoantibodies of insulin-dependent diabetes mellitus (IDDM), which confirms that they are indeed type 2.[2] On many reservations, it is not uncommon to see patients in their teens diagnosed with type 2 diabetes.

Pathogenesis

Much of the information on the pathogenesis of diabetes comes from ongoing National Institutes of Health studies of the Pima Indians of Arizona. Current theories on the etiology of type 2 diabetes suppose an interaction between genetic and environmental factors. Crucial to understanding of the development of type 2 diabetes in Native Americans is the concept of insulin resistance. Insulin resistance is defined as the inability to clear glucose from the blood with normal levels of insulin. In an effort to maintain euglycemia, the pancreas hypersecretes insulin, resulting in higher-than-normal insulin levels.

Insulin resistance appears to be one of the earliest defects in a sequence of events leading to overt hyperglycemia. The interaction between weight gain, diets rich in fat, and a decrease in physical activity appear to worsen insulin resistance until the pancreatic beta cells (which are already overproducing insulin) "fatigue." The result of this fatigue is a relative decrease in insulin production and an increase in blood glucose.

Glucose elevations rise from normal ranges to glucose-intolerant ranges and finally diabetic ranges. With rising blood sugars, the pancreatic beta cells experience glucose toxicity with further decreases in insulin secretion. This vicious cycle can lead to significant hyperglycemia.[3]

The genetics of diabetes are under intense study. One popular theory about the high prevalence of diabetes in Native Americans is the "thrifty gene theory." This supposes that the genotype that permitted Native Americans to thrive in areas where food was scarce has

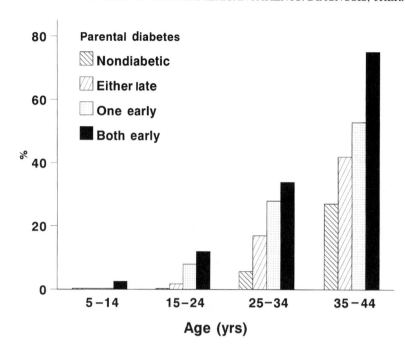

Figure 22-1. Prevalence of diabetes in Pima Indians, by presence and age of onset of diabetes in the parents. Persons for whom both parents had been examined were grouped into four groups according to parental diabetes: both early, one early, either late, or nondiabetic, according to whether the parents had diabetes and whether the parental diabetes was diagnosed before or after age 45 years. (Reprinted with permission from WC Knowler, DJ Pettit, MF Saad, PH Bennett. Diabetes mellitus in the Pima Indians: incidence, risk factors and pathogenesis. Diabetes Metab Rev 1990;6:1–27.)

led to excessive weight gain and diabetes now, in times of plentiful food and decreased activity. Type 2 diabetes appears to be polygenic, which makes genetic investigation difficult and a simple thrifty gene theory implausible.

Risk Factors

Full-blooded Native Americans are clearly at high risk for type 2 diabetes. Strong Heart Study data showed that the prevalence of diabetes increased significantly as the percentage of Native American heritage increased. Family studies in the Pima population suggest that diabetes risk increases with the declining age of diagnosis of parental diabetes (Figure 22-1). Patients with a family history of diabetes also have substantially increased risk of diabetes with increasing body mass index (Figure 22-2). Central obesity (which correlates with waist-to-hip ratio), decreased physical activity, high-calorie diets, hyperinsulinemia, history of mother with diabetes in pregnancy, and history of impaired glucose tolerance or gestational diabetes are all risk factors for development of type 2 diabetes.[4]

Diagnosis

The diagnosis of diabetes has been revised. A July 1997 publication by the Expert Committee on the Diagnosis and Classification of Diabetes Mellitus states that, to be diagnosed with diabetes, a patient must have any of these

criteria on two different days (in the absence of unequivocal hyperglycemia)[5]:

1. Symptoms of diabetes plus a random blood glucose of 200 mg/dl or higher
2. Fasting glucose of 126 mg/dl or higher (fasting = no calorie intake for at least 8 hours)
3. Fasting 75-g glucose tolerance test with a 2-hour value of 200 mg/dl or higher

Impaired glucose tolerance is defined as 2-hour post–75-g glucose tolerance test value of 140–199. A new category, impaired fasting blood glucose, is defined as fasting blood glucose of 110–126.[5]

Use of hemoglobin A_{1c} (Hgb A_{1c}) to diagnose diabetes is not a part of the diagnostic criteria, although it may be more useful in the future as the test becomes more standardized. Some studies have shown that Hgb A_{1c} greater than 7.0 (measured by high-performance liquid chromatography) strongly suggests diabetes.

Metabolic Management

Treatment of type 2, or non–insulin-dependent diabetes mellitus (NIDDM), can be difficult and frustrating for patients and providers. Although the mainstay of therapy should always include diet and exercise, social issues, such as low income with lack of food choice, absence of exercise facilities, and dearth of family support, can make these difficult to adhere to. Nutrition intervention should

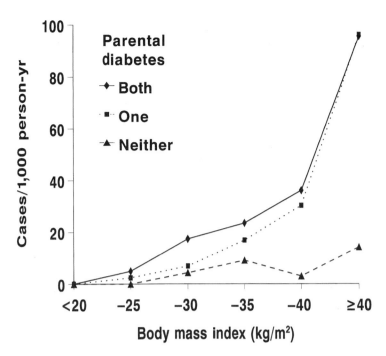

Figure 22-2. Incidence of type 2 diabetes in offspring of Pima Indians by body mass index and parental diabetes. (Reprinted with permission from WC Knowler, DJ Pettit, PJ Savage, PH Bennett. Diabetes incidence in Pima Indians: contributions of obesity and parental diabetes. Am J Epidemiol 1981;113: 144–156.)

include knowledge of local dietary habits. Patients should be encouraged to change things one step at a time to allow their palates to become accustomed to altered food tastes and because sustainable behavior changes occur gradually. Because many Native Americans live with larger family units, in which a mother or grandmother cooks, nutrition counseling to individual patients may not be fruitful unless other family members participate. Emphasis on reduction of dietary fat and total calories is essential because many newly diagnosed persons with diabetes assume that reducing table sugar or "sweet foods" is all that is required.

Exercise is clearly beneficial for diabetes treatment; moderate aerobic exercise (walking) is preferable. Exercise improves insulin sensitivity. The amount of time spent exercising per day is more important than the intensity. Heavy weightlifting is discouraged, particularly in patients with hypertension and diabetic retinopathy.

Medications are an important part of therapy. No particular medications have been studied in Native American groups, so assumptions about efficacy are extracted from other trials of NIDDM patients.

The sulfonylureas, the least expensive and oldest of the oral agents, are a good first-line choice. Sulfonylureas appear to act via a specific receptor on the beta cell, presumably stimulating insulin release. Patients on sulfonylureas typically have decreases in blood sugars while their insulin levels increase. Glimepiride, the newest sulfonylurea, may act via a separate receptor to reduce overall insulin secretion without decreasing control, which presumably provides benefits in terms of atherosclerosis, but this is unproved.

Patients typically gain weight on initiation of sulfonylureas. Hypoglycemia is a common side effect with these drugs and can be long-lasting in the case of the first-generation agents (e.g., chlorpropamide), particularly in those with decreased creatinine clearance. Despite the drugs' proved efficacy, 30% of patients fail sulfonylurea therapy over 5 years.

Metformin, approved for use in the United States in 1995, appears to act by enhancing hepatic sensitivity to insulin; patients on metformin have decreases in blood glucose and decreases in serum insulin levels. Hypoglycemia does not occur with metformin alone. Metformin also appears to have beneficial effects on blood pressure, lipids, and weight. Its use is limited by its cost, the need for multidosing, gastrointestinal side effects, and the need to avoid it in patients with the potential for decreased drug clearance (significant pulmonary, cardiac, or renal problems). Lactic acidosis, a more common feature of the drug's forerunner phenformin, is rare, but when it occurs, often happens in the setting of decreased clearance. Providers and pharmacists should review guidelines for prescribing to familiarize themselves with its contraindications. Metformin should also be stopped when patients are severely ill and before surgeries and cardiac catheterizations.

Acarbose, an alpha-galactosidase inhibitor, works by binding carbohydrates in the proximal intestine, thereby decreasing absorption proximally and increasing absorption distally. The effect is to decrease postprandial hyperglycemia. The side effects of acarbose are its limiting feature; nearly one-third of patients discontinue it because

Table 22-1. Prioritization of Glucose Control in the Clinical Setting by Duration

Clinical Setting	Treatment Priorities
No complications	Tight glucose control
DM <10 yrs	Complication screening
Early complications	Glucose control
DM >10 yrs	HTN, lipid control as important as glucose control
Significant complications (e.g., renal insufficiency, s/p CVA coronary disease)	Glucose control—perhaps not as tight
	Avoid hypoglycemia
	HTN, lipid control are crucial

DM = diabetes mellitus, HTN = hypertension, CVA = cerebrovascular accident; s/p = status post.

of increased flatus. Acarbose also requires multiple doses per day; it is best taken with the first bite of the meal.

Troglitazone, the first in a class of agents known as *thiazolidenediones*, appears to work as an insulin sensitizer. Patients on high doses of insulin are able to reduce their insulin dose on this drug. The drug can be used as monotherapy, but it appears to be effective only in patients with measurable C-peptide concentrations.[6] Troglitazone has been implicated in several episodes of severe hepatic dysfunction; current recommendations are to monitor liver function tests monthly for 6 months on beginning the medication. Troglitazone has the advantage of once-a-day dosing with few side effects, but it is extremely expensive, even compared to other newer agents.

Insulin therapy for NIDDM for those with continued poor control on oral agents is highly individualized. Split mixed preparations, combinations of neutral protamine Hagedorn (NPH) and regular insulin, and multidose regimens are acceptable. Insulin dosage for NIDDM patients is typically much higher than for IDDM patients and can approach 1–2 U/kg because of underlying insulin resistance.

Combination Therapy

Combination therapy is becoming more and more popular for NIDDM treatment as more drugs become available. However, not enough data are available to allow comment on the usefulness of many of the different combinations.

For patients on maximum-dose sulfonylureas with suboptimal control (a common scenario), there are several options. Adding metformin improves Hgb A_{1c} significantly, whereas switching from a sulfonylurea to metformin does not improve control.[7] Addition of troglitazone also seems to improve control in these patients.

The other well-studied option for these patients is a combination of insulin and oral agents. The combination of NPH at bedtime with a sulfonylurea improves control over the use of NPH alone at bedtime. The so-called bedtime insulin, daytime sulfonylurea (BIDS) therapy, has also been compared to daytime sulfonylureas with morning NPH and found to have less hypoglycemic effect. Control seems to be equal between BIDS therapy, daytime sulfonylurea with daytime NPH, and multidose insulin in 2 or 4 injections per day. Weight gain was also significantly less in the combination groups.[8] For patients more than 30% above ideal body weight, a dose of 70 over 30 insulin before dinner (as opposed to bedtime) may be more effective because NPH insulin seems to last longer in obese patients.

Acarbose has also been shown to improve glycemic control modestly in patients on a wide variety of regimens. It can be used as adjunctive treatment with insulin, metformin, or sulfonylureas, assuming that side effects are not limiting.[9]

For patients on high-dose insulin therapy, small studies have found that addition of metformin is beneficial in reducing amounts of insulin needed and improving control. Troglitazone has shown similar promising results.

Treatment Goals

It is important to tailor therapy to individual patients, keeping in mind duration of diabetes, degree of complications, and age (Table 22-1). The American Diabetes Association (ADA) guidelines, based largely on the Diabetes Control and Complications Trial (DCCT), suggest that a Hgb A_{1c} of 7.0 mg/dl or less (equaling an average blood sugar of 150 mg/dl or less) is the goal for control.[10] The ADA suggests that acceptable fasting blood glucose be less than 140 mg/dl and ideally above 115 mg/dl, and postprandial values be less than 180 mg/dl and ideally less than 120 mg/dl. Although these may be worthwhile treatment goals in relatively young type 2 patients without end-organ disease, patients who already have significant complications, particularly cardiovascular and cerebrovascular disease, may not benefit from such intensive control. Other parameters, such as hypertension and lipids, may be more important, and focusing on control may distract provider and patient from these important issues. "Loosening control" somewhat in these patients may prevent hypoglycemic events, which can be catastrophic for these patients and the elderly.

Judging the effectiveness of therapy is equally challenging. Using isolated finger-stick measures in a clinic setting can be misleading, and treatment decisions should not be made on this one value. Blood glucose self-monitoring, although very useful, has limitations in assessing control and requires more motivated patients, but home monitoring can give the patient and provider the crucial information to make changes in the treatment regimen. Glycosylated hemoglobins, particularly the Hgb A_{1c} by high-performance liquid chromatography, are especially useful to judge control. Based on DCCT data, correlation can be made between Hgb A_{1c} values and blood sugar values, thereby making it easier for patients to understand the relationship of the Hgb A_{1c} to blood glucose (Table 22-2).

Complications Management

Renal

Between 1982 and 1994, the number of diabetics on dialysis increased fivefold; diabetic nephropathy is now the number one cause of end-stage renal disease (ESRD). From 1987 to 1990, diabetic ESRD incidence for Native Americans was six times the rate for whites.

As research into diabetic nephropathy has given insight into early changes involved in the advance to ESRD,[11] more attention is being paid to early detection and treatment as a means of delaying or preventing dialysis. Understanding terms that pertain to the albumin excretion rate is crucial to effective screening (Table 22-3). Screening for microalbuminuria is now recommended by the ADA. Dipsticks to detect microalbuminuria are relatively inexpensive and have a good positive predictive value (Table 22-4), but a patient must have two positive tests to have true microalbuminuria.[12] Although data on whether targeted treatment of microalbuminuria delays or prevents ESRD is lacking, the progression of diabetic nephropathy from microalbuminuria to macroalbuminuria to renal insufficiency to ESRD is well documented. Investigations into treatments in each phase report decreases in albuminuria and, in the later stages, a delay in doubling of creatinine and the need for dialysis.

Screening for microalbuminuria can be expensive and confusing. Many factors can confound the screening process. A careful combination of dipsticks for microalbumin and urine for albumin-creatinine ratio can be used to implement a cost-effective program (Figure 22-3). If a patient has microalbuminuria, treatment with an angiotensin-converting enzyme (ACE) inhibitor can be considered even in normotensive individuals,[13, 14] and intensification of glycemic control appears to slow disease progression. Microalbuminuria also appears to be an independent risk factor for cardiovascular disease.

Diabetic patients with gross proteinuria or macroalbuminuria have positive protein on a routine urine dipstick. Most routine urine dipsticks begin to detect proteinuria when it reaches 360 mg of albumin excreted per day. The diagnostic question that often arises in this clinical situation is how to confirm that this is indeed diabetic nephropathy. Diabetic nephropathy is a diagnosis of exclusion; some screening tests to rule out other disease are

appropriate. A good eye examination is crucial in this situation because diabetic nephropathy is usually accompanied by diabetic retinopathy. The absence of diabetic retinopathy should prompt consideration of alternate diagnosis or referral to a nephrologist. For those with isolated proteinuria (i.e., no other urine sediment, such as RBCs or casts) and diabetic retinopathy, a screening serum protein electrophoresis, urine electrophoresis, antinuclear antibody testing, and renal ultrasound are usually sufficient to exclude other possible kidney diseases. If these are without abnormalities, then the diagnosis is usually secure. Quantification of how much protein a patient is spilling is also important; this can be done with a 24-hour urine for protein and creatinine or a spot urine for protein-creatinine ratio. The spot urine test correlates well with the 24-hour urine and can be done more readily.[15] Patients with greater degrees of proteinuria, especially with nephrotic features, appear to progress faster.

Treatment for diabetic nephropathy involves strict control of hypertension, with an eye toward improving intraglomerular hemodynamics. ACE inhibitors are the drugs of choice for this; numerous studies have shown that ACE inhibitors reduce micro- and macroalbuminuria, slow the doubling time of creatinine, and delay ESRD, often independent of blood pressure effects.[16, 17] Although some of these studies were performed in IDDM patients,

Table 22-2. Correlation Between Hemoglobin A_{1c} (Hgb A_{1C}) and Blood Glucose*

Hgb A_{1c} (%) by HPLC	Blood Glucose (mg/dl)
5	90
6	120
7	150
8	180
9	210
10	240
11	270
12	300

HPLC = high-performance liquid chromatography.
*Please note that there is variation between laboratory tests. Standardization of the Hgb A_{1c} assay is ongoing.

Table 22-3. Quantification of Albuminuria in Diabetic Kidney Disease

	μg/min	mg/g of Creatinine	mg/L
Normoalbuminuria	<20	<30	<20
Microalbuminuria	20–200	30–300	20–200
Macroalbuminuria	>200	>300	>200

Table 22-4. Sensitivity and Specificity of Micral Dipsticks Using Cutoff Value of ≥20 mg/L

Sensitivity	97%
Specificity	72%
Positive predictive value	94%
Positive predictive value of negative test	84%

Source: Adapted from CE Morgensen, E Vestbo, PL Paulsen, et al. Microalbuminuria and potential confounders. Diabetes Care 1995;4:577–581.

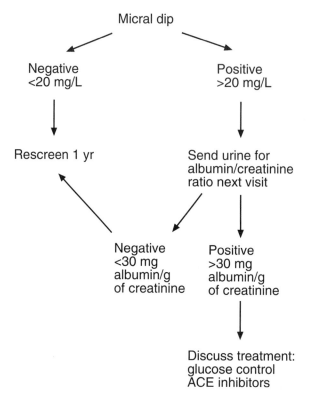

Figure 22-3. Suggested protocol for microalbuminuria screening. (dip = dipstick; ACE = angiotensin-converting enzyme.)

the pathophysiology appears to be close enough to extrapolate to NIDDM patients.

For patients who cannot tolerate ACE inhibitors, verapamil, diltiazem, nicardipine, or losartan may be reasonable alternatives because they have been shown to decrease proteinuria. These agents, however, have not been as well studied as ACE inhibitors.

As diabetic nephropathy advances, blood pressure control emerges as the most important parameter. Blood pressure goals below the usual target of 140/90 mm Hg may be appropriate in this situation. Any agent that lowers blood pressure is appropriate. Control of hyperlipidemia also appears to be important. As creatinine starts to rise above 1.5 mg/dl, patients may have a paradoxical improvement in blood sugar levels because of decreased insulin clearance. In later stages of disease, attention should be paid to calcium and phosphate metabolism and anemia. Many nephrologists begin dialyzing diabetics when their creatinine rises above 5.0 mg/dl or their creatinine clearance drops to less than 15 ml/minute.

Foot Care

The combination of macrovascular and neurologic insults in diabetes can make the foot particularly vulnerable to complications. Diabetes is the most common underlying reason for amputations, and care for diabetic foot ulcers requires multiple visits and prolonged hospital stays. The emphasis in diabetic foot care should be on prevention.

Components of a diabetic foot examination should include inspection for calluses, corns, abnormal rubbing from improper shoe wear, and deformities; palpation of peripheral pulses; and monofilament testing. Trimming corns and calluses and correcting footwear can often prevent ulcers. Monofilament screening is crucial to identifying high-risk patients. Screening should be done with a 5.07 Semmes-Weinstein filament (approximating 10 g of pressure) on nine points on the foot (Figure 22-4). Failure to sense this monofilament, except in the heel area, where skin thickness may interfere, denotes loss of protective sensation in that area. Studies suggest that risk of foot ulcer in these patients is 10 times the rate in sensate patients.

Treatment of the diabetic foot should include counseling on footwear (for normal sensate feet, running shoes are ideal) and advising patients to check feet daily, to avoid going barefoot, and to use moisturizing creams without alcohol or perfume. For patients who lack protective sensation, consideration should be given to providing extra-depth shoes. These are molded to the patient's feet to reduce abnormal pressures and prevent ulceration. Patients who lack protective sensation should have their feet checked by a provider monthly.

Care for ulcer is beyond the scope of this chapter, but identification of high-risk versus low-risk ulcers can help determine who needs hospitalization and surgical care and who can be treated as an outpatient (Table 22-5). Follow-up of ulcers should be active, especially as insensate patients may ignore lesions until the infection becomes severe.

Diabetic neuropathy symptoms can be painful. Typical symptoms include hyperesthesia, lancinating or burning pain, and muscle cramping. Symptoms are often made worse by bedclothes or sheets and are typically worse at night (as opposed to ischemic pain).Treatment is directed at pain relief. A nonsteroidal anti-inflammatory drug or acetaminophen is a reasonable first choice, but for patients with more severe symptoms, amitriptyline, desipramine, or nortriptyline adjusted to doses of 100–150 mg qhs can provide significant relief. Capsaicin cream is also useful.

Neuropathy

Diabetic neuropathy can manifest in a variety of ways, but peripheral neuropathy in the lower extremities is the most common form. Diabetic gastroparesis, erectile dysfunction, chronic diarrhea and constipation, orthostatic hypotension, and neurogenic bladder are examples of autonomic neuropathies. Mononeuropathies can affect the third, fourth, and sixth cranial nerves or spinal nerves, simulating disk disease.

Eye Disease

Poorly controlled persons with diabetes often complain of blurry vision. This is a result of osmotic swelling of the lens and an inability to focus. Glasses prescriptions for these patients should be deferred until the patient has reached steady-state glycemic control.

Patients with diabetes do have higher rates of cataracts and glaucoma, but retinopathy is the biggest threat to vision. Because type 2 patients may have been hyperglycemic for 5 years before diagnosis, screening for retinopathy should begin at diagnosis. Screening should be continued yearly by a qualified provider (usually an optometrist or ophthalmologist) with a dilated examination. Background or nonproliferative retinopathy, characterized by small excretions of proteins and aneurysmal (dot and blot) hemorrhage, is relatively stable and heralds possible progression. Proliferative retinopathy, marked by neovascularization, often requires intervention because new vessels are weak and can lead to retinal detachment or hemorrhage with vision loss. Laser photocoagulation therapy can often prevent these complications.

Macrovascular Disease

It is important to realize that the number one cause of mortality in people with diabetes is macrovascular disease. The type 2 diabetic's risk of coronary disease is two to five times normal. There is considerable debate as to

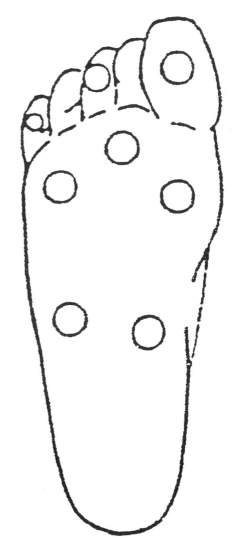

Figure 22-4. The nine-point monofilament examination includes the areas shown plus the dorsum of the foot. When calluses are present, the area of normal skin next to the callus should be tested, not the callus itself. To prevent biased results, examination should be performed with the patient's eyes closed; the patient says yes when he or she feels the monofilament. The monofilament should be pressed against the skin enough to bend it.

the role of hyperglycemia in the development of macrovascular (particularly coronary) disease.[18] Although it was not specifically designed to answer the question of glycemic control and macrovascular disease risk, the DCCT did show a nonsignificant trend toward lower low-density lipoprotein (LDL) levels with tight glycemic control. Data from the United Kingdom Prospective Diabetes Study, which was designed to look at the role of glycemic control with various treatment regimens and the risk of macrovascular disease, should be available in 1998.

Table 22-5. Factors in Determining Foot Ulcer Management

Clinical Picture	Management
Superficial ulcer, no infection	Strict nonweightbearing, wound care
Superficial ulcer	Strict nonweightbearing
< 2 cm of cellulitis	Antibiotics
No ischemia	Wound care
No bone or joint involvement	
Adequate social support	
Full-thickness ulcer	Hospitalize
> 2 cm of cellulitis	Antibiotics
Systemic toxicity	Metabolic control
Ischemia	Surgical intervention with
Joint or bone involvement	debridement or amputation
Poor social situation	Revascularization as needed
	Wound care

Source: Adapted from GM Caputo, PR Cavanagh, JS Ulbrecht, et al. Assessment and management of foot disease in patients with diabetes. N Engl J Med 1994;331:854–860.

Because of neuropathy, coronary artery disease may present more atypically, so an increased level of clinical suspicion can lead to earlier diagnosis. Control of other risk factors, such as tobacco use, hypertension, and lipids, is also crucial. Screening for lipid abnormalities should be performed on a yearly basis with a fasting lipid panel to assess total cholesterol, high-density lipoprotein (HDL), triglycerides, and LDL. High triglyceride levels accompanied by low HDL is typical in NIDDM patients. Intervention for lipid abnormalities in diabetic patients should occur when LDL exceeds 130 mg/dl, triglycerides exceed 150 mg/dl, or HDL is less than 35 mg/dl. Start by attempting to improve glucose control and diet. For those with LDL above 130 mg/dl, triglycerides above 250 mg/dl, or HDL less than 35 mg/dl, medical therapy should be considered. Patients with known coronary disease should have target LDL at less than 100 mg/dl and triglycerides below 150 mg/dl.[19]

Although it is not as well studied, the presence of peripheral vascular or carotid disease also should prompt aggressive lipid treatment in the hope of disease regression and on the assumption that macrovascular disease in one area probably signals disease in other areas.

Periodontal Disease

Diabetes is associated with an increased risk of periodontal disease. Periodontal disease can lead to gum line recession and eventual tooth loss. Appropriate dental care can prevent or treat many of these problems and avoid

Table 22-6. Minimum Standards of Care for Patients with Diabetes in the Indian Health Service

Baseline studies
  Height
  Date of diagnosis
Each clinic visit
  Blood pressure
  Weight
  Blood glucose
  Foot check
Immunizations
  Flu vaccine, annual
  Pneumovax, once
  Diphtheria-tetanus, every 10 yrs
  Purified protein derivative status
Self-care education
  Nutrition education regularly; nutritionist every 6 mos to 1 yr
  Diabetes education
  Exercise education
  Blood glucose self-monitoring
  Diabetes prevention education
Annually
  Creatinine
  Complete urinalysis; include microalbuminuria if available
  Cholesterol and triglyceride levels
  Eye examination
  Dental examination
  Complete foot examination
  Screen for neuropathy
Health maintenance
  Physical examination as baseline
  Pap smear and pelvic examination, annual
  Breast examination, annual
  Mammogram every 1–2 years for ages 40–49 yrs, yearly older than 50 yrs
  Rectal examination and stool guaiac, annually for adults older than 40 yrs
Other
  ECG baseline; repeat every 1–5 yrs as needed
Special tests
  Hemoglobin A_{1c}
  C-peptide

ECG = electrocardiogram.

tooth loss. Patients with diabetes should see their dentist at least once and ideally twice a year.[20]

Public Health Aspects of Diabetes

As with tuberculosis in the early 1900s, diabetes is an epidemic. The Indian Health Service has developed minimum standards of care for patients with diabetes to aid providers in caring for these patients (Table 22-6). The Indian Health

Service also conducts yearly audits of service units to assess aspects of diabetes care and give local providers a sense of which areas need improvement.[21] These data are available from the local area office. Education materials on a wide variety of topics specifically developed for Native Americans are also available free of charge.

Local hospitals and clinics are encouraged to develop their own flow sheets to keep track of yearly screening examinations for diabetics and their own education programs. Service units, such as Sacaton and Claremore, have developed ADA-accredited education programs.

Conclusion

Diabetes is a complicated and frustrating disease for patients and providers. Systematic approaches to screening and acceptance of any improvement in glycemic control as progress (while maintaining ideal goals) can make treatment of these patients more satisfying.

Summary Points

1. Type 2 diabetes is the type overwhelmingly found among Native Americans.
2. Prevalence varies from tribe to tribe, with the highest prevalence found in the Pimas of Arizona.
3. Insulin resistance precedes the development of diabetes.
4. Risk factors for NIDDM include family history, obesity, decreased physical activity, hyperinsulinemia, and history of impaired glucose tolerance or gestational diabetes.
5. Specific diagnostic criteria exist for the diagnosis of diabetes.
6. Diet and exercise are the mainstays of therapy; exercise therapy is directed at duration rather than intensity of exercise.
7. Combination therapy is useful in the management of NIDDM; well-studied examples include BIDS therapy, and combined use of sulfonylureas and metformin.
8. Hemoglobin A_{1c} is more useful in judging glucose control than random blood sugars in clinic.
9. Goals for diabetic therapy should be tailored to individual patients.
10. Screening for microalbuminuria can be done cost effectively.
11. Diabetic nephropathy is a diagnosis of exclusion, usually in the presence of retinopathy; ACE inhibitors are the first choice for therapy.
12. Prevention is key for diabetic foot care; use of monofilament testing can identify high-risk patients.
13. Eye examinations should be done annually by a trained provider.
14. Macrovascular disease is still the number one cause

of death in diabetics; fasting fractionated lipid screens should be part of routine care.
15. The Indian Health Service does a yearly audit of diabetes care; the local area office can furnish providers with these results.

Acknowledgments

The authors would like to thank Dorothy Gohdes, M.D., F.A.C.P., for her help in preparing this chapter.

References

1. Knowler WC, Bennett PH, Botazao LF, Doniach D. Islet cell antibodies and diabetes mellitus in Pima Indians. Diabetologia 1979;17:161–164.
2. Lee ET, Howard BV, Savage PR, et al. Diabetes and impaired glucose tolerance in three American Indian populations aged 45–74 years. Diabetes Care 1995;18: 599–610.
3. Polonsky KS, Sturis J, Bell G. Non-insulin dependent diabetes mellitus—a genetically programmed failure of the beta cell to compensate for insulin resistance. N Engl J Med 1996;334:777–783.
4. Gohdes D. Diabetes in North American Indians and Alaska Natives. Diabetes of America (2nd ed). NIH publication no. 95-1468. Bethesda, MD: National Institutes of Health, NIDDK, 1995;683–701.
5. Gavin JR, Alberti KGMM, Davidson MB, et al. Report of the Expert Committee on the Diagnosis and Classification of Diabetes Mellitus. Diabetes Care 1997;20: 1183–1197.
6. Saltiel AR, Olefsky JM. Thiazolidinediones in the treatment of insulin resistance and type II diabetes. Diabetes 1996;45:1661–1670.
7. Defronzo RA, Goodman AM. Multicenter Metformin Study Group. Efficacy of metformin in patients with non-insulin dependent diabetes mellitus. N Engl J Med 1995;333:541–549.
8. Yki-Jarvinen H, Kauppila M, Kujansu E, et al. Comparison of insulin regimens in patients with non-insulin dependent diabetes mellitus. N Engl J Med 1992;327: 1426–1433.
9. Chiasson JL, Josse RG, et al. The efficacy of acarbose in the treatment of patients with non-insulin dependent diabetes mellitus. Ann Intern Med 1994;121:928–935.
10. The Diabetes Control and Complications Trial Research Group. The effect of intensive treatment of diabetes on the development and progression of long term complications in insulin-dependent diabetes mellitus. N Engl J Med 1993;329:977–984.
11. Neslon RG, Bennett PH, Beck GJ, et al. Development and progression of renal disease in Pima Indians with non–insulin-dependent diabetes mellitus. N Engl J Med 1996;335:1636–1642.
12. Mogensen CE, Vestbo E, Paulsen PL, et al. Microalbuminuria and potential confounders. Diabetes Care 1995;18:572–581.

13. Ravid M, Savin H, Jutrin I, et al. Long-term stabilizing effect of angiotensin-converting enzyme inhibition on plasma creatinine and on proteinuria in normotensive type 2 diabetic patients. Ann Intern Med 1993;118: 577–581.
14. Ahmad J, Siddiqui MA, Ahmad H. Effective postponement of diabetic nephropathy with enalapril in normotensive type 2 diabetic patients with microalbuminuria. Diabetes Care 1997;20:1576–1581.
15. Rodby RA, Rohde RD, Sharon Z, et al. The urine protein to creatinine ratio as a predictor of 24-hour urine protein excretion in type 1 diabetic patients with nephropathy. The Collaborative Study Group. Am J Kidney Dis 1995;26:904–909.
16. Kasiske BL, Kalil RS, Ma JZ, et al. Effect of antihypertensive therapy on the kidney in patients with diabetes: a meta-regression analysis. Ann Intern Med 1993;118: 129–138.
17. Lewis EJ, Hunsicker LG, Bain RF, et al. The effect of angiotensin-converting enzyme inhibition on diabetic nephropathy. N Engl J Med 1993;329:1456–1462.
18. Barret-Connor E. Does hyperglycemia really cause coronary disease? Diabetes Care 1997;20:1620–1623.
19. Garber AJ, Vinik AI, Crespin SR. Detection and management of lipid disorders in diabetic patients. Diabetes Care 1992;15:1068–1074.
20. Dennison DK, Gottsegen R, Rose LF. Diabetes and periodontal disease. J Periodontol 1996;67:166–176.
21. Gohdes D, Rith-Najarian S, Acton K, Shields R. Improving diabetes care in the primary health setting. The Indian Health Service experience. Ann Intern Med 1996;124: 149–152.

Part V
Oncology

Chapter 23
Epidemiologic Patterns of Cancer

Nathaniel Cobb

At the end of the nineteenth century, cancer was considered a rare disease among Native Americans.[1] Infectious diseases and accidents were the leading health problems, and few people lived long enough to develop cancer. As we near the end of the century, under the influence of changing patterns of smoking, diet, environmental exposures, and the aging of the population, the incidence of cancer has increased steadily. By the 1980s, cancer was the third leading cause of death for American Indians and Alaska Natives, after heart disease and injuries. Indian Health Service (IHS) statistics show that in 1993, the number of cancer deaths exceeded accidental deaths, moving into second place.[2] This chapter reviews the available cancer mortality and incidence data, discusses the reasons for variations in cancer rates, and recommends approaches to cancer screening.

Mortality

Death certificates are the most reliable source of information about causes of death among Native Americans. Each state records deaths through a system of coroners and medical examiners. The National Center for Health Statistics then compiles death certificates from state reports into a single file, which is the source of data for most mortality studies. Race is recorded in this file as American Indian or Alaska Native. Several studies have shown that death certificates frequently identify native people as white or Hispanic,[3, 4] however, which can result in significant undercounting of cancer deaths.

In the 1950s, the Bureau of Indian Affairs used death certificate data to publish statistics showing that cancer death rates among Native Americans were considerably lower than among whites.[5] Researchers at the National Cancer Institute confirmed these findings in a series of publications. They demonstrated that the low rates were only partially explained by short life expectancy (in 1964, American Indians lived an average of 20 years less than whites), competing causes of death, and lack of diagnosis. Several researchers at the time also noted that the types of cancer observed differed significantly from the pattern observed in other U.S. populations.[6]

More recent studies have continued to find that the overall cancer mortality rate among Native Americans is lower than that of other U.S. races,[7, 8] even when sampling is designed to minimize racial misclassification (Figures 23-1 through 23-3). The overall Native American rate of death from cancer in 1993 was 148 per 100,000 (adjusted for age), which is 14% lower than the U.S. death rate of 172 per 100,000. The pattern of occurrence observed in the 1950s still applies in most areas. Women die less frequently of cancer of the lung and breast and more frequently of cancer of the cervix, gallbladder, and kidney than the U.S. all races population (Figures 23-4 through 23-6). Men have lower death rates from cancer of the lung, prostate, colon, and pancreas and higher rates of death from cancer of the stomach, liver, and kidney. When death rates are broken down regionally, it is apparent that there are marked geographic differences, most notably for lung and breast cancer.

Incidence

Historically, there have been only a few reliable sources for cancer incidence (newly diagnosed cases) among American Indians.[9] The first and best source for incidence data is the New Mexico Tumor Registry (NMTR), which has been in existence since 1966 and is now part of the National Cancer Institute's Surveillance, Epidemiology, and End Results (SEER) program. Established by

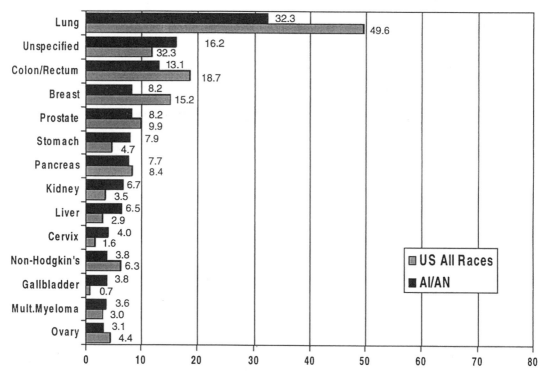

Figure 23-1. Age-adjusted death rates for the leading causes of cancer mortality among Native Americans compared with death rates for all U.S. races. Native American death certificate data are from U.S. counties containing Indian lands or reservations. U.S. all races death rates are from National Cancer Institute data for 1988–1992. Rate per 100,000, adjusted to the 1970 U.S. population. (AI = American Indian; AN = Alaska Native; Mult. = multiple.) (Adapted from N Cobb, RE Paisano. Cancer Mortality among American Indians and Alaska Natives in the United States, 1989–1993. IHS Pub. No. 97-615-23. Rockville, MD: Indian Health Service, 1997; and CL Kosary, LAG Ries, BA Miller, et al. [eds]. SEER Cancer Statistics Review, 1973–1992: Tables and Graphs. NIH Pub. No. 96-2789. Bethesda, MD: National Cancer Institute, 1995.)

the National Cancer Act of 1971, the SEER system is responsible for monitoring the impact of cancer on the general population. The five state registries (Connecticut, Hawaii, Iowa, New Mexico, and Utah) and six metropolitan registries (Atlanta, Detroit, Los Angeles, San Francisco/Oakland, San Jose/Monterey, and Seattle/Puget Sound) that are SEER reporting sites were selected to represent the diversity of American people.

From its inception, the NMTR was concerned with accurate counting of cases in a multiracial and multiethnic state. It has developed procedures, such as data linkage with IHS and abstractor training, that result in more accurate racial classification than is found in other registries. Since 1969, the NMTR has collected data from all Navajo-area IHS sites, including those in Arizona. To increase the representation of American Indians in SEER, in 1980 the NMTR began collecting cancer cases from all IHS sites in Arizona. Since 1994, a data-sharing agreement with the Arizona Cancer Registry and the IHS has improved collection of cases among American Indians who do not receive their health care through IHS.

In 1974, the Alaska Native Cancer Surveillance Project began efforts to collect cancer incidence and mortality data for Alaska Natives, and since 1984, the data collected has conformed with the SEER format. Retrospective case findings have extended the database for Alaska Natives back to 1969. This valuable registry is now known as the Alaska Native Tumor Registry (ANTR), and is funded in part by the National Cancer Institute. Although it is not technically a SEER registry, data from the ANTR are used by the SEER program to report on cancer incidence for Alaska Natives.[10] Currently, the SEER program sites, including Alaska, cover 27% of the Native American population. This combined database is extremely useful for some purposes, but combining Alaska Natives with southwestern tribes may not give a cancer picture that is representative of either region because of very different dietary and tobacco use patterns.

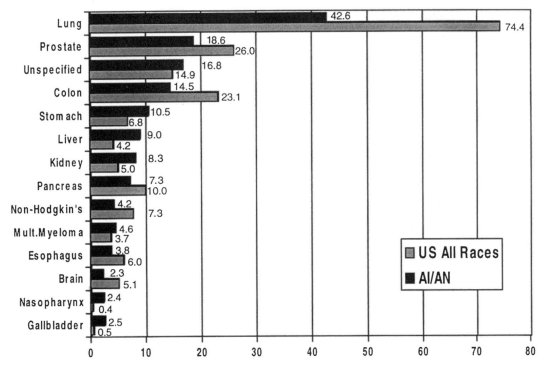

Figure 23-2. Age-adjusted death rates for the leading causes of cancer mortality among Native American men compared with death rates for men of all U.S. races. Native American death certificate data are from U.S. counties containing Indian lands or reservations. U.S. all races death rates are from National Cancer Institute data from 1988–1992. Rate per 100,000, adjusted to the 1970 U.S. population. (AI = American Indian; AN = Alaska Native; Mult. = multiple.) (Adapted from N Cobb, RE Paisano. Cancer Mortality among American Indians and Alaska Natives in the United States, 1989–1993. IHS Pub. No. 97-615-23. Rockville, MD: Indian Health Service, 1997; and CL Kosary, LAG Ries, BA Miller, et al. [eds], SEER Cancer Statistics Review, 1973–1992: Tables and Graphs. NIH Pub. No. 96-2789. Bethesda, MD: National Cancer Institute, 1995.)

Many states have cancer registries; the number has been increasing since the Centers for Disease Control and Prevention (CDC) started a national registries program in 1994. Most state registries receive their data from hospital reporting and do not capture all cancer cases from the state, often missing federal facilities, such as Veteran's Administration hospitals and the IHS. Racial misclassification is also a common problem in many state registries. In an attempt to improve classification of race, several state cancer registries have begun sharing data and matching agreements with the IHS. Few states other than Alaska, New Mexico, and Arizona find that they have enough American Indian or Alaska Native cancer cases to report incidence rates separately from the general population.

Cancer incidence for Alaska Natives, New Mexico Indians, and U.S. whites is shown in Tables 23-1 and 23-2. The dramatic differences between the three groups are evident in these tables. Of particular interest are the low rates of lung, colon, and breast cancer among New Mexico Indians and the high stomach and colon cancer rates among Alaska Natives. Rather sparse data from other areas indicate that other American Indian groups have cancer incidence rates that fall somewhere between these extremes.

There is no evidence at this time that these differences are due to genetic factors. To understand the variation in cancer rates, it is important to remember that Native American populations are diverse, with a wide range of diets, environmental exposures, and personal customs. Alaska Natives have a high-fat diet and tend to smoke more than southwestern tribes, who use less tobacco than any group in the United States. Tribes from the Great Plains and northern states also have high smoking rates, which is reflected in their lung cancer statistics.

To explain the colon cancer rates, it should be noted that Alaska Natives have a diet that includes a heavy preponderance of meat and fat, whereas southwestern Indians until quite recently had a diet of corn,

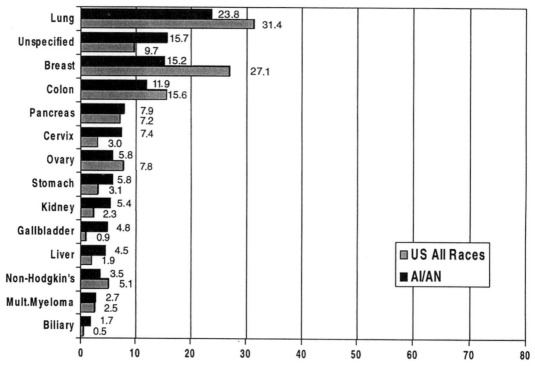

Figure 23-3. Age-adjusted death rates for the leading causes of cancer mortality among Native American women compared with death rates for women of all U.S. races. Native American death certificate data are from U.S. counties containing Indian lands or reservations. U.S. all races death rates are from National Cancer Institute data for 1988–92. Rate per 100,000, adjusted to the 1970 U.S. population. (AI = American Indian; AN = Alaska Native; Mult. = multiple.) (Adapted from N Cobb, RE Paisano. Cancer Mortality among American Indians and Alaska Natives in the United States, 1989–1993. IHS Pub. No. 97-615-23. Rockville, MD: Indian Health Service, 1997; and CL Kosary, LAG Ries, BA Miller, et al. [eds]. SEER Cancer Statistics Review, 1973–1992: Tables and Graphs. NIH Pub. No. 96-2789. Bethesda, MD: National Cancer Institute, 1995.)

beans, squash, and wild meat that was relatively low in fat.

The remarkably low incidence of breast cancer among southwestern Indian women clearly deserves further investigation. Known risk factors for breast cancer, such as reproductive factors and family history, can only explain approximately one-fourth of breast cancer cases. It seems likely that the difference in breast cancer rates between white and Indian women has other determinants, possibly environmental.[11]

The difference in lung cancer rates is explained by regional differences in smoking habits. Lung cancer among New Mexico Indian men is extremely rare and almost always associated with a history of working in uranium mines in the 1950s.[12]

The reason for high stomach cancer rates is a subject of considerable research interest. Chronic infection with *Helicobacter pylori* is thought to be a contributing cause.

Liver cancer is more common among Native Americans because of a higher rate of chronic hepatitis B infection and alcohol-related liver disease.

A Note on Calculating Rates

In calculating rates, whether of incidence or mortality, the count of the population at risk (also known as the *denominator*) is a critical part of the equation. For American Indian and Alaska Native health statistics, there are several choices of denominator. The most commonly used source for population counts is the U.S. census. Census figures are easily available, and they are the most accurate population counts available for most purposes. Several issues are important when using census data for Native Americans. First, race is self-identified, so a person is counted as American Indian or Alaska Native if they check that box, regardless of ancestry or tribal enrollment. This can lead to the *Dances with Wolves* phenomenon: When being Indian is considered a positive thing, census counts may increase, whereas at other times, some Indian people may choose not to identify themselves as such because of concerns about discrimination. The other problem is that census counts are often much larger than the "service population" count of the IHS, which includes only enrolled members of federally recognized

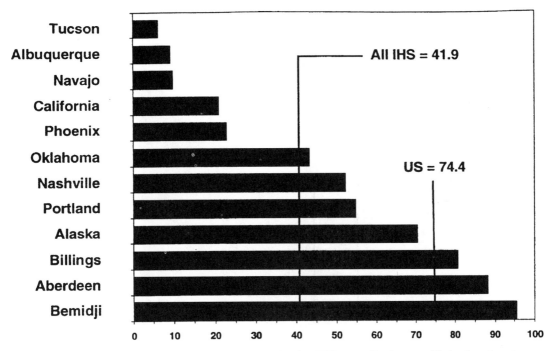

Figure 23-4. Male lung cancer death rates for Indian Health Service (IHS) areas. Southwestern Native Americans have markedly lower lung cancer rates, whereas northern plains and Alaska Natives are comparable to U.S. all races death rates. Rate per 100,000 per year, adjusted to the 1970 U.S. population. (Reprinted with permission from N Cobb, RE Paisano. Cancer Mortality among American Indians and Alaska Natives in the United States, 1989–1993. IHS Pub. No. 97-615-23. Rockville, MD: Indian Health Service, 1997.)

tribes who live on or near reservations. This count almost totally excludes the large urban Indian groups in many cities as well as members of tribes that are not federally recognized. A third problem is that the U.S. census has often been criticized for undercounting poor and homeless populations, which may include significant numbers of urban Native Americans. It is important to consider these issues when choosing a source of population data and when looking at health statistics for this population.

Screening and Clinical Practice

The unusual pattern of cancer occurrence in Native American communities suggests some modifications to the standard approach to screening and treatment.

The low rates of breast cancer among Indian women make mammography an expensive screening tool, and until recently it was available at only a few IHS sites. Since 1991, funding from the CDC has allowed many IHS sites to obtain mammography, and the standard of care now includes routine mammography (every 1 or 2 years) for all women older than age 50 years. A relatively high proportion of premenopausal breast cancers among Indian women reinforces the need for careful clinical breast examination for women of all ages.

The most common risk factor for cancer of the gallbladder is cholelithiasis. The high rate of gallbladder cancer indicates that clinicians should consider cholecystectomy for Indian people with gallstones, even if asymptomatic. Indeed, the recent decline in gallbladder cancer rates is probably caused by the increase in cholecystectomy for other indications. However, there is no screening test for gallbladder cancer.

Cervical cancer rates remain high both among young and elderly Native American women. The IHS policy calls for annual Pap screening for all women older than 18 years (or on becoming sexually active). Child sexual abuse may be a risk factor for cervical cancer, and such a history should trigger earlier screening.

There is no good screening test for stomach cancer, but a high index of suspicion should be maintained whenever

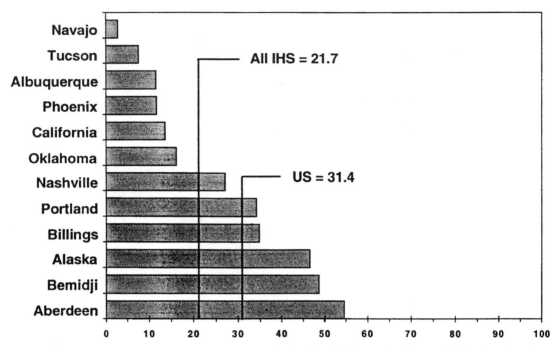

Figure 23-5. Female lung cancer death rates for Indian Health Service (IHS) areas. Southwestern Native Americans have markedly lower lung cancer rates, whereas those for northern plains and Alaska Natives are comparable to U.S. all races death rates. Rate per 100,000 per year, adjusted to the 1970 U.S. population. (Reprinted with permission from N Cobb, RE Paisano. Cancer Mortality among American Indians and Alaska Natives in the United States, 1989–1993. IHS Pub. No. 97-615-23. Rockville, MD: Indian Health Service, 1997.)

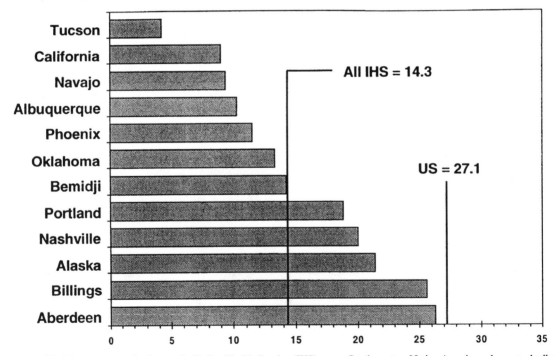

Figure 23-6. Breast cancer death rates for Indian Health Service (IHS) areas. Southwestern Native Americans have markedly lower breast cancer rates, whereas those of northern plains and Alaska Natives are comparable to U.S. all races death rates. Rate per 100,000 per year, adjusted to 1970 U.S. population. (Reprinted with permission from N Cobb, RE Paisano. Cancer Mortality among American Indians and Alaska Natives in the United States, 1989–1993. IHS Pub. No. 97-615-23. Rockville, MD: Indian Health Service, 1997.)

Table 23-1. Cancer Incidence, Men, 1988–1992[a]

Cancer Site	Alaska Native Rate[b]	American Indian Rate[c]	White Rate
All sites	372.0	196.0	469.0
Lung	81.1	14.4	76.0
Colon	65.6	13.0	38.9
Prostate	46.1	52.5	134.7
Stomach	27.2	—[d]	10.2

[a]Rates per 100,000. Age-adjusted to U.S. 1970 population.
[b]From Alaska Native Tumor Registry.
[c]New Mexico Indians only.
[d]Rates not calculated when less than 25 cases.
Source: Adapted from BA Miller, LN Kolonel, L Bernstein, et al. (eds). Racial/Ethnic Patterns of Cancer in the United States 1988–1992. NIH Pub. No. 96-4104. Bethesda, MD: National Cancer Institute, 1996.

there is unexplained gastrointestinal blood loss or stomach symptoms. There is not yet enough information to recommend routine screening for or treatment of *H. pylori* infection as a measure to prevent stomach cancer.

A high rate of occult gastrointestinal blood loss among Alaska Natives frustrates the clinician who wants to screen for colon cancer. Research indicates that chronic gastritis related to *H. pylori* infection is often the cause of such blood loss. Given the expense and morbidity associated with colonoscopy, a reasonable algorithm may be to treat first for *H. pylori* and proceed with the full gastrointestinal workup only if fecal occult blood is still found. This is an area of medicine that is changing rapidly, and the clinician should consult the most recent literature available.

Social Context

Most Native American languages do not have a word for cancer in their vocabulary, presumably because it was such a rare disease in the past. Many now refer to cancer as "the sore that does not heal" or some variation on that theme. This name reflects a fatalistic attitude that is found in many communities. The reluctance to talk about negative outcomes is common, and it can be a real deterrent to adequate care and informed decision making with patients and their families. The clinician should be aware of the social isolation and hopelessness that a cancer patient may experience. If the patient has a cancer that might be curable, it is important to be very clear in communicating that fact. Many patients automatically believe that their disease is incurable and may refuse what they perceive as palliative treatment. Referral to a cancer support group or to another community member who is a cancer survivor can be very helpful. If the patient is interested in traditional healing methods, the physician should point out that it is possible to have both traditional and modern treatments, often simultaneously. Logistic difficulties often interfere with cancer treatment because the recommended course may involve frequent long drives to a radiation oncology center or cancer center. Issues of child care, travel expenses, and fear of the medical center environment combine to reduce the likelihood of compliance with treatment for cancer. The gender of the provider can also be a barrier to screening and care, especially among older women.

Table 23-2. Cancer Incidence, Women, 1988–1992[a]

Cancer Site	Alaska Native Rate[b]	American Indian Rate[c]	White Rate
All sites	348.0	180.0	346.0
Breast, invasive	78.9	31.6	111.8
Colon	52.2	—[d]	28.2
Lung	50.6	—[d]	41.5
Ovary	—[d]	17.5	15.8

[a]Rates per 100,000. Age-adjusted to U.S. 1970 population.
[b]From Alaska Native Tumor Registry.
[c]New Mexico Indians only.
[d]Rates not calculated when less than 25 cases.
Source: Adapted from BA Miller, LN Kolonel, L Bernstein, et al. (eds). Racial/Ethnic Patterns of Cancer in the United States 1988–1992. NIH Pub. No. 96-4104. Bethesda, MD: National Cancer Institute, 1996.

Summary

Compared with other U.S. races, American Indians and Alaska Natives have higher rates of cancer of the stomach, gallbladder, cervix, kidney, and liver and lower rates of cancer of the lung, breast, and prostate. There are marked regional differences in the frequency of some cancers, especially lung and breast. Tobacco abuse is the major preventable cause of cancer among Native Americans. Clinicians should maintain a high index of suspicion for the more common cancers and should adjust their screening practices accordingly. Adequate social and emotional support is essential to completing a difficult course of cancer treatment.

References

1. Hrdlicka A. Physiological and Medical Observations. Washington, DC: U.S. Government Printing Office, 1908.
2. Indian Health Service. Trends in Indian Health, 1996. Washington, DC: U.S. Department of Health and Human Services, Indian Health Service Office of Planning, Evaluation, and Legislation, Division of Program Statistics, 1997.
3. Frost F, Tollestrup K, Ross A, et al. Correctness of racial coding of American Indians and Alaska Natives on the Washington State death certificate. Am J Prev Med 1994;10:290–294.
4. Sorlie PD, Rogot E, Johnson NJ. Validity of demographic characteristics on the death certificate. Epidemiology 1992;3:181–184.
5. Smith RL. Recorded and expected mortality among the Indians of the United States with special reference to cancer. J Natl Cancer Inst 1957;18:385–396.
6. Dunham LJ, Bailar JC III, Laquer GL. Histologically diagnosed cancers in 693 Indians of the United States, 1950–65. J Natl Cancer Inst 1973;50:1119–1127.
7. Valway S, Kileen M, Paisano RE, Ortiz E. Cancer Mortality among Native Americans in the United States, 1984–88. Albuquerque, NM: U.S. Public Health Service, Indian Health Service, 1992.
8. Cobb N, Paisano RE. Cancer Mortality among American Indians and Alaska Natives in the United States, 1989–1993. IHS Pub. No. 97-615-23. Rockville, MD: Indian Health Service, 1997.
9. Nutting PA, Freeman WL, Risser DR, et al. Cancer incidence among American Indians and Alaska Natives, 1980 through 1987. Am J Public Health 1993;83: 1589–1598.
10. Miller BA, Kolonel LN, Bernstein L, et al. (eds), Racial/Ethnic Patterns of Cancer in the United States 1988–1992. NIH Pub. No. 96-4104. Bethesda, MD: National Cancer Institute, 1996.
11. Cobb N. Environmental causes of cancer among Native Americans. Cancer 1996;78:1603–1606.
12. Samet JM, Kutvirt DM, Waxweiler RJ, Key CR. Uranium mining and lung cancer in Navajo men. N Engl J Med 1984;310:1481–1484.

Part VI
Hematology

Chapter 24
Anemias

Ana Mariá López

Anemia in the Native American population in North America appears to be as common as it is in general primary care. Anemia in an adult is defined as a hematocrit below 37% in a female and below 41% in a male. Nutritionally based anemias, especially due to iron deficiency, are commonly diagnosed in the Native American population. Although specific differences in the presentation, evaluation, and treatment of the specific anemia in the Native American population have not been fully elucidated, such differences may exist. In addition, the term *Native American* embraces a wide variety of people, with different genetic, cultural, and geographic origins. Although these differences are blurred for the purposes of this discussion, additional study may allow for a more textured understanding of the separate nations and their specific health issues. This chapter reviews the general approach to the patient with anemia and highlights specific considerations for the Native American patient.

Epidemiology

The epidemiology of anemia in the Native American population in North America has not been completely studied. Anthropologic data demonstrate that anemia may have been a long-standing problem in Native American populations in North America. Analyses of bone protein in skeletal remains reveal porotic skeletal lesions, which may be related to iron-deficiency anemia.[1–4] Diets lacking ferrous iron, such as a diet high in maize, promote porotic bone lesions because iron is a necessary enzyme cofactor for the early phase of bone mineralization.[4] In a sample of 454 skeletons from the British Columbia coast, cribra orbitalia, an abnormality similar to porotic hyperostosis, was present in 19% of infants and toddlers, 33% of growing children, 13% of adult females, and 5% of adult males.[1] The early onset of iron-deficiency anemia may be more strongly associated with an endemically

inadequate diet in pregnant females, which adversely affects the fetus, than with the weaning diet.[2] In addition, the effects of diet on the fetus may act synergistically with the early onset of parasitic infections in promoting iron-deficiency anemia.[2, 5]

Clinical Presentation

History

In general, the patient presents with symptoms that arise from the decreased oxygen capacity of the red blood cell: easy fatigability, dyspnea with exertion, tachypnea, tachycardia at rest or with exertion, and palpitations. A dietary history is important to assess nutritional deficiencies. The possibility of a congenital anemia should be considered, and a thorough personal and family history should be taken. Any prior therapy for the anemia and its effects should also be noted. A history of blood loss should always be considered. In women of reproductive age, anemia may be related to heavy menses. The patient with iron-deficiency anemia may develop pica (a craving for unusual foods, such as ice). In advanced situations, the patient may complain of dysphagia.

For the patient with vitamin B_{12} deficiency, the anemia may be severe, with hematocrit levels of 10–15%. The megaloblastic state may produce several changes, including glossitis, diarrhea, and anorexia nervosa. In addition, vitamin B_{12} deficiency may lead to a complex set of neurologic symptoms. Initially, the peripheral nerves are affected and the patient complains of paresthesias. When the posterior columns are affected, the patient has difficulty with balance. As the disease progresses, cerebral function can be affected. Occasionally, dementia precedes the hematologic problem.

In hemolytic disorders, the patient may present with jaundice and a profound anemia, which may be associated with cardiac failure. Chronic diseases, such as cancer, chronic inflammation or infection, and liver disease, often result in anemia.

Physical Examination

On examination, the patient may appear pale and fatigued. The respiratory rate may be elevated, and the heart rate may be increased. The conjunctivae and oral mucosa are often pale. The patient may have icterus with pruritus, brittle nails, a smooth tongue, and cheilosis. In iron-deficiency anemia, dysphagia may be present and may be associated with the formation of an esophageal web (Plummer-Vinson syndrome). A systolic flow murmur may be present, and capillary refill of the nail beds may be slow. In very late cases, the patient may present with signs and symptoms of high-output cardiac failure. The examination should also assess possible underlying hematologic disease by evaluating for bone pain, lymphadenopathy, and splenomegaly. If the patient has a megaloblastic anemia due to vitamin B_{12} deficiency, diminished position and vibratory sense may be found on neurologic examination. Patients with a macrocytic anemia due to folic acid deficiency have a similar presentation to those with vitamin B_{12} deficiency, except for the neurologic symptoms.

Diagnostic Studies

Several laboratory studies are used to delineate the etiology of the anemia. The studies should be obtained in a thoughtful manner, taking into account the potential diagnostic possibilities.

Anemia may be suspected after a complete history and physical examination and confirmed with a complete blood count. Aside from the hemoglobin and hematocrit, the mean corpuscular volume (MCV) and red blood cell distribution width are the most significant red blood cell indices because they provide information about red cell size. The peripheral smear offers additional information. In microcytic anemias, the peripheral smear may demonstrate anisocytosis, poikilocytosis, hypochromia, target cells, and nucleated red blood cells. If thalassemia is suspected, hemoglobin electrophoresis is necessary to make the diagnosis. In macrocytic anemias due to vitamin B_{12} or folate deficiency, anisocytosis and poikilocytosis are noted, along with hypersegmented neutrophils. Pancytopenia may also be seen because vitamin B_{12} affects all cell lines. Erythropoietin is usually elevated in persons with anemia, except for anemia associated with renal disease. The reticulocyte count differentiates the anemias due to decreased production from the anemias due to increased destruction. Iron levels, total iron-binding capacity, and ferritin are useful in the evaluation of a microcytic anemia. Ferritin is usually the most sensitive

of these studies, reflecting depletion of iron stores. Vitamin B_{12} (normal range: 150–350 pg/ml) and folate (normally >6 ng/ml) levels determine a nutritional cause for macrocytic anemias. The red blood cell folate level is more reliable because it reflects folic acid intake over the past few months. In anemias due to vitamin B_{12} deficiency, the lactate dehydrogenase level may be elevated, along with the indirect bilirubin, thereby reflecting intramedullary destruction of developing erythroid cells. These levels should be obtained before replacing the suspected deficient nutrient. A Coombs' test is useful in identifying a hemolytic anemia. Examination of the bone marrow helps define the primary bone marrow abnormalities that result in anemia.

Diagnostic Approach and Differential Diagnosis

The first step in managing anemia is evaluation and correction of the volume status. Next, a reticulocyte count should be obtained to assess clinically effective red blood cell production. Under normal conditions, the reticulocyte count is approximately 100,000/µl. When the normal individual requires increased amounts of red blood cells, the reticulocyte count increases to a maximum level of approximately 400,000/µl. To assess effective erythropoiesis, the reticulocyte count should be corrected by multiplying the actual reticulocyte count by the observed hematocrit and dividing by a normal hematocrit of 45%.

If anemia is present in association with decreased or normal red blood cell production, the erythrocyte size may help to elucidate the cause of the anemia. The erythrocyte may be small (microcytic), normal (normocytic), or large (macrocytic).

Microcytic Anemia

A microcytic anemia may be due to iron-deficiency anemia, thalassemia, or anemia of chronic disease. A severe microcytic anemia (MCV <70 fl) is always due to either iron deficiency or thalassemia. Iron-deficiency anemia is the most common cause of anemia in the world and is often seen in the Native American population.[6] Although African-American children matched for ferritin and iron with white children appear to have slightly lower hematocrits, no such difference appears to exist between similarly matched Native American and white children. Based on these data, the same diagnostic criteria for anemia can be used for both the Native American and white population.[7]

The major cause of iron deficiency is blood loss: menstrual, gastrointestinal, or due to blood donation. Blood loss must always be evaluated in a patient with iron-deficiency anemia. Dietary iron deficiency is a common cause of anemia in children, but it is usually not seen in adults. Iron malabsorption is usually due to gastric surgery. Increased iron requirements occur with repeated pregnancy, especially if accompanied by lactation. Other causes of iron-deficiency anemia are chronic hemoglobinuria and idiopathic pulmonary hemosiderosis, in which iron is sequestered in pulmonary macrophages.

Iron is required for heme formation. Up to 95% of total body iron is present in the hemoglobin of circulating red blood cells. Iron deposits exist as ferritin or hemosiderin. Iron-deficiency anemia demonstrates a low serum iron, increased total iron-binding capacity, and reduced serum ferritin.

Thalassemias would be unusual in the Native American population. In general, they result in a greater degree of microcytosis (i.e., lower MCV), for any given level of anemia compared to iron-deficiency anemia. The erythrocyte usually appears abnormal at an earlier stage of anemia, and iron studies are normal. Thalassemia minor is usually associated with a mild microcytic anemia or microcytosis without anemia. Thalassemia major is characterized by a more severe anemia, which may be accompanied by marrow expansion, resulting in skeletal abnormalities and organomegaly.

Anemia of chronic disease is characteristically associated with a low serum iron but normal or increased bone marrow iron stores, low total iron-binding capacity, and increased serum ferritin. If anemia of chronic disease and iron-deficiency anemia coexist, the serum ferritin level may be normal.

Normocytic Anemias

Normocytic anemias may be associated with anemia of chronic disease, a metabolic problem (such as uremia or protein malnutrition), or a primary bone marrow problem. If anemia of chronic disease is not identified as characterized above and the patient does not have evidence of a metabolic problem, then evaluation of the bone marrow is necessary. Bone marrow evaluation could reveal decreased production of red cell precursors or abnormal production of red cell precursors. If the marrow is hypoplastic, the patient may have aplastic anemia. If the marrow is being replaced, then the production of red cell precursors is impaired. Common causes of a myelophthisic marrow include solid tumors, myelodysplasia, and leukemia.

Macrocytic Anemias

Macrocytic anemias are most commonly due to vitamin B_{12} or folic acid deficiencies and are diagnosed by reduced serum levels, vitamin B_{12} level less than 100 pg/ml, folic acid level less than 3 ng/ml, or red blood cell folate level of less than 150 ng/ml. In addition, macro-ovalocytes and hypersegmented neutrophils may be present on the peripheral smear. A severe macrocytic anemia (MCV >125 fl) is usually due to vitamin B_{12} or folic acid deficiency.

Vitamin B_{12} deficiency is rarely due to diet alone, except in strict vegetarians. It is usually due to a primary or secondary malabsorption of vitamin B_{12}. Pernicious anemia results in primary vitamin B_{12} malabsorption. Secondary causes of vitamin B_{12} malabsorption include gastric or ileal resection or bile salt deficiency.

Folic acid deficiency is often due to diet alone. Folic acid is present in most fruits and vegetables but especially in citrus and green, leafy vegetables. Those at risk for folic acid deficiency are persons who drink alcohol excessively, anorectic cancer patients, and others who either do not eat fruits and vegetables or overcook them. Folic acid deficiency may also be related to malabsorption due to tropical sprue, increased requirements due to pregnancy, increased losses due to dialysis, or drug metabolism. Trimethoprim impairs folic acid metabolism, and phenytoin impairs folic acid absorption. Methotrexate inhibits the reduction of folic acid to its active form.

If a macrocytic anemia is present and normal B_{12} and folic acid levels are obtained, then drug toxicities or a primary bone marrow problem must be considered. The bone marrow may reveal myelodysplasia or a congenital dyserythropoietic anemia.

If anemia is present in the face of increased red blood cell production, then causes of red cell destruction must be explored. A significant cause of red cell destruction is hemolysis. Haptoglobin level is depressed in hemolysis of intravascular or extravascular origin. (Haptoglobin is the main plasma protein that binds hemoglobin.) If intravascular hemolysis is present, free hemoglobin may be present in the plasma, and urinary hemosiderin may be found due to iron entering the renal system.

The Coombs' test detects antibody or complement of the red cell surface and helps distinguish immune from nonimmune causes of hemolysis. If the Coombs' test is positive, the patient should be evaluated for warm or cold antibodies. If warm antibodies are present, an autoimmune hemolytic anemia or drug toxicities should be considered. If cold antibodies are present, the patient may have primary or secondary cold agglutinin disease or paroxysmal cold hemoglobinuria, and hematologic consultation is necessary.

If the Coombs' test is negative, nonhemolytic causes of anemia should be pursued. If splenomegaly is present, it must be considered as the cause of red blood cell destruction. Splenomegaly has multiple causes, such as sickle-cell disease and thalassemia, which can themselves lead to anemia.

If splenomegaly is absent, other causes of red blood cell destruction must be considered. Mechanical trauma is a common cause of red blood cell destruction and correlates with the presence of schistocytes on the peripheral smear. Trauma is commonly due to a mechanical heart valve. In addition, the presence of an abnormal hemoglobin, such as in sickle cell anemia, or an abnormal red blood cell membrane, such as in hereditary spherocytosis, promotes red cell destruction.

Therapy

Iron-deficiency anemia is rarely life threatening. The first step in the treatment process is identifying and correcting the cause of the anemia (i.e., identifying and treating the source of excessive blood loss). Oral iron therapy is often necessary and effective. Increasing dietary iron is rarely effective. Plain, nonenteric, and nonextended release tablets should be prescribed at a dose of 65 mg of elemental iron, up to three times a day between meals. The usual form of elemental iron used is ferrous sulfate 325 mg three times per day. If the patient is unable to swallow pills, ferrous sulfate syrup is available and contains 32 mg of elemental iron per 4 ml. Although it is recommended that iron supplements be taken on an empty stomach, compliance may improve if the supplement is taken with food. In addition, it may be difficult for the patient to initiate therapy at the three-times-daily dosage; therefore, working up to that dose may also improve compliance to treatment. Therapy should begin at the time of diagnosis and should continue for 6 months after the hemoglobin has normalized to build up reserves. The average length of therapy is 8 months. Although poor iron absorption is occasionally found, the most common cause of lack of response to iron therapy is poor compliance.

Patients may report constipation, heartburn, or abdominal cramps while on iron supplements. These side effects often decrease after reducing the iron intake. Patients should be made aware that their stools will be black while on iron therapy. If the patient is taking liquid iron, teeth discoloration may occur and can be avoided by using a straw and rinsing the mouth after each dose of iron. All oral iron preparations should be kept out of the reach of small children because severe, acute iron poisoning can occur easily.

Parenteral iron is available and is indicated if the patient is unable to take oral medications or is unable to absorb oral iron. Iron dextran may produce fever, rash, arthralgias, aseptic meningitis, lymphadenopathy, splenomegaly, anaphylactic shock, and death. A test dose should be given initially, and the patient should be closely observed for anaphylaxis. The use of parenteral iron is risky; it should be initiated only after oral iron has been attempted and failed. In the severely anemic patient at risk for ischemic injury, red blood cell transfusion is indicated.

Vitamin B_{12} or folic acid deficiency is treated by specifically replacing the deficient nutrient. Vitamin B_{12} is generally first replaced at a dose of 200 µg intramuscularly daily for the first week, weekly for the first month, and then monthly for life. If the patient stops therapy, the vitamin deficiency will recur. Patients usually respond quickly to treatment with an increased reticulocyte count within the first week. The neurologic symptoms are usually reversible as long as they have not been long-standing (i.e., more than 6 months).

Folic acid is replaced orally at a dose of 1 mg per day. In addition, persons with increased physiologic requirements should be supplemented at this dose. Patients usually respond promptly with improved reticulocyte counts within a week. The hematologic problems generally resolve by 3 months. Because patients with vitamin B_{12} deficiency may have coexisting folic acid deficiency, folic acid supplementation may improve the hematologic condition while the neurologic symptoms progress. If vitamin B_{12} deficiency is suspected, its serum levels must be tested.

Anemia of chronic disease rarely requires treatment. If the patient becomes symptomatic or is transfusion dependent, erythropoietin three times per week may help to alleviate the anemia.

Thalassemia patients may not require treatment, may need folic acid, or may require regular red blood cell transfusions, especially at times of increased hematologic requirements, such as pregnancy. Occasionally, splenomegaly contributes to transfusion needs, and splenectomy may decrease transfusion needs. Iron-chelating agents are necessary to avoid hemosiderosis. Allogeneic bone marrow transplantation may be effective in young children with β-thalassemia major without organ damage due to iron overload.[8]

Conclusion

Anemia is a common clinical problem in general medical practice. The nutritional anemias are likely the most prevalent in this population. Specific differences associated with the Native American population have not been well delineated. At this time, standard clinical, laboratory, and therapeutic criteria should be applied to Native American patients.

Summary Points

- *Iron deficiency anemia*: microcytic anemia with a low serum ferritin and absent iron stores; it responds to iron supplementation.
- *Anemia of chronic disease*: microcytic anemia that occurs in the presence of a chronic illness and is characterized by a low serum iron, low total iron-binding capacity, normal or high ferritin levels, and normal or increased bone marrow iron stores.
- *Anemia due to vitamin B_{12} deficiency*: macrocytic anemia, which is associated with a low vitamin B_{12} level and, occasionally, with neurologic symptoms.
- *Anemia due to folic acid deficiency*: macrocytic anemia with a normal vitamin B_{12} level and a low folic acid or red cell folate level, or both.
- *Hemolytic anemia*: decreased haptoglobin level. If the Coombs' test is positive and warm antibodies are

present, consider drug toxicities or autoimmune hemolytic anemia. If the Coombs' test is positive and cold antibodies are present, primary or secondary cold agglutinin disease or paroxysmal cold hemoglobinuria should be considered.

- *Nonhemolytic causes of red cell destruction that result in anemia* include trauma due to a mechanical heart valve, splenomegaly, abnormal hemoglobin (sickle cell anemia), or abnormal red cell membrane (hereditary spherocytosis).

References

1. Whalen EA, Caulfield LE, Harris SB. Prevalence of anemia in First Nations children of northwestern Ontario. Can Fam Physician 1997;43:659–664.
2. Cybulski JS. Cribra orbitalia, a possible sign of anemia in early historic native populations of the British Columbia Coast. Am J Phys Anthropol 1977;47: 31–39.
3. Palkovich AM. Endemic disease patterns in paleopathology: porotic hyperostosis. Am J Phys Anthropol 1987;74:527–537.
4. Von Endt DW, Ortner DJ. Amino acid analysis of bone from a possible case of prehistoric iron deficiency anemia from the American Southwest. Am J Phys Anthropol 1982;59:377–385.
5. El-Najjar MY, Ryan DJ, Turner CG, Lozoff B. The etiology of porotic hyperostosis among the prehistoric and historic Anasazi Indians of Southwestern United States. Am J Phys Anthropol 1976;44:477–487.
6. Gonzales-Richmond JA, Madrigal Fritsch H, Naranjo Banda A, Moreno-Terrazas O. Food consumption, nutritional status and intestinal parasitosis in a native community. Salud Publica Mex 1985;27:336–345.
7. Corbett TH. Iron deficiency anemia in a Pueblo Indian village. JAMA 1968;205:186.
8. Yip R, Schwartz S, Deinard AS. Hematocrit values in white, black and American Indian children with comparable iron status. Evidence to support uniform diagnostic criteria for anemia among all races. Am J Dis Child 1984;138:824–826.

Part VII
Renal Disease

Chapter 25

Caring for the Patient with Progressive Renal Disease

Andrew S. Narva

Burden of Renal Disease among American Indians and Alaska Natives

American Indians (AIs) and Alaska Natives (ANs) have high rates of end-stage renal disease (ESRD), kidney failure requiring dialysis, or transplantation for survival. National data from the U.S. Renal Data System (USRDS) show that at the end of 1995, 3,807 ESRD patients were identified as AI or AN.[1] The 1995 prevalence and incidence rates of ESRD among AIs and ANs were more than three times greater than those of whites and only slightly below those of blacks. AI and AN incidence rates show a rate of increase resulting in a *doubling of new cases of ESRD every 4.5 years.* Sixty-three percent of new cases of ESRD among AIs and ANs were due to diabetes. Incidence rates for ESRD due to diabetes among AIs and ANs were six times the rate of white Americans and are increasing 17% per year. A systems model developed by the Indian Health Service (IHS) Kidney Disease Program predicts that the number of AIs and ANs with ESRD due to diabetes in 2010 will more than quadruple the number treated in 1990 (unpublished data, IHS Kidney Disease Program).

The rates cited describe the burden of ESRD among all persons identified by their treatment facility as AIs or ANs. However, these national rates mask significant regional variation as well as differences among the 540 tribes that make up the AI community. ESRD Network 15 (Arizona, New Mexico, Colorado, Utah, Wyoming, and Nevada) includes more than 40% of the AIs and ANs identified in the USRDS database and the majority of AIs and ANs with ESRD living on reservations, primarily in Arizona and New Mexico. Ninety-two percent of these ESRD patients are full-blooded AIs or ANs. Analyzed data shows that the burden of kidney failure is much higher among the AIs of the Southwest who receive their care from IHS. Two AI communities of the Southwest, Zuni Pueblo, New Mexico, and Sacaton, Arizona, may have the highest

treated rates of ESRD in the world, respectively 12.6 and 14.0 times the U.S. all races rate (Table 25-1) (unpublished data, IHS Kidney Disease Program).

For each patient currently being treated, several patients wait in the wings. Thus, virtually all providers in the IHS are seeing significant numbers of patients with renal disease. This chapter outlines an approach to the management of patients with progressive renal disease.

Evaluation and Monitoring of Patients with Renal Disease

Identification: The Deceptive "Normal Creatinine"

Identification of patients with early renal disease is a problem because many providers may be falsely reassured by a patient's "normal creatinine." Creatinine is a product of muscle metabolism and is produced at a fairly constant rate of 15–20 mg/kg per day in women and 20–25 mg/kg per day in men, with decreasing production after age 50 years. Baseline creatinine is a function of muscle mass and can vary significantly. Thus, a serum creatinine of 1.2 mg/dl in a muscular male may reflect normal glomerular filtration rate (GFR), but the same value in an elderly woman may reflect 50% loss of renal function. Also misleading is the natural history of renal disease in diabetics, the initial phase of which is associated with an increase in GFR, followed by a slow decline to normal GFR and below. Proteinuria begins at approximately the time normal GFR is achieved as it declines from hyperfiltration levels. This may explain the diabetic patient with significant proteinuria and normal creatinine clearance. Additional difficulties arise from the physiology of serum creatinine itself. The value of creatinine as an indicator of GFR derives from the assumed lack of renal tubular reabsorption or secretion. Creatinine is a less-than-perfect

Table 25-1. Prevalence of End-Stage Renal Disease Among American Indians (AIs), 1994

	U.S. All Races	U.S. All AIs and ANs	Southwest AIs and ANs	Southwest AI and AN Risk Ratio	Zuni Service Unit	Zuni Risk Ratio	Sacaton Service Unit	Sacaton Risk Ratio
Prevalence (treated cases/100,000 population)	94.9	206.5	433.0	4.6	1,192.7	12.6	1,326.5	14.0

AN = Alaska Native.

marker, however, and is, in fact, secreted in increasing quantities as renal function deteriorates. Thus, serum creatinine and the creatinine clearance both *overestimate* GFR in the injured kidney.

How do you confirm your suspicion that a patient with a "normal creatinine" has renal insufficiency? In a diabetic patient, dipstick-positive proteinuria confirms significant renal injury. A 24-hour collection for creatinine clearance will support this *if* the urine collection is complete. Because of variation in urine collection, a simpler method of calculating GFR based on age, weight, and serum creatinine may be a more reliable estimate of GFR in the typical outpatient.[2] The formula (the Cockcroft-Gault formula) is stated thus:

$$\frac{\text{Creatinine}}{\text{clearance}} \approx \frac{(140 - \text{age}) (\text{body weight in kg})}{\text{Plasma creatinine} \times 72}$$
$$\text{for women, multiply by } 0.85$$

Screening Evaluation

It is not necessary to comprehensively review the evaluation of patients with renal disease. Extensive reviews are included in most standard texts. However, it is important to tailor the evaluation to the particular population being screened. Most AI and AN patients with renal disease have diabetic nephropathy. However, being diabetic does not immunize the patient from coexisting glomerulonephritis, myeloma, membranous nephropathy, or other causes of nephrotic syndrome. Thus, in the diabetic patient with nephrotic-range proteinuria, a brief workup is indicated to rule out other renal diseases, some of which may be treatable. Such a workup should include, in addition to history and physical examination (including dilated retinal examination), complete blood count, erythrocyte sedimentation rate (ESR), antinuclear antibody (ANA), rheumatoid factor, hepatitis B surface antigen, hepatitis C antibody, serum protein electrophoresis, urine protein electrophoresis, complement studies (C3, C4), creatinine, blood urea nitrogen, electrolytes, liver function tests, albumin, renal ultrasound, and urine culture. An assessment of postvoid residual by catheter or bladder ultrasound is particularly important in diabetics to

rule out neurogenic bladder. Patients with proteinuria, diabetic retinopathy, and the absence of evidence of other processes on the screening tests described can be considered to have diabetic nephropathy. Biopsy is not indicated. If there is evidence of a second process (e.g., positive ANA and hypocomplementemia), referral to a nephrologist for possible biopsy should be considered.

Diabetes is not the only renal disease that is more prevalent among AIs and ANs. The burden of glomerulonephritis is also increased, at least in southwestern tribes.[3] Much of this is due to immunoglobulin A glomerulonephritis (IgA GN) or similar mesangial processes involving the deposition of immunoglobulins. Henoch-Schönlein purpura (seen with increased frequency in AI and AN children) and IgA GN appear identical on renal biopsy. Because IgA GN may occur in association with upper respiratory tract infection (URI), it is sometimes confused with poststreptococcal glomerulonephritis (PSGN). Distinction of IgA GN from PSGN is probably the most common diagnostic issue in evaluating nondiabetic renal disease in AIs and ANs. IgA GN occurs concurrently with URI, is sometimes associated with gross hematuria, and may be associated with an increased IgA fibronectin level. Complement levels remain normal. PSGN occurs 10–21 days after the pharyngitis and is associated with hypocomplementemia.

Monitoring Patients with Renal Disease

It is rarely necessary to obtain a 24-hour urine collection to monitor patients. The Cockcroft-Gault formula provides an adequate estimate of creatinine clearance. In a patient with established proteinuria, it is also not necessary to do repeated 24-hour urine collections. The ratio of protein to creatinine calculated from a spot urine approximately reflects in grams the amount of protein excreted per day.[4] This relationship derives from the excretion rate of creatinine, which is approximately 1 g in 24 hours. Thus, if the ratio of protein to creatinine in a spot urine is 3, the patient excretes approximately 3 g of protein in 24 hours. Although this ratio does not give a precise indication of 24-hour protein excretion (underestimating in persons with large muscle mass and overestimating in patients with small muscle mass), it is an accurate reflection of changes in protein excretion and is quite useful for following most patients. It may be less reliable in diabetic patients with nephrotic proteinuria.[5] The Cockcroft-Gault formula for estimating creatinine clearance and the protein-to-creatinine ratio for estimating proteinuria have been validated for use in pregnant women with renal disease (including preeclampsia) as well.[6]

Predicting when a patient will require renal replacement therapy is difficult, but it can be estimated by plotting the reciprocal of the plasma creatinine against time.[7] This generally plots as a straight line for any individual. For a nondiabetic, extrapolating to the time when the serum creatinine will be 8 mg/dl (the reciprocal of which is 0.125) is a reasonable estimate of the time of initiation of dialysis. For a diabetic, a creatinine of 6 mg/dl (reciprocal = 0.15) would be appropriate.

Diabetic Nephropathy

As a result of the explosive growth of ESRD due to diabetes, IHS clinicians are highly motivated to optimize the medical management of diabetic patients to prevent the complications of renal failure and to postpone for as long as possible the need for ESRD treatment. Several modalities, including blood pressure reduction, low-protein diets, and attainment of near-normoglycemia, have received attention in the general medical literature, but it is not always clear how to apply these in the clinical setting.

Mechanism of Injury: The Hemodynamic Hypothesis

Studies in animals suggest that damage to the diabetic kidney is mediated by elevated glomerular capillary blood pressure. This *hemodynamic hypothesis*[8] suggests that hyperglycemia results in volume expansion, which *elevates* GFR and glomerular capillary pressure. These increased pressures and flows cause glomerular injury. GFR is initially maintained by the hypertrophy of the remaining nephrons. The elevated flows and pressures over time cause further injury, however, resulting in the inexorable decline in kidney function. This model of injury, although it cannot be proved directly in humans, does suggest a theoretical basis for therapy; if the pressure in the glomerular capillary can be reduced, perhaps the progression of renal disease can be slowed.

Predicting Risk

One-third to one-half of patients with type 1 diabetes develop overt renal disease. Data from the Pima study[9] indicate that virtually all patients with type 2 diabetes eventually develop nephropathy. Early predictors of nephropathy in type 1 include microalbuminuria (i.e., elevated albumin excretion but below the level that can be detected by dipstick) and rise in systolic blood pressure. Both of these changes occur early in the course of disease, when GFR is *increased*, before nephrons begin to drop out. Patients with type 2 also manifest these changes. Once proteinuria is clinically detectable (dipstick positive or 300 mg/L), renal disease is generally considered irreversible.

Five stages in the evolution of diabetic renal disease have been described. *Stage I* is characterized by hypertrophy of the kidney and *elevation* in GFR. Pathologic changes in the glomerulus, including glomerular basement membrane thickening, are present in *stage II*. Microalbuminuria (30–300 mg/day) is detected in *stage III* (also known as *incipient nephropathy*), along with an increase in blood pressure from baseline (though not necessarily to hypertensive levels). Renal disease becomes clinically detectable in *stage IV* (overt nephropathy) with dipstick-positive proteinuria (more than 300 mg/L) and hypertension. Stage V is ESRD. Stages I and II may be reversible; stage III may be arrestable.

Therapeutic Approaches

The major interventions that have been investigated are tight glucose control using multiple injections or insulin pump, blood pressure control, and protein-restricted diet. Many of these studies have been conducted in type 1 patients. Although the response to treatment of diabetic kidney disease may be exactly the same in patients with type 2 diabetes, this has not been proved.

Glucose Control

Early in the course of diabetic nephropathy (stages I, II, and III), near-normalization of blood glucose has significant benefit on renal function. Use of insulin pumps in type 1 patients has reduced microalbuminuria and the elevated GFR of early diabetes. Pump therapy over 6–24 months preserves renal function in type 1 patients with incipient disease. Achievement of near-normoglycemia normalizes the GFR and slows the rate of progression of renal disease. Studies using frequent insulin injections instead of a pump showed results nearly as good. The Diabetes Control and Complications Trial study[10] demonstrated that intensive glucose control slowed the development of microalbuminuria and the progression to dipstick-positive proteinuria in type 1 diabetes. The implications of these studies for type 2 diabetes are unclear. It seems likely that improvement in glycemic control in type 2 patients by weight loss, exercise, or drug therapy would also be beneficial early in the course of diabetes. Because of a prolonged asymptomatic phase, however, clinicians may not have the opportunity to intervene at this early stage.

Once nephropathy is established, evidenced by dipstick-positive proteinuria, tight glycemic control provides less benefit to the kidneys. *Insulin pump therapy with near-normalization of blood glucose in type 1 patients has not been shown to reverse or arrest progression of overt renal disease.*

Blood Pressure Control

Progression of diabetic renal disease and blood pressure are inextricably linked. Elevations in blood pressure, though not necessarily to hypertensive levels, are detectable (along with a drop in GFR) well before the serum creatinine changes. "Normal" blood pressure can be associated with progression of renal disease; our criteria for initiation of treatment of diabetic patients may be revised in the future.

Several long-term studies have demonstrated that antihypertensive therapy is beneficial in early and late stages of nephropathy. In untreated hypertensive patients, GFR declines approximately 1 ml per minute per month; antihypertensive treatment slows the rate of decline by approximately two-thirds. Antihypertensive therapy reduces proteinuria, presumably by lowering glomerular capillary pressure. Angiotensin-converting enzyme (ACE) inhibitors (e.g., lisinopril and captopril) lower glomerular capillary pressure by dilation of the efferent arteriole. These agents have been shown to ameliorate the renal injury even when systemic blood pressure is not affected.[11] In hypertensive patients, ACE inhibitors provide a significant additional benefit compared to other antihypertensive medications with the same level of blood pressure control. A National Institutes of Health (NIH)-sponsored management conference recommended that ACE inhibitors be initiated in patients with any one of the following: hypertension (more than 140/90 mm Hg), creatinine more than 1.5, or proteinuria exceeding 300 mg per day.[12] There is evidence that normotensive type 2 patients with microalbuminuria may benefit from treatment with ACE inhibitors.[13] Although there have been consensus statements from several groups endorsing the practice, the NIH conference did *not* agree that the data justified the use of ACE inhibitors in normotensive type 2 patients with microalbuminuria at this time.

Not only are conventional drugs being replaced with ACE inhibitors, but also, published studies justify a lower therapeutic goal for blood pressure than the traditional 140/90 mm Hg. The Modification of Diet in Renal Disease (MDRD) study showed that maintaining a mean arterial pressure of 90 mm (equivalent to 125/75 mm Hg) slows progression of renal disease to a greater degree than do higher blood pressure levels. Benefit is greatest in patients with more severe disease.

Dietary Protein Restriction

Protein restriction was advocated in the past to reduce the metabolic work of the failing kidney and to reduce symptoms of uremia. With the advent of dialysis and transplantation, the role of protein in the diet was largely ignored. The importance of protein restriction is re-emerging with evidence that protein loading elevates glomerular flows and pressures, augmenting similar

changes associated with hyperglycemia.[14] In newly diagnosed diabetic patients, changing to a low-protein diet normalizes GFR. Several studies up to 2 years in duration have shown that the decline of renal function is significantly slowed in patients with overt nephropathy who are placed on a low-protein diet[15]; proteinuria is reduced and rate of GFR decline slows. The definitive study of protein restriction, however, MDRD,[16] showed an insignificant benefit from severe protein restriction. This study included only a handful of diabetic patients. Although aspects of protein restriction remain controversial, the American Diabetes Association recommends reduction in protein intake to 0.8 g/kg body weight for patients who have or are at risk for nephropathy.

Therapeutic Strategy for Diabetic Nephropathy

Blood glucose control should be optimized at all times but probably is most beneficial before vascular complications develop. Selecting patients for other preventive interventions is difficult because dipstick testing is not sensitive enough to detect levels of albuminuria associated with incipient nephropathy. Methods for the detection of microalbuminuria are available, and routine screening is recommended by both the American Diabetes Association and the National Kidney Foundation. Given the high risk of virtually the entire AI and AN community and the cost and time involved in screening for microalbuminuria, however, it is not unreasonable to reserve screening for microalbuminuria for settings where a *specific* intervention is planned. Otherwise, the cost may not be justified. Serum creatinine is an extremely insensitive indicator of renal disease and can be particularly misleading in older people with small muscle mass. Retinopathy is associated with nephropathy in only two-thirds of patients.

The first sign of renal injury that a clinician might notice is a slight elevation of blood pressure (e.g., from 100/70 mm Hg to 130/85 mm Hg). The potential benefits of aggressive treatment of such elevations of blood pressure with ACE inhibitors is currently being evaluated. For hypertensive patients, there is good justification for aggressively achieving and maintaining a mean blood pressure of 90 mm Hg (equivalent to 125/75). Moderate protein restriction (0.8 g/kg/day) may also be indicated.

Once dipstick-positive proteinuria is present, blood pressure control and protein restriction should be stressed. There is no evidence that tight glucose control alters the progression of stage IV nephropathy. Vigorous therapy of blood pressure (mean blood pressure of 90 mm Hg) is certainly justified, and ACE inhibitors are probably the agents of choice. Alternative drugs include the calcium channel blockers, a heterogeneous group of drugs with mixed results in clinical studies. The nondihydropyridine calcium channel blockers, verapamil and diltiazem, probably have kidney-protective properties similar to ACE inhibitors.[17] The dihydropyridine drugs (e.g., nifedipine) probably offer little renal protection beyond the lowering of systemic blood pressure.

In summary, for patients with established diabetic nephropathy and proteinuria, blood pressure control is the most important determinant of rate of progression. Antihypertensive therapy, probably with an ACE inhibitor as the initial drug of choice, should be pursued aggressively. Modification of protein intake may be helpful as well.

Managing the Complications of Chronic Renal Failure

Goals for the primary care physician in the management of chronic renal failure leading to ESRD are as follows[18]:

1. Optimize the conservative management of patients with early kidney disease.
2. Facilitate early orientation to renal replacement therapy for improved patient education, better-informed choice of treatment, and a reduced need for emergent initiation of dialysis.
3. Provide care to hemodialysis, peritoneal dialysis, and transplant patients that complements the care provided by the consulting nephrologist.
4. Assist tribes in their efforts to establish or improve reservation-based dialysis facilities.

To meet these goals, the primary care physician should be prepared to address the clinical issues described in the following section. Management recommendations are summarized in Table 25-2.

Avoiding Additional Renal Insults

Injured kidneys are particularly vulnerable to additional damage from drugs, hypotension, and infection. Most clinicians are aware of the nephrotoxicity of aminoglycosides and other commonly used drugs. Nonsteroidal anti-inflammatory drugs (NSAIDs), however, which can harm the kidney through a variety of mechanisms,[19] are not always recognized as a significant threat. Because AI and AN patients have high rates of rheumatologic disease, NSAIDs are frequently prescribed and probably cause significant renal morbidity, often not recognized. Sulindac and nonacetylated salicylates are only *relatively* safer than other NSAIDs.[20] If it is necessary to use a NSAID, be certain the patient is not intravascularly volume depleted (e.g., from congestive heart failure or cirrhosis) or hyperkalemic, and follow renal function carefully. Contrast agents, ionic and nonionic, are nephrotoxic and are most likely to cause clinically detectable injury to patients with serum creatinine more than 2 mg/dl.[21] Ultrasound examinations are widely available, and contrast studies are rarely required in evaluation of renal disease. If a patient with renal insufficiency must receive contrast, use of volume expansion before the study and furosemide at the time of the study may be protective.[22] Finally, ACE inhibitors, widely advocated as the antihypertensive of choice in patients with progressive renal disease,[23] should be used cautiously in

Table 25-2. Suggested Guidelines for Management of Progressive Renal Disease*

No renal disease (primary prevention)
  Community education
    Hypertension control
    Progressive nature of renal disease
    Organ donation or transplantation
Early renal failure (GFR >50% normal)
    Identification of patients with significant GFR loss with "normal" creatinine and entry into chronic disease registry
    Use of nomogram to calculate GFR for all diabetics yearly
  Early intervention
    Hypertension control
    ACE inhibitors
    Diet
Moderate renal failure (GFR 20–50% normal)
  Early education about ESRD
  Maximal conservative therapy
  Early treatment of complications of renal failure
    Bone disease: follow Ca and P; initiate use of phosphate binders
    Hepatitis B vaccine
    Isoniazid prophylaxis if indicated
    Avoid venipuncture in nondominant arm
Severe renal failure (GFR 10–20% of normal)
  Education about options for renal replacement therapy in consultation with nephrologist
  Appropriate elective access placement
  Optimal management of complications
    Hypertension
    Volume overload
    Bone disease; follow calcium and phosphorus regularly and PTH yearly
    Acidosis
End-stage renal disease
  Continue routine care for comorbid diseases (e.g., routine diabetic care for eyes and feet)
  Continue routine health maintenance (e.g., Pap smears, rectal examination)
  Encourage participation in patient group

*Because serum creatinine values can be misleading, these guidelines are described in terms of percentage of normal GFR. Normal renal function can be estimated at 120 ml/min/1.73 m^2 body surface area (BSA) in women and 130 ml/min/1.73 m^2 BSA in men.
GFR = glomerular filtration rate; ACE = angiotensin-converting enzyme; ESRD = end-stage renal disease; PTH = parathyroid hormone.

patients with creatinine more than 3 mg/dl because of an increased risk of marked deterioration in renal function.

Preventing Bone Disease

One of the most dangerous complications of chronic renal disease is renal osteodystrophy. Although bone disease probably begins early in the course of renal failure, when 50% of GFR has been lost, it has not usually been treated until it becomes obvious with hyperphosphatemia and hypocalcemia. Initiation of phosphate binding with calcium carbonate early in the course of disease may be helpful. $CaCO_3$ can serve as a phosphate binder or as a calcium supplement, the former when given with meals, the latter when given between meals. Aluminum-based phosphate binders should be avoided because of the central nervous system and bone toxicity associated with long-term use and should only be used when the $Ca \times PO_4$ product exceeds 60. The early use of vitamin D (calcitriol) may be indicated in the patient who remains hypocalcemic despite $CaCO_3$ or who has an elevated intact parathyroid hormone level.

Preventing Infection

Patients with renal disease, as people with other chronic diseases, should receive yearly influenza vaccination and pneumococcal vaccine. Isoniazid prophylaxis should be given to renal patients with positive tuberculin tests, regardless of age. Dialysis patients are routinely immunized with hepatitis B vaccine; however, only approximately 50% develop immunity. Vaccination earlier in the course of their disease might be more effective.

Treating Anemia

Randomized, double-blinded, placebo-controlled studies have shown that erythropoietin (EPO) increases the hematocrit in predialysis patients and results in improved quality of life, specifically increased sense of well-being, ability to perform work better, less angina, and increased appetite.[24] Clinical experience supports these findings and the possibility that dialysis can be delayed in some cases. Although EPO is an expensive drug, the reality is that providers serving AI and AN populations provide care to communities with the highest rates of treated renal failure in the world. Approximately two-thirds of these patients have diabetic nephropathy with associated vasculopathy of coronary arteries, peripheral vessels, and other vessels. Many of these patients develop significant anemia with resulting symptoms. Use of EPO has been delayed in some settings due to concern about cost. In reality, the cost is much less than some have anticipated for several reasons: The cost of EPO has decreased to approximately $65 per 10,000 units (U). The dose required is in the range of 10,000 U per week for 2–3 weeks followed by a rapid taper to 2,000–4,000 U per week. Duration is rarely longer than a few months. Thus, the total cost for EPO for an average patient is $400–$500. The minimum cost of 1 week of dialysis is $500.

Before initiating EPO, other causes of anemia should be ruled out with a stool guaiac for occult blood as well as vitamin B_{12} and folate levels. Iron saturation (iron/total iron-binding capacity ratio) of more than 20% and fer-

ritin level greater than 100 are necessary for the marrow to respond to EPO. All patients should be placed on supplemental iron. Initial dosing of 10,000 U per week subcutaneously is usually adequate. Hematocrit should be followed every 2 weeks, and the dose should be tapered as the goal hematocrit (32–36%) is approached.

Diet

In general, a low-protein (0.8 g/kg/day or less), low-phosphorus diet is appropriate to maintain existing renal function and avoid metabolic bone disease. This should be individualized with the help of a nutritionist.

Preparation for Renal Replacement Therapy

Vascular Access

Creation of vascular access is necessary to provide the high blood flows used in hemodialysis (300–400 ml/min). The timely establishment (creatinine of 5–6 mg/dl) of vascular access can significantly improve the patient's quality of life by minimizing "access grief." Creation of a native-vein arteriovenous fistula in the wrist or forearm, if possible, is the access of first choice because it does not require the use of artificial material, which may act as a nidus of infection. However, these fistulae may require up to 2 months to mature. A synthetic graft connecting artery and vein may be used in patients with smaller vessels and can be used earlier postoperatively. Access is usually placed in the nondominant arm; this allows the patient to eat and perform manual tasks while on dialysis. If access is not placed before the patient requires dialytic treatment, temporary access, usually a subclavian catheter, can be used. These lines carry the risk of infection, thrombosis, and pneumothorax, however, complications that are best avoided in a patient already ill with uremia. Patients who intend to be treated with peritoneal dialysis do not need placement of vascular access.

Patient Education

The goals of renal patient education are as follows:

1. Maximize the patient's understanding of and cooperation with a regimen to maintain existing renal function.
2. Fully explain the different modalities of renal replacement therapy (hemodialysis, peritoneal dialysis, and transplantation) so that the patient may make informed decisions before reaching ESRD.
3. Provide information to the patient on renal replacement therapy to enhance understanding of the treatment.
4. Provide community education to support primary prevention, decrease fear, and increase understanding of dialysis and transplantation.

Sources of information include the nursing and social work staff of the nearest dialysis unit and the local affiliate of the National Kidney Foundation. The NIH produces an excellent pamphlet entitled "Choosing a Treatment That's Right for You" (NIH Pub. No. 96-2412). An AI- and AN-oriented educational video is available from the IHS Kidney Disease Program.

Collaborating with the Dialysis Provider

The role of the primary provider does not end with the initiation of dialysis. ESRD patients, particularly diabetic patients, rarely receive comprehensive primary care through the dialysis unit. For many reservation-based dialysis facilities, the nephrologist is present on site 1 day per week or less. As a result, it is beneficial for the ESRD patient to continue to have a primary provider, and it is incumbent on these providers to maintain their commitment to the comprehensive care of these patients. Several excellent handbooks describe the evaluation and management of health problems of ESRD patients[25] and should be available to providers in hospitals and outpatient facilities.

References

1. U.S. Renal Data System. USRDS 1997 Annual Data Report. Bethesda, MD: National Institutes of Health, 1997.
2. Cockcroft DW, Gault MH. Prediction of creatinine clearance from serum creatinine. Nephron 1976;16:13.
3. Narva A, Beaver S, Blackman D, et al. Descriptive study of renal disease at Pueblo of Zuni [Abstract]. Am J Kidney Dis 1992;8.
4. Schwab SJ, Christensen RL, Dougherty K, Klahr S. Quantitation of proteinuria by the use of protein-to-creatinine ratios in single urine samples. Arch Intern Med 1987;147:943.
5. Rodby RA, Rohde RD, Sharon Z, et al. The urine protein to creatinine ratio as a predictor of 24-hour protein excretion in type 1 diabetic patients with nephropathy. Am J Kidney Dis 1995;26:904.
6. Quadri KHM, Bernardini J, Greenberg A, et al. Assessment of renal function during pregnancy using a random urine protein to creatinine ratio and Cockcroft-Gault formula. Am J Kidney Dis 1994;24:416–420.
7. Mitch WE, Walser M, Buffington GA, Lemann J. A simple method of estimating progression of chronic renal failure. Lancet 1976;2:1326.
8. Zatz R, Brenner BM. Pathogenesis of diabetic microangiopathy. Am J Med 1986;80:443–453.
9. Nelson RG, Kunzelman CL, Pettitt DJ, et al. Albuminuria in type 2 (non-insulin–dependent) diabetes mellitus and impaired glucose tolerance in Pima Indians. Diabetologia 1989;32:870–876.
10. DCCT Research Group. The effect of intensive treatment of diabetes on the development and progression of long-term complications in insulin-dependent diabetes mellitus. N Engl J Med 1993;329:977–986.
11. Lewis EJ, Hunsicker LG, Bain RP, Rohde RD. The effect of angiotensin-converting-enzyme inhibition on diabetic nephropathy. N Engl J Med 1993;329:1456–1462.
12. Jacobsen H, Striker G. Report on a workshop to develop management recommendations for the prevention of progression in chronic renal disease. Am J Kidney Dis 1995;25:103–106.
13. Ravid MR, Savin H, Jutrin I, et al. Long-term stabilizing effect of angiotensin-converting enzyme inhibition on plasma creatinine and on proteinuria in normotensive type 2 diabetic patients. Ann Intern Med 1993;118:577–581.
14. Brenner BM, Meyer TW, Hostetter TH. Dietary protein intake and the progressive nature of kidney disease. N Engl J Med 1982;307:652–659.
15. Zeller K, Whittaker E, Sullivan L, et al. Effect of restricting dietary protein on the progression of renal failure in patients with insulin-dependent diabetes mellitus. N Engl J Med 1991;324:78–84.
16. Klahr S, Levey AS, Beck GJ, et al. The effects of dietary protein restriction and blood-pressure control on the progression of chronic renal disease. N Engl J Med 1994;330:877–884.
17. Bakris GL, Barnhill BW, Sadler R. Treatment of arterial hypertension in diabetic humans: importance of therapeutic selection. Kidney Int 1992;41:912.
18. Morbidity and mortality of renal dialysis: an NIH consensus conference statement. Ann Intern Med 1994;121:62–70.
19. Clive DM, Stoff JS. Renal syndromes associated with nonsteroidal antiinflammatory drugs. N Engl J Med 1984;563–572.
20. Whelton A, Stout RL, Spilman PS, Klassen DK. Renal effects of ibuprofen, piroxicam, and sulindac in patients with asymptomatic renal failure. Ann Intern Med 1990;112:568–576.
21. Parfrey PS, Griffiths SM, Barrett BJ, et al. Contrast material-induced renal failure in patients with diabetes mellitus, renal insufficiency, or both. N Engl J Med 1989;320:143–149.
22. Solomon R, Werner C, Mann D, et al. Effects of saline, mannitol, and furosemide on acute decreases in renal function induced by radiocontrast agents. N Engl J Med 1994;331:1416.
23. Giatras I, Lau J, Levey AS. Effect of angiotensin-converting enzyme inhibitors on the progression of nondiabetic renal disease: a meta-analysis of randomized trials. Ann Intern Med 1997;127:337–345.
24. US Recombinant Human Erythropoietin Predialysis Study Group. Double-blind, placebo-controlled study of the therapeutic use of recombinant human erythropoietin for anemia associated with chronic renal failure in predialysis patients. Am J Kidney Dis 1991;18:50–59.
25. Daugirdas JT, Ing TS. Handbook of Dialysis. Boston: Little, Brown, 1994.

Part VIII
Musculoskeletal Disease

Chapter 26
Rheumatic Diseases

Bridget T. Walsh, Michael L. Tutt, and David E. Yocum

Diagnosing and caring for the Native American patient with rheumatic diseases is both challenging and very rewarding. Native Americans have a rich culture and belief system that are often very different from those of Western society (which most physicians are taught). Learning these beliefs and understanding their philosophies about seeking medical care and taking medications with the expectation of disease cure can help improve health care delivery to these individuals. This is especially true when dealing with the rheumatic diseases, which, for the most part, have no cure and for which medications require weeks, sometimes months, to take effect and may only partially treat the disease. Therapies typically must be continued for years, and most have significant toxicities, which must be explained in detail before prescribing. It is imperative that the Native American patient understand that the goals of therapy for most rheumatic diseases are controlling pain and inflammation, maintaining function, and often suppressing the immune system to control disease rather than to cure it totally. There are limited data on rheumatic diseases in Native Americans, and what has been published is predominantly epidemiologic rather than therapy-based study. This chapter summarizes what has been published and gives guidelines on evaluation and care (based both on prior studies and personal experience caring for more than 700 Native Americans with rheumatic diseases in Arizona and New Mexico since the early 1990s).[1]

Prevalence of Rheumatic Conditions in the Native American

Rheumatoid arthritis (RA), seronegative spondyloarthropathies (SpAs) and systemic lupus erythematosus (SLE or lupus) are present at much higher rates in many but not all of the Native American populations that have been compared to whites (Table 26-1). RA, for example, is expected to be seen in the general white population at a rate of 1–2% but has been found with a prevalence as great as 4.5–5.3% for the Pima in Arizona (and as high as 6.95% in these women),[2–4] 4.1% in the Blackfeet tribe in Montana,[5] 2.4% in the Alaskan Indian,[6] 5.3% in the Chippewa,[7] and 3.4% in the Yakima of the Pacific Northwest.[8] Other tribes have not shown an increased prevalence, however, such as the Alaskan Eskimo (0.6%),[9, 10] the Nuu-Chah-Nulth of the Pacific Northwest (1%),[11] and the Inuit of Canada (0.7%).[12]

SLE has also been found with a prevalence exceeding 40 per 100,000 (that expected for whites) in the Nuu-Chah-Nulth (348 per 100,000)[11] and in Tlingit women (more than 90 per 100,000).[6] SLE has also been seen with a greater annual incidence than in whites (expected annual incidence of 7 per 100,000) in three tribes: Sioux (16.6 per 100,000), Crow (27.1 per 100,000), and Arapaho (24.3 per 100,000).[13] Other tribes have not shown similar trends: SLE prevalence for the Pima, Navajo, and Cheyenne is 4 per 100,000[4, 13, 14]; for the Cherokee, 1.5 per 100,000[13]; and for the Hopi and Kiowa, 5 per 100,000.[4, 13]

Seronegative SpAs, especially Reiter's syndrome (RS), ankylosing spondylitis (AS), and sacroiliitis (SI), have also been found at significantly greater prevalence rates in the Native American than in the white. The Canadian Haida had a 4.7% overall rate (6.2% AS [men only] and 9.86% SI),[15–17] Pima had a 3.85–11.00% prevalence of SI,[2, 4, 18, 19] the Blackfeet reported prevalence of 2.67% for SI,[4, 16] and the Inuit reported prevalence of 1.2% (men overall) for SpA in general[12] compared to 1% or less for whites.[20]

The term *Navajo arthritis* was first described by Muggia et al.[21] in 1971, characterizing individuals with an acute, self-limited, asymmetric inflammatory arthritis. When Rate et al.[22] looked more closely at medical records, including HLA-B27 status, it was clear that these individuals most likely had a reactive arthritis or a variant of one of the seronegative SpAs related to the high rates of HLA-B27 positivity seen in many of these tribes.[23] The rate in

Table 26-1. Rheumatic Diseases in Selected Native American Tribes

Tribe/Location (references)	Rheumatoid Arthritis	Seronegative Spondylo-arthropathy (AS, RS, SI*)	Systemic Lupus Erythematosus	HLA-B27	HLADR4	RF	ANA
Apache/Arizona[25]	ND	ND	ND	~33%	ND	ND	ND
Arapahoe[13]	ND	ND	24.3/100,000	ND	ND	ND	ND
Blackfeet[4,16]	4.1% (≥ age 30 yrs)	SI 2.67%	4/100,000	ND	ND	5.6%	ND
Cherokee[13]	ND	—	1.5/100,000	—	—	—	—
Cheyenne[13]	ND	—	4/100,000	—	—	—	—
Chippewa/Minnesota[7]	6.8%	—	5/100,000	11%	68%	15%	—
Crow[13]	ND	—	27.1/100,000	—	—	—	—
Eskimo/Alaska							
Inupiat[9]	0.7%	1%	3/100,000	—	—	—	—
Yupik[10]	0.6%	—	—	—	—	—	—
Hopi[14]	—	—	5/100,000	9%	—	—	—
Haida/Canada[15–17,24]	—	AS 6.2% (men) SI 9.86%	ND	50%	—	—	—
Inuit/Canada[12]	0.65% (1.8% women)	0.84 (1.24 men) AS 0.19% (0.28% men) RS 0.12% (0.34% men)	0	25–36%	36.8%	—	—
Kiowa	—	—	5/100,000	—	—	—	—
Navajo/Arizona[13,14,22]	—	0.5% ReA	5/100,000	36%	—	—	—
Pima/Arizona[2,4,18,19]	4.5 (age >30 yrs) 5.3% (age >20 yrs)	SI 3.85%	4/100,000	18%	—	7% 19%	—
Sioux[13]	ND	ND	16.6/100,000	—	—	—	—
Tlingit, Haida, Tsimshian/southeastern Alaskan Indians[6]	2.4%	1% (age >20 yrs), AS 0.33%, RS 0.33%	7/100,000 Prevalence 0.09%	—	—	16%	—
Tohono-Oodem[40]	ND	ND	ND	9%	—	—	—
Yakima/Washington[8,36]	3.4% (women)	—	—	21%	38%	7.4% (women)	—

AS = ankylosing spondylitis; ND = no data; RS = Reiter's syndrome; SI = sacroiliitis; RF = rheumatoid factor; ANA = antinuclear antibody; ReA = reactive arthritis.

the Haida is 50%[17,24]; in Alaskan Eskimos, 25–40%[9,10]; Navajo, 36%[14]; Apache, 30%[25]; Pima, 18%[26]; Zuni, 13%[27]; and Hopi, 9%; compared to 7% in whites.[14] It is clear from studies in whites and other populations that seronegative SpAs are associated with HLA-B27 positive status. Besides this association, reactive arthritis (the likely process involved in Navajo arthritis) is associated with specific genitourinary and enteric pathogens (*Chlamydia trachomatis*, *Yersinia enterocolitica*, *Shigella flexneri*, and *Salmonella*), which are endemic in several Native American tribes. It is likely that the combination of the HLA-B27 prevalence and these pathogens result in the excess disease seen in some of these populations.

General Approach to Rheumatologic Problems

The approach to most rheumatic conditions in Native Americans is similar to that in whites, although a few differences bear mentioning. First, there is considerable overlap of various rheumatic diseases in this population, which makes comparisons and following strict criteria difficult.[1] Many individuals with an RA-like polyarticular inflammatory arthritis involving the small joints of the hands and feet and with a positive rheumatoid factor (RF) also have sacroiliitis or a positive HLA-B27 (more common in the SpA). Many individuals with SpA have severe peripheral erosive disease and a positive RF (28%),[1] which are more characteristic of RA. Describing the clinical pattern of joint involvement, attempting to evaluate for erosive disease and SI radiographically, identifying extraarticular manifestations, and evaluating the patient serologically (including RF, antinuclear antibody [ANA], and HLA-B27) are the essential parts of a rheumatic evaluation. When there is uncertainty about the diagnosis, describe the findings and reserve a specific diagnosis for when it is completely clear. In this way, a more complete characterization of rheumatic diseases in Native Americans can be achieved.

The following is designed to be a guide for the clinician caring for the Native American patient. The reader is referred to a general textbook on rheumatology for an in-depth review of these topics.

Monoarticular Arthritis

Acute monoarticular arthritis is common in the Native American population. The Native American individual presenting with an acute monoarticular arthritis should be treated like anyone with the condition—that is, for possible septic joint. Without prompt treatment, a septic joint can lead to significant joint destruction and, in some cases, mortality. The joint should be tapped and fluid sent for cell count, culture (with Gram's stain), and crystals. Septic joints typically have white blood cell (WBC) counts above 50,000, with a predominance of polymorphonuclear neutrophil leukocytes. Urethral or cervical cultures (and, if suspected, throat and rectal cultures) for gonorrhea should be obtained for young adults, along with routine synovial, blood, and urine cultures. The patient should be admitted and the joint tapped daily, checking cell counts and culture for improvements. Empiric antibiotics should be initiated based on expected pathogens (ceftriaxone for suspected gonococcal arthritis for the young adult, and *Staphylococcus aureus* coverage for the immune suppressed, the elderly, and those with open wounds). Adjust antibiotics based on culture results. Antibiotics should be continued for 2–4 weeks for septic arthritis, except for the RA patient, for whom 6 weeks of antibiotics are typically recommended.

Many presenting with an acute monoarticular arthritis will not grow any organisms from the synovial fluid or blood cultures. When this is the case and there is an inadequate response to appropriate antibiotics or the patient develops other inflamed joints, a reactive arthritis should be considered (as discussed under Reactive Arthritis [Navajo Arthritis and Reiter's Syndrome]). Nonsteroidal anti-inflammatory drugs (NSAIDs) can be initiated after evaluation of an initial antibiotic response or if reactive arthritis is suspected. Indomethacin, ibuprofen, and naproxen are well tolerated and effective in most Native American patients. An intraarticular injection of a corticosteroid (Table 26-2) can be considered only after an exhaustive search for infection has failed to yield positive results and the patient does not respond to the measures mentioned in preceding paragraphs.

Crystalline arthritis (e.g., gout, pseudogout) often presents as a monoarticular inflammatory process. Synovial fluid analysis for crystals can identify gout and pseudogout, and radiographic analysis can help to diagnose pseudogout (chondrocalcinosis) (Figure 26-1) and calcium hydroxyapatite (calcific tendonitis). These diagnoses are common in men and can be seen in postmenopausal women.

Chronic monoarticular arthritis is most often osteoarthritis (OA). The synovial fluid in OA is noninflammatory (WBC <2,000), and radiographs reveal sclerosis, osteophyte formation, subchondral cystlike changes, and joint space narrowing. When the synovial fluid is inflammatory (i.e., WBC count exceeding 2,000), one must consider either a crystalline arthritis or an atypical, indolent infectious process, such as tuberculosis or fungal infection. Occasionally, a synovial biopsy must be done if the cultures of the fluid are sterile and the suspicion is high.

Oligoarticular or Polyarticular Arthritis

Acute oligoarticular or *polyarticular arthritis* can be due to a number of conditions, including the onset of a chronic condition. Although most of the chronic inflammatory disorders begin at some point, the process should go on for at least 6 weeks before the patient is labeled with a chronic rheumatic condition. Acute self-limited processes are often due to infections, as in the following examples:

- Disseminated gonorrhea often presents as a polyarticular arthritis with tenosynovitis, fevers, and skin rash.
- Viral infections (including hepatitis) often present as a polyarticular inflammatory arthritis mimicking RA.
- Lyme arthritis (prevalent in certain parts of the United States and not well studied in the Native American population) is associated with a tick bite, a typical skin rash (erythema chronica migrans), and oligoarticular arthritis, with the knee being the most common joint involved.

Table 26-2. Joint and Soft Tissue Steroid Injections

Joint	Total Volume	Needle Gauge	Triamcinolone (Aristospan) (20 mg/ml)	Prednisolone (Hydeltra) (20 mg/ml)	Lidocaine (Xylocaine) (1% W/O)	Bupivacaine (Marcaine)
Knee	3–4 ml	18–25*	1–2 ml	1–2 ml	1 ml	1 ml
Ankle	1–2 ml	22–25	1 ml	1 ml	0.5 ml	0.5 ml
Shoulder	2–3 ml	20–25	1–2 ml	1–2 ml	0.5–1.0 ml	0.5–1.0 ml
AC	1.0–1.5 ml	22–25	0.5 ml	0.5 ml	0.5 ml	0.25 ml
Elbow	1–2 ml	22–25	1 ml	1 ml	0.5 ml	0.5 ml
Wrist	1.0–1.5 ml	22–25	0.5–1.0 ml	1 ml	0.5 ml	0.5 ml
MCP or PIP	0.5 ml	22–25	0.25 ml	0.25 ml	0.25 ml	0.25 ml
Soft Tissue Tendinitis						
Biceps	2–3 ml	22–25	1 ml	1 ml	0.5–1.0 ml	0.5–1.0 ml
Epicondylitis						
Lateral	2–3 ml	22–25	1 ml	1 ml	0.5–1.0 ml	0.5–1.0 ml
Medial	2–3 ml	22–25	1 ml	1 ml	0.5–1.0 ml	0.5–1.0 ml
de Quervain	2–3 ml	22–25	1 ml	1 ml	0.5–1.0 ml	0.5–1.0 ml
Subdeltoid	2 ml	22–25	1 ml	1 ml	0.5–1.0 ml	0.5–1.0 ml
Olecranon	2 ml	22–25	1 ml	1 ml	0.5–1.0 ml	0.5–1.0 ml
Trochanter	2 ml	22–25	1 ml	1 ml	0.5–1.0 ml	0.5–1.0 ml
Anserine	1 ml	22–25	0.5 ml	0.5 ml	0.25–0.50 ml	0.25–0.50 ml
Prepatellar	1 ml	22–25	0.5 ml	0.5 ml	0.5 ml	0.5 ml
Trigger points	1–2 ml	25–27	1 ml	1 ml	0.5–1.0 ml	0.5–1.0 ml
Carpal tunnel syndrome	0.5 ml	22	0.5 ml	0.5 ml	0.5 ml	0.5 ml

Steroid Preparations		
Generic	**Trade Name**	**Quantity**
Triamcinolone hexacetonide	Aristospan	20 mg/ml
Triamcinolone acetonide	Kenalog	10–40 mg/ml
Methylprednisolone acetate	Depo-Medrol	20, 40, 80 mg/ml
Betamethasone acetate	Celestone	3–6 mg/ml
Prednisolone tertiary butylacetate	Hydeltra	20 mg/ml

*Gauge of needle: use larger gauge to withdraw fuild; can use smaller gauge to do just injection.
AC = acromioclavicular; MCP = metacarpophalangeal; PIP = proximal interphalangeal; W/O = water (in) oil (emulsion).

• Allergic reaction to a drug presents as polyarticular arthritis processes; vasculitis and malignancies can present with an inflammatory arthritis.

Nonarticular manifestations can give clues to the underlying disease, especially skin changes, inflammatory eye disease, or other major organ involvement. Although one can check RF and ANA in this population, it is sometimes preferable to wait until the acute process subsides (unless there is a clear suggestion of lupus or RA) because these can often be positive with infectious processes and confuse the picture. Acute rheumatic fever must still be considered in the individual with a recent streptococcal infection, migratory oligoarticular or polyarticular arthritis involving the medium to large joints (ankles, wrists, knees), and skin rash or carditis. In one study, Native Americans in New Mexico had twice the mortality due to rheumatic fever and chronic rheumatic heart disease compared to Hispanics and whites, although the mortality rate was decreasing.[28]

With any acute oligoarticular or polyarticular arthritis condition, a search for an underlying cause should be sought, the offending agent should be withdrawn, or the underlying infection should be treated, if identified. Monitoring over time is typically required, and one should expect resolution of the problem within 4–6 weeks. Supportive therapy should be initiated (e.g., NSAIDs). Rarely are steroids or other agents needed.

Chronic oligoarticular or polyarticular arthritis is identified when the process has gone on for more than 6 weeks. The main diseases that result in a chronic process are discussed in the following sections. The reader is referred to a rheumatology text for full discussion of more rare conditions.[20]

Figure 26-1. Radiograph of a Native American with acute wrist arthritis demonstrating chondrocalcinosis at ulnar styloid.

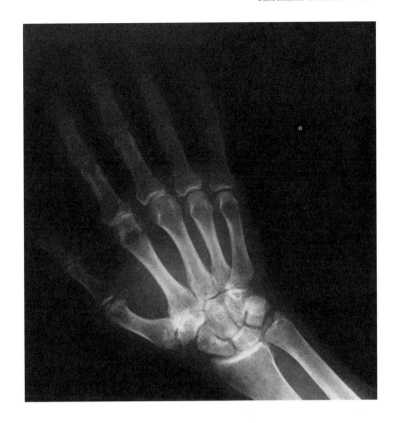

Rheumatoid Arthritis

Although much is written about Navajo arthritis and the seronegative SpA, RA is actually seen more commonly in Native Americans, especially women. Although there is a controversy about its origin, many think that RA is a New World disease, in part because archaeologic remains in Europe do not demonstrate bony changes consistent with RA until the 1800s. In contrast, characteristic erosive changes in skeletal remains of Native Americans in Alabama, Kentucky, and northern Ohio, dating back many thousands of years, have been reported.[29–31] The exploration of the New World and commerce with Europe suggests a possible infectious trigger and may have assisted in this condition now being seen worldwide.

Clinical Features and Diagnosis of Rheumatoid Arthritis in the Native American

Patterns of Joint Involvement

RA in Native Americans is similar to that in whites in most ways but has some differences. It is typically a polyarticular arthritis involving the small joints of the hands and feet (as well as any other synovial joint). It is often an erosive process. It can be associated with SI, which is rare in whites with RA.

Extraarticular Manifestations

Extraarticular manifestations are also common in Native Americans, but a full characterization has not been done. Subcutaneous nodules (seen in 20–25% of white patients) have been reported in as many as 35–44% of Native Americans,[7, 8, 32] are usually seen with seropositive individuals, and are typically found on the extensor surfaces of the elbow and the hand, and occasionally on the Achilles tendon. Rheumatoid vasculitis has been seen in Native Americans (both mild and severe vasculitis). Ulcerations of the lower extremity or neurologic symptomatology (numbness, burning, weakness, foot drop) are the most common manifestations of vasculitis, and patients may require cytotoxic agents and high-dose corticosteroids to control the disease. Felty's syndrome, typically seen in individuals with long-standing disease and positive RF, is manifest by frequent infections, an enlarged spleen, and a low WBC count.

Cardiopulmonary involvement (pericarditis, pleurisy, interstitial lung disease) is seen in anywhere from 1% to as many as 20% of white individuals, but little is known about its manifestation in Native Americans with RA. The pleural fluid associated with RA is typically an exudative process with low glucose. Corticosteroids in doses of 20–40 mg per day are often needed to control cardiopulmonary involvement if NSAIDs fail. It is sometimes difficult to differentiate pulmonary involvement due specifically to the RA from that due to methotrexate (MTX) or gold salts. Occasionally, medications must be stopped.

Ophthalmologic manifestations can be very severe and occasionally threaten vision loss. The most common ophthalmologic manifestation we have seen in the Native American is sicca syndrome, with dry eyes (and dry mouth).[1] Rose bengal or Schirmer's testing can help document keratoconjunctivitis and decreased tear production, respectively. Artificial tears or saliva can help with symptoms, and oral pilocarpine tablets (Salagen 5.0–7.5 mg orally qid) have been shown to increase tear and saliva production and may be of benefit. Episcleritis (mild inflammation of superficial scleral vessels, typically without pain) and scleritis (severe vasculitis involving deep layers of the sclerae, associated with severe pain and threat to vision) are potential problems and warrant an ophthalmologic evaluation. Topical steroid for episcleritis and systemic steroids or even cytotoxics may be needed for scleritis.

Generalized osteoporosis and periarticular osteopenia are common in RA. Individuals on steroids have an increased risk for osteoporosis and fracture, especially postmenopausal women, and should be on calcium (1,500 mg/day), vitamin D (400 IU/day), and an antiresorptive agent (e.g., estrogen, alendronate sodium [Fosamax], or calcitonin nasal spray [Miacalcin]). Some attempt to measure bone density to stratify fracture risk (e.g., with dual energy x-ray absorptiometry [DEXA] scan, calcaneal ultrasound, peripheral DEXA) is strongly encouraged. Until more is known about the average bone density in Native Americans, it is prudent to treat prophylactically.

Laboratory tests in the Native American patient with RA reflect a positive RF in 26–97%[2, 4, 7, 8, 11, 12, 32] and a positive ANA in 53–86%.[7, 32, 33] A normochromic normocytic anemia is often seen in these individuals due to the chronic inflammation. Macrocytic anemia may be seen in those on MTX, azathioprine, and sulfasalazine (SSA). Blood loss due to NSAIDs and marrow suppression from medications must also be considered. An elevated sedimentation rate or C-reactive protein reflects inflammation; either test can be used to monitor therapy.

Synovial fluid analysis is similar to that in whites, demonstrating more than 2,000 WBCs, predominantly mononuclear cells (consistent with an inflammatory process) and often very low glucose levels.

Radiographs of the hands and feet are useful at baseline to determine if erosions exist and for future comparison to evaluate effectiveness of therapy. Periarticular osteopenia is one of the earliest manifestations of an inflammatory process. Marginal erosions (especially of the ulnar styloid), metacarpophalangeal joints, proximal interphalangeal joints, and joint destruction requiring replacement are common in the Native American population (Figure 26-2). Figure 26-3 demonstrates protrusio acetabuli, a progression of inflammatory arthritis at the hip, in which there is symmetric joint space narrowing and axial migration of the femoral head. In patients with RA and hip pain, a plain x-ray should be obtained.

Diagnosis

The American College of Rheumatology (ACR) has developed criteria for diagnosing RA and identifying those in remission (Table 26-3).[34] These have not been validated in the Native American patient and therefore should only be used as a guide. If the diagnosis is unclear, it is best to describe the process and wait until more definitive criteria manifest. If the RF is negative at the initial evaluation, it should be repeated in the future because it often turns positive with time, but one must also consider the possibility of a seronegative SpA in this population.

Besides the diagnosis, an attempt should be made to determine the severity of disease and presence of poor prognostic indicators. When present, these indicators raise one's risk of developing erosive disease (e.g., more than 20 active joints, positive RF, elevated sedimentation rate, rheumatoid nodules, and a positive HLA-DR4 in whites). The HLA-DR4 alleles, seen with great frequency in severe active RA in whites, are seen in some but not all Native American tribes.[7, 32, 35] The more severe the disease and the more poor prognostic indicators there are, the earlier the disease should be treated and with more aggressive medication.

Treatment of Rheumatoid Arthritis in Native Americans

General

Information specific to treating the Native American patient with RA is included, where known, or from our own experience using certain medications in these patients. The goals of treatment for all RA patients include (1) slowing or halting disease progression, (2) relieving inflammation, (3) maintaining function, (4) relieving pain, and (5) improving systemic symptoms. An assessment of the extent of disease, including extraarticular manifestations, should be done to categorize the patient according to disease severity and to assist in determining therapy. See Table 26-4 for details about dosing, toxicity, and monitoring therapy of specific medications.

Most patients benefit from having an NSAID initiated early. The selection of the NSAID depends on concomitant medications, concomitant diseases, and the patient's age, in addition to cost of therapy. No one NSAID agent has been shown to be superior to all others. Most Native American patients tolerate ibuprofen, naproxen, and indomethacin and receive symptomatic relief from these agents. For mild disease, the milder disease-modifying antirheumatologic drugs (DMARDs) (e.g., hydroxychloroquine [Plaquenil], SSA, and oral gold) should be instituted first, especially for milder disease. The first two are well

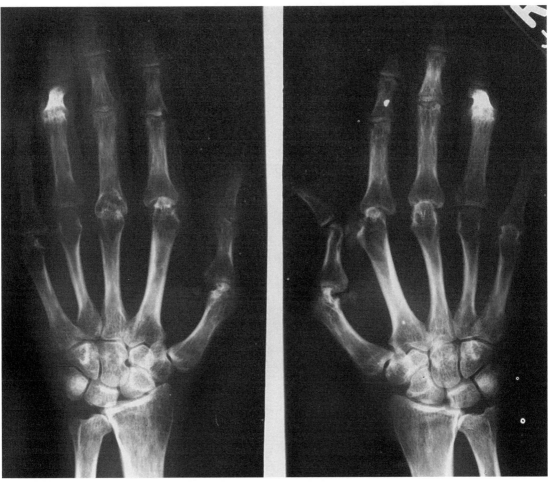

Figure 26-2. Radiographs of a Native American with rheumatoid arthritis. Note periarticular osteopenia, ulnar styloid erosions, loss of joint space, and marginal erosions of metacarpophalangeal joints and proximal interphalangeal joints.

tolerated and effective in the Native American patient.[1] When these agents fail to control disease, adding another agent is often necessary. More severe disease often requires the more potent DMARDs (MTX, azathioprine [Imuran], gold salts, cyclosporin, and rarely cyclophosphamide). MTX is by far the most widely used of these next-line agents and is well tolerated and very effective in our experience. Gold salts have been used for years to treat RA and were used to treat many Native Americans with RA in the 1970s and 1980s. Increased proteinuria and rash were frequent reasons for its discontinuation in one study of Yakima Indians.[36] We found similar experiences when reviewing records of RA patients who had been on gold (most had a good response to the medication, though). We therefore defer using gold until a failure of other DMARDs occurs. Some investigation in whites supports a trial of tetracycline-type antibiotics (e.g., minocycline) for early or mild RA. There are no data on this therapy in Native Americans. The U.S. Food and Drug Administration has approved cyclosporin for use in RA, and it has been used in

several Native American patients, especially those with more severe disease or with rheumatoid vasculitis.[1] It appears to be well tolerated.

These DMARDs can also be called slow-acting antirheumatic drugs because the onset of action typically takes anywhere between 6 and 8 weeks and sometimes 3–4 months. Many Native American individuals stop the medication if they do not understand this.

Should one agent not work or a side effect develop, switch to an alternative agent. If a partial response has been achieved, adding a third agent to control disease may be more beneficial than starting all over with a new agent. Once remission has been achieved (morning stiffness <30 minutes, no swollen or painful joints, and normalization of the sedimentation rate) and maintained for a period of 6 months to a year, a very slow tapering of medicine (by 10–25% every 3–4 months) could be considered, with close monitoring for a flare of disease. The more severe the disease, the more reluctant one should be to discontinue medications completely (unless there is a

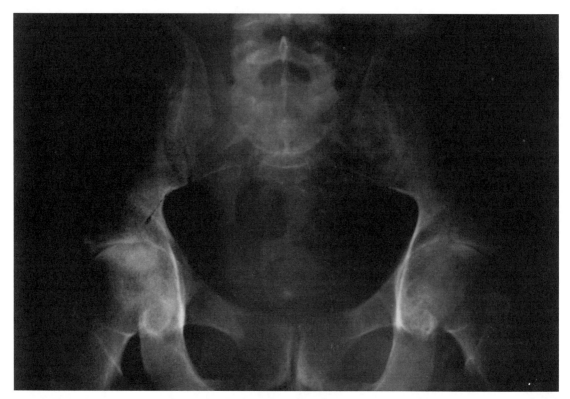

Figure 26-3. Radiograph of a Native American with rheumatoid arthritis and bilateral hip pain. Note severe loss of joint space and axial migration of the femoral heads with rear protrusion through acetabuli (protrusio acetabuli). Also note suspicious sacroiliac joint (*right*).

Table 26-3. American College of Rheumatology Criteria for Diagnosing Rheumatoid Arthritis*

Morning stiffness of at least 30–60 mins before maximal improvement

At least three active inflamed joints simultaneously with soft tissue swelling or joint fluid; at least one area of involvement must include the joints of the hands (i.e., wrists, MCPs or PIPs)

Symmetric arthritis

Rheumatoid nodules over bony prominences or over extensor surfaces

Positive rheumatoid factor

Radiographic demonstration of erosions or unequivocal bony decalcification localized in the periarticular region

*The patient must fulfill four of the six criteria to be given the strict diagnosis (primarily for research).
MCPs = metacarpophalangeal (joints); PIPs = proximal interphalangeal (joints).
Source: Adapted from FC Arnett, S Edworthy, DA Block, et al. The 1987 revised ARA criteria for rheumatoid arthritis. Arthritis Rheum 1987;30:S17.

toxicity). This is because occasionally, once a medication is discontinued, a flare of disease can occur, and the medication may no longer be effective when restarted.

Corticosteroids may be needed in the severe rheumatoid patient, although chronic use remains controversial. When needed, they should be used in the lowest possible dose (<10 mg/day), with risk-benefit ratio considered and toxicity reviewed. We typically recommend avoiding frequent bursts of prednisone (i.e., 60, 40, 20, 10 mg/day) because in the occasional rheumatoid patient it can trigger rheumatoid vasculitis, especially in those with more long-standing disease. Doses of 20–40 mg/day may be needed to control extraarticular manifestations, such as pericarditis, pleurisy, or inflammatory eye disease. Very high-dose steroids (i.e., 1,000 mg methylprednisolone [Solu-Medrol] intravenously for 3 days) may be needed when all other DMARDs have failed to control disease, or with severe complications of disease, but this should be done in consultation with a rheumatologist. Intramuscular injections (e.g., triamcinolone acetonide, 20–40 mg, or prednisolone, 20–40 mg) can be used as a bridge to help control the disease until other agents begin working.

Table 26-4. Antirheumatic Medications

Drug	Indications	Dosing	Toxicity	Monitoring
HCQ	Alone: mild RA, SLE; can try with CPPD and SpA except psoriasis. Combine with most other medications for severe delayed sensitivity	Start: 200 mg bid; Goal: ≤5 mg/kg/day	Skin rash, hyperpigmentation. Eye rare, heme rare in G6PD deficiency	CBC, renal, LFTs q6mos. Ophthalmologic examination q6-12mos
SSA	Alone: Mild RA, SpA. Avoid in SLE. Combine with other medications for severe delayed sensitivity	Start: 500 mg/day, ↑ q wk by 500 mg (bid) Goal: 2-4 g/day split	Severe rash, allergic reaction. Marrow suppression rare	CBC q2wks × 2 mos, then q1-3mos, LFTs, renal, and urinalysis in 1 mo; then q3mos
MTX	Moderate to severe RA, SLE, SpA, vasculitis	Start: 7.5-10.0 mg/wk. Advance: q mo by 2.5 mg. Maximum: ~ 25 mg/wk	GI, oral ulcers, headache, rash. Pulmonary early or after chronic use, hepatic (cirrhosis), marrow suppression	Baseline hepatitis B and C, CBC, LFTs, CXR, (? HIV). Follow-up: LFTs with albumin q4-8wks, CBC q1-2mos Renal q4mos
Gold (IM)	Moderate to severe RA; can try with SpA	Test dose: 10 mg IM. Weekly: 25 mg/wk up to 50 mg/wk; extend to q2wks after 6 mos if able	Skin rash, GI, pulmonary (rare), renal, heme	Urinalysis (dipstick) q wk before medication (hold if protein) CBC, LFTs, renal q1- mos
Gold (oral)	Alone: mild RA	Start: 3 mg bid ↑ 3 mg tid in 3-6 mos prn	Skin rash, GI, heme	CBC, LFTs, renal, urinalysis after 1 mo; then q1-3mos
Minocycline	Mild RA	Start: 100 mg bid	Skin rash/photosensitivity. Autoimmune induction	CBC q6mos. Periodic renal, LFTs
Imuran	Moderate to severe RA, SLE, vasculitis	Start: 50 mg/day. Advance: 25-50 mg/day q mo. Maximum: 150-200 mg/day	GI, marrow suppression	CBC q2wks × 1-2 mos; then q mo LFTs, renal q1-3mos
Cyclosporin	Alone or combine with MTX for moderate to severe RA; possibly SLE, psoriasis	Start: 2-3 mg/kg/day split bid. Maximum: 3-4 mg/kg/day	Renal, hypertension, gingival hyperplasia, hirsutism	Baseline: renal Follow-up: renal q2wks × 1-2 mos; then q mo CBC, LFTs q1-3mos
CTX	Severe RA, SLE (renal, CNS), vasculitis	Orally: start 50 mg/day. Advance: 25-50 mg/day q mo. Maximum: 150-200 mg/day. Intravenously: start 750 mg/m²; subsequent dose based on nadir white blood count. Administer: monthly × 6 mos then q2-3mos for 2 yrs (variable)	Marrow suppression, hemorrhagic cystitis, ovarian suppression. Pulmonary (rare)	CBC, urinalysis 7-14 days after CTX, Periodic LFTs, renal

HCQ = hydroxychloroquine; SSA = sulfasalazine; CTX = cytoxan; CBC = complete blood count with differentials and platelets; G6PD = glucose-6-phosphate dehydrogenase; RA = rheumatoid arthritis; MTX = methotrexate; IM = intramuscular; CPPD = calcium pyrophosphate dihydrate; SLE = systemic lupus erythematosus; SpA = seronegative spondyloarthropathies; CNS = central nervous system; LFTs = liver function tests; CXR = chest x-ray; HIV = human immunodeficiency syndrome; GI = gastrointestinal; prn = as required; ? = possible. ↑ = increase; ? = possible.
Source: Adapted from JH Klippel (ed). Primer on the Rheumatic Diseases. Atlanta: Arthritis Foundation, 1997; and The American College of Rheumatology Ad Hoc Committee on Clinical Guidelines. Guidelines for monitoring drug therapy in rheumatoid arthritis. Arthritis Rheum 1996;39:723-731.

Intraarticular injections (e.g., triamcinolone acetonide, 20–40 mg, or prednisolone, 20–40 mg, with lidocaine 1% without epinephrine and bupivacaine; see Table 26-2) are very useful adjuncts and may help limit the amount of oral steroid needed. The possibility of underlying infection must be considered, especially if one joint is much more active than the others. In this situation, consider arthrocentesis and sending the fluid for culture before injecting the steroid. It means an extra trip for the patients but in the long run avoids serious sequelae, should an infection be present.

Supportive Measures

No matter which category the patient falls into, mild or severe, physical therapy and possibly occupational therapy with splinting should be considered. Wrist splints worn at night help to decrease pain, swelling, and symptoms of carpal tunnel syndrome and help to keep the wrist in a more functional position. Strengthening exercises for periarticular musculature also are valuable but must be done in a controlled setting, especially when there is significant active swelling. For the Native American, bread making, basket weaving, and rug making may be continued, but when significant swelling of the joint jeopardizes the supporting ligaments and tendons, overuse must be avoided. Analgesics are often necessary, especially to keep individuals functioning. Cyclobenzaprine or tricyclic antidepressants at night are well tolerated by most Native Americans, helping those who have difficulty sleeping.

Seronegative Spondyloarthropathies

The seronegative SpAs are an interesting group of diseases that are seen with high prevalence in many of the Native American tribes, probably related to the high prevalence of HLA-B27 in many tribes (as discussed under Prevalence of Rheumatic Conditions in the Native American). The SpAs include AS, reactive arthritis (including RS, a specific type of reactive arthritis), and Navajo arthritis. Psoriatic arthritis and arthritis associated with inflammatory bowel diseases are rare in Native Americans. SpA are characterized by inflammatory arthritis, most typically of the axial spine (sacroiliac joints and spine) or other peripheral joints, depending on the specific disease. Extraarticular manifestations include enthesitis (inflammation where the tendons and ligaments insert into the bone), inflammatory eye disease, and characteristic dermatologic changes (keratoderma blennorrha'gica). Individuals usually have a negative RF and thus are seronegative.

Characteristics of Disease

AS is the prototype for the seronegative SpAs. It is a chronic, systemic inflammatory disorder primarily affecting the axial skeleton, particularly in the form of bilateral SI (Figure 26-4). Besides bilateral SI, there is inflammation along the anterior and posterior longitudinal ligaments, resulting in squaring of the vertebral bodies (Figure 26-5) and calcification, with ultimate ossification of the ligaments and posterior elements. The end result is an inflexible, ankylosed spine. The amount of flexibility in the lumbar spine (or lack thereof) can be assessed by marking off 10 cm above the sacroiliac joints, then measuring this area as the individual bends forward (Schober test). Normally, this area should increase by 6 cm on forward bending, but in the individual with AS, it often does not increase by more than 1–2 cm, if that. An x-ray of the lumbosacral spine with sacroiliac views confirms the diagnosis; it should be done whenever ankylosis is suspected. The arthritis often involves the proximal joints (hips and shoulders) but can involve the peripheral joints as well.

Extraarticular Disease

Acute anterior uveitis (iritis) (seen in up to 30% of whites with AS) is seen in many Native Americans, although exact prevalence is unknown. Pain, photophobia, blurred vision, and increased lacrimation are common symptoms. Corticosteroids, either topical or systemic, are needed to control the inflammation and prevent synechiae formation. Other extraarticular manifestations (i.e., ascending aortitis, aortic valve incompetence, conduction abnormalities, and pulmonary fibrosis in the upper lobes) may be seen. Neurologic involvement may result from the cauda equina syndrome (narrowing about the cord) or fracturing through the ankylosed spine, which creates a pseudoarthrosis, resulting in an unstable spine. Caution must be used during intubation and endoscopy to avoid hyperextension of the neck if it is fused.

Diagnosing Ankylosing Spondylitis

Bilateral SI is key to the diagnosis of AS. Ankylosis of the spine, progressing up from the sacrum, supports the diagnosis as well. The HLA-B27 antigen is positive in more than 90% of AS patients, and in Native Americans the RF and ANA can be positive.

Therapy for Ankylosing Spondylitis

Presently, there is no cure for AS. Extension exercises are essential for maintaining an erect posture. Swimming seems to be the best overall exercise but is generally not available to most Native Americans. The pain and stiffness can often be controlled by NSAIDs. Indomethacin appears to be the most effective NSAID, and it is generally well tolerated by most of the Native Americans we follow. For those with peripheral arthritis, we have initiated SSA with good results. Corticosteroids have little place in treating this disease, except when there is severe iritis. When arthritis of the hip is severe enough, total joint replacement is often needed. Perioperative radiation therapy is used in whites to prevent heterotopic ossification of the surrounding tissues, but we have little experience with this therapy in Native Americans.

Figure 26-4. Bilateral sacro-iliitis in a Native American patient with early ankylosing spondylitis.

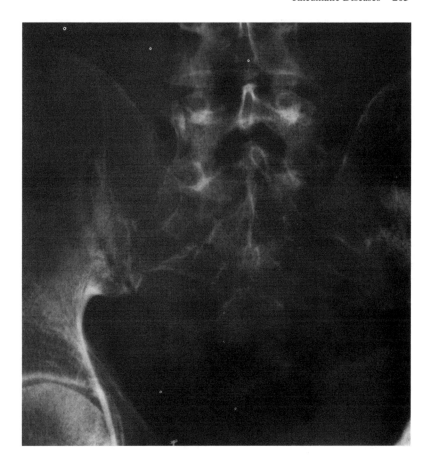

Reactive Arthritis (Navajo Arthritis and Reiter's Syndrome)

Reactive arthritis (ReA) is the overall heading under which Navajo arthritis and RS fall. ReA is a sterile inflammatory process involving peripheral joints after certain gram-negative enteric pathogens or genitourinary infections. These infections can trigger a monoarticular, oligoarticular, or even a polyarticular arthritis in 2–10% of patients in the general population,[37] but they can be seen in as many as 20% or more in genetically susceptible individuals (i.e., those that are positive for HLA-B27).[38]

Extraarticular symptoms are more common with ReA than with AS and include inflammatory eye disease, SI, balanitis, keratoderma blennorrha'gica, and enthesopathies (an inflammation in which the tendon inserts into the bone that is often associated with calcification).

Diagnosis

The diagnosis of ReA or RS is primarily clinical. Classic RS includes inflammatory eye disease (conjunctivitis), arthritis, and urethritis, although other features (as mentioned in the preceding section) may be seen. The RF is negative by definition in the seronegative SpA, but in Native Americans, a positive RF can be seen in up to 28%,[1] thus complicating the clinical evaluation. A positive HLA-B27 is seen in the majority of Native Americans with ReA. A lumbosacral spine radiograph should be considered in any young patient with inflammatory-sounding back pain (i.e., pain and stiffness worse in the morning and better with activity).

Therapy

NSAIDs are the first line of therapy. Indomethacin is often the most effective. Often, NSAID therapy is not enough. SSA is the next choice of therapy and is very effective in the Native American population.[1] Because severe, active disease is commonly seen in these individuals, MTX is often needed to control disease. Occult human immunodeficiency virus infection must be considered before starting MTX, and baseline hepatitis serology (B and C antigens) should be checked as well. MTX should not be given to those who use regular or excessive alcohol. Occasionally, steroids are used for recalcitrant disease. Local steroid injections are preferred.

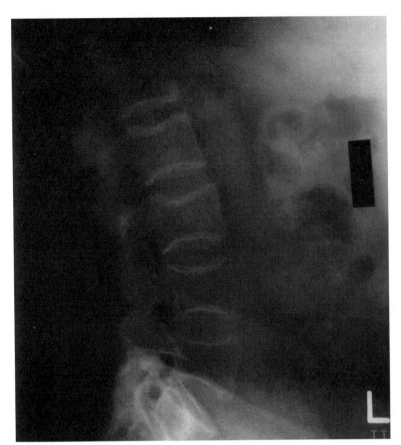

Figure 26-5. Native American with inflammatory low-back symptoms. Note squaring of lumbar vertebrae.

Systemic Lupus Erythematosus

SLE is an autoimmune disease of uncertain etiology. It has, however, clear links to estrogen (increased frequency in women), certain genetic factors (class III major histocompatibility complex alleles C4 null allele and 21 hydroxylase in many ethnic groups), ethnic predisposition (black, Hispanic, and Native American), and likely environmental triggers. The pathogenesis is related to induction of autoimmunity, polyclonal B cell activation, and faulty downregulation of the immune response with immune complex activation, resulting in tissue inflammation and injury. The disease manifestations can be diverse between individuals and even within an individual at various times (i.e., in flares of disease). The 1982 ACR criteria presently used were derived from the study and evaluation of numerous lupus patients, primarily whites, so their applicability to Native Americans has not been studied.

We know that there appears to be an increased incidence rate of SLE in the Sioux, Arapaho, and Crow tribes,[13] but little data are available on the characteristics of disease in these or other tribes. Much of the detailed data we have on SLE in the Native American comes from

the Boyer and Templin group's work with the Alaskan Indian population.[6, 32] In this population, arthritis was seen at a much higher rate than in whites (92% vs. 63%), as was serositis (62% vs. 40%) and serious neurologic disease (31% vs. <20%). Skin manifestations were seen in up to 46% and mucositis in 15%. Renal disease was seen in approximately 40%, and hematologic manifestations (neutropenia, lymphopenia, or hemolytic anemia) were seen in just more than 50%. Immunologic abnormalities (i.e., positive anti-dsDNA, false-positive syphilis test) were found in 77%, and 100% were ANA positive.

Diagnosis

The diagnosis of SLE is based on symptoms, clinical manifestations, and positive serologies. The ACR criteria are merely guidelines for study, and not all patients fulfill all criteria. An ANA is typically positive, which should prompt a check for more specific autoantibodies (dsDNA and anti-Smith). Anti-Ro (SS-A) and anti-La (SS-B) antibodies can be checked if there are sicca symptoms, suggesting Sjögren's syndrome. A complete blood count (CBC) with differential and platelets and a urinalysis with a microscopic evaluation should be done on all individuals. Symptoms and clinical findings should guide further evaluation. For example, pleuritic chest pain should prompt a chest x-ray or echocardiogram, or both. Hypertension, proteinuria, elevated creatinine, or abnormal urinalysis should prompt a 24-hour urine analysis and a renal biopsy. Psychosis, severe headaches, and seizures are indications for computed tomography or magnetic resonance imaging brain scanning, antineuronal and antiribosomal P antibodies, and a lumbar puncture with oligoclonal bands and immunoglobulin G synthesis rate. A C3 and C4 (third and fourth complement components) are often done to evaluate activity of disease because they are measures of immune complex production. C3 and C4 are typically low in active SLE.

Treatment

The treatment of SLE varies with the activity of disease and the specific organ systems involved. Because lupus is a chronic disease with flares and remissions, two levels of medications may be needed: one to control the chronic disease and prevent flares, and one to treat flares as they come. One first must determine the activity of disease and which organ systems it involves.

Generally, for more mild disease involving the joints, skin, mucosa, or constitutional symptoms, supportive measures (e.g., sunscreen, rest, aphthous ulcer mix), NSAIDs, or antimalarial compounds (e.g., hydroxychloroquine) are very effective and well tolerated. It must be remembered that NSAIDs may cause neurologic side effects and even aseptic meningitis, which may confuse the picture and must be taken into account in the setting of central nervous system (CNS) lupus. Some data suggest that hydroxychloroquine may be beneficial in suppressing flares of lupus.[39] Therefore, once started, the drug is usually continued unless there are intolerable side effects or pregnancy. Occasionally, MTX or azathioprine can be used for recalcitrant joint or skin disease not controlled with these measures. Glucocorticoids should be reserved for the more severe, major organ involvement because of the risk-benefit ratio. If needed, doses less than 0.5 mg/kg per day should be used. Topical or intralesional steroid for the skin can be used, but caution must be exercised.

Moderately active disease with involvement of the lung (pleurisy), heart (pericarditis), or hematologic abnormalities (severe hemolytic anemia or thrombocytopenia) typically require corticosteroids given at 0.5–1.0 mg/kg per day in single or divided doses. This dosage is best maintained for at least 4 weeks or until the disease is well controlled before tapering. Tapering should be done slowly (e.g., 10–20% decrements) every 2–4 weeks, as dictated by disease activity and toxicity. Should untoward side effects develop or the disease flare as the corticosteroid is tapered, adding an immune suppressant as a steroid-sparing agent (e.g., MTX, azathio-

prine, or cyclophosphamide [in severe cases]) should be considered.

Severe organ-threatening or life-threatening disease (e.g., CNS lupus, diffuse proliferative glomerulonephritis, pulmonary hemorrhage) must be treated aggressively with both corticosteroids in doses of 1–2 mg/kg per day (single or divided) and cytotoxics. Cyclophosphamide intravenous pulse therapy used monthly for 6 months and then every 3 months for 18 months is recommended for severe lupus nephritis. Azathioprine can be used as well if toxicity develops. Less data are available on cerebritis, so the length of treatment is not known. Six monthly pulses of cyclophosphamide is the typical starting regimen. High-dose corticosteroids (1 g intravenously for 3 days) may be needed in severe cases, and plasmapheresis and immunoglobulin therapy (considered investigational) may be needed in refractory cases or when active SLE with infection complicates the picture.

Monitoring Patients

Monitoring patients depends on the severity and activity of disease and the medications being used to control disease. Generally, following disease activity requires a thorough history and physical examination, basic laboratory parameters (i.e., a CBC with differential and platelets, a creatinine, and a urinalysis) approximately every 1–2 months initially (when disease is very active or cytotoxics are being used) and then every 3–4 months. Some people advocate checking C3, C4, and dsDNA antibodies regularly, but this is more controversial. The C3 and C4 can help in the evaluation of disease activity if they are shown to be very low in active disease and improved or normalized when the disease is treated.

References

1. Arizona Arthritis Center Native American Clinic Data Base, 1991–present.
2. Del Puente A, Knowler WC, Pettitt DJ, Bennett PH. High incidence and prevalence of rheumatoid arthritis in Pima Indians. Am J Epidemiol 1989;19:1170–1178.
3. Henrad JC, Bennett PH, Burch TA. Rheumatoid arthritis in Pima of Arizona; an assessment of the clinical component of the New York criteria. Int J Epidemiol 1975;4:119–126.
4. Lichtenstein MJ, Pincus T. Rheumatoid arthritis identified in population based cross sectional studies: low prevalence of rheumatoid factor. J Rheumatol 1991;18:989–993.
5. Bunin JJ, Burch TA, O'Brien WN. Bull Rheum Dis. 1964;15:349–350.
6. Boyer GS, Templin DW, Lanier AP. Rheumatic diseases in Alaskan Indians of the southwest coast: high prevalence of rheumatoid arthritis and systemic lupus erythematosus. J Rheumatol 1991;18:1477–1484.

7. Harvey J, Lotz M, Stevens MB, et al. Rheumatoid arthritis in a Chippewa band. Arthritis Rheum 1981;24: 717–721.

8. Beasley RP, Wilkens RF, Bennett PH. High prevalence of rheumatoid arthritis in Yakima Indians. Arthritis Rheum 1973;16:743–748.

9. Boyer GS, Lanier AP, Templin DW. Prevalence rates of spondyloarthropathies, rheumatoid arthritis, and other rheumatoid disorders in an Alaskan Inupiat Eskimo population. J Rheumatol 1988;15:678–683.

10. Boyer GS, Lanier AP, Templin DW, Bulkow L. Spondyloarthropathy and rheumatoid arthritis in Yupic Eskimos. J Rheumatol 1990;17:489–496.

11. Atkins C, Reuffel L, Roddy J, et al. Rheumatic disease in the Nuu-Chah-Nulth native Indians of the Pacific Northwest. J Rheumatol 1988;15:684–690.

12. Oen K, Postle B, Chalmers IM, et al. Rheumatic diseases in an Inuit population. Arthritis Rheum 1986;29:65–74.

13. Morton RO, Gershwin EM, Brady C, Steinberg AD. The incidence of systemic lupus erythematosus in North American Indians. J Rheumatol 1976;3:186–190.

14. Morse HG, Rate RG, Bonnell MD, Kuberski T. High frequency of HLA-B27 and Reiter's syndrome in Navajo Indians. J Rheumatol 1980;7:900–902.

15. Gofton JP, Robinson HS, Trueman GE. Ankylosing spondylitis in a Canadian Indian population. Ann Rheum Dis 1966;25:525–527.

16. Gofton JP, Lawrence JS, Bennett PH, Burch TA. Sacroiliitis in eight populations. Ann Rheum Dis 1966; 25:528–532.

17. Gofton JR, Chalmers A, Price GE, Reeve CE. HLA-B27 and ankylosing spondylitis in BC Indians. J Rheumatol 1975;2:314–318.

18. Cohen LM, Mittal KK, Schmidt FR, et al. Increased risk of spondylitis stigmata in apparently healthy HLA-B27 men. Ann Intern Med 1976;84:1–7.

19. Lisse JR, Kuberski TT, Bennett PH, Knowler WC. High risk of sacroiliitis in HLA-B27 positive Pima Indian men. Arthritis Rheum 1982;25:236–238.

20. Kelly WA, Harris ED, Ruddy S, Sledge CB. Textbook of Rheumatology. Philadelphia: Saunders, 1993; 681–1060.

21. Muggia AL, Bennahum DA, William RC Jr. Navajo arthritis: an unusual, acute, self-limited disease. Arthritis Rheum 1971;14:348–355.

22. Rate RG, Morse HG, Bonnell MD, Kuberski T. Navajo arthritis reconsidered, relationship to HLA-B27. Arthritis Rheum 1980;23:1299–1302.

23. Kahn MA. HLA-B27 and its subtypes in world populations. Curr Opin Rheumatol 1995;7:263–269.

24. Gofton JP. Epidemiology, tissue type antigen and Bechterew's syndrome (ankylosing spondylitis) in various ethnic populations. Scand J Rheumatol 1980;9 (suppl 132):166–168.

25. Walsh BT, Hamstra AS, Hamstra T, et al. Correlation between HLA-B27, *Shigella* enteritis and development of arthritis in Native American populations. Arthritis Rheum 1997;40(suppl):144.

26. Spees EK, Kostyu DD, Elston RC, et al. HLA profiles of the Pima Indians of Arizona. In Dausset J, Colombani J (eds), Histocompatibility Testing 1972. Copenhagen: Munsgaard, 1973:345–349.

27. Searles RP, Voyles WF, Billowitz E, et al. Prevalence of HLA-B27 and sacroiliitis in a prospective study of Zuni Indians. Tissue Antigens 1979;14:174–176.

28. Becker TM, Wiggins CL, Key CR, Samet JM. Ethnic differences in mortality from acute rheumatic fever and chronic rheumatic heart disease in New Mexico, 1958–1982. West J Med 1989;150:46–50.

29. Rothschild BM, Woods RJ. Symmetrical erosive disease in archaic Indians: the origin of rheumatoid arthritis in the New World. Semin Arthritis Rheum 1990;19:278–284.

30. Rothschild BM, Turner KR, DeLuca MA. Symmetrical erosive peripheral polyarthritis in the late archaic period of Alabama. Science 1988;241:1498–1501.

31. Woods RJ, Rothschild BM. Population analysis of symmetrical erosive arthritis in Ohio woodland Indians 1200 years ago. J Rheumatol 1988;15:1258–1263.

32. Templin DW, Boyer GS, Lanier AP, et al. Rheumatoid arthritis in Tlingit Indians: clinical characterization and HLA associations. J Rheumatol 1994;21:1238–1244.

33. Scofield RH, Fogle M, Rhoades ER, Harley TB. Rheumatoid arthritis in a United States Public Health Service hospital in Oklahoma. Arthritis Rheum 1996; 99:283–286.

34. Arnett FC, Edworthy S, Block DA, et al. The 1987 revised ARA criteria for rheumatoid arthritis. Arthritis Rheum 1987;30:S17.

35. Willkens RF, Hansen TA, Malongren TA, et al. HLA antigens in Yakima Indians with rheumatoid arthritis. Lack of association with HLA-DW4 and HLA-DR4. Arthritis Rheum 1982;25:1435–1439.

36. Wilkens RF, Blandau RL, Aoyana OT, Beasly P. Studies of rheumatoid arthritis among a tribe of North West Indians. J Rheumatology 1976;3:9–14.

37. Keat A. Reiter's syndrome and reactive arthritis in perspective. N Engl J Med 1983;309:1606.

38. Calin A, Fries JF. Experimental epidemic of Reiter's disease. Ann Intern Med 1976;84:564–566.

39. The Canadian Hydroxychloroquine Study Group. A randomized study of the effects of withdrawing hydroxychloroquine sulfate in systemic lupus erythematosus. N Engl J Med 1991;324:150–154.

Chapter 27

Developmental Dysplasia of the Hip

Eric Henley and Richard M. Schwend

In this chapter, we present practical information on the screening and diagnosis of developmental dysplasia of the hip (DDH), its epidemiology, natural history, basic treatment principles, and specific relevance to Native American populations.

Definition

DDH was formerly known as *congenital dislocation of the hip*. It refers to the abnormal formation of the hip joint occurring between organogenesis and maturity as a result of instability.[1] The terminology has changed to encompass the variability in presentation, depending on time and severity. Not all dysplasia of the hip can be diagnosed at birth, and a spectrum exists in infants and children, ranging from laxity to true dislocation. DDH includes the conditions of laxity (loose capsular structures), acetabular dysplasia (inadequate development of the acetabulum), subluxation (partial contact of the femoral head with the acetabulum), and dislocation (the femoral head completely out of the hip socket). The functional consequences can range from a normal lifestyle to severe arthritis in young adulthood, resulting in pain, disability, and repeated operative procedures. It is currently the most common reason for a Native American adult to require a total hip replacement.

Epidemiology

The rate of hip dysplasia in Scandinavia, England, and North America varies from 2 to 19 per 1,000 live births. Several North American Native populations have demonstrated higher rates: 40–60 per 1,000 in Navajo[2, 3] and 35–600 per 1,000 in Cree-Ojibwa of Island Lake, Manitoba.[4] There is little literature on studies of DDH in other tribes. In non-Native adults, a study of 474 patients with end-stage hip disease showed that 43% had dysplasia as the underlying etiology.[5]

Risk factors for DDH (Table 27-1) include those associated with intrauterine position: breech position, torticollis, and metatarsus adductus. Although only 2–3% of babies are breech presentations, 16–25% of DDH patients are born breech. There is a fourfold increase in females, and the left side is affected 60% of the time. DDH is present in 2–10% of siblings and 1–2% of biological parents.[1] Thus, although all newborns and infants should be screened carefully for DDH, particular attention should be paid to those with significant or multiple risk factors (see Screening).

Natural History

Hip laxity, acetabular dysplasia, subluxation, and dislocation each has its own natural history. Hip laxity is often present at birth. The femoral head is positioned in the socket. With the Barlow test (a stress maneuver), a sensation movement is noticeable as the femoral head comes out of the socket. These hips should be observed for persistent instability but usually improve spontaneously.

Acetabular dysplasia is often associated with laxity. As the laxity improves, the acetabular dysplasia generally improves, albeit more slowly, over several months or years. If still present in the walking child, acetabular dysplasia improves much more slowly. Bones do not reliably remodel after 4 years of age, so acetabular dysplasia does not spontaneously improve after this age. Adults with acetabular dysplasia can develop osteoarthritis and require total hip replacement in their 60s and 70s.

Subluxation in an infant can remain unchanged, gradually improve, or worsen. Due to its unpredictable natural history, it is generally treated in infancy. In the older child, it is less likely to improve spontaneously because the deformity becomes more fixed and remodeling less

Table 27-1. High-Risk Factors for Developmental Dysplasia of the Hip

Intrauterine position factors
  Breech position
  Torticollis
  Metatarsus adductus
Positive family history
Lower-limb deformity

likely. Persistent subluxation in the infant or child requires treatment and, in the adult, usually leads to arthritis, often in the patient's 30s.

Hip dislocation in the newborn can improve spontaneously, but this is not predictable, and the untreated, dislocated hip can become fixed in that position. On examination of the newborn, the hip is in a dislocated position but can be gently pushed back into the acetabulum (Ortolani sign). If the hip remains dislocated for several months, the iliopsoas, adductor, and hamstring muscles develop contractures, and the hip has limited abduction. Later in infancy, the hip may become irreducible. The young infant can often be treated without surgery, but the walking child usually requires operative treatment. Treated dislocations do not always have successful outcomes, and approximately half of the children needing closed reduction have acetabular dysplasia as adults.[6] Early diagnosis and treatment leads to better outcomes.[7]

Etiology and Cradle Boards

Salter[8] has shown that the primary problem in developmental dysplasia is capsular and ligamentous laxity present at birth. The dislocation is usually not present until shortly after birth, although it can develop later; this is why the term *developmental* rather than *congenital* hip dysplasia is used. After birth, the infant continues to remain in the protective flexed, abducted, and externally rotated position. Salter demonstrated on a stillborn infant that if the anterior capsule and ligamentum teres were removed, the hip was stable in the flexed position but dislocated with extension. External stressors, such as swaddling or the cradle board, can force the hip into the unstable position of extension and adduction. Combining this with capsular laxity can result in dislocation.

In the first few weeks of life, capsular laxity usually resolves, and the hip spontaneously becomes more stable. Barlow[9] found the prevalence of instability to decrease from 1 in 60 infants on the first day of life to 1.5 in 1,000 by the end of the second month. This spontaneous improvement is assisted by the infant's muscle activity and is prevented by the hip being held in extension and adduction.

In his study of the Cree and Ojibwa, Walker[4] found bilateral hip involvement more often than unilateral.

Infant swaddling and care and transportation on cradle boards was common. He believed that the position of hip extension and abduction during early infancy (when the hip ligaments are lax), vertical propping in the cradle board, and a small gene pool all contributed to the high prevalence of hip disease.

Swaddling and the cradle boards are still used in Navajo populations. In 1994, Harcke and Schwend (unpublished data) found that 80% of infants still spent time in the cradle board. Mothers thought that the cradle board was a tradition and the infant was calmer in the device. Diapers are universally worn, however, which help to place the hips in the safer position of abduction and flexion in the cradle board. Increased use of child car seats further lessens the time in the cradle board.

Developmental Dysplasia of the Hip in Native Americans

From 1956 to 1962, the Navajo-Cornell Field Health Research Project of Cornell University Medical College investigated the prevalence of DDH in Navajo children from Many Farms, AZ, near Ganado. All families refused treatment. Of 548 children born between 1955 and 1961, 87% received a pelvic radiograph. Four children (7 per 1,000) had dislocation and 18 (33 per 1,000) had subluxation or hip dysplasia.[2] In 1982, Pratt et al.[10] reviewed the 18 patients with acetabular dysplasia and found marked improvement in the radiographic appearance of the hip: 15 were judged to be normal. In 1995, Schwend et al.[11] revisited 10 of these 18 patients with acetabular dysplasia as young children. They were now approximately 35 years old, and all were doing well except for one patient with occasional, minor hip pain. Despite overall radiographic improvement, eight hips in 5 of these 10 patients had residual abnormalities. Patients with subluxation during infancy were less likely to be normal as adults.

Coleman studied Navajo infants from Shiprock, NM, and found that of 23 untreated hips, only five became radiographically normal. In contrast, 11 of 12 hips treated with abduction splinting became normal. He advocated treatment because "it is impossible to predict with any degree of accuracy what the ultimate fate of a dysplastic hip will be if treatment is denied."[3]

In 1995, Schwend and Pratt[12] reviewed screening anteroposterior pelvic radiographs done as part of an intravenous pyelogram examination in a sample of 200 Navajo patients with average age of 49 years. A total of 12 patients (60 per 1,000) had radiographic abnormalities suggestive of DDH, including one dislocated hip, although the criteria for diagnosis may have been more sensitive than that used in previous studies. In 1994, Harcke and Schwend studied a small group of healthy Navajo infants from Shiprock, NM, with ultrasound screening and found a prevalence of hip dysplasia of 20 per 1,000 (R. Schwend and T. Harcke, personal com-

Figure 27-1. The Ortolani test. As hip abduction is attempted by the examiner, the examiner's long finger over the patient's greater trochanter pushes anteriorly to try to lift the femoral head over the posterior lip of the acetabulum and reduce the hip (*arrow*). A positive Ortolani test is present when the examiner hears a palpable "clunk" as the patient's hip reduces. A high-pitched "click" at full abduction should not be considered a positive Ortolani test and is probably due to fascia lata slipping over the greater trochanter in this position. (Reprinted with permission from V Tolo, B Wood. Pediatric Orthopaedics in Primary Care. Baltimore: Williams & Wilkins, 1993;149.)

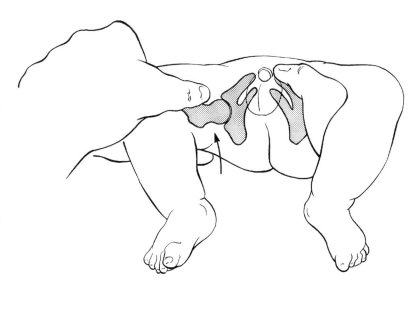

munication). Eighty percent of these infants spent some time in a cradle board, although only for short periods of the day.

Walker[4] made some fascinating observations based on a retrospective survey of the Cree and Ojibwa of Island Lake in 1977. Despite the high rate of DDH, including significant numbers of children and adults with limps, the population at that time did not view this as a functional disability. They resisted efforts to decrease cradle-board use because it was the most practical way to transport babies in an area without level walkways that could support a baby carriage. The sole disability referred to was the difficulty in portaging a canoe with a man who limps: "He dips and you don't."[4] This paper serves as a reminder of the importance of cultural sensitivity.

Similarly, the Cornell project on the Navajo Reservation noted that the vast majority of Navajo adults and children for whom hip surgery had been recommended refused the surgery.[2] This was attributed to the Navajo not desiring to correct what they saw as a nonhandicapping condition and having seen several of their people have corrective surgery that produced a disability in terms of mobility (from the Navajo point of view) that had not previously existed.

Screening

All newborns should have their hips examined by a reliable, experienced clinician. The history should be reviewed for risk factors associated with an increased incidence of DDH (see Table 27-1). In newborns, hip flexion, abduction, and external rotation are normal. From

birth until 4–6 months of age, the primary way to detect DDH is through correct performance of the Ortolani reduction maneuver (the "O" means hip is "out") and Barlow provocative test.

The principle of the Ortolani test (Figure 27-1) is that the femoral head is resting in a dislocated or subluxed position. The test answers the question, "Is this hip out of its normal location, and is the hip reducible?" The infant should be quiet and comfortable, and the test is done gently. While the patient's pelvis is stabilized, his or her hip is gently abducted and, as the patient's thigh is raised, the examiner perceives the sensation of movement of the femoral head back into the hip socket (see Figure 27-1). This is described as a low-pitched sensation or clunk. A high-pitched click is due to extraarticular soft tissues and has no association with dysplasia. The Barlow maneuver (Figure 27-2) is the opposite of the Ortolani. The examiner adducts the patient's limb, causing the located femoral head to dislocate. Although the Barlow maneuver can tell the examiner if the hip has laxity, it can also increase laxity and, at least theoretically, lead to instability. For this reason, we recommend that the Ortolani test be performed first. If it is normal, one can then *very gently* do the Barlow maneuver.

As the infant becomes older, the instability seen with the Ortolani or Barlow tests often resolves. Because DDH may not be detected in the first months of life, all infants should continue to have their hips examined at each well child visit until they are walking appropriately. After 4–6 months of age, findings that suggest a problem in the infant include asymmetric skinfolds, limitation of hip abduction (Figure 27-3), and the Galeazzi sign (relative shortening of the femoral segment). If there is a delay in

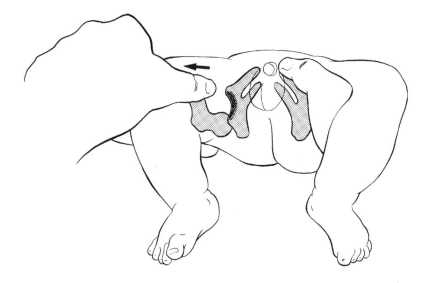

Figure 27-2. The Barlow test is a provocative test to detect any tendency of the hip to dislocate. At rest, the patient's hip is reduced and abduction is near normal or normal. With the patient's leg in a flexed and adducted position, the examiner pushes laterally with his or her thumb (*arrow*). If the patient's hip dislocates, as shown in the illustration, the Barlow test is positive. Reduction usually occurs readily with hip abduction after a positive Barlow test. (Reprinted with permission from V Tolo, B Wood. Pediatric Orthopaedics in Primary Care. Baltimore: Williams & Wilkins, 1993;149.)

walking, especially beyond 18 months, hip dislocation should be a primary consideration and an anteroposterior pelvis radiograph taken. Bilateral dislocated hips in the older infant are often very difficult to detect because the instability may have resolved and the contractures, though present, are symmetric and not very obvious.

Ultrasound imaging is extremely sensitive to instability. It is not accepted as a universal screening tool, however, because of the technical expertise required, low cost-effectiveness, favorable natural history of minor abnormalities, and a high false-positive rate, given the relatively low prevalence of DDH. Ultrasound has been used as a screening tool for certain high-risk infants (i.e., positive family history of dysplasia, history of breech delivery, congenital deformities, or positive findings on examination). It is most useful in the first 5 months of life. Ultrasound is best performed at 4–6 weeks of age, when mild degrees of instability should have resolved and arrangements can be made to have the procedure done by an experienced ultrasonographer.

Radiographs are not useful to diagnose DDH in young infants because of the absence of the ossific nucleus until after 5 months of age. After that time, the radiograph can be more useful.

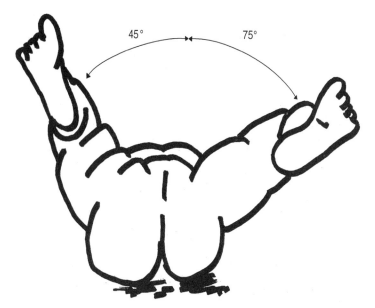

45°   75°

Figure 27-3. If hip abduction is asymmetric and limited to less than 60 degrees on one side, developmental dysplasia of the hip is likely.

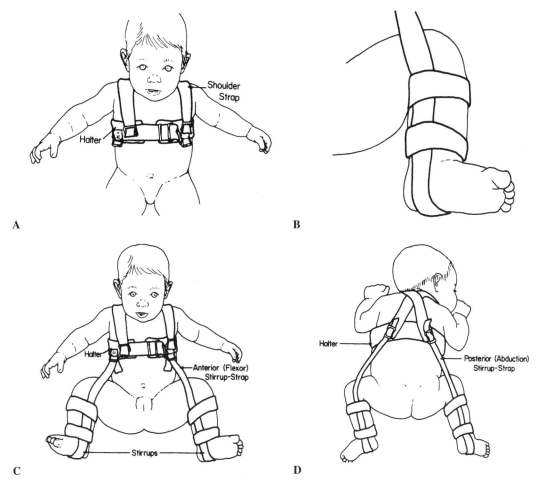

Figure 27-4. The Pavlik harness. A. The chest halter is positioned at the patient's nipple line and fastened with Velcro closures. B. The patient's leg and foot are set into the stirrups and fastened with Velcro straps. C. The anterior (flexion) stirrup straps are connected to the halter. D. The posterior (abduction) stirrup straps are attached to the halter. (Reprinted with permission from S Mubarak, S Garfin, R Vanee, et al. J Bone Joint Surg Am 1981;63:1244.)

Treatment

The hip with some laxity (Barlow positive) can be observed, and an ultrasound may be performed at 4–6 weeks to determine if it has normalized. Hips with a positive Ortolani sign, indicating that the hip is out of the socket, should be referred immediately; if subluxation or dislocation is confirmed, treatment is indicated. Most referrals are for high-pitched soft tissue clicks about the hip; most of these resolve by the end of the first year. In one study of infants with clicks, none were from a high-risk group, and all ultrasounds were normal.[13]

The standard of care in the United States for treating a dislocated or subluxed hip in the infant younger than 6 months old is the Pavlik harness (Figure 27-4). This device encourages hip flexion beyond 100 degrees and allows passive abduction. One study showed that timing

of treatment can be important: There was a 63% success rate if treatment was initiated by 3 weeks and a 20% success rate if treatment began after 3 weeks.[7] Ultrasound imaging is used to follow the hip being treated to ensure that it has been reduced. If reduction has not been accomplished after 3 weeks in the harness, a different treatment is indicated, usually an arthrogram with closed reduction in the operating room and casting. The harness is usually used for several months if treatment is successful.

For mild laxity and acetabular dysplasia, it remains unclear if treatment provides any additional benefit, given the natural history of these conditions. For severe acetabular dysplasia with a located femoral head, treatment with the harness in infants younger than 6 months of age or an abduction brace in older infants is commonly used. Osteonecrosis rates of up to 7% in the harness have been reported; therefore, it should only be used when the benefits clearly outweigh the risks.

With the introduction of ultrasound, more infants with stable, dysplastic hips are being treated with the Pavlik harness. Because the natural history of this condition is gradual improvement, ultrasound evaluation and harness treatment appear to be extremely successful. The small but real risk of osteonecrosis as well as the comfort of the infant and interaction with the family make it important to be careful to not overdiagnose and overtreat.

After 6 months of age, the Pavlik harness is not used. Infants are generally treated with a spica cast after reduction under anesthesia. As the child ages, closed reduction becomes more difficult, and surgical techniques are employed.

Summary Points

- Be aware of risk factors for DDH.
- Carefully screen all children at birth and at each well child visit until they are walking normally. Use the Ortolani and Barlow tests in early infancy and other signs of DDH, particularly limited abduction, after 4 months.
- Refer all young infants with a positive Ortolani test urgently. You may schedule infants with positive Barlow test or other significant risk factors for ultrasound at 4–6 weeks of age.
- After 4–5 months of age, infants should be evaluated with radiograph or by consultant if the examination is abnormal.
- Be aware of accepted indications for the use of the Pavlik harness to avoid unnecessary use.
- Cultivate a relationship with a capable orthopedist, ideally, one with an interest in and experience with DDH.
- Remain sensitive to parents' and families' cultural beliefs about DDH and medical treatment in general.

References

1. Novacheck T. Developmental dysplasia of the hip. Pediatr Clin North Am 1996;43:829–848.
2. Rabin D, Barnett C, Arnold W, et al. Untreated congenital hip disease. Am J Public Health 1965;55:1–44.
3. Coleman S. Congenital dysplasia of the hip in Navajo infants. Clin Orth 1968;56:179–193.
4. Walker JM. Congenital hip disease in Cree-Ojibwa population. Can Med J 1977;116:501–504.
5. Aronson J. Osteoarthritis of the Young Adult Hip. Etiology and Treatments. In Instructional Course Lectures, The American Academy of Orthopaedic Surgeons (Vol 35). St. Louis: Mosby, 1986: 119–128.
6. Malvitz TA, Weinstein SL. Closed reduction for congenital dysplasia of the hip. J Bone Joint Surg Am 1994;76A:1777–1792.
7. Harding M, Harcke HT, Bowen JR, et al. Management of dislocated hips with Pavlik harness treatment and ultrasound monitoring. J Pediatr Orthop 1997;17:189–198.
8. Salter RB. Etiology, pathogenesis, and possible prevention of congenital dislocation of the hip. Can Med Assoc J 1968;98:933–945.
9. Barlow TG. Early diagnosis and treatment of congenital dislocation of the hip. J Bone Joint Surg Br 1962;44:292.
10. Pratt WB, Freiberger RH, Arnold WD. Untreated congenital hip dysplasia in the Navajo. Clin Orth 1982;69–77.
11. Schwend R, Pratt W, Fultz J. Untreated acetabular dysplasia of the hip in the Navajo. Presented at the American Academy of Orthopaedic Surgens Annual Meeting. February 1996.
12. Schwend R, Pratt W. Hip morphology in the Navajo adult. Presented at the John Hall Symposium, Children's Hospital, Harvard Medical School. October 1996.
13. Bond CD, Hennrikus WL, DellaMaggiore ED. Prospective evaluation of newborn soft-tissue hip "clicks" with ultrasound. J Pediatr Orthop 1997;17:199–201.

Part IX
Obstetrics and Gynecology

Chapter 28
Delivery of Prenatal Care

Alan G. Waxman

The desire to ensure the physical and emotional well-being of women during pregnancy transcends cultural differences. Prenatal care is motivated by the desire for a healthy newborn. Women also want a pregnancy, labor, delivery, and puerperium that is safe for the new mother and baby and that contributes to a physically and emotionally healthy family unit. This chapter looks at the role played by prenatal care for Native American women. The components of prenatal care are also reviewed, especially as they relate to the clinical practice unique to Indian country.

Before European contact, Native American societies had customs and taboos to ensure a healthy pregnancy and newborn that were specific to their individual belief systems, geography, and economies. In pueblo cultures of the Southwest, for example, women were encouraged to take frequent warm baths and to restrict their activity during pregnancy.[1] Among the Navajos, on the other hand, pregnancy was considered a normal process; therefore, excessive rest was discouraged and maternal activity encouraged.[2] Taboos proscribing certain behaviors were common, often across tribal lines. Both the Zunis and their neighbors the Navajos, for example, were warned against viewing the dead while pregnant. Often, such taboos involved the husband and the pregnant woman. For example, the Zunis believed that congenital anomalies could result if a father-to-be shot a rabbit or prairie dog.[3] For either Navajo parent to view a ceremonial sand painting during pregnancy would result in illness for the unborn child.[4]

Many of these beliefs are still held, and traditional ceremonies remain important. Navajo women are advised by their elders to think positive thoughts during the pregnancy to facilitate an easy pregnancy, labor, and delivery. The tying of knots during pregnancy is thought to result in an obstructed labor. Making specific preparations for the arrival of the baby in advance of the birth (e.g., making a cradle board, buying baby clothes, or naming the baby) may bring bad luck to the baby or its parents. On the other hand, performing a Blessingway ceremony is believed to bring harmony to the pregnant woman, place her in tune with the holy people who created mankind, and facilitate the childbirth process.[4] In the early 1980s, Milligan[2] found that a large proportion of Navajo women still adhered to most of these beliefs. As recently as 1992, 31% of prenatal patients surveyed at the Gallup Indian Medical Center indicated that they planned to have a Blessingway in preparation for their current pregnancy (Waxman, unpublished data).

The modern biomedical approach to prenatal care was initially a response to the high rates of maternal mortality before the latter half of the twentieth century. Pregnancy-induced hypertension was a major and largely preventable cause of maternal death among American Indians and the rest of the United States population.[5] The commonly used medical model for prenatal care focuses on the early detection and prevention of pregnancy-induced hypertension. This model has been shown to reduce maternal and neonatal mortality by reducing premature birth.

The federal government's target for its Healthy People 2000 health promotion program is that 90% of pregnant American Indian and Alaska Native women begin prenatal care in the first trimester of pregnancy.[6] In 1991–1993, 62% of Native American women living in counties on or near reservations met this objective. Rates ranged from 75.8% for Alaska to 47.8% for those on or near the Navajo reservation.[7] This compares with 77.7% in the general U.S. population. Gilchrist et al.[8] found that approximately one in five Navajo and Sioux women did not begin prenatal care until the third trimester or had no prenatal care. This study did not determine why women did not seek care earlier, even with the barrier of direct cost of care removed. The investigators suggested that part of the reason may lie with cultural beliefs (i.e., the Navajo reluctance to prepare for childbirth and the traditional beliefs that pregnancy is a natural process and that doctors and hospitals are associated with illness and death).

Content of Prenatal Care

In 1986, the U.S. Public Health Service convened an expert panel on the content of prenatal care. The panel's report expanded the focus of prenatal care beyond the prevention of specific complications of pregnancy, such as prematurity or pregnancy-induced hypertension, to include the promotion of the health and well-being of the mother, her infant, and family from conception through infancy.[9] The panel divided the content of prenatal care into three principal activities:

1. Risk assessment
2. Health promotion and education
3. Medical and psychosocial follow-up

These three functions should be ongoing and integrated, beginning with a preconceptional visit and continuing through the pregnancy and in many cases, the puerperium.

Risk Assessment

Risk assessment includes ongoing evaluation for medical, obstetric, and psychosocial risks. It begins with a complete history and physical examination at the preconceptional visit or the first prenatal visit. Particular attention is paid to conditions that may affect the pregnancy (e.g., baseline weight and blood pressure; pre-existing diabetes or cardiac disease; last menstrual period [LMP] and uterine size; alcohol, tobacco, and other substance abuse; and history of domestic violence). Certain laboratory tests are effective as part of the initial risk assessment. Some should be repeated in at-risk patients; others are timed to correspond with particular gestational ages (see Laboratory Testing). Risk assessment continues with each subsequent visit to include evaluation for new medical or psychosocial risk factors, weight gain, blood pressure, fundal growth, fetal heart rate assessment and, in the third trimester, fetal lie and engagement.[9]

The organizational structure of most prenatal services in Indian country revolves around a clinic with multiple providers. In many cases, the clinics are part of a larger network of health care facilities. Clinical management must ensure that a uniform standard of care is maintained in settings with multiple providers, possibly of differing professional disciplines, such as family physicians, obstetrician-gynecologists, nurse practitioners, nurse midwives, and physician assistants. This is best accomplished by using a set of written practice guidelines or protocols reinforced with periodic quality improvement monitoring.

Health Promotion and Education

Three components of health promotion and education are recommended by the U.S. Public Health Service Expert Panel on the Content of Prenatal Care:

1. Counseling to promote and support healthful behavior
2. Pregnancy and parenting education
3. Information on health care during the prenatal period, labor, delivery, and the puerperium

Prenatal and parenting education should be uniform and comprehensive and should continue through the course of prenatal and postpartum care. Some facilities achieve this by providing prenatal and parenting classes as part of the prenatal care package. Others use one-on-one education by the providers augmented with written materials. In either case, the principle of one standard of comprehensive education is important. The most important positive lifestyle measures should be discussed at the preconceptional or first prenatal visit and be reinforced at subsequent visits. This should include avoidance of substance abuse (i.e., tobacco, alcohol, teratogens, and illegal drugs). Care in the use of over-the-counter medications should also be reviewed. Education about safe sex practices is easily incorporated into counseling before offering human immunodeficiency virus (HIV) testing. Nutrition and optimal weight gain in pregnancy should be reviewed. Discussion of the importance of seat belts is important in the first trimester. In the middle and third trimesters, follow-up information should include how to adjust the belts as the uterus grows (i.e., tight across the lap, with the shoulder belt coming over the uterus). Among American Indian and Alaska Native women of reproductive age, mortality from motor vehicle accidents is two to three times that of the general U.S. population.[10] A more detailed discussion of prenatal and parenting education is beyond the scope of this chapter.

A word about the language used in counseling is in order. Although it is not true of all Native American cultures, in some societies, such as the Navajo, positive thoughts are associated with physical and spiritual harmony. Words are thought to have power to influence health and well-being. Health education counseling is often best offered in the third person. When discussing fetal alcohol syndrome, for example, it is preferable to say, "Some women who drink during pregnancy have babies with birth defects" rather than "If *you* drink during pregnancy, *your baby* will be born with birth defects."[11]

Medical and Psychosocial Follow-Up

Conditions identified during risk assessment should be appropriately managed by the health care provider, consultants, or community intervention services. Management may involve a single visit, such as treatment of a urinary tract infection, or may continue throughout the entire pregnancy (e.g., for pregestational diabetes mellitus).

Periodic case-management conferences for women with at-risk pregnancies ensure that appropriate consultation has been obtained. Management plans should be written on the medical record so that each provider who may interact with the patient follows the same plan. Consultation may involve social services, nutritionists, mental health workers, and specialty consultants. The use of special-focus programs should also be emphasized. Examples include diabetes team, alcohol and substance abuse programs, and community-based fetal alcohol syndrome prevention activities.

Laboratory Testing

Two aspects of prenatal risk assessment that deserve special attention are laboratory testing and gestational age assessment. The rest of this chapter concerns the role and timing of several laboratory tests and appropriate assessment of gestational age, using both clinical and ultrasound parameters.

A number of laboratory tests should be performed during the preconceptional or first prenatal visit. Some should be repeated or timed to correspond with certain gestational ages.[12]

Complete Blood Count

Anemia, especially iron-deficiency anemia, is common in Native American women. A complete blood count should be assessed at the preconceptional or first prenatal visit and repeated at 24–28 weeks.[13]

Blood Type and Rh Factor

A much greater proportion of the Native American population is Rh (D) positive than the 87% expected of American women of European descent. This is especially true of those in the Southwest, Northern Plains, and Alaska. The relative infrequency of D-negative patients requires a greatly increased vigilance on the part of prenatal care providers. To prevent D isoimmunization, D immunoglobulin must be given postpartum to unsensitized D-negative mothers. It must also be given to unsensitized women early in the third trimester (28–29 weeks), except when the father of the baby is known to also be D negative. Failure to give Rh (D) immune globulin prophylaxis in the third trimester is associated with a 1.7% risk of D isoimmunization.[14]

Prenatal Antibody Screen

Certain antibodies, such as Kell, Duffy, or Kidd, can cause erythroblastosis fetalis and should be screened for early in pregnancy. If a woman tests positive for one of these antibodies, her partner should also be tested. Kell, for example,

is most commonly transmitted by transfusion, and it has been estimated that the partners of 90% of Kell-immunized women are Kell negative. The fetus is therefore at no added risk from its mother's antibody status.[15]

Immunity to Rubella

Women who are not immune to rubella should be vaccinated postpartum.[12]

Hepatitis B Surface Antigen

All women should be tested for hepatitis B surface antigen at the first prenatal visit. Those who are initially negative should be tested again in the third trimester and offered vaccination if they are exposed to hepatitis B during pregnancy or if they engage in high-risk behavior, such as intravenous drug use. Hepatitis B has been endemic in Alaska Native communities.[13]

Urinalysis and Culture

If urinalysis is done at a preconceptional visit, it need not be repeated. Urine dipstick for protein and glucose need not be repeated at subsequent visits because there are better tests to diagnose pregnancy-induced hypertension and diabetes. Asymptomatic bacteriuria is common in pregnancy and is associated with an increased risk for pyelonephritis, prematurity, and low birth weight.[13]

Purified Protein Derivative

One percent of reported cases of tuberculosis in the United States occurs in American Indians and Alaska Natives. Skin testing for tuberculosis is indicated in communities where tuberculosis is endemic.[13]

Tests for Syphilis, Gonorrhea, Chlamydia, and Human Immunodeficiency Virus

Screening for syphilis is generally recommended. Although screening of high-risk women for gonorrhea in the first and third trimesters is recommended by the American College of Obstetricians and Gynecologists, the Centers for Disease Control and Prevention recommends first-trimester screening of all pregnant women. Screening of high-risk women is recommended for Chlamydia. Risk factors include age younger than 25 years, multiple sex partners, previous positive Chlamydia test, or friable cervix with mucopurulent discharge. The prevalence of these infections in the community should also be considered. HIV testing should be offered to all pregnant women. The risk of vertical transmission can be reduced by two-thirds with treatment during pregnancy. Thorough, sensitive counseling of all pregnant women is essential.[13]

Cervical Cytology

The mortality from cervical cancer in Native American women is approximately twice that of the general popu-

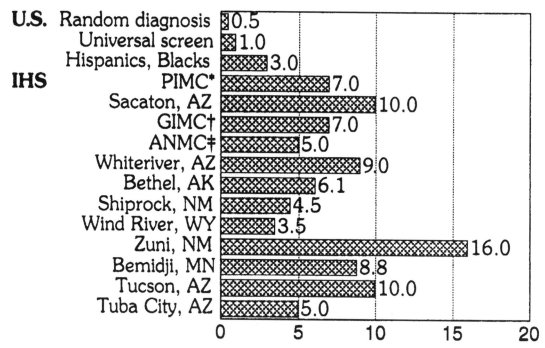

Figure 28-1. Rates (per 100 deliveries) of diabetes in pregnancy reported by various Indian Health Service (IHS) and tribal hospitals. *Phoenix Indian Medical Center, Phoenix, Arizona (an IHS referral center). †Gallup Indian Medical Center, Gallup, New Mexico (an IHS referral center). ‡Alaska Native Medical Center, Anchorage, Alaska (an IHS referral center). (Reprinted with permission from NB Attico, KC Smith, AG Waxman, et al. Diabetes mellitus in pregnancy: views toward an improved perinatal outcome. IHS Provider 1992;17:154.)

lation.[16] The preconceptional or first prenatal visit is an ideal opportunity for cervical cytology screening.

Diabetes Screening

Native American women are at risk for gestational diabetes. All Native American women, regardless of other risk factors, should be screened at 24–28 weeks with a 1-hour plasma glucose test after a 50-g oral glucose load. Those with values of 140 mg/dl or greater should be followed up with a 3-hour glucose tolerance test using a 100-g glucose challenge. (Diagnosis is made if two or more plasma glucose values equal or exceed the following: fasting, 105 mg/dl; 1-hour, 190 mg/dl; 2-hour, 165 mg/dl; or 3-hour, 145 mg/dl.[17]) Those with additional risk factors for type 2 diabetes should be tested at the preconceptional or first prenatal visit for pre-existing type 2 diabetes.

The rates of diabetes in pregnancy reported by Indian Health Service hospitals are many times higher than the rate in the U.S. general population (Figure 28-1).[17] Pima Indians have the highest rates of non–insulin-dependent diabetes mellitus of any ethnic group in the world. Studies of this group show that the offspring of women with abnormal glucose tolerance in pregnancy are more likely to be overweight and ultimately develop diabetes

themselves.[18] These and other studies have led the authors of a Technical Bulletin of the American College of Obstetricians and Gynecologists to suggest that "in certain Native American populations, the prevalence of gestational diabetes mellitus is so high that pregnant women in these populations can be considered to have a positive screen. They may proceed directly to diagnostic testing."[19]

Screening for Neural Tube Defects and Down Syndrome

Multiple-marker screening (i.e., maternal serum alpha-fetoprotein, estriol, and human chorionic gonadotropin) should be offered to all women presenting before 20 weeks gestation. This test screens for open neural tube defects, ventral wall defects and, in women younger than age 35 years, Down syndrome. Women older than 35 years should be offered genetic amniocentesis based on age-specific risk alone; the multiple-marker screen cutoff for recommending amniocentesis is equal to the age-specific risk at age 35 years. The test may also identify women at risk for prematurity, intrauterine growth restriction, pregnancy-induced hypertension, abruptio placentae, and stillbirth.[20] Counseling must be done with delicacy and cultural sensitivity. Follow-up of a positive multiple-marker screening test often requires expensive subspecialty diagnostic procedures, including targeted ultrasound and amniocentesis. These procedures are not readily available at most primary care Indian Health Service, urban Indian, or tribal facilities.

The early diagnosis of a neural tube defect or Down syndrome may be useful to the infant's family by affording time to learn how to care for and seek resources for an infant with special needs. Other families may decide to seek an abortion on the basis of these findings. Abortion cannot be paid for with federal dollars. Indian Health Service, urban Indian, or tribal facilities may elect not to pay for the screening test. Even in this event, patients must be informed of the availability of these tests should they wish to purchase them elsewhere.

Gestational Age Assessment

An important aspect of ongoing risk assessment is monitoring fetal growth. Accurate knowledge of gestational age is essential to prevent the morbidity and mortality associated with premature delivery and postdate dysmaturity. It is also important to schedule screening tests, which must be performed at specific times during the pregnancy (e.g., screening for neural tube defects at 16–18 weeks and for diabetes at 24–28 weeks). A number of techniques may be used to assess gestational age.

History of Last Menstrual Period

A woman with regular menstrual cycles, especially if associated with menstrual or premenstrual symptoms, such as cramps, breast tenderness, or irritability, has a high likelihood of ovulating 2 weeks before the onset of menses. In the usual 28-day cycle, this equates to 2 weeks after the first day of the LMP. The average duration of pregnancy is 280 days after the LMP. The estimated due date (EDD) may be calculated from the LMP by subtracting 3 months and adding 7 days (i.e., if the LMP began on April 6, the EDD is January 13). Women must be counseled that delivery may safely be anticipated within a range of 3 weeks before their assigned due date to 2 weeks afterward).

Clinical Landmarks

Many women do not keep track of their menstrual periods with precision, and cycle lengths may vary considerably from the idealized 28 days. Pregnancy may be dated with some reliability by clinical landmarks if evaluated in the first and early second trimester.

1. *Uterine size.* First-trimester examination by a skilled examiner can predict gestational age within 1–2 weeks. From approximately 20–30 weeks, the fundal height in centimeters corresponds 1 to 1 with the gestational age in weeks, with an accuracy of 1–2 weeks. A tape measure should be used to measure from the top of the patient's symphysis pubis to the top of the fundus, and her bladder should be empty.
2. Fetal heart sounds can generally be first heard at 16–19 weeks using a DeLee-Hillis fetal stethoscope or at 9–10 weeks using a Doppler stethoscope.[21]

Ultrasound

Currently, 60–70% of women in the United States have at least one ultrasound during pregnancy. Routine ultrasound is not currently indicated in low-risk pregnancies. The large multicenter Routine Antenatal Diagnostic Imaging with Ultrasound Sudy (RADIUS) trial found no improvement in perinatal mortality when ultrasound was used routinely early in the second trimester and repeated in the third trimester rather than only for specific obstetric indications. The sensitivity of ultrasound screening for major congenital anomalies in low-risk populations varies widely (17–47%) depending on clinical setting, gestational age, and skill of the sonographer. Although early ultrasound does increase the accuracy of gestational age assessment, it does not appear to decrease the incidence of obstetric interventions. Investigators in several studies were not consistent in showing a decrease in induction of labor for postdate pregnancy. The RADIUS study, on the other hand, showed an increase in induction of labor for presumed intrauterine growth restriction but with no accompanying decrease in low–birth-weight infants.[22]

Ultrasound is most accurate in determining gestational age when used early in pregnancy. A first-trimester crown-rump length should be accurate to within 5 days (2 standard deviations). By the mid- to late second trimester, the standard deviation for gestational age by measurement of biparietal diameter or femur length is 7–10 days. Accuracy can be improved by averaging gestational age measurements. Accuracy of third-trimester measurements is within 21 days.[23] Gestational age and EDD should be assigned by the earliest reliable measurement and should not be changed subsequently. For example, if the EDD based on a first-trimester ultrasound is within 5 days of the due date based on the LMP, the menstrual date should prevail. If a discrepancy of more than 5 days exists, however, the ultrasound should be considered more accurate. In this instance, should a subsequent ultrasound in the third trimester favor the menstrual date, it should be disregarded in favor of the EDD based on the first-trimester scan.

Key Points

- Efforts should be made to increase the use of prenatal care in Native American communities. These health promotion efforts should be sensitive to the cultural variations in how each Native American group views preventive medicine and the preparation for childbirth. Traditional beliefs must be appreciated and respected and, if possible, incorporated into risk-reduction and health education efforts.

• The components of prenatal care, risk assessment, health promotion and education, and medical and psychosocial follow-up should begin with the pre-conceptional or first prenatal visit and continue throughout the prenatal course and through the postpartum visit.

• The timing and content of prenatal laboratory assessment should take into consideration the prevalence of various conditions in the community.

• Gestational age can usually be assessed with clinically acceptable precision by either clinical or ultrasound parameters. An EDD based on late ultrasound measurements should not supersede a differing due date based on several consistent clinical parameters obtained early in the pregnancy.

References

1. Speert H. Obstetrics and Gynecology in America: A History. Chicago: American College of Obstetricians and Gynecologists, 1980;24.
2. Milligan BC. Nursing care and beliefs of expectant Navajo women: development and implementation of an experimental nursing intervention study. American Indian Quarterly 1984;8:83–101.
3. Parsons EC. Zuni Conception and Pregnancy Beliefs. In Babcock BA (ed), Pueblo Mothers and Children: Essays by Elsie Clews Parsons 1915–1924. Santa Fe, NM: Ancient City Press, 1991;32.
4. Waxman AG. Navajo childbirth in transition. Med Anthropol 1990;12:187–205.
5. Waxman AG. Maternal mortality in a southwest American Indian Population. Presentation, Fourth Annual IHS Research Conference, Tucson, AZ, 1991.
6. National Center for Health Statistics. Healthy People 2000 Review. Hyattsville, MD: U.S. Public Health Service, 1997;135.
7. Indian Health Service. Regional Differences in Indian Health, 1996. Washington, DC: U.S. Department of Health and Human Services, Government Printing Office, 1996;29.
8. Gilchrist AP, Smith AN, Saftlas AF, et al. Patterns of prenatal care utilization among Sioux and Navajo women. IHS Provider 1993;18:177–181.
9. Public Health Service, U.S. Department of Health and Human Services. Caring for Our Future: The Content of Prenatal Care, A Report of the Public Health Service Expert Panel on the Content of Prenatal Care. Washington, DC: Public Health Service, 1989.
10. Indian Health Service. Trends in Indian Health, 1993. Washington, DC: U.S. Department of Health and Human Services, Government Printing Office, 1993;57.
11. Carresse JA, Rhodes LA. Western bioethics on the Navajo reservation: benefit or harm? JAMA 1996;274:826–829.
12. American College of Obstetricians and Gynecologists. Guidelines for Perinatal Care (4th ed). Elk Grove, IL: American Academy of Pediatrics, and Washington, DC: American college of Obstetricians and Gyneocologists,1997;65–90.
13. U.S. Preventive Services Task Force. Guide to Clinical Preventive Services (2nd ed). Baltimore: Williams & Wilkins, 1996;231–347.
14. American College of Obstetricians and Gynecologists. Prevention of D Isoimmunization. Technical Bulletin No. 147. October 1990.
15. American College of Obstetricians and Gynecologists. Management of Isoimmunization in Pregnancy. Educational Bulletin No. 227. August 1996.
16. Cobb N, Paisano RE. Cancer Mortality among American Indians and Alaska Natives in the United States: Regional Differences in Indian Health, 1989–1993. IHS Publication No. 97-615-23. Rockville, MD: Indian Health Service, 1997;33.
17. Attico NB, Smith KC, Waxman AG, et al. Diabetes mellitus in pregnancy: views toward an improved perinatal outcome. IHS Provider 1992;17:153–163.
18. Pettitt DJ, Bennett PH, Saad MF, et al. Abnormal glucose tolerance during pregnancy in Pima Indian women: long-term effects on offspring. Diabetes 1991;40(suppl 2):126–130.
19. American College of Obstetricians and Gynecologists. Diabetes and Pregnancy. Technical Bulletin No. 200. December 1994.
20. American College of Obstetricians and Gynecologists. Maternal Serum Screening. Educational Bulletin No. 228. September 1996.
21. Cunningham FG, MacDonald PC, Gant NF (eds). Williams' Obstetrics (20th ed). Stamford, CT: Appleton & Lange, 1997;232.
22. American College of Obstetricians and Gynecologists. Routine ultrasound in low-risk pregnancy. ACOG Practice Patterns. August 1997.
23. American College of Obstetricians and Gynecologists. Ultrasonography in Pregnancy. Technical Bulletin No. 187. December 1993.

Chapter 29
Teenage Pregnancy

Dorothy J. Meyer and Colleen Williams

In the 1970s, teenage pregnancy emerged as a national problem with several negative social outcomes, including increased health care costs, school dropout rates, and lost wages. By available data, the proportion of adolescent American Indian (AI) women giving birth has remained approximately 20% of total AI births (Table 29-1) since 1980.

Many articles about adolescent pregnancy have been published, but few publications address adolescent pregnancy in Indian country. Between 1988 and 1990, the Indian Health Service (IHS) provided a grant to the Adolescent Health Program of the University of Minnesota for a survey of AI adolescents.[1] Almost 14,000 teenagers from 50 tribes across the United States completed the survey, which explored feelings about school, family, health status and practices, emotional health, sexual behavior, and risk-taking behaviors. This survey revealed some unique information about AI adolescents but generally identified more commonalities than differences from other adolescent groups.

Obviously, the primary reason that an adolescent becomes pregnant is sexual activity without the use of contraception. Consistent with other adolescent populations, 56.8% of AI adolescent girls and 65% of boys said that they had sexual intercourse by grade 12. Of the sexually active teens, the average age of first intercourse was 14.2 years for girls and 13.6 for boys. Fifty percent of the sexually active females and 40% of the males reported that they "always" used a birth control method. When asked where they would feel most comfortable obtaining birth control, 51.9% of females and 27.8% of males gave their community clinic as their primary choice. Therefore, according to the adolescents themselves, tribal and IHS clinics have an important role in adolescent pregnancy prevention.

Adolescent Pregnancy Prevention

In public health terms, prevention focuses on three levels: primary, secondary, and tertiary.

Primary Prevention

Primary prevention targets children and adolescents before the onset of sexual activity and promotes delaying the initiation of sexual activity. Primary prevention is grounded in the attitude, behavior, teaching, and example of every child's family, community, and culture. Community-based primary prevention interventions generally consist of church, school, and other initiatives that focus on education of the child and adolescent.

Primary Prevention in Schools

In reservation schools, it is common for primary care providers to assist in teaching school-based educational courses. These courses can provide an excellent opportunity for positive interaction with teens and school staff to promote the primary prevention of teen pregnancy. Presentations usually consist of basic health information, such as anatomy and physiology, but also can address other issues, such as the unrealistic view of sexuality promoted by the media. Teens should be made aware that not everyone is "doing it" and that attraction does not necessitate sexual activity, although both seem to be common media messages. These presentations can also provide the opportunity to discuss healthy relationships and ways to be intimate without having sex.

The IHS, with the support of the Centers for Disease Control and Prevention, has helped schools to establish comprehensive health education programs in schools. A comprehensive health curriculum often includes a discussion of the sexuality of adolescents. In the United

Table 29-1. Percentage of Teen Births among American Indians and Alaska Natives in Reservation States

Calendar Years	Total Births	Teen Births	Percentage of Teen Births
1980–1982	105,802	24,159	22.8
1981–1983	112,017	24,418	21.8
1982–1984	117,495	24,661	21.0
1983–1985	120,110	24,088	20.1
1984–1986	121,623	23,759	19.5
1985–1987	124,832	23,832	19.1
1986–1988	127,219	24,201	19.0
1987–1989	97,649	18,835	19.3
1990–1992	101,320	19,996	19.7
1991–1993	101,226	20,305	20.1

Source: Adapted from Indian Health Service. Trends in Indian Health. Washington, DC: U.S. Department of Health and Human Services, Indian Health Service, 1986–1996.

States, the idea that sex education promotes sexual activity in teens continues to be expressed, although studies do not support this.

Primary Prevention in Clinical Settings

Opportunities for primary prevention efforts also occur in direct care clinical situations. Many health organizations, including the IHS, recommend periodic (e.g., Early and Periodic Screening, Diagnosis, and Treatment) or annual physicals, including "sports" physicals. The discussion of sexual issues should begin at the neonatal examination with parents and progress to direct conversations with the teen during medical visits. When adolescent physicals are performed, the practitioner can raise topics such as physical changes and sexual activity. If the adolescent is not sexually active, reinforcement and support for abstinence should be provided. If sexually active, methods of preventing pregnancy and sexually transmitted diseases (STDs) can be discussed. At times, the preteen or teen is brought to the clinic by a parent for counseling on physical changes, pregnancy, and STD prevention. This type of visit should be encouraged and provides an excellent time to educate both child and parent as a family. Talking about sexuality requires skill that is generally learned by experience. It helps to remember that, although shy, almost all adolescents want to talk about sexual issues. For teens to share their concerns, it is essential that the practitioner listen, remain nonjudgmental, and address the adolescent's questions seriously and sincerely. It may take a number of visits for a teen to feel comfortable enough with the practitioner to discuss his or her specific concerns.

Confidentiality

When dealing with adolescents, issues of confidentiality are often raised by adolescents and their families. Obviously, parents often do not know everything about their adolescent's concerns and activities. This is normal developmentally because the adolescent is in the process of seeking individuation and emancipation from the family.

At the time of the initial teen visit, the issue of confidentiality should be discussed with the adolescent. He or she should be told that every effort to maintain confidentiality will be made, but there are exceptions. These include situations in which physical harm to self or others is possible, in which legal obligations are involved (e.g., sexual abuse), or in which family involvement is essential to the solution of the problem.[2] If the parent is present at the visit, time should be provided to speak with the teen alone. This not only reinforces that the visit is confidential but also recognizes that the teen is an individual with her own responsibility.

Secondary Prevention

Secondary prevention activities primarily focus on avoiding pregnancy for sexually active teens. Adolescents presenting to clinics for pregnancy testing, menstrual problems, or pelvic or vaginal complaints should be provided the opportunity for counseling on pregnancy prevention and STDs.

Pregnancy Testing

Pregnancy testing should be readily available and accessible to every teen. Clinics and other health care venues, such as public health nurses, can do the testing. One study in the *Journal of the American Medical Association*[3] found that 34.2% of teens who had ever conceived had a prior negative pregnancy test. When a pregnancy test is done, if it is negative, the adolescent should be offered counseling on pregnancy prevention and a follow-up appointment as desired.

Barriers to Clinic Care

There can be a number of barriers to adolescents seeking care at clinics. In IHS and tribal facilities, primary care providers and nursing staff consistently raise concerns about whether a teen can be seen for health care services without parental permission.

Legal Guidelines.   Legal guidelines vary greatly by individual states and tribes, from no legislation to specific laws prohibiting adolescent care services. A number of legal opinions have supported the minor's right to nonsurgical methods of family planning without parental permission at federally funded facilities.[4] To best address this issue, each facility should develop a policy on providing services to adolescents.

Negative Attitudes Toward Adolescents.   In addition to legal questions, other barriers to clinic accessibility include, at times, the perceived negative attitude of providers and other staff members to adolescents. Ideally, only staff who appreciate teens should be assigned to work with them. Realistically, in most smaller clinics, all staff members interact with teens and sometimes must be reminded about the special qualities and needs of teens, especially in relation to their psychosocial development. If possible, allowing the teen to see a consistent practitioner of his or her choice is desirable.

Confidentiality.   A common barrier to obtaining care is the adolescent's concern for confidentiality. The issue of confidentiality should be discussed directly with the adolescent. If the parent asks questions about the adolescent, the practitioner should simply indicate that information cannot be released and the parent should talk with the adolescent. Secondary to issues of confidentiality, especially in small communities, it is important to provide situations in which the adolescent can obtain care. For instance, if pregnancy tests or prenatal visits are provided only at certain specified times or in specific clinics, the adolescent may delay seeking care. It is important to incorporate visits among multiple or general visitations and at convenient times for the adolescent.

Sometimes, dealing with the issue of confidentiality can be difficult, as in the case of an adolescent pregnancy. Teens know that their parents need to (and eventually will) know of the pregnancy, but many have difficulty in the initial telling. It is not uncommon for a teen's first request to be not to notify her parents. The practitioner should honor the teen's request but also encourage her to tell her parents. In this case, it may be helpful for the provider to offer to assist the adolescent by informing the family in her presence. It is common for parents to react negatively to the announcement of a teen's pregnancy at first. Revealing it in a neutral environment, such as the clinic and in the presence of the practitioner, often helps to dissipate this negative parental reaction. In most AI families, all infants are welcomed into the family at birth. In the adolescent health survey, eight of 10 teens said that their family cares a great deal about them. It is essential to reassure the teen that, no matter what the initial reaction, there will be family support.

Maturity.   Another potential difficulty in working with teens is psychological maturation. Adolescence is generally divided into three periods: early (10–14 years), middle (15–17 years), and late (18–20 years). The physical changes of adolescence generally occur in early and middle adolescence. Psychological and cognitive development occur in middle and late adolescence, with the major task being separation from parents and assuming independence. The way adolescents think and solve problems also undergoes considerable development. Especially in early and middle adolescence, it is common for adolescents to have low self-esteem, deny their fertility, lack long-range goals, and be preoccupied with boyfriend or girlfriend and peer pressures. With middle and late adolescents, the primary theme should be developing responsibility for one's own behavior.

As part of the normal psychosocial development, many teens feel invulnerable (e.g., pregnancy and STDs "can't happen to me"), which leads to delay in seeking care. Limited understanding of explanations is especially common in the early adolescent period, and consistent repetition of information is required. In working with adolescents, it is important to accept the teen as an adult and treat with appropriate respect. Yet, it is also important to not show disappointment when adult behaviors are not forthcoming.

Teens have limited decision-making skills, which leads to inappropriate conclusions. This also extends to making decisions about birth control methods, such as overestimating the magnitude of birth control side effects, including weight gain, acne, and cancer risks. In the adolescent health survey, more than 8% of girls and 4% of boys in grades 10–12 did not use birth control methods because of worry about side effects. When providing information about family planning methods, both positives and negatives should be openly and evenly presented. The risks of pregnancy should always be presented for comparison as part of weighing the risks and benefits of contraceptive use. More frequent follow-up with a regular practitioner helps to promote compliance.

In the AI adolescent health survey, 20% of adolescents said that they would first go to their parents for information on birth control. When contraceptive services are provided, all adolescents should be encouraged to discuss these issues with their parents, and this encouragement should be documented in the medical notation.

Fear of Pelvic Examination.   The first pelvic examination can be very stressful for the adolescent female. Secondary to inappropriate expectations or lack of knowledge, it is common for the teen to express fear, or even tears, when presenting for her first pelvic examination. Extra time must be allotted when performing this examination. It is essential to explain what will happen, using pictures to illustrate anatomy as well as the procedure. It also is helpful to have the girl make a tubelike structure with her hand, into which the practitioner inserts the speculum, just as in the examination. At this time, the need for pelvic muscle relaxation can be illustrated, and issues of discomfort discussed. The speculum used should be an appropriate size. Usually, a Peterson speculum or long, thin-bladed speculum is best to use at the first examination. (Word imagery is extremely important, and the use of strong words, such as *blades*, should be avoided.) The procedure is explained in the presence of the parent or guardian (if available); then the adolescent is asked to select who will be present, if anyone. Sometimes the mother wants to be present and the girl refuses. In this case, a proactive policy can support the adolescent's request. More often, the adolescent wants the mother to be present but the mother is uncomfortable with this request. In this situation, a nurse can be asked to support the adolescent. Pelvic examinations should never be performed by a male practitioner without a chaperone or assistant. This is also desirable when a female practitioner performs a woman's health examination. After the examination is complete, the pictures should be used to review what was done and any findings, including normal findings. It also is important to recognize the adolescent's cooperation, her ability to control her reactions and body, and the normalcy of the examination. Finally, the gynecologic examination should be presented in a positive light—that is, as something that all females do as part of taking care of themselves.

At times, a teen presents by requesting family planning methods but refuses a pelvic examination. In 1993, the U.S. Food and Drug Administration Fertility and Maternal Health Advisory Committee voted in favor of giving patients seeking oral contraceptives the option of deferring physical examination without being denied a prescription. This has been reflected in package inserts. Although the examination may be deferred, it should be performed at the earliest opportunity. Delaying the examination does not negate the need for counseling about what the pelvic examination entails, the need for a pelvic examination, and an explanation of risks and benefits of birth control. Delaying the pelvic examination is an important option when the adolescent may avoid asking for contraception because of fear of the pelvic examination. This option also can be considered when the patient is having her period or when there is a delay in scheduling the examination in clinic. A limited prescription (1–2 months) can be provided with the understanding that a pelvic examination is required before the prescription can be renewed. The presently available urine pregnancy tests are extremely sensitive and should be performed before the initiation of any method of family planning, even in the event of a menstrual period (which could also be implantation bleeding

or other types of discharge). If an STD is suspected, a pelvic examination is necessary.

Obesity and Irregular Menses

With the increasing rates of obesity in adolescent females, irregular menses are a common complaint. Waiting for a period to start a family planning method can lead to a pregnancy or a 2- to 3-month wait, which the teen perceives as a long time. In this situation, an acceptable clinical practice has been to obtain a urine human chorionic gonadotropin test, have the adolescent preferably abstain or use condoms for 1–2 weeks, and then return for a repeat test. If negative, the method can be initiated.

Offer Choices in Counseling

When offering counseling to adolescents, it is more acceptable to offer choices and allow the teen to make his or her own decision. For instance, in avoiding pregnancy, it is best to offer a number of choices: abstain, have intercourse, or maybe have intercourse. The "maybe" is an important choice to give to adolescents because sexual activity may be an infrequent occurrence for the teen. In the AI adolescent health survey, nearly half of sexually active teens reported that they had intercourse only a couple of times a year or less. In sexually active AI teens, almost 30% did not use a birth control method because sex was unexpected or there was no time to prepare. This third "maybe" option must be considered and addressed in counseling: "maybe" methods (condoms, diaphragms, and, previously, sponges) and other ways to deal with "maybe" situations.

Link to Alcohol and Drug Use

Some studies have shown a linkage between sexual activity and alcohol and drug use in adolescents. Although data are not available for AI adolescents, it is a common clinical impression that this linkage also holds for AI adolescents. Not only are adolescents who use alcohol and drugs more often sexually active than those who do not, but also infrequent sexual activity often occurs around the casual use of drugs and alcohol. This association may be explored with the teen, with methods of avoidance presented. It is important for the adolescent girl to understand the risks associated with alcohol use, including possibly placing herself in situations in which there are increased chances for unprotected sex or rape.

Sexually Transmitted Diseases

When discussing STDs, it may be useful to use picture information, such as Figure 29-1, which shows that each partner is exposed to STDs from previous partners during intercourse. Teens appreciate frank and honest discussions about STDs. Patience is required, especially with adolescents who have recurrent STDs. Only presenting worst-case scenarios can lead to less cooperation, for when the scenario does not occur, the adolescent may

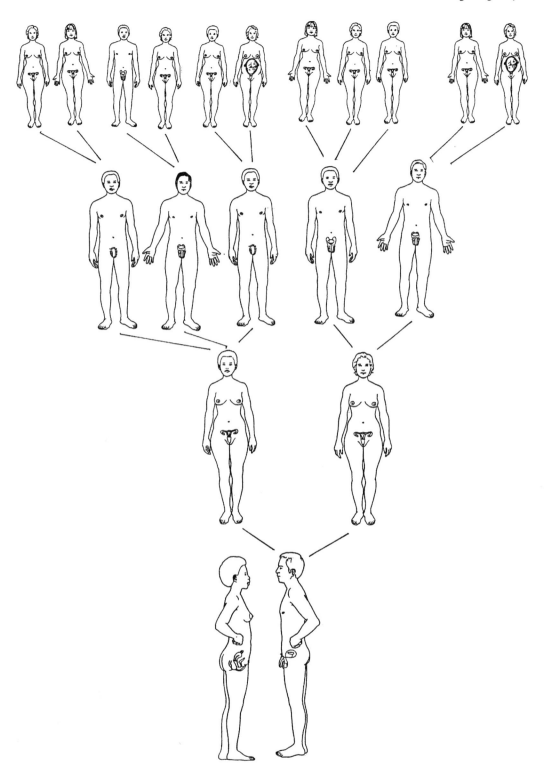

Figure 29-1. Picture information shows that each sexual partner is exposed to sexually transmitted diseases from previous partners.

become distrustful and not believe in further counseling. When possible, better compliance and understanding can be obtained when counseling teens as a couple rather than individually.

Sexual Abuse

Especially when sexual activity is initiated in early adolescence, concern about possible abuse is raised and should be discussed with the adolescent. In the AI adolescent survey, adolescents who said they were physically or sexually abused were more likely to have had sexual intercourse than were nonabused youths. Almost 50% of those who reported having been physically abused had intercourse, compared with 28% of AI adolescents who were not physically abused. The same pattern holds for victims of sexual abuse, with 50% reporting sexual activity compared to 28% of peers. When approached appropriately, many adolescents do reveal previous abuse. With others, the abuse may be revealed at a later visit. When raising this issue with adolescents, the practitioner should explain the reasons for obtaining this history.

Male Responsibility

Secondary adolescent pregnancy prevention efforts should also include the promotion of male responsibility. In the AI adolescent health survey, 48.7% of sexually active boys stated that they used condoms for contraception, which is similar to other groups of adolescent boys. Latex condom use should be encouraged for sexually active teens for STD protection and contraception. There can be multiple barriers to obtaining and using condoms, such as concerns about confidentiality, access, cost, and the perception that the risk of pregnancy and STDs is low. In school programs and in clinical counseling, abstinence should be stressed as the only way to avoid pregnancy and infection completely. Yet, sexually active teens should be taught how to use condoms properly, effectively, and consistently.[5] Both the American College of Obstetricians and Gynecologists and the American Academy of Pediatrics support making condoms available to teens by their families, clinics, school health programs, and other youth-serving agencies through medical professional organizations.[6, 7] Many adults are concerned, however, that condom availability promotes sexual activity. A number of studies of school-based clinics do not show that distribution of contraceptives promotes sexual activity.[8]

Tertiary Prevention

Tertiary prevention addresses pregnant adolescents. In this situation, there are two goals: providing appropriate prenatal services and avoiding further pregnancies until adulthood. The provision and components of obstetric care for the adolescent is the same as for any

other woman, with the exception that teens, especially early adolescents, generally require more time per visit and more frequent visits for explanations and teaching. Again, it is essential to verbally repeat important messages and to have pictures available to reinforce this teaching. Additionally, seeing a regular practitioner for care can promote compliance.

Every effort should be made to include the father and family members in both prenatal care and intrapartum services. In Indian country, every pregnancy is a "family" pregnancy, but this is especially true of the adolescent pregnancy. Pregnancy is also a time in which both the pregnant woman and the partner look toward their coming roles as parents. For the pregnant adolescent, reestablishing her relationship with her mother is important to the normal psychological process of pregnancy. Her mother's supportive role becomes especially important to the pregnant teen in the latter half of pregnancy. This important maternal role should be recognized, discussed, and supported. If the mother is not available, an alternate maternal figure should be identified. In Indian country, in supportive and open intrapartum services, it is common to have teens request that special adults, such as the mother, grandmother, aunts, or sisters, be present to welcome the newborn at the birth. Attending births involving the extended family can be one of the more enjoyable experiences for a clinician. Multiple concerns are commonly raised regarding the medical consequences of teenage pregnancy at this time. A number of studies have shown that age by itself is not a major determinant of medical risks, especially in middle and late adolescence. Adolescents who receive early and consistent prenatal care do not seem to be at greater risk for medical problems associated with pregnancy. Many teens do not receive such care, however, and age becomes an associated risk factor for a poor outcome. Data do seem to support a risk of low birth weight in adolescents, especially in early adolescent pregnancy, although these data have not been replicated in Native Americans. The negative consequences of adolescent pregnancy seem to be more apparent in psychosocial data (i.e., lower educational levels, increased school dropout rates, fewer employment opportunities, and economic disadvantage).

Since 1980, 25–28% of pregnancies in AI teens have been repeat pregnancies (Table 29-2). Studies have shown a greater increase in morbidity in second and higher-order pregnancies in adolescents than in first pregnancies. In addition, the adverse social consequences of adolescent pregnancy increase, such as greater unemployment and school dropout.

The period of pregnancy often entails much clinical care, family and community support, and inclusion in other social programs. This support must continue after the birth to enhance parenting skills, support pregnancy

Table 29-2. Teen Births and First Child among American Indians and Alaska Natives in Reservation States

Calendar Years	Total Teen Births	First Child	Percentage First Child	Percentage Second or Higher-Order Child
1983–1985	24,088	17,946	74.5	25.5
1984–1986	23,759	17,618	74.2	25.8
1985–1987	23,832	17,612	73.9	26.1
1986–1988	24,201	17,771	73.4	26.6
1987–1989	18,835	13,661	72.5	27.5
1990–1992	19,996	14,534	72.7	27.3
1991–1993	20,305	14,845	73.1	26.9

Source: Adapted from Indian Health Service. Trends in Indian Health. Washington, DC: U.S. Department of Health and Human Services, Indian Health Service, 1986–1996.

spacing, continue the building of the adolescent's self-esteem and development, and encourage continued educational attainment.

School-based programs for adolescents continue to be supported in the general population and in Indian country. Because school is the place where adolescents spend the majority of time, accessibility and availability of care is ensured. When allowed to function without restrictions, these programs can and should provide primary, secondary, and tertiary preventive services. When adolescents are actively included in the process, acceptability of services increases. There are many examples of established and successful school-based programs that provide comprehensive and accessible services to AI youth. One example is the adolescent program established by the IHS and University of New Mexico, which developed a number of successful teen health centers providing accessible, comprehensive, multidisciplinary services to adolescents.

Summary

Adolescent pregnancy is a societal problem related to the normal physical and psychosocial changes of adolescence. As primary care providers, we must be sensitive to and respectful of our adolescent patients by giving them choices and supporting their assumption of responsibility for their actions.

References

1. University of Minnesota Adolescent Health Program. The State of Native American Youth Health. Minneapolis, MN: University of Minnesota Adolescent Health Program, February 1992.
2. Greydanus DE, Patel DR. Consent and confidentiality in adolescent health care. Pediatr Ann 1991;20:80–84.
3. Zabin LS, Emerson MR, Ringers PA, Sedivy V. Adolescents with negative pregnancy test results, an accessible at-risk group. JAMA 1996;275:113–117.
4. Wever N. Consent for treatment of minors. Legal opinion, April 29, 1991.
5. Baylor College of Medicine. Contraceptive Counseling for Adolescents. In D Grimes (ed), The Contraception Report. 1991;1.
6. American College of Obstetricians and Gynecologists. The adolescent obstetric-gynecologic patient. ACOG Technical Bulletin No. 145. September 1990.
7. American Academy of Pediatrics. Condom availability for youth. AAP Policy Statement. Pediatrics 1995;95.
8. Baylor College of Medicine. Adolescent Pregnancy Prevention Programs. In D Grimes (ed), The Contraception Report 1994;5.

Chapter 30
Diabetes Mellitus in Pregnancy

N. Burton Attico

Diabetes mellitus is occurring in epidemic proportions in American Indians (AIs) and Alaska Natives (ANs). Diabetes mellitus is commonly considered a disease of aging, with prevalence rates commonly expressed as rates for individuals older than age 45 years. There is a significant prevalence in the younger AI and AN reproductive population (Figure 30-1), however, with the reproductive age usually considered as ending at age 45 years. The incidence of gestational diabetes mellitus (often a precursor to overt diabetes mellitus) is also increasing in AI and AN women.[1] Diabetes during pregnancy carries the potential for adverse perinatal outcomes, but with close attention to screening, diagnosis, and management, good perinatal outcomes are usually probable. The elements of diagnosis and management of diabetes in pregnancy that are being used successfully in several Indian Health Service (IHS) programs are outlined in this chapter.

Diagnosis

Although gestational diabetes by definition is "carbohydrate intolerance of variable severity with onset or first recognition during pregnancy,"[2, 3] for practical clinical purposes, diabetes in pregnancy in AI and AN women can be divided into *pregestational* (existing before pregnancy) and *gestational* (present only during pregnancy).[4] This clinical and functional distinction helps to define the perinatal risks for both fetus and mother. This obstetric classification and distinction does not depend on whether the diabetes is of the insulin-dependent (IDDM), insulin-managed, or non–insulin-dependent (NIDDM) type.

The placental contrainsulin hormones (mainly somatomammotropin) and other factors that tend to induce or incite pure gestational diabetes become most active during the latter half of pregnancy. Therefore, diabetes diagnosed before 20 weeks gestation probably represents a pregestational type of diabetes. This also means

that final "classification" (either pregestational or gestational) for the individual patient may be a retrospective clinical diagnosis made only after interconceptional testing has been done to rule out a latent diabetes mellitus existing in the nonpregnant state.[3, 5] There is normally a slight improvement in glucose tolerance in the gravida before 20 weeks gestation.

There is an important distinction to be made between *screening* tests and actual *diagnostic* tests for the diabetic condition, as well as differences between nonpregnancy and pregnancy tests and screens. In medicine, screens are used because of their convenience (both to the patient and the provider), the occurrence of few false-negatives, rare missed positives, and reduced or minimal cost, whereas tests are used to make an actual definitive diagnosis. The preprocedure preparation (fasting vs. nonfasting), the test doses used in pregnancy (50 and 100 g vs. 75 g), the time after the specified test dose that blood samples are drawn (multiple vs. single), and the blood sugar values that indicate further action is needed are very different, as is the significance of the various test values obtained. Capillary blood sugar testing and values are to be used only for screening, never for making a diagnosis of diabetes in pregnancy.

On a first prenatal visit, a random blood sugar value greater than 120 mg/dl should be followed by a standard *pregnancy* oral glucose tolerance test (OGTT). Because early diagnosis is so important in establishing the diagnosis of high-risk pregnancy, all pregnant women (and especially AI and AN women[1, 4, 6, 7]) should have a diabetes screen between 24 and 28 weeks gestation.[8] Individuals who are at higher risk should be screened (if possible) in each trimester. This *gestational diabetes screen* (O'Sullivan screen) consists of 50 g of glucose, administered orally, nonfasting (and without regard to the timing of the last meal), with a blood sugar drawn 1 hour later (Table 30-1). Any gravida with a blood sugar screen value in excess of 140 mg/dl should have a standard

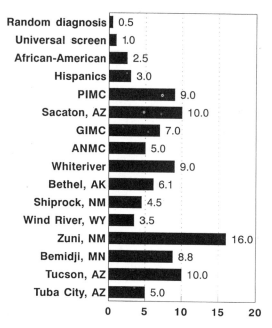

Random diagnosis   0.5
Universal screen   1.0
African-American   2.5
Hispanics   3.0
PIMC   9.0
Sacaton, AZ   10.0
GIMC   7.0
ANMC   5.0
Whiteriver   9.0
Bethel, AK   6.1
Shiprock, NM   4.5
Wind River, WY   3.5
Zuni, NM   16.0
Bemidji, MN   8.8
Tucson, AZ   10.0
Tuba City, AZ   5.0

0   5   10   15   20

Figure 30-1. Incidence rates (per 100 deliveries) for diabetes in pregnancy, various locations and groups. (PIMC = Phoenix Indian Medical Center, Phoenix, Arizona; GIMC = Gallup Indian Medical Center, Gallup, New Mexico; ANMC = Alaska Native Medical Center, Anchorage, Alaska [all are Indian Health Service referral centers].) (Reprinted with permission from NB Attico, KC Smith, AG Waxman, RL Ball. Diabetes mellitus in pregnancy: views toward an improved pregnancy outcome. The IHS Primary Care Provider 1992;7:153–164.)

Table 30-1. Standard Pregnancy Oral Glucose Tolerance Test: Blood Sugar Values (mg/dl) for Pregnant and Non-pregnant Persons after 100 g Glucose Load (given fasting)*

| Time | Whole serum or (blood plasma) | |
	Pregnant	Nonpregnant
Fasting	90 (105)	105 (120)
1 hr	165 (190)	170 (195)
2 hrs	145 (165)	120 (140)
3 hrs	125 (145)	110 (125)

*Any two elevated values (or fasting blood sugar [FBS] elevation alone) are diagnostic of diabetes in pregnancy. A single elevated value (aside from the FBS) represents gestational carbohydrate intolerance. Values within 15% of the diagnostic levels are considered borderline.

Source: Adapted from American College of Obstetricians and Gynecologists. Management of Diabetes Mellitus in Pregnancy. ACOG Technical Bulletin No. 200 1994;1–8. [Reprinted in Diabetes Spectrum 1992;5:22.]

OGTT. The OGTT consists of 100 g of glucose administered fasting, and blood is drawn fasting and at 1, 2, and 3 hours. (It has been noted that some IHS laboratories also draw blood at 30 minutes. There is no diagnostic value associated with this time interval in pregnancy, and thus the 30-minute blood draw should not be done.) Two elevated values (two of four) indicate gestational diabetes. An elevated fasting blood glucose (more than 105 mg/dl) is virtually diagnostic of gestational diabetes and probably requires insulin for management. Although one elevated value (other than the fasting value) indicates gestational carbohydrate intolerance (GCI), that condition should be managed just like class A diabetes because most studies show a higher incidence of macrosomia in these pregnancies (however, these women should not be labeled diabetic) (Table 30-2). Values within 15% of the diagnostic levels are considered borderline and may indicate a need for further testing during that pregnancy.

The present home blood glucose monitors should not be used for diagnostic testing or screening, only for post-diagnostic patient management. Glycosylated hemoglobin (HbA$_{1c}$) values, although useful in predicting possible macrosomia if elevated, are usually not sensitive enough

for diagnosis unless the elevation is consistently more than 1% above normal values. Coordination with other necessary prenatal laboratory work avoids excessive venipunctures and enhances patient compliance and cooperation in testing.

Because of the high incidence, health care providers for AI and AN women have an obligation to prove that the individual woman does not have diabetes associated with each pregnancy, rather than finding out if she has diabetes. Skip pregnancies (pregnancies without diabetes between pregnancies with gestational diabetes) have occurred. In addition, some gestational diabetes does not become manifest until 32 weeks gestation or later (reportedly as many as 15–20%). Thus, in high-risk individuals (including those with GCI and borderline diabetes), retesting with the standard pregnancy OGTT (not the screen) should occur at 32 weeks. Using high-risk factors alone as trigger criteria for screening may miss almost 50% of cases of diabetes in pregnancy.[9] The American College of Obstetricians and Gynecologists (ACOG) Technical Bulletin[4] lists Native American women as a special high-risk group in whom the clinician should consider going directly to a gestational diabetes test rather than beginning with a gestational diabetes screen because of demonstrated high AI and AN population prevalence (see Figure 30-1). At a special IHS-ACOG consultation presentation in 1992, AI and AN pregnancy incidence values were shown to be multiples of those in the general population.

Alternatives are being explored for both the screening and testing phases. The standard glucose test solutions are highly concentrated and hygroscopic and, when administered to pregnant women, even when given cold and flavored, frequently precipitate nausea or vomiting (in

5–15% of patients). In spite of the importance of the test, many women do not complete or repeat the test if they become nauseated, especially if nausea and vomiting have been a major pregnancy problem before that time. Alternatives to the O'Sullivan screen test are the jelly bean screen[10] and screening or testing with glucose polymer solutions (Polycose), reported by Murphy and colleagues,[11, 12] and presently used by many staff at the Anchorage Medical Center. The WHO test has been adopted in some IHS locations because it requires fewer venipunctures (two vs. four) and it can be administered as a simple single test (simultaneous screen and test). Thus, the patient does not need to return for retesting (significant because the test requires fasting).

Perinatal Risks and Classifications

Those caring for AI and AN patients have an obligation to look actively for diabetes in pregnancy and to maintain a high index of suspicion. The reasons for this are that treatment carries essentially no risk to the mother or offspring, whereas undiagnosed and therefore untreated cases may yield extremely morbid outcomes. Although 99% of cases of diabetes in pregnancy in AI and AN women represent either type 2 (pregestational) or type 4 diabetes (gestational), early detection and tight management (i.e., maintaining normal pregnant blood sugars) remain key factors in fostering a good outcome of pregnancy. Diabetes-related morbidity in the mother may include a need for management with insulin (with the risk of possible hypoglycemic reactions), an increased incidence of preeclampsia and hydramnios (polyhydramnios), and a higher rate of cesarean section or other operative deliveries. Most obstetric complications are more frequent or more severe in the pregestational diabetic woman.

Perinatal morbidity is still extremely high in the offspring. Morbidity includes high rates of congenital anomaly (trebled in the pregestational diabetic), late stillborns, macrosomia, birth injury (usually related to macrosomia), hypocalcemia and neonatal tetany, hyperbilirubinemia, and delayed lung maturity with increased rates of neonatal respiratory distress syndrome. With early diagnosis and tight management, morbidity decreases dramatically.

Despite the introduction of the now familiar National Diabetes Data Group (NDDG) classification in 1979, most obstetricians continue to use the Priscilla White classification (Table 30-2) from the Joslin Diabetes Clinic because it offers a clinical prognostic and management value not found in the NDDG schema. The newest schema is an etiologic one, introduced in July 1997.[7] The White classification allows the provider to anticipate potential complications by further defining the patient's diabetes by age at onset, duration, existing complications, or adverse perinatal complications during previous pregnancies. For example, before the use of retinal laser ther-

Table 30-2. Modified Priscilla White Classification Schema for Diabetes in Pregnancy (1989)[a]

Class	Age of onset	Duration of diabetes
A[b]	Any	Any
B	>20 yrs	10 yrs
C	10–19 yrs	10–19 yrs
D	<10 yrs	Older than 20 yrs, or hypertension
E[c]	Any	Pelvic vessel calcifications
F	Any	Nephropathy
R	Any	Retinopathy
RF	Any	Nephropathy and retinopathy
H	Any	Heart disease
G[d]	Any	Adverse pregnancy history
T	Any	Transplant

[a]This classification schema is the system preferred by most obstetricians and gynecologists because it is clinically relevant. It has been endorsed by the American College of Obstetricians and Gynecologists. Macrosomia is more common in class A and B diabetic women than in other classes.
[b]By definition, the class A patient is diabetic only when pregnant, regardless of the method of management (either with diet alone or combined with insulin).
Class A subclasses: A-1 = Blood sugars normalized with diet alone; A-2 = Insulin required for normalization.
[c]Class E is not commonly used clinically at present (signifies a restrictive pelvic circulation).
[d]Added to another diagnosis.
Source: Reprinted with permission from JW Hare (ed). Diabetes Complicating Pregnancy: The Joslin Clinic Method. New York: Alan R. Liss, 1989.

apy, women with class R diabetes (proliferative retinopathy) were known to have a high likelihood (50%) of rapid acceleration of retinal disease during pregnancy that could result in loss of sight, despite a successful fetal outcome. The White classification system identifies women at risk for retinal damage, which enables the health care provider to refer them for screening and, if needed, treatment (retinal photocoagulation). Those with class A/G (diabetes with a history of previous adverse pregnancy outcome, see Table 30-2) are usually treated similar to class B or C diabetes because of the significantly higher risks to their fetuses. The NDDG classification should be considered a medical etiologic schema, whereas the White classification should be considered a clinical management and risk assessment schema. Most diabetes in pregnancy in AI and AN women falls into White's classes A through C, although with increased childhood-onset diabetes occurring, more class D diabetics are anticipated.

Clinical Antepartum Management

Pregnancy care begins with the standards set for any pregnant patient. Diet should be regularized for normal weight gain, and supplemental prenatal vitamins, calcium, and iron should be included, along with folic acid. Teaching should focus on pregnancy expectations and the additional risks of a diabetic pregnancy, with the need for monitoring for potential complications. The mother should be given information about nutritional goals and expectations during pregnancy. Lifestyle changes are in order.

The key to management of the pregnant diabetic is attaining and maintaining normal pregnant blood sugar levels (pregnancy normoglycemia or euglycemia) throughout the pregnancy. Blood sugar goals in the pregnant diabetic are the same as in the normal pregnant woman, in whom there is a tendency toward a fasting hypoglycemia (10–15 mg/dl lower than nonpregnant glucose levels) and a slight postprandial hyperglycemia (15–25 mg/dl higher). Target blood glucose values in the pregnant diabetic are therefore 60–90 mg/dl before breakfast and 120 mg/dl at 2 hours after meals.[2] Some reports have recommended measuring preprandial blood sugar levels, but these have not become standard. Attempts to achieve normoglycemia with diet alone should not be prolonged more than 7–10 days. Hospitalization should be used freely in the new diabetic or in difficult-to-manage situations (e.g., persistent hyperglycemia; infections, such as pyelonephritis; and ketoacidosis) and when rapid or intense intervention is desired. As in the nonpregnant diabetic, diet, exercise, and hypoglycemic agents remain key management components, but insulin is the only hypoglycemic agent that should be used during pregnancy. Most oral hypoglycemic agents do cross the placenta and may induce fetal hyperinsulinemia or islet cell hypertrophy. Insulin does not cross the placenta; therefore, mother and fetus function with their own glucoregulation mechanisms. Management must be individualized, coordinated, and multidisciplinary, with all members of the team (physician, diabetes educator, clinic nurse, dietitian or public health nutritionist, public health nurse, and others) contributing within their specialty areas in a complementary way, as described under Diet, Exercise, and Home Blood Glucose Monitoring. Because much depends on patient compliance, proper patient education and motivation are critical. Additionally, the patient should be cautioned (intergestationally) to report or look for possible pregnancy early so that early diagnosis and proper management intervention are possible.

Diet

Intensive counseling should be done by a dietitian or public health nutritionist, regulating the patient's diet to a level of 15 kcal/lb per day (30–35 kcal/kg) using the patient's ideal, nonpregnant body weight. An additional 200–400 kcal per day should be allowed for pregnancy needs; thus, a total of 2,000–3,000 kcal per day is usually prescribed. The patient must be monitored to ensure a normal pregnancy weight gain (22–30 lb). Although the patient might be obese, pregnancy is not the time to attempt weight reduction. At least a 15-lb weight gain in the grossly obese is advised. Because of the pregnant diabetic's high incidence of hydramnios (25–40%), care must be taken that weight gain does not mask (or represent) excess amniotic fluid. In planning the diet, calories (nutrients) for snacks are to be displaced from an antecedent or subsequent meal, so that the total prescribed calories remain the same. Complex carbohydrates, with high dietary fiber, are a mainstay of the diet; simple sugars and "empty calories" should be avoided. Protein should provide 20% of calories, and dietary fat goals should be 30% or less. This is an ideal time to initiate education for proper eating habits.

Several small meals rather than three big meals per day should be encouraged, especially in the patient taking insulin. Dietary consultation, instruction, and modification should occur at 6- to 8-week intervals, or more often. Counseling should include education on the proper balance of fat, protein, fiber, and carbohydrates (especially using complex carbohydrates and avoiding simple sugars) in the daily diet. Additional dietary sessions (either individual or group) should be scheduled for the new diabetic because she is managing a new disease, coupled with the pregnancy and its needs. Whatever dietary counseling is given, some retrospective estimate of the actual caloric intake should be attempted. A permissive yet understanding attitude must be expressed so as to maintain some measure of trust and encourage voluntary compliance.

Exercise

Increased exercise is another key to management of the nonpregnant diabetic. Strenuous exercise has been demonstrated to cause abnormal fetal heart rate patterns (even in athletes), and thus strenuous exercise in pregnancy is not encouraged. Brisk walking for 15–30 minutes after each meal lowers blood sugar, however, is known to be safe in pregnancy, stimulates fluid return from the lower extremities, provides muscle activity for most major muscle groups, promotes cardiovascular stimulation, and is a start (or a continuation) of a good habit. Exercise should be curtailed if either preterm labor or uterine contractions start.

Hypoglycemic Agents

Oral hypoglycemic agents are not to be used (are contraindicated) in pregnancy in the United States, although they are sometimes used in other parts of the world. Virtually all oral hypoglycemic agents cross the placenta. If a pregestational diabetic has been previously managed with oral hypoglycemic agents, these medications should be stopped and the patient switched to insulin during the pregnancy. If normoglycemia (both fasting and postprandial) cannot be attained and maintained with diet alone in any patient with diabetes in pregnancy (class A-1), insulin is indicated. Insulin should be started if the fasting blood glucose exceeds 105 mg/dl or the 2-hour postprandial glucose consistently exceeds 120 mg/dl; the patient should then be reclassified as class A-2 (see Table 30-2). Macrosomia is more frequent in gravida with prolonged hyperglycemia.

Insulin is usually given in split (multiple) doses, at least twice daily, especially if more than 25–30 units of insulin are needed daily for control. Usually, the insulin dose is divided as follows: (1) Two-thirds of the total daily dose is given before breakfast (two-thirds of it as neutral protamine Hagedorn [NPH] and one-third as regular insulin) and (2) one-third of the total daily dose is given before supper (half of this as NPH and half as regular insulin). For example, if the total daily dose is 60 U, the patient takes 40 U before breakfast (26 U of NPH and 14 U of regular insulin) and 20 U before supper (10 U of NPH and 10 U of regular insulin). *The calculated insulin dosage is then adjusted as necessary to best maintain pregnancy normoglycemia for the individual patient.* A starting guide is 0.5–0.7 U/kg daily. Most providers do not prescribe 70/30 insulin mixtures in the pregnant patient.

Presently, only human insulin should be used for managing diabetes in pregnancy to avoid potential insulin antibody production and sensitization; do not use beef or beef and pork insulin mixtures in the pregnant patient. This is especially so for women who have been on intermittent insulin therapy. A plan can be devised with the patient for potential self-modification of the insulin dosage, between visits, for persistent deviations from the euglycemic goal. A better plan, however, may be to facilitate easy patient access to a knowledgeable and understanding provider.

Hospitalization

Hospitalization should be readily used when needed for rapid control, or if any pregnancy- or diabetes-related complications develop (e.g., hypertension, pyelonephritis, ketoacidosis, hydramnios, persistent hyperglycemia, infection, preterm labor, preeclampsia). When hospitalization is used for blood sugar regulation, the customary rule of not changing insulin dosage more often than every other day need not be observed. Dosage is changed as often as necessary to obtain rapid glucose control and to avoid prolonged hospitalization. The aim should be a hospitalization of no longer than 5–7 days when used for glycemic stabilization. Scheduling other needed procedures during that hospitalization (e.g., ultrasound examinations, patient teaching, nonstress or stress testing, fetal profiles, repeat urine cultures, creatinine clearance, dietary education, eye examination) attains maximal hospital benefit and cost-effectiveness. Fine-tuning the insulin dosage should be done on an outpatient basis, using the patient's home or regular diet and routine. Many patients like the camaraderie they find during hospitalization on the larger services. This may be a patient's first exposure to the well-demonstrated value and function of support groups.

Hospitalization should also be used before delivery (1–3 days) for re-evaluation and restabilization.

Home Blood Glucose Monitoring

Home blood glucose monitoring (also called *blood glucose self-monitoring*) is essential to obtaining glycemic control today. More than 95% of pregnant diabetics elect to use home blood glucose monitoring. It should not be forced. At one time, visual strips were used, but virtually all strips available today are electrochemical and cannot be read visually. Most monitors now have an enclosed memory chip. Some monitors even interact with computer programs and "dump" the contents of their memory chips into a personal computer for graphic review and analysis. It should be recognized that monitors read capillary blood glucose, the values of which are within 15% of laboratory determinations of venous blood glucose levels. Although most home blood glucose monitors are becoming increasingly foolproof and automatic, these monitors can be fooled.

Other Factors, Studies, and Considerations

Because many pregnancies with diabetes may be terminated early, proper gestational dating is essential and should always be meticulous. Although menstrual dating is used as a standard, gestational dating should include at least one objective measure, usually diagnostic ultrasonic fetometry (before 18–20 weeks), but perceived fetal movement and fetoscope fetal heart tones are also important.[13] Ultrasound can be used to determine hydramnios, which is found in almost 40% of diabetic pregnancies, although only half that number are clinically significant. Ultrasound can also be used for early detection and monitoring of fetal anomaly. On many obstetric services, an additional ultrasound is routinely performed at 36–38 weeks to attempt calculation of fetal weight to rule out macrosomia.

Because of the danger of late intrauterine fetal demise (stillbirth), periodic electronic fetal monitoring is started at 34–36 weeks on a twice-weekly schedule (especially in class A-2 or higher). Many centers do not perform electronic fetal monitoring on class A-1 patients until 39–40 weeks. Additionally, daily home fetal movement monitoring and charting should be started at the same stage of pregnancy on all diabetics. Any decrease in fetal movement demands an immediate nonstress test. There is usually a progressive increase in insulin requirement as the pregnancy nears term. Maternal insulin requirement tends to increase steadily during pregnancy; rarely does it decrease in a well-progressing pregnancy. Any sudden decrease in maternal insulin requirements should be carefully evaluated (including a nonstress test in the evaluation) because this may be an early sign of decreasing placental function. Maternal hypoglycemia should be avoided because fetal hypoglycemia usually occurs simultaneously. Long-term glycemic control should be monitored by obtaining HbA_{1c} levels at 4- to 8-week intervals; elevated levels can help to predict macrosomia.[14] The explanation for this is that as glucose, amino acids, and free fatty acids cross the placenta, the fetal islet cells hypertrophy, producing high levels of fetal insulin, which promote excessive glycogen and fat storage in the fetus and macrosomia.

Because of the frequency and importance of urinary tract infections in the diabetic, a urine culture (not just a dipstick) should be obtained each trimester (and probably monthly in those with a previous history of urinary tract infections) to look for asymptomatic bacteriuria or silent pyelonephritis.[15] Urinary tract infections should be treated promptly and vigorously, with close follow-up to detect recurrences or resistant infections. The choice of antibiotic must always consider the pregnancy status. Pyelonephritis in pregnancy always warrants hospitalization, at least for initiation of therapy.

Patients with known retinopathy require comanagement by an ophthalmologist. All other diabetic patients should have a baseline eye examination in early pregnancy to rule out proliferative retinopathy; this is a rare occurrence in the gestational diabetic.

To provide proper oversight of the pregnant diabetic, prenatal visits should be at least twice as often as usual for the patient's stage of gestation. Discussing intercurrent events (related either to the diabetes or to the pregnancy) with the patient and anticipating possible complications (anticipatory guidance) can simplify care (expectant intervention and oversight rather than reactive management). Patients should be given a special sheet or log book to write down their blood glucose results, times of determinations, and any reactions or variations in usual meal schedules or other intercurrent events. With computer-assisted blood glucose management, this oversight becomes very graphic and less difficult, thereby facilitating demonstration of the degree of control (or noncontrol) to the patient. Some computer programs even visually demonstrate the degree of control according to the time of day or the day of the week, so that trends can be sought.

As hyperglycemia is a proven teratogen that can alter the well-being of the fetus, the goal of the provider must be to manage blood sugars closely, so as to not let the fetus know that it is in a potentially hazardous location. All women with diabetes in pregnancy should have blood sugars that are as close as possible to those of the normal nondiabetic pregnant woman; in other words, intensive diabetes management. Control of diabetes in pregnancy means that blood sugar values should be the same as those in the nondiabetic pregnant woman.[2, 9, 16, 17]

It is obvious from this discussion that a team approach is necessary to manage a diabetic pregnancy successfully. No single health care discipline can manage all these factors. Established protocols facilitate care and ensure uniformity in application by team members, with continuity of care, consistency in information given to the patient, and empathy and compassion for the patient. Interdisciplinary consultation and review also facilitates care of the diabetic pregnancy. Nonetheless, this does not mean a "many-cooks" type of management. Algorithms can help to ensure that all (or most) providers at a facility are reacting and prescribing alike (Figure 30-2). Consultation should be used liberally in unusual situations or for complications. Patient instructional materials are available from IHS Area Diabetes Control Officers and are adapted, tested, and updated for suitability in each IHS area. Patient instructional materials are also available from ACOG, the American Diabetes Association, the American Dietetic Association, and the March of Dimes Birth Defects Foundation (at varied levels of reading ability).

Intrapartum Management

What represents a term pregnancy in the pregnant diabetic? Class A diabetics are presently allowed to go to 40 weeks without intervention, uncomplicated class B and C can go to 38–39 weeks, and others (complicated) are terminated 1 week earlier, as soon as amniocentesis indicates fetal lung maturity. A class G pregnancy must be intensively evacuated on an individual basis, but it is usual to terminate earlier than the previous poor pregnancy outcome. Use of antenatal electronic monitoring has allowed more pregnancies to go to term or to await spontaneous onset of labor. In general, diabetic pregnancies should not be allowed to go beyond 42 weeks.

Patients should be admitted for evaluation and stabilization 1–3 days before induction is planned. Amniocentesis to assess fetal lung maturity is mandatory if pregnancy is to be terminated before 40 weeks (a positive phosphatidylglycerol is more reliable than the lecithin-sphingomyelin ratio). Ripening of the cervix by use of prostaglandin gel (or prostaglandin analogues), as well as use of serial inductions, has made medical induction easier and more predictably favorable. Although cesarean section rates of 50% in pregnant diabetics are not uncommon in most facilities, many IHS facilities have substantially lower rates. Cesarean section rates in pregnant diabetics are 28% at the Phoenix Indian Medical Center (vs. 12–14% in its general obstetric population), 21.7% at the Gallup Indian Medical Center (vs. 13% in its general obstetric population), and 26.2% at the Public Health Service Indian Hospital in Shiprock, New Mexico (vs. 12.3% in its general obstetric population). These low rates are largely attributable to the use

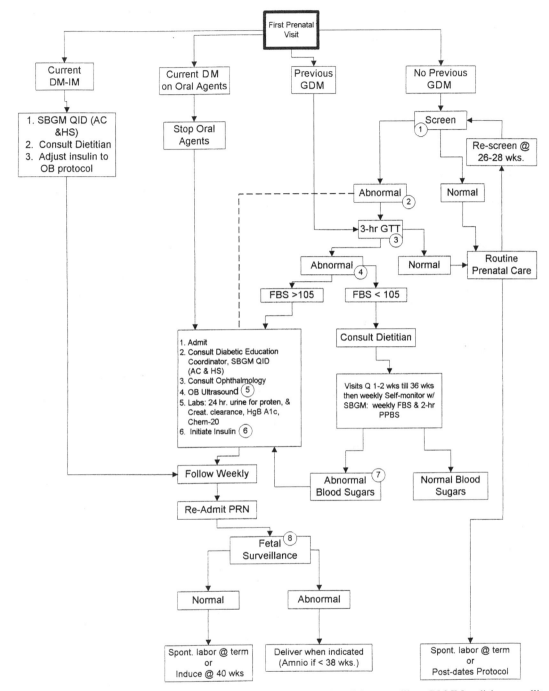

Figure 30-2. Algorithm for gestational diabetes mellitus (GDM). (DM = diabetes mellitus; DM-IM = diabetes mellitus, insulin managed; GTT = glucose tolerance test; FBS = fasting blood sugar; PPBS = postprandial blood sugar; OB = obstetrical; AC = before meals; HS = bedtime; HbA$_{1c}$ = glycosylated hemoglobin; creat. = creatinine; Amnio = amniocentesis; prn = as necessary; QID = for times a day.)

of serial inductions and the hospitals' wide experience in managing diabetes in pregnancy. Cesarean section should be done only for standard obstetric indications in the diabetic pregnancy (e.g., macrosomia, arrested labor, cephalopelvic disproportion, fetal distress), not because of the diabetes.

Induction (or cesarean section) should be scheduled so that delivery occurs while patient and staff are fresh, not late in the day, and so that critical management decisions can be made while adequate medical and nursing staff are immediately available. Up to one-third to one-half of the morning dose of insulin is usually given on induction day and the blood sugar monitored with capillary blood sugars. If the 6 A.M. blood sugar is <80 mg/dl, then fractional coverage only should be considered, omitting the intermediate-duration insulin that morning. Regular insulin should be used to control intrapartum hyperglycemia (aim at 80–120 mg/dl intrapartum). Subcutaneous insulin should be given no more than every 4 hours, if possible (the action of regular insulin is 1–6 hours, and thus accumulation is possible with shorter intervals). Alternatively, particularly if the total insulin requirement is low, complete intrapartum coverage might be attempted with small fractional doses of regular insulin (some obstetricians use intravenous admixtures of insulin and dextrose). Total insulin requirements tend to be low on the day of delivery (muscle may be able to use glucose on a bypass system) and tend to drop dramatically as soon as the infant and placenta are delivered because of loss of the placental contrainsulin factors. As lispro insulin (a new, very rapidly acting insulin analogue) becomes more widely available and used, this management regimen is expected to change, both antepartum and intrapartum.

The obstetric team should be alert to the possibility of shoulder dystocia, which is common in the infant of a diabetic pregnancy, and be skilled in its management. A pediatrician should be available at the delivery and the nursery staff prenotified. Neonatal monitoring should be available and early prophylactic feeding of the neonate planned to prevent possible hypoglycemia (milk is usually better than glucose solution, which may actually cause a rebound hypoglycemia). Because of the size of the team and the possibility of delivery complications, most staff recommend that delivery rooms be used rather than smaller birthing rooms for the diabetic pregnancy. Although the infant may be large, it may also be preterm and may have the problems of thermoregulation, poor suck, difficulty in glycemic regulation, and neural changes. Early neonatal discharge (<48 hours) is not recommended by most pediatricians because of the potential for persistent or delayed neonatal hypoglycemia, hypocalcemia, and hyperbilirubinemia. There is no standard as to what level of capillary blood sugar represents hypoglycemia in the neonate. Home blood glucose monitors (commonly used in the nursery) may be inaccurate in these lower ranges.

After birth, insulin is usually not required for at least 4–5 days (except for occasional small doses of regular insulin). This "honeymoon" period often extends to 2–3 weeks. In the gestational diabetic, blood sugars should continue to be monitored until the provider is sure that the diabetic (or glucose-intolerant) state is no longer present. The tight control required during pregnancy can be loosened to allow levels of 110–150 mg/dl and to avoid hypoglycemia. There is no contraindication to breast-feeding in diabetes. If the woman elects not to breast-feed, then her diet should be immediately reduced by at least 300–400 kcal per day, to the levels usually prescribed in the nonpregnant, hypocaloric diabetic diet (1,500–1,800 kcal/day), so that interconceptional weight reduction can begin. For the woman who is grossly obese and breast-feeding, caloric restriction should be strongly considered. Such caloric restriction in the mother usually does not degrade the quality of breast milk because her fat stores are mobilized. If needed in the pregestational diabetic, oral hypoglycemic agents (or insulin) may usually be resumed at the pregestational level after approximately 10 days.

Interconceptional Care

Interconceptional care involves attaining any needed weight loss, institution of family planning to ensure that any future pregnancies are planned (because of the woman's high-risk status, there should be few unintended pregnancies), and periodic testing to evaluate for possible onset of the overt diabetic state in women who have had gestational diabetes. All newly diagnosed cases of gestational diabetes should be retested and reclassified in the intergestational period (using the standard 75-g OGTT) to determine whether they were truly gestational diabetics, rather than pregestational diabetics who were unmasked by the special pregnancy testing.[2, 5, 18] The children born of diabetic pregnancies also require special monitoring (see Interconceptional Diabetes Testing).

Family Planning

Preconceptional counseling of diabetic women is an important part of family planning. Although there are relative contraindications to most family planning methods, no single family planning method is absolutely contraindicated in the diabetic or in women with a history of gestational diabetes. Patients should be informed of the definite risk for congenital anomalies if blood sugars are elevated during the early weeks of a pregnancy and given the knowledge, responsibility, and methods for planning and spacing their future pregnancies. Preconceptional counseling is an integral part of family planning, and it is very effective in this condition. Although oral contraceptives are known to interfere with glucose tolerance, those effects can be easily monitored.[16] The newer, lower-dose oral contraceptives, especially those with third-generation progestins, are reported to have less effect on blood lipids, and the triphasics are reported to have even less effect on both blood lipids and carbohydrate metabolism.[19-21]

Intrauterine devices (IUDs) should have restrictions similar to those for the nondiabetic, but with a much earlier trigger to remove the device if problems (especially infection) develop. IUDs are safe, especially in mutually monogamous couples, and with the Dalkon Shield now long off the market (since 1976), IUDs do not present the difficulties published in the popular press. Subcutaneous implants (e.g., levonorgestrel [Norplant System]) are not contraindicated in the diabetic, and they may be the ideal method in suitable patients. Many women now choose "the shot" (medroxyprogesterone [Depo-Provera]), which is fast becoming one of the most popular effective contraceptives available to and chosen by AI and AN women (studies show no interference with glucose metabolism in diabetics).[19, 22] Most important, pregnancies in these women should be planned and not unintentional or unexpected. In many women who may have completed their childbearing, sterilization may be a desired option and should be offered. It is vital that the value of preplanning pregnancy be stressed in counseling. Women should also be advised and encouraged to seek care if at any time they suspect they may be pregnant.

Interconceptional Diabetes Testing

The diagnosis of pure gestational diabetes should be confirmed by an OGTT at the 6-week postpartum visit (the nonpregnancy 75-g test, not the 100-g pregnancy test). Because the woman has already demonstrated a risk factor or predilection for developing overt diabetes, this testing (the 75-g OGTT) should be repeated periodically (probably annually or biennially), between pregnancies. If a diagnosis is to be made from a fasting plasma glucose, the nonpregnant values should be used.

Fifty percent of women who have had gestational diabetes develop overt diabetes within the succeeding 5–7 years, and 60% develop it within 16 years.[9] Periodic interconceptional diabetes testing for early diagnosis of overt diabetes remains a problem and is a public health, preventive care issue. Because active, preventive intervention may delay the onset of overt diabetes, each locale should work out a system that best suits the patient population and the local health care delivery system. Because women often do not "recall" the need for their own periodic testing (convenient or inadvertent denial), the following are some ideas for flagging these women for active, periodic intervention:

1. Develop an active patient register, and send out appointment slips at appropriate times for retesting.
2. Place a notation on the problem list of the patient's chart, and when the patient comes in for other reasons, discuss or mention the need to undergo periodic retesting.
3. Flag the infant's chart as "infant of diabetic mother" or "offspring of diabetic mother." When the child comes in, discuss the need for the mother's returning for her retesting, or order retesting at that time, without making her feel self-conscious. Both mother and child need follow-up.
4. Use the IHS sticker for flagging maternal charts, which is available from the IHS Area Diabetes Control Officers.

Interconceptional management and control of the diabetic woman is important to management of any subsequent pregnancy. Normoglycemia in early pregnancy, the stage of organogenesis, is believed to be essential to preventing or reducing congenital anomalies in the offspring.[17]

Offspring of the Diabetic Pregnancy

The longitudinal studies of the National Institute of Diabetes, Digestive and Kidney Diseases at Gila River[23] show that offspring of a diabetic mother (ODM) are likely to be macrosomic at birth, and most individuals stay that way throughout life. These ODM have a significantly higher incidence of diabetes themselves (45% by age 20–24 years) than their siblings born during their mother's nondiabetic pregnancy (8.6% by age 20–24 years). The mechanism of vulnerability of the ODM is not yet known; the possibilities of disturbances in lipid metabolism or pancreatic islet beta-cell hyperactivity are currently being investigated in animal models. Regardless of the cause, it is clear that the ODM requires lifelong monitoring for obesity as a trigger factor and for potential onset of overt diabetes mellitus; the ODM already has the most important risk factor, which is heredity. Diabetes has been observed to occur at a younger age in the ODM than in the parents.[6]

Summary

The desired outcome in pregnancy is a healthy mother with a healthy newborn. Diabetes in pregnancy represents a known high-risk condition, with good perinatal outcome highly possible and probable today for AI and AN women.[10, 17] A high index of suspicion, universal screening of pregnant AI and AN women (repeated if necessary), tight management of blood sugars to normal pregnant values, and a search for early manifestations of any complications (either in the pregnancy itself or in the diabetic condition) can assist with predictable attainment of good outcomes. This chapter is not an exhaustive study but, rather, a status update and summary with the aim of improving perinatal outcome. The reader is referred to the works cited (see References) for more detail on managing diabetes in pregnancy, with attention to the fact that concepts in this disease are constantly evolving. Constant chart reviews, using the quality assurance philosophy, should be done.

Acknowledgments

I wish to thank colleagues in the IHS for their assistance on this project. This was indeed a cooperative project, and without their help and ideas, would not have been completed.

References

1. Attico NB, Smith KC, Waxman AG, Ball RL. Diabetes mellitus in pregnancy: views toward an improved pregnancy outcome. The IHS Primary Care Provider 1992; 17:153–164.
2. American College of Obstetricians and Gynecologists. Management of Diabetes Mellitus in Pregnancy. ACOG Technical Bulletin No. 92 1986;1–5.
3. National Diabetes Data Group. Classification and diagnosis of diabetes mellitus and other categories of glucose intolerance. Diabetes 1979;28:1039–1057.
4. American College of Obstetricians and Gynecologists. Management of Diabetes Mellitus in Pregnancy. ACOG Technical Bulletin No. 200 1994;1–8.
5. Metzger B, Organizing Committee. Summary and recommendations of the Third International Workshop Conference on Gestational Diabetes Mellitus. Diabetes 1991;40(suppl 2):197–201. [Reprinted in Diabetes Spectrum 1992;5:22.]
6. Indian Health Service Physician's Introduction to Type II Diabetes [Instructional Pamphlet]. Albuquerque, NM: IHS Diabetes Program, 1991.
7. The Expert Committee on the Diagnosis and Classification of Diabetes. Report of the Expert Committee on the Diagnosis and Classification of Diabetes. Diabetes Care 1997;20:1183–1197.
8. Gabbe SG, Landon MB. Diabetes Mellitus in Pregnancy. In Quilligan EJ, Zuspan FP (eds), Current Therapy in

Obstetrics and Gynecology (3rd ed). Philadelphia: Saunders 1990;213–218.
9. Hare JW (ed). Diabetes Complicating Pregnancy: The Joslin Clinic Method. New York: Alan W. Liss, 1989.
10. Boyd KL, Ross EK, Sherman SJ. Jelly beans as an alternative to a cola beverage containing fifty grams of glucose. Am J Obstet Gynecol 1995;173:1889–1892.
11. Bergus GR, Murphy NJ. Screening for gestational diabetes mellitus: comparison of a glucose polymer and a glucose monomer test beverage. J Am Board Fam Pract 1992;5:241–247.
12. Murphy NJ, Meyer BA, O'Kell RT, Hogard MF. Carbohydrate sources for gestational diabetes screening: a comparison. J Reprod Med 1994;39:977–981.
13. Attico NB, Meyer DJ, Bodin HJ, Dickman D. Gestational age assessment. Am Fam Physician 1990;41:553–560.
14. American College of Obstetricians and Gynecologists. Macrosomia. ACOG Technical Bulletin No. 92 1986;1–5.
15. Attico NB, Meyer DJ, Ball RL. An update on UTI in pregnancy. Family Practice Recertification 1995;17:28.
16. Perkins R. Maternal Diabetes. In Haffner WHJ, Harris TR (eds), Obstetric, Gynecologic, and Neonatal Care: A Practical Approach for the Indian Health Service (6th ed). Washington, DC: American College of Obstetricians and Gynecologists, 1990;E15–E22.
17. Attico NB, Bodin HJ, Goodin TL, et al. Diabetes mellitus in pregnancy: a 1986 update of the PIMC recipes. The IHS Primary Care Provider 1992;11:146–151.
18. Hollingsworth DR. Pregnancy, Diabetes and Birth: A Management Guide (2nd ed). Baltimore, MD: Williams & Wilkins, 1992.
19. Attico NB. Contraception update: oral agents, implants, and investigational methods. Family Practice Recertification 1992;14:87.
20. Mishell DR. Oral contraception: past, present, and future perspectives. Int J Fertil 1992;37(suppl 1):7–18.
21. Tavob Y. Oral contraceptives: an epidemiological perspective. Int J Fertil 1992;37(suppl 1):199–203.
22. Attico NB. Contraception update: barrier methods, IUDs, and sterilization. Family Practice Recertification 1992;14:45.
23. Pettitt DJ, Aleck KA, Baird HR, et al. Congenital susceptibility to NIDDM: role of intrauterine environment. Diabetes 1988;37:622–628.

Chapter 31
Patterns of Natality and Infant and Maternal Mortality

Alan G. Waxman

The knowledge of certain vital events is essential to program planning and evaluation in maternal and child health. Knowing the birth rate, trends in birth rate, and determinants of fertility in a population helps in planning the allocation of resources for health and social service programs. Examples include obstetric services, family planning services, immunization and health programs for children, schools, and Head Start programs. Maternal and infant deaths, although relatively infrequent events, should be systematically reviewed. Reporting of infant and maternal deaths is required by all states.[1] Maternal and infant deaths are sentinel events that point to sources of morbidity in a population and often serve as quality indicators of a health care system. Case finding, combined with detailed review of each case singly and in the context of similar cases in the community, serve to identify risk factors involved. When the findings are shared with health care providers and program managers, the risk factors and systems factors may be acted on to improve the health and well-being of children and childbearing women in the community. Review of these vital events becomes more important as the management of health care in Indian country moves from a nationwide system to local tribal control, from a system composed of many hospitals and clinics to an administrative unit that is often a single hospital or clinic. The ability to identify and review deaths in conjunction with other health care agencies that provide for Native Americans regionally or nationally provides a contextual framework for otherwise isolated events.

In this chapter, I review trends in births and maternal and infant deaths in Indian country. Current data are reviewed, as are some of the factors influencing these vital statistics.

Sources of Data

The population data presented in this chapter, except where otherwise specified, are computed by the Indian Health Service (IHS) based on the U.S. census and state birth and death certificates. It represents the IHS service population, which consists of American Indians and Alaska Natives living in counties on or adjacent to federal Indian reservations in the United States, also referred to as the IHS "service area."[2] Individuals are included in the service population whether they have used the services of the IHS. (Before 1972, the IHS measured its service population based on the American Indian and Alaska Native population of reservation states rather than counties.) The terms *Native American*, *Native*, *American Indian*, and *Alaska Native* refer to this population. IHS data are used because they are the most complete health data available on Native Americans. It is estimated that approximately 60% of the approximately 2.38 million Native Americans living in the United States reside within the IHS service area.[2] IHS data also include Native Americans who live in major cities adjacent to reservations, such as Albuquerque, Phoenix, Oklahoma City, Rapid City, and Anchorage. Their data may not accurately represent members of tribes not recognized by the federal government, Native Hawaiians, or American Indians and Alaska Natives living away from reservations, including those in cities with large American Indian populations, such as Los Angeles, Denver, and Chicago. As new tribes are "recognized" by the federal government, the IHS service area expands. For example, in 1983 and 1984, the states of Connecticut, Rhode Island, Texas, and Alabama were added as reservation states. Between 1980 and 1990, 58 counties were added to the IHS service area.[3]

Population estimates that serve as the denominators for birth rates in this chapter are based on the decennial U.S. census, with extrapolations for intercensus years based on calculations from projected 10-year trends of natural increase for each county. The use of census data is problematic as they are based on self-assignment of race. For the many individuals of mixed race, this may result in underreporting of Native American ethnicity. Studies of the 1980 and 1990 censuses, however, suggest that this may be less of a problem than it was in previous censuses.[4]

Assignment of race in the vital events described in this chapter (birth, maternal death, and infant death) is based on various criteria. The IHS identifies a newborn as American Indian or Alaska Native if either parent is so identified on the birth certificate. The National Center for Health Statistics (NCHS), by contrast, identifies an infant as Native American only if the mother is Native. Before 1989, the NCHS used a complex formula for mixed race that gave precedence to the parent of nonwhite race. In cases in which both parents were of different nonwhite races, the father's race was assigned to the child unless either parent was Hawaiian, which was then given precedence.[5]

Assignment of race at death, on the other hand, is generally based on the observations of the funeral director or other individual completing the death certificate. It may be based on the decedent's last name, the certifier's impression of racial characteristics, or the report of a relative, who may consider him- or herself to be of different race than the decedent or than the parents considered him or her. Several studies have shown inconsistencies when infant mortality rates for minority races are based on death certificate data alone. More accurate assignment of race can be made if death certificates are linked with birth certificates.[5] For example, Hahn et al.[6] found that 36.6% of infants dying in the first year of life who had been classified as American Indian or Alaska Native at birth were assigned a different race at death, usually white. When linked birth and death certificate information is used to calculate infant mortality rates, the rates of minority deaths usually increase. This is especially true for Native American infant deaths. Several authors using linked birth and death certificate data have recalculated American Indian and Alaska Native infant mortality rates upward by 17–40% over the rates based on death certificates alone.[5]

Because of relatively small numbers of Native American births and maternal and infant deaths, birth and death rates in this chapter are based on vital events occurring over 3 years and are presented for the middle year (e.g., a rate designated for 1992 would be the average of the 3-year rate for 1991–1993).[2]

Birth Rates

The birth rate for American Indians and Alaska Natives is almost twice that of the general U.S. population. For 1992, the birth rate for Native Americans in the IHS service area was 26.6 births per 1,000 population. This compares with 15.9 per 1,000 for the U.S. population, including all races, and 15.0 for whites.[2] This relatively high Native American birth rate holds true for all parts of the country. Although the IHS does not break down these data by individual tribes, it does tabulate it by region. The birth rates are highest for tribes residing in the north central plains, especially North and South Dakota (33.9 per 1,000 population) and lowest for the combined tribes of the East Coast and Southeast (21.3 per 1,000).[7]

Accurate nationwide birth rates for Native Americans have been available since 1955, when the United States. Public Health Service assumed management of the health care of American Indians and Alaska Natives. Between 1955 and 1971, birth rates declined for the population of the United States in general, including Native Americans. Over this period, the birth rate for Native Americans living in reservation states declined 16.8%, from 37.5 to 31.2 per 1,000 population, while the U.S. all races rate decreased by 30.1%, from 24.6 to 17.2. Between 1973 and 1992, however, the birth rate for the U.S. general population gradually increased, from 14.8 to 15.9 per 1,000. At the same time, American Indians and Alaska Natives (now counted as those living in counties on or near reservations) experienced a continuation of the decline in birth rate documented since 1955, with birth rates decreasing from 31.7 to 26.6 per 1,000 population (Figure 31-1).[2]

The higher Native American birth rate may be explained in part by several observations:

1. The American Indian and Alaska Native population is younger than the general U.S. population. According to the 1990 census, the median age for American Indian and Alaska Native females was 25 years, compared with 34 years for women of all races.
2. Native women begin their childbearing at a younger age. Forty-five percent of Native mothers deliver their first child before age 20 years, as opposed to 23.7% of all mothers in the U.S. population.
3. In addition to starting childbearing younger, Native women have more children on average. Of children born in 1992, 22.7% of those born to American Indian or Alaska Native mothers were the fourth or higher in birth order, compared with 10.8% of U.S. newborns of all races.[2]

Many factors determine the fertility of a population, some biological (e.g., age at menarche), some social and economic. One important factor is the ease of access to contraceptive methods. Family planning methods other than abortion are readily available to American Indians and Alaska Natives at no cost through the IHS system. There is regional variation, however, in availability of some of the more expensive family planning methods. For example, although oral contraceptive pills are greatly discounted to the federal government and are readily available through-

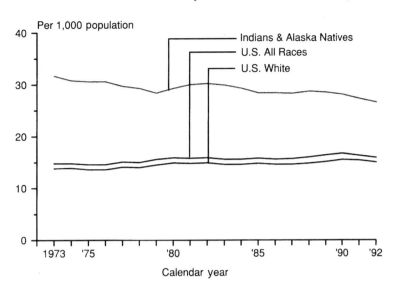

Figure 31-1. Declining Native American birth rate since 1973 compared with birth rates for U.S. all races and U.S. whites, which have shown a relative increase over the same years. The birth rate for American Indians and Alaska Natives remains 67% higher than the U.S. all races rate and 77% above the U.S. white rate. (Reprinted with permission from Indian Health Service. Trends in Indian Health, 1996. Washington, DC: U.S. Department of Health and Human Services, Indian Health Service, Office of Planning, Evaluation, and Legislation, Division of Program Statistics, 1997;35.)

out the IHS system, intrauterine devices (IUDs) and the progesterone implants must be purchased essentially at cost by IHS and tribal facilities. The choice of methods available is sporadically limited by budgetary constraints and market forces. For example, before 1985, the IUD was the most widely used contraceptive among Navajo women.[8] In 1985, most IUDs were removed from the U.S. market due to product liability litigation pressures. The Navajo birth rate, which had been decreasing steadily from the mid-1960s, showed a small increase from 1986 through 1989, some of which has been attributed to the disappearance of the IUD.[8] Since 1990, however, after the return of the IUD and the introduction and increasing popularity of other long-term contraceptive methods, the birth rate of Navajos living on or near their reservation resumed its downward trend (Michael Everett, Navajo Area Division of Program Planning and Evaluation, personal communication). The availability of sterilization is also restricted in some IHS areas, where the procedure must be paid for with limited contract care dollars.

Maternal and Infant Mortality

Surveillance and review of maternal and infant deaths are an important part of any program that provides for the health of Native American communities. The U.S. Department of Health and Human Services targeted the reduction of maternal and infant mortality among its national health objectives for the year 2000. Reduction in the infant mortality rates of American Indian and Alaska Natives was particularly identified. The year 2000 objective calls for reduction of the overall infant mortality rate to 8.5 per 1,000 live births and the postneonatal death rate (deaths of infants between 28 days and 1 year of age) to 4 per 1,000 live births.[9]

Maternal Mortality

Maternal mortality is defined as the death of a woman from any cause related to or aggravated by pregnancy or its management, regardless of the duration of the pregnancy. Deaths from accidental or incidental causes are generally excluded.[1]

Maternal mortality is expressed as a ratio of the number of pregnancy-associated deaths to 100,000 live births. Although frequently called a "rate," maternal mortality "ratio" is a more accurate designation. A true rate would include in the denominator only the events from which the numerator could be taken (i.e., maternal deaths as a proportion of all pregnancies). The deaths identified in the maternal mortality ratio, however, include those related to abortions, ectopic pregnancies, and other pregnancy outcomes that are not reported on state vital records and therefore are excluded from the denominator of live births.

Maternal mortality case findings in Indian country are more accurately achieved by active surveillance (i.e., mandatory reporting augmented by frequent inquiries by maternal-child health officials) than by reliance on vital records, IHS data tapes, or matched birth and fetal death records.[10]

The U.S. maternal mortality ratio declined steadily into the mid-1980s. For all races, its nadir was in 1987, at 6.6 deaths per 100,000 live births; for whites, the lowest ratio was 4.9, recorded the previous year. Since then, rates have risen slightly, and the slope has plateaued, with annual ratios of 7.8–8.4 for all races and 5.0–5.9 for whites.[2]

Maternal mortality has declined for Native Americans as well. The decline since the middle of the twentieth century has been much more dramatic than for the general U.S. population. In part, this decline was related to

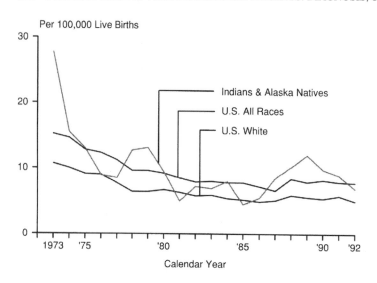

Figure 31-2. The maternal mortality ratio for American Indians and Alaska Natives, although previously more than twice the U.S. all races ratio, has been comparable since the mid-1970s. The short-term fluctuations in the graph result from the relatively small number of births each year. The addition or subtraction of one or two deaths changes the ratio dramatically. (Reprinted with permission from Indian Health Service. Trends in Indian Health, 1996. Washington, DC: U.S. Department of Health and Human Services, Indian Health Service, Office of Planning, Evaluation, and Legislation, Division of Program Statistics, 1997;39.)

hospital deliveries becoming the norm for women living on reservations.[11] In 1958, there were 16 maternal deaths of Native American women living in reservation states, giving a maternal mortality ratio for 1957–1959 of 82.6 per 100,000 live births. In 1972, when counties on or near reservations defined the IHS service area, there were nine Native American maternal deaths. In the years between 1973 and 1994, the annual average was 2.3 American Indian or Alaska Native maternal deaths per year with a range of 0–5. The maternal mortality ratio for Native Americans had fallen to 27.7 in 1973 and to 13.0 by 1975, essentially the same level as the U.S. all races rate. Since then, with the exception of a small increase between 1987 and 1992, the ratio has been consistent with the U.S. all races rate (Figure 31-2).[2]

The Navajo area of IHS accounts for a disproportionate number of maternal deaths in Indian country. Between 1986 and 1994, there were 22 maternal deaths of Native American women living in the IHS service area nationwide, with a maternal mortality ratio of 7.44 deaths per 100,000 live births. During this period, the Navajo area recorded eight maternal deaths, for a ratio of 15.67, more than double that of the entire IHS (from data provided by the IHS Demographic Statistics Team, Office of Public Health).

Between 1981 and 1990, there were 13 maternal deaths among users of the Navajo-area IHS.[10] These were subject to systematic, detailed review. Eleven of the women were Navajo, one was Ute, and one Hopi. None of the deaths was related to abortion, ectopic pregnancy, or gestational trophoblastic disease. Pregnancy-induced hypertension (PIH) was the underlying cause of death in seven cases, sepsis in four, and hemorrhage in two. This distribution of mortality mirrors that of developing nations. In the general U.S. population from 1979–1986,

the most common cause of maternal death was pulmonary embolus, followed by PIH and hemorrhage with almost equal frequency, then infection (approximately one-third as often as PIH or hemorrhage) (Figure 31-3).[12]

Infant Mortality

In 1955, the infant mortality rate for American Indians and Alaska Natives living in states with federal Indian reservations was 62.7 per 1,000 live births.[2] This was 2.4 times the U.S. all races rate (26.4) and 2.7 times that for whites (23.6). By 1972, the rate for Native Americans had dropped to 22.2 per 1,000 live births. This was still 25% higher than the rate for U.S. all races (17.7). The U.S. white rate that year was 15.8. The infant death rates for the U.S. population and the two subsets, white and Native American, have continued to decline through the early 1990s. Although the rate for whites has been lower than for all races by a relatively constant proportion since the early 1970s, the difference between the Native American population and all races steadily narrowed until 1983, at which time the American Indian and Alaska Native rate was only 3% higher. Over the 1980s, the Native infant mortality rate remained within only 1 death per 1,000 live births of the U.S. all races rate. In 1992, it reached 8.8 (Figure 31-4).[2]

Infant mortality of Native Americans living in cities may reflect different health problems, access to care, and health-seeking behavior than is seen on reservations. Grossman et al.,[4] reporting on the American Indian and Alaska Native residents of King County (Seattle), Washington, found that although the infant mortality rate was 80% higher than the white rate, it was lower than Washington's rural Native population rate, but the latter difference did not reach statistical significance.

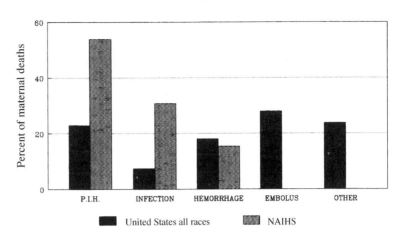

Figure 31-3. The distribution of maternal deaths in the Navajo area Indian Health Service (NAIHS), 1981–1990, compared to the U.S. all races rate, 1979–1986, is more characteristic of less industrialized nations than the United States. Pregnancy-induced hypertension (PIH) was the most common cause of death, followed by infection and hemorrhage. (Adapted from AG Waxman. Maternal mortality in a southwest American Indian population. Presentation at the Fourth Annual IHS Research Conference, Tucson, AZ, 1991; and HK Atrash, LM Koonin, HW Lawson, et al. Maternal mortality in the United States, 1979–1986. Obstet Gynecol 1990;76: 1055–1060.)

Neonatal and Postneonatal Mortality

Demographers and public health officials divide the infant death statistic into deaths occurring within the first 28 days of birth (neonatal deaths) and those occurring from 28 days to 1 year of age (postneonatal deaths). The neonatal death rate tends to reflect deaths related to congenital anomalies and conditions related to the pregnancy, such as prematurity. It reflects the health care system's ability to prevent such conditions and to treat them successfully when they arise. Deaths occurring after the first 28 days also include some infants with congenital and obstetric-related conditions who survived the first month but not the first year. Postneonatal mortality is more heavily influenced by conditions in the home and social environment, whose influence is felt after the infant leaves the hospital.

Since at least 1972, the Native American neonatal mortality rate has been consistently lower than the U.S. all races rate. Since 1981, it has been below that of the white race as well. For 1991–1993, the neonatal mortality rate for American Indians and Alaska Natives was 4.0 per 1,000 live births, which is 26% below the 1992 U.S. all races rate of 5.4 and 7% lower than the rate for whites (4.3). In spite

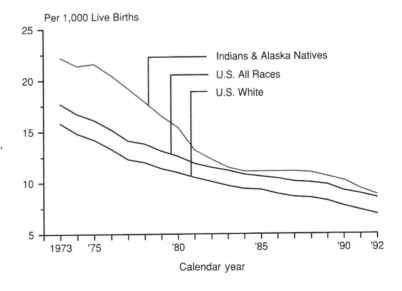

Figure 31-4. Infant death rates of Native Americans were comparable to rates of the U.S. population in general by the mid-1980s. A small difference remains, composed mostly of postneonatal deaths. (Reprinted with permission from Indian Health Service. Trends in Indian Health, 1996. U.S. Department of Health and Human Services, Public Health Service, IHS. Washington, DC: Government Printing Office, 1996:40.)

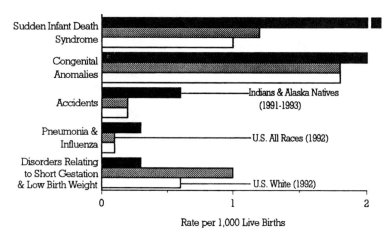

Figure 31-5. The leading cause of infant death in Native Americans is sudden infant death syndrome (SIDS). For U.S. all race and white populations, congenital anomalies are a more common cause of death than SIDS. (Reprinted with permission from Indian Health Service. Regional Differences in Indian Health, 1996. U.S. Department of Health and Human Services, Public Health Service, IHS. Washington, DC: Government Printing Office, 1996;23.)

of a lower neonatal mortality rate, the overall infant mortality rate for American Indians and Alaska Natives remains above that of all races and of whites; the difference lies in the postneonatal fraction. In 1973, the Native postneonatal mortality rate was 12.0 per 1,000 live births, which is 2.6 times the rate for the U.S. general population and three times that of whites. Although it declined to 4.9 per 1,000 live births by 1992, the Native American postneonatal mortality rate still exceeded the U.S. all races rate by 60% and the white rate by 90% (i.e., 3.1 and 2.6, respectively). Looked at another way, postneonatal mortality accounts for 55.7% of the Native American infant mortality rate, whereas it makes up only 36.5% and 37.7% of the infant mortality for U.S. all race and white populations, respectively.[2]

In 1992, the five leading causes of infant deaths in the United States, in order of decreasing frequency, were (1) congenital anomalies, (2) sudden infant death syndrome (SIDS), (3) disorders relating to short gestation and low birth weight, (4) respiratory distress syndrome,

and (5) newborn effects of maternal complications of pregnancy[2] (Figures 31-5 through 31-7). This ranking holds true for whites and all races in the United States. For American Indians and Alaska Natives living on or near reservations, SIDS, which is largely a condition of the postneonatal period, exceeds congenital anomalies as the most common cause of infant death. As is often the case when trying to generalize about Native Americans, however, there are tribal and regional differences. Congenital anomalies are a greater contributor to infant death in some southwestern tribes than SIDS.[7] The higher rate of smoking among Alaska Natives and the northern plains tribes (a risk factor for SIDS) has been proposed as one explanation for the regional difference.[13] Prematurity, on the other hand, is responsible for infant death only 40% as often in American Indians and Alaska Natives as in the U.S. all races population.[2]

The Centers for Disease Control and Prevention reviewed the most common congenital anomalies, both lethal and nonlethal, among various minority groups for

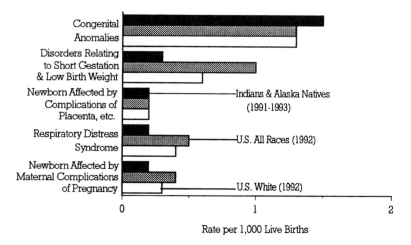

Figure 31-6. Among causes of neonatal death in American Indians and Alaska Natives, congenital anomalies are relatively more common than among all races and whites in the United States. On the other hand, complications of prematurity account for relatively fewer Native deaths. (Reprinted with permission from Indian Health Service. Regional Differences in Indian Health, 1996. U.S. Department of Health and Human Services, Public Health Service, IHS. Washington, DC: Government Printing Office, 1996;23.)

Figure 31-7. Postneonatal mortality in Native American infants is more likely to be caused by sudden infant death syndrome, accidents, homicides, and respiratory infections than in U.S. all race or white populations. (Reprinted with permission from Indian Health Service. Regional Differences in Indian Health, 1996. U.S. Department of Health and Human Services, Public Health Service, IHS. Washington, DC: Government Printing Office, 1996;24.)

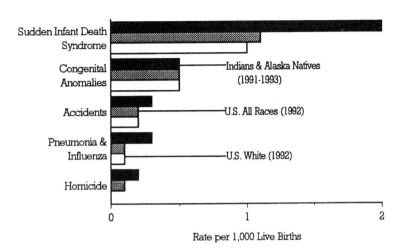

1981–1986. They found higher rates of several potentially lethal anomalies in American Indians than in whites, blacks, Asians, or Hispanics. These included hydrocephalus without spina bifida, atrial septal defect, valve stenosis and atresia, rectal atresia and stenosis, and autosomal abnormalities (excluding Down syndrome).[14] The incidence, frequency, and lethal potential of various birth defects vary with different regions and tribal groups. Specific autosomal recessive disorders, for example, tend to cluster in restricted genetic pools. The Navajo population has a higher-than-expected incidence of several autosomal recessive conditions, some of which cause infant death. These include severe combined immunodeficiency syndrome, congenital harlequin-type ichthyosis, and Navajo neuropathy. Navajo neuropathy is rare, unique to the Navajo population, and fatal in the first year of life in approximately one-third of cases (Diana Hu, chief clinical consultant for pediatrics, Navajo Area Indian Health Service, personal communication).[15]

Accidents are three times as likely and homicides twice as likely to kill American Indian and Alaska Native infants as white infants or infants in the overall U.S. population. In a study of accidental infant deaths among Native American infants in 10 northwestern states, a panel from the American Academy of Pediatrics found that environmental and socioeconomic factors, including unemployment and substance abuse, played a major role.[16]

Pneumonia and influenza, infections mostly presenting in the postneonatal period, are also far more frequent causes of death in American Indians and Alaska Natives than in whites or the U.S. total population.[2] This may be related in part to geographic isolation, poverty, and late care seeking.

The impact of SIDS represents arguably the most striking cause of excess infant mortality in Native Americans. These otherwise unexplained deaths affect proportionately almost twice as many Native American infants as infants in the general U.S. population. In

1992, SIDS accounted for 42% of American Indian and Alaska Native postneonatal mortality. In most cases, the diagnosis of SIDS is appropriately assigned. The diagnosis was based on autopsy findings at a very high rate in Washington,[17] Oklahoma,[18] and on the Warm Springs reservation in eastern Oregon.[19] In North and South Dakota, on the other hand, Oyen et al.[20] reported, the overall autopsy rate for infants suspected of SIDS was only 63%.

Risk factors for SIDS include a number of socioeconomic and medical conditions endemic in Indian communities: (1) low socioeconomic status and education, (2) young maternal or paternal age, (3) low birth weight, (4) single mother, (5) smoking and substance abuse, and (6) late or no prenatal care.[3] The association of these factors with SIDS in Indian communities has been documented. In a study of SIDS deaths in Washington, Irwin et al.[17] eliminated racial differences in SIDS rates between Indians and whites by adjusting for several of these socioeconomic and medical factors. On the other hand, the higher prevalence of SIDS in boys that is reported for most other ethnic groups does not hold true for Native American infants.[17, 18, 20]

As has been noted by Honigfeld and Kaplan and other investigators,[16, 21] most of the excess postneonatal mortality in Native American communities is associated with preventable factors in the home environment, such as child safety, abuse and neglect, smoking, substance abuse, and poor parenting skills (e.g., late recognition of illnesses and inadequate care-seeking behavior). These factors provide a focus for public health intervention.

Summary Points

- Trends in natality and infant and maternal mortality are important indicators of the health of populations and the success of health care systems. The study of individual cases and clusters of infant and maternal deaths helps to identify risk factors and provides direction for program modification in maternal and infant health, injury prevention, and environmental health.

- As Native American health care moves from federal to tribal control, national and regional review of many cases may give way to sporadic reviews of isolated deaths. Joint intertribal mortality review conferences could provide a larger number of cases for evaluation. Such reviews would help to identify conditions that place women and children at risk that are not limited by boundaries of tribal custom or geography.

- The birth rate of American Indians and Alaska Natives living in the IHS service area declined from 31.7 to 26.6 per 1,000 population between 1973 and 1992. It remained 67% higher than the U.S. all races birth rate.

- Maternal mortality among Native American women occurs with roughly the same frequency per 100,000 live births as in the U.S. population in general.

- The neonatal mortality rate of American Indians and Alaska Natives is less than those of the U.S. all races and white populations. Postneonatal mortality, on the other hand, is sufficiently excessive to pull the overall Native American infant mortality rates to levels that exceed the U.S. white and all races rates. High rates of SIDS, congenital anomalies, and causes related to social and environmental factors are responsible for the high incidence of postneonatal death.

References

1. American Academy of Pediatrics, American College of Obstetricians and Gynecologists. Guidelines for Perinatal Care (4th ed). Elk Grove, IL: American Academy of Pediatrics, and Washington, DC: American College of Obstetricians and Gynecologists, 1997;325.
2. Indian Health Service. Trends in Indian Health, 1996. Trends in Indian Health, 1996. Washington, DC: U.S. Department of Health and Human Services, Indian Health Service, Office of Planning, Evaluation, and Legislation, Division of Program Statistics, 1997;8–45.
3. Rhoades ER, Brenneman G, Lyle J, et al. Mortality of American Indian and Alaska Native infants. Annu Rev Public Health 1992;13:269–285.
4. Grossman DC, Krieger JW, Sugerman JR, et al. Health status of urban American Indians and Alaska Natives; a population-based study. JAMA 1994;271:845–850.
5. Indian Health Service. Final Report: Methodology for Adjusting IHS Mortality Data for Inconsistent Classification of Race-Ethnicity of American Indians and Alaska Natives between State Death Certificates and IHS Patient Registration Records. U.S. Department of Health and Human Services, Public Health Service, IHS. Washington, DC: Government Printing Office, 1996.
6. Hahn FA, Mendlein JM, Helgerson SD. Differential classification of American Indian race on birth and death certificates, U.S. Reservation states, 1983–1985. IHS Provider 1993;18:8–11.
7. Indian Health Service. Regional Differences in Indian Health, 1996. U.S. Department of Health and Human Services, Public Health Service, IHS. Washington, DC: Government Printing Office, 1996;27–41.
8. Williams RL. Effects on Navajo birth rate from loss of the intrauterine device. J Health Care Poor Underserved 1994;5:47–54.
9. National Center for Health Statistics. Healthy People 2000 Review 1995–96. U.S. Department of Health and Human Services, Public Health Service, CDC, NCHS. Washington, DC: Government Printing Office, 1996;16.
10. Waxman AG. Maternal mortality in a southwest American Indian population. Presentation at the Fourth Annual IHS Research Conference, Tucson, AZ, April 1991.
11. Waxman AG. Navajo childbirth in transition. Med Anthropol 1990;12:187–205.
12. Atrash HK, Koonin LM, Lawson HW, et al. Maternal mortality in the United States, 1979–1986. Obstet Gynecol 1990;76:1055–1060.
13. Bulterys M. High incidence of sudden infant death syndrome among northern Indians and Alaska Natives compared with southwestern Indians: possible role of smoking. J Community Health 1990;15:185–194.
14. Chavez GF, Cordero JF, Becerra JE. Leading major congenital malformations among minority groups in the United States, 1981–1986. MMWR Morb Mortal Wkly Rep 1988;37:17–24.
15. Clericuzio CL. Autosomal recessive disorders among the Navajo [Abstract]. Proceedings of the Greenwood Genetic Center, 1996;16.
16. Fleshman CV. Injury deaths among American Indian and Alaska Native Infants. IHS Provider 1992;10:186–190.
17. Irwin KL, Mannino S, Daling J. Sudden infant death syndrome in Washington State: why are Native American infants at greater risk than white infants? J Pediatr 1992;121:242–247.
18. Kaplan DW, Bauman AE, Krous HF. Epidemiology of sudden infant death syndrome in American Indians. Pediatrics 1984;74:1041–1046.
19. Nakamura RM, King R, Kimball EH, et al. Excess infant mortality in an American Indian population, 1940–1990. JAMA 1991;226:2244–2248.
20. Oyen N, Bulterys M, Welty TK, et al. Sudden unexplained infant deaths among American Indians and whites in North and South Dakota. Paediatr Perinat Epidemiol 1990;4:175-183.
21. Honigfeld LS, Kaplan DW. Native American postneonatal mortality. Pediatrics 1987;80:575–578.

Chapter 32
Gynecologic Health Care

Ora Botwinick

Health is defined by the World Health Organization as not simply the absence of disease but the state of complete physical, mental, and social well-being. Western medicine focuses on the organic, physical model and, often, artificially divides the spiritual and physical. Traditional Native American communities recognize the intertwining of the physical and spiritual world.

A woman contributes to the development, nurturing, and function of her family and community whether she is a biological mother. To maintain and promote women's health, the health care provider must view the patient as an individual in a web of interconnected relationships. Relationships include those with her partner, nuclear and extended family, community, tribe, Western world, and spiritual world.[1]

The primary care practitioner is often the only person who provides regular health care to women as they move through the circle of life. Therefore, primary care practitioners have the opportunity to assess a woman's personal health characteristics and to counsel her on preventive care. Both the U.S. Preventive Services Task Force (USP-STF)[2] and the Indian Health Service (IHS) have developed guidelines that promote effective interventions based on the individual woman's personal health practices and characteristics. In this chapter, guidelines are reviewed and suggestions are given for the provision of health care to women. Although Native American women experience the full spectrum of gynecologic conditions, this discussion focuses on selected, relevant topics. These include taking the history, with an emphasis on questioning that is inclusive and respectful of all patients; prevention of cervical cancer, a potentially preventable neoplasm; breast cancer screening (because early detection can save lives); urinary incontinence (UI), an often undiagnosed but treatable problem; and estrogen replacement, a therapy requiring patient-specific decisions. Domestic violence, a common problem with tremendous

impact on the lives of women and their families, is discussed in Chapter 14.

Taking the History

The relationship between practitioner and patient must be one of mutual respect. To develop such an atmosphere, the practitioner must be nonjudgmental and open to caring for patients of all sexual orientations. Often, practitioners assume that all patients are heterosexual or that the elderly patient is not interested in sex.[3] Our patient population includes heterosexual, gay, lesbian, and bisexual individuals of all ages. To deliver effective preventive health care, personal characteristics and behavior must be determined.

When taking a sexual history, the practitioner should use direct questions. Words such as "partner" are preferable to "he" or "husband." "Sexual activity" is preferable to "intercourse." One approach is to ask patients (1) "Are you sexually active?" (2) "Do you have sex with men, women, or both?" (3) "Over the past year, have you had a new sexual partner?" and (4) "Do you have any concerns about your sexual life?"

UI and domestic violence are prevalent but often unrecognized problems. To address these issues, the practitioner might ask all women the following questions routinely. (1) "Tell me about problems you have with your bladder" or "How often do you leak urine?"[4] (2) "Violence is common in many women's lives. I now routinely ask about it. Have you ever been, or are you now being hurt by your partner?"[5]

The history should be repeated at future examinations because a patient's partners and her comfort in discussing personal issues may vary over time. Responses to such questions guide the clinician in counseling women about preventive health measures, such as immunization for hepatitis B, screening for gynecologic cancers, estrogen replacement therapy (ERT), and in decreasing risk factors for unintentional pregnancy and for sexually transmitted diseases, including human immunodeficiency virus (HIV).

Cervical Cancer

Despite an overall decreased rate of neoplasm, Native American women have a significantly higher rate of squamous cell cervical cancer than that of U.S. women of other races. The age-adjusted mortality rate among Native Americans from cervical cancer for 1991–1992 was 5.2, or nearly double that of the U.S. all races rate of 2.7. The rate was notably higher (14.2) in the Aberdeen area of the Indian Health Service.[6] The mortality from this disease is tragic because cervical cancer is potentially preventable.

In 1989, the USPSTF recommended screening Pap smears with the onset of sexual activity and, subsequently, at least every 3 years. Women at high risk are urged to have more frequent Pap smears. The USPSTF advises that women older than 65 years may choose to discontinue regular Pap smear testing, if previous regular screening yielded normal results.[2] In contrast, due to the high risk of cervical cancer among Native Americans, the IHS guidelines recommend indefinite yearly screening. Efforts by the IHS to expand cervical cancer screening have resulted in a shift of stage detected, from invasive cervical cancer to precursor lesions, such as in situ squamous cell carcinoma.[7] However, rates of invasive cervical cancer continue to increase with advancing age. The bimodal distribution of cervical cancer, with a second peak among elderly women, suggests insufficient screening of the elderly. In Healthy People 2000, objective 16.4 is to reduce the age-adjusted mortality rate from this disease to 1.3.[8] To meet this objective, increased screening must be provided to patients least likely to present for care, such as the elderly or those living at a distance from medical facilities.

Diagnosis

Risk factors for cervical cancer include Native American and Hispanic ethnicity; low socioeconomic status; history of multiple sexual partners; partners who have multiple sexual partners; cigarette smoking; prior or current infection with human papillomavirus (HPV) types 16, 18, and 31, herpes simplex, or HIV; and history of prior cervical dysplasia or cancer.[9] Low intake of vitamins C, E, and folate has been associated with cervical dysplasia in southwestern Native American women.[10]

Native American women require annual Pap smears at the onset of sexual activity or from age 18 years to the indefinite future. Because Pap smears are the primary screening test for cervical cancer, proper specimen col-

lection is critical to minimize false-negative rates. An endocervical brush is advisable for sampling because it increases the yield of endocervical cells sevenfold. Although many providers traditionally have not used the endocervical brush during pregnancy, several studies suggest that the brush can be used safely. Pap smears should be collected by first using a spatula to scrape the portio and then using the endocervical brush to sample the endocervix, due to the bleeding that often occurs with the brush. This technique is likely to include the transformation zone, the site of origin of most cervical cancers. Rapid fixation of samples is critical. Next, test for sexually transmitted diseases, such as gonorrhea and chlamydia. If profuse vaginal discharge is noted, it should be gently removed before the Pap smear.[9]

Specimens should be sent to laboratories with adequate quality control measures, which use the 1988 Bethesda system for reporting cervical and vaginal cytologic diagnoses. This system describes the adequacy of the sample along with descriptive diagnoses. Pap tests may be termed normal or as having benign cellular changes due to infection with an organism such as *Trichomonas*, *Chlamydia*, fungus, or herpes simplex. The term *atypical squamous cells of undetermined significance* (ASCUS) is used in limited cases and is clarified with descriptions of either benign changes or neoplasia. HPV, mild dysplasia, and cervical intraepithelial neoplasia (CIN I) are grouped together under the category of low-grade squamous intraepithelial neoplasia (LGSIL). *High-grade squamous intraepithelial lesion* is a term encompassing the full spectrum of carcinoma precursors, ranging from moderate dysplasia (CIN II) or severe dysplasia (CIN III) to cancer in situ.

Prevention and Management

The primary health care practitioner must work with patients to decrease modifiable risk factors, such as cigarette smoking, multiple sexual partners, and diets lacking in micronutrients.

Most abnormal Pap smears can be managed by the primary care practitioner.[11]

1. Pap smears that are normal should be repeated at 1-year intervals, except for women with high-risk factors, such as HIV, who require Pap tests every 6 months.
2. Pap smears with benign cellular changes, either reactive or due to infection, should be treated as indicated and then repeated in 1 year.
3. Paps with ASCUS favoring benign changes should be treated as appropriate and repeated in 6 months. Persistence of ASCUS necessitates colposcopy, directed biopsy, and endocervical curettage (ECC). If Pap tests at 6-month intervals provide normal results three times, the patient can be screened with annual Paps.

4. Paps with ASCUS favoring neoplasia are evaluated with colposcopy-directed biopsy and ECC.
5. Although two-thirds of LGSIL lesions often spontaneously regress, colposcopic evaluation and ECC are preferred to the option of interval Pap smears due to the high rate of cervical cancer in Native American women.
6. Paps with high-grade squamous intraepithelial lesion require colposcopic evaluation, biopsy, and ECC.
7. Paps with atypical glandular cells of undetermined significance require colposcopy, ECC, and endometrial biopsy to rule out preinvasive or invasive adenocarcinoma.

To enable early treatment of premalignant intraepithelial cervical lesions and reduction in cervical cancer rates, colposcopy must be accessible, done within a reasonable time interval and, ideally, done on site. This goal is facilitated by the IHS Colposcopy Course for Primary Care Providers, a program directed by Alan Waxman, Senior IHS Clinician for Obstetrics and Gynecology, in consultation with other IHS physicians and the American College of Obstetricians and Gynecologists.[12] Approximately 50 physicians, nurse practitioners, nurse midwives, and physician assistants have been trained in colposcopic evaluation and in managing patients with cytologically lower-grade lesions, such as LGSIL or less. The course includes a minimum of 50 directly supervised examinations with colposcopy-directed biopsy, ECC, or cryosurgery, and stresses recognition of high-grade lesions by colposcopy. Patients with high-grade lesions or positive ECCs are referred for treatment.

Almost all Native American women must be considered at risk for cervical cancer. To actualize the objectives of Healthy People 2000,[8] care must be accessible. It is critical to educate women as to the value of cancer screening. Culturally appropriate methods must be used to recruit and screen women. A randomized study at a large health maintenance organization revealed that a simple reminder system for Pap smears and mammography involving a letter mailed to patients' homes and a chart reminder boosted screening rates significantly.[13]

Collaborative work by health care practitioners facilitates the aspiration to prevent cervical cancer. The number of providers available to deliver preventive care must be increased. Care must be extended to women who are uninterested in family planning or prenatal care. Such patients could be screened in satellite health, preventive health, diabetic, or urgent care clinics.[14] Screening systems using intensively trained nurses to conduct high-quality breast and cervical examinations were found to be successful in the program developed by Kottke and Trapp.[15] Involvement of trained and supervised nurses of Native American heritage who have committed to long-term work with the IHS can help to address two barriers

to obtaining care: (1) the embarrassment that patients experience when discussing personal issues and (2) the poor continuity of care at some IHS facilities due to a high rate of physician turnover.

Breast Cancer

Breast cancer is the second leading cause of death due to cancer among women in the United States.[16] Although the age-adjusted breast cancer mortality rate among Native American women is nearly half that of U.S. women of all races, it remains the cancer with the highest incidence among Native American women.[17] Research indicates that early detection and treatment are beneficial in decreasing mortality from breast cancer. At present, mammography is the only screening method to detect subclinical breast cancer. Despite this evidence, many Native American women have not been screened. Late detection of breast cancer is implicated as a reason that breast cancer is diagnosed more often in the invasive rather than the in situ stage among Native Americans.[16] As breast cancer incidence increases with age and as life expectancy has increased among Native American women, it is reasonable to assume that morbidity and perhaps mortality from breast cancer will become more significant as the "baby boom" population ages.

Objective 21.2 of Healthy People 2000 is to increase to 70% the proportion of Native American women who receive timely screening tests appropriate for age and gender, as recommended by the USPSTF.[9] Recommendations include screening for breast cancer in women ages 50–69 years on a 1- to 2-year basis with mammography and annual clinical breast examination or with mammography alone. Women at high risk ages 40–49 years or healthy women ages 70 years and older are advised to consider following the same recommendations.[2]

Diagnosis

Risk factors for breast cancer include female gender, older age, and residence in North America. Strong risk factors include presence of the gene mutations BRCA1 and BRCA2,[18] personal history of contralateral breast cancer, and history of breast cancer in a first-degree relative, particularly if the cancer occurred at a premenopausal age. Associated factors include early menarche, nulliparity, birth of first child after age 35 years, menopause after age 55 years, and atypical breast hyperplasia on biopsy. These risk factors suggest that female hormones, specifically estrogen and progesterone, are causally related to breast cancer incidence.

Identification of modifiable risk factors is critical. High levels of dietary fat, low levels of antioxidant vitamins, and high levels of alcohol use are associated with breast cancer.[18] Data from a large Norwegian study indicates that regular exercise is associated with risk reduction. The risk reduction is greater in premenopausal women and those younger than age 45 years than in postmenopausal women or those older than age 45 years.[19] Analysis of the Nurses Health Study data indicates that weight gain after age 18 years is associated with the risk of postmenopausal breast cancer in women who have never used ERT.[20] Use of postmenopausal hormones for longer than 10 years is causally associated with a 43% increase in the rate of breast cancer, although overall mortality is decreased.[21]

The annual gynecologic examination provides an opportunity to screen for breast diseases and to instruct the patient in breast self-examination. Physical examination is critical, especially in the younger woman with dense breast tissue, for whom mammographic screening has limited efficacy. Ten percent of breast cancers can be detected by physical examination alone. The ideal time for examination is after menstruation because engorgement is minimal. Visual inspection is followed by palpation in the seated and supine position. The breast and axilla should be examined digitally by applying varying amounts of pressure with the index and middle fingers. To increase detection rates, a systematic and time-intensive method is advised. Studies reveal that only search duration is consistently associated with increased detection rates.[22] Palpable breast masses should be evaluated, as indicated, with diagnostic procedures, such as mammography, ultrasonography, or breast aspiration. Asymptomatic women without palpable masses require screening as suggested by the USPSTF.[2]

Prevention

Although women with risk factors have a higher incidence of breast cancer, most women with breast cancer have lacked the traditionally identified risk factors. Therefore, all women should be considered at risk and screened appropriately. Recruitment systems are needed, as discussed in the section on cervical cancer.[13, 15] Detection of preclinical breast cancer requires meticulous breast examination at convenient medical clinics and mammography. Mobile mammography vans can improve access to mammography in rural areas. Healthy lifestyles that include exercise, low-fat and high-fiber diets, and adequate intake of fruits and vegetables should be promoted. Modifiable risk factors must be addressed. Patients should be counseled to avoid excessive alcohol and carcinogens, such as cigarettes and ionizing radiation. The clinician can counsel the perimenopausal woman about the use and length of duration of ERT.[18]

Urinary Incontinence

UI, defined as the involuntary loss of urine sufficient to be a problem, is a common but often unaddressed med-

ical problem.[4] UI can affect a woman's emotional and functional well-being, whether she is a homemaker, business executive, sheepherder, or elderly woman at risk for institutionalization. It is estimated that only half the people with UI report the problem to physicians due to both patients' and physicians' belief that UI is an unfortunate but unavoidable part of aging. Although prevalence increases with age, UI is not a normal part of aging.[8] Estimates of prevalence range from 10–30% of women younger than age 65 years to more than 50% of nursing home residents. Although commonly viewed as a problem affecting older multiparous women, it is common in young, nulliparous women, especially during vigorous physical exercise. There is a paucity of data specific to Native Americans, but clinical experience with the Navajo population at Gallup Indian Medical Center in the 1990s mirrors that of other U.S. races. As health care practitioners began to focus on the issue and offer treatment, patients acknowledged the problem.

The high prevalence of UI, coupled with the limited education of most health care practitioners in this area, stimulated the formation of the Urinary Incontinence in Adults Update Panel. In 1996, the panel challenged all primary health care practitioners to increase knowledge about UI and to initiate evaluation and basic treatment. Research indicates that noninvasive treatment results in either significant improvement or remission of symptoms in many women.[4]

Diagnosis

The annual gynecologic examination presents an opportunity to screen for UI. The patient interview is the most critical part of the evaluation. Useful approaches are to make open-ended requests, such as, "Tell me about problems you have with your bladder," or a more specific question, such as, "How often do you leak urine when you don't want to?" To overcome cultural barriers to care, the subject can be broached respectfully by trained nursing staff who might share the cultural heritage of the patient population.

Past medical, neurologic, surgical, and obstetric history should focus on assessment of risk factors, characteristics of the patient's incontinence, and medication review. Causes of systemic or neuromuscular disorders, such as diabetes, stroke, multiple sclerosis, and prior pelvic surgery, should be identified. Mobility restrictions or arthritis can result in functional incontinence. Low fluid intake associated with bowel habits suggesting constipation, as well as obesity, can strain the pelvic floor. Obstetric history, including parity, mode of delivery, and largest birth weight, might suggest direct injury to the pelvic floor. Menopausal and estrogen statuses are important. The urethra, trigone, and vagina are hormonally responsive. Hypoestrogenic changes result in decreased vascularity and atrophy of the periurethral and urethral tissue, thereby increasing risk of stress incontinence

(SUI). Circumstances of the patient's incontinence suggest the type of UI. *SUI*, defined as the involuntary loss of urine associated with an increase in intra-abdominal pressure, may be provoked by coughing, laughing, changing position, or vigorous exercise. Urge incontinence is defined as the involuntary loss of urine associated with the abrupt and strong desire to void. Because the condition is often associated with contraction of the detrusor, the smooth muscle wall of the bladder, the term *detrusor instability* (DI) is also used. Characteristics of DI include urgency (often stimulated by the sight of water), urinary frequency of more than seven times in 24 hours, nocturia, and nocturnal enuresis. A voiding diary is helpful. This is completed over a 24- to 48-hour period and shows the time and volume of voiding, fluid intake, and precipitating factors. Medication history is needed. Culprits may include diuretics, alpha-antagonists, such as prazosin, which can produce undesired urethral relaxation, or anticholinergics, which can lead to urinary retention and overflow incontinence.

Physical examination includes a neurologic examination of the lower body and pelvic and rectal examination. Urine analysis is critical to rule out infection, hematuria, or glycosuria. Postvoid residual (PVR) is needed. PVR less than 50 ml implies normal bladder emptying. PVR greater than 200 ml is abnormal and suggests overflow incontinence. Urodynamics or imaging studies are not part of the basic evaluation but are indicated if needed to clarify diagnosis or in the patient who fails initial treatment.[4]

Therapy

Therapy includes behavioral, medical, and surgical techniques.[4]

1. All patients must be educated about the physiology of the urinary tract.
2. Pelvic muscle exercises, also known as *Kegel exercises*, are indicated for both SUI and DI. Although Kegels alone may promote continence, the success of this technique depends on the patient's ability to contract the correct muscles and her commitment to perform the exercises. It is necessary to contract the perivaginal and periurethral muscles for 10 seconds 40–80 times a day for at least 8 weeks. The repetitive guidance of the health care practitioner over time is invaluable in teaching Kegels. Such exercises may be augmented by therapies used to improve pelvic floor musculature and anatomic positioning, such as biofeedback, electrical stimulation, vaginal cones, and contraceptive diaphragms.
3. Bladder training is used primarily for patients with DI but is also useful in SUI and mixed incontinence. The technique requires voiding according to a preset timetable rather than by urinary urges. Using the patient's pretreatment voiding diary, a voiding interval is chosen that is more frequent than the incontinent episodes. Over time, the voiding interval is increased until 2- to 3-hour intervals are achieved.
4. Smoking cessation is helpful in patients with chronic cough. Weight control is recommended for the obese. Avoidance of caffeinated beverages is advisable due to their irritant and diuretic effects.
5. ERT, either oral or vaginal, should be considered in menopausal women with either SUI or DI.
6. Other medications helpful in treatment of selected patients with DI include antispasmodics, such as oxybutynin (2.5–5.0 mg tid or qid), or anticholinergics, such as propantheline (7.5–30 mg three to five times daily). SUI can be helped by alpha-agonists, such as phenylpropanolamine (25–100 mg, sustained release, bid) or pseudoephedrine (15–30 mg tid). Tricyclics, such as imipramine (10–25 mg tid) are used to treat both SUI and DI because of their combined alpha-adrenergic and anticholinergic properties.
7. Overflow incontinence is often treated by clean, intermittent self-catheterization. This technique does not require antiseptic urethral preparation and is preferable to long-term indwelling catheterization.
8. Functional incontinence, a diagnosis of exclusion, is minimized by promoting mobility.
9. Surgery is reserved primarily for women who fail conservative management.

Estrogen Replacement Therapy

Because life expectancy for Native American women has increased to 77.1 years, primary care practitioners will provide health care to more perimenopausal women.[6] There is little information on Native American women in the perimenopausal years or the cultural acceptance of ERT. Research indicates that the incidence of coronary heart disease, osteoporosis, UI, and breast cancer all increase with age. ERT is one therapy with the potential to affect morbidity and mortality from these diseases.

ERT has documented beneficial health benefits. It decreases vasomotor symptoms and the severity of UI. It is cardioprotective and reduces the relative risk of coronary heart disease to 0.60. Osteoporotic fractures are prevalent in the elderly and can result in decreased functional independence. ERT reduces the relative risk of hip fracture to 0.46 after 10 years of therapy. ERT alone increases endometrial cancer rates, but combination therapy with progestins results in cancer rates that are similar to that of the general population. Adversely, 10 years of ERT are associated with a 1.46 relative risk of breast cancer.[23] The fear of breast cancer often prevents women from using ERT, but the mortality from coronary heart disease is significantly greater than the mortality from breast cancer. In fact, heart disease is the second leading cause of death in Native American women ages 55–64 years and the leading cause of mortality in women ages 65 years and older.[24]

Health care practitioners must promote health and independence among women of all ages, including the perimenopausal and elderly woman. ERT is an important preventive health measure, but the decision to use ERT is often a difficult choice. Risks, benefits, and contraindications must be reviewed. Absolute contraindications to ERT include undiagnosed vaginal bleeding, estrogen-dependent neoplasms, breast cancer in most cases, and active thromboembolic disorders. Relative contraindications include liver disease, migraines, thrombophlebitis, and gallbladder disease.

ERT is thought to increase overall life expectancy, especially in women with risk factors for coronary heart disease. Women who lack risk factors for coronary heart disease or osteoporosis but who have strong risk factors for breast cancer may not benefit significantly from ERT in the long term because their risk of mortality due to breast cancer will increase.[21, 23] The practitioner can guide patient-specific decisions about ERT through dialogue with the patient about her personal health characteristics and preferences. The decision to use ERT should be re-evaluated over time, with particular attention to the optimum duration of therapy.[25]

Both women who opt for and those who decline ERT should be counseled on other preventive health measures, such as exercise, maintaining a stable weight, calcium supplementation, and the reduction of cardiovascular disease risk factors. If a patient chooses to use ERT, progestins are needed concurrently to prevent endometrial hyperplasia, except in women without a uterus. Overall benefits of mortality reduction are maintained with continuous or cyclic therapy and with ERT alone. Commonly prescribed regimens are

1. *Continuous therapy*: daily 0.625 mg conjugated estrogen or 0.625 mg estrone sulfate or 1.0 mg estradiol with daily 2.5 mg medroxyprogesterone acetate (MPA). This regimen is simple in that the daily dose is standardized throughout the month. It is more often associated with breakthrough bleeding within the first 6–12 months of usage, however, especially in the recently menopausal woman. Ultimately, most women achieve amenorrhea.

2. *Cyclic therapy*: daily 0.625 mg conjugated estrogen or 1.0 mg estradiol with 5–10 mg MPA on days 1–10 of each month. Many women have cyclic withdrawal bleeding with this regimen. The 5-mg dose of MPA is preferred in women who are at risk for fluid retention or depression. Transdermal estrogen preparations with oral progestins are alternatives.

Summary

It is the collective task of health care workers to provide high-quality gynecologic care to Native American women.[26]

To achieve the goals of Healthy People 2000, the primary health care practitioner must focus on the woman as an individual with unique health characteristics and on the woman as part of a community.[8] Practitioners who begin a dialogue with patients can open a pathway to wellness. They must overcome the hesitation to discuss medical issues that have social and public health impact. Primary health care workers have the responsibility to routinely ask about unspoken but prevalent problems of domestic violence and UI. Efforts should be made to screen all Native American women for cervical cancer annually, including the elderly and women who do not enter doctor's offices. Mammographic screening for breast cancer and clinical breast examination must be offered on a 1- to 2-year basis to all women ages 50–69 years and to high-risk women ages 40–49 years or healthy women ages 70 years or older. The perimenopausal patient deserves our respect and consideration of preventive health measures, such as ERT, that can maximize independence and function.

References

1. Leppert PC. Uniqueness of Women's Health. In PC Leppert, FM Howard (eds), Primary Care for Women. Philadelphia: Lippincott–Raven, 1997;1.
2. U.S. Preventive Services Task Force. Guide to Clinical Preventive Services (2nd ed). Baltimore: Williams & Wilkins, 1996.
3. Roberts SJ, Sorenson L. Lesbian health care: a review and recommendations for health promotion in primary care settings. Nurse Pract 1995;20:43–47.
4. Fantyl JA, Newman DK, Colling J, et al. Urinary Incontinence in Adults: Acute and Chronic Management. Clinical Practice Guideline No. 2, 1996 Update. Rockville, MD: U.S. Department of Health and Human Services, Public Health Service, Agency for Health Care Policy and Research. AHCPR Publication No. 96-0682, 1996.
5. American College of Obstetricians and Gynecologists. Domestic Violence. ACOG Technical Bulletin No. 209. Washington, DC: ACOG, 1995.
6. Indian Health Service. Regional Differences in Indian Health, 1996. Rockville, MD: U.S. Department of Health and Human Services, 1996;Charts 4.30 and 4.34.
7. Chao A, Becker TM, Jordan SW, et al. Decreasing rates of cervical cancer among American Indians and Hispanics in New Mexico (United States). Cancer Causes Control 1996;7:205–213.
8. U.S. Public Health Service. Healthy People 2000: National Health Promotion and Disease Prevention Objectives. DHHS Publication No. PHS 91-50212. Washington, DC: U.S. Department of Health and Human Services, 1991.
9. American College of Obstetricians and Gynecologists. Cervical Cytology: Evaluation and Management of

Abnormalities. ACOG Technical Bulletin No. 183. Washington, DC: ACOG, 1993.

10. Buckley DI, McPherson S, North CQ, Becker TM. Dietary micronutrients and cervical dysplasia in southwestern American Indian women. Nutr Cancer 1992; 17:179–185.

11. New Mexico Breast and Cervical Cancer Detection and Control Program. Pap test algorithm. Santa Fe, NM: New Mexico Department of Health, Public Health Division, 1996.

12. Waxman AG. Colposcopy training for IHS providers. The IHS Primary Care Provider 1992;17:41–43.

13. Somkin CP, Hiatt MA, Hurley LB, et al. The effect of patient and provider reminders on mammography and Papanicolaou smear screening in a large health maintenance organization. Arch Intern Med 1997;157:1658–1664.

14. Landen ML. Cervical cancer screening: at the patient's or the health system's convenience? The IHS Primary Care Provider 1992;17:174–179.

15. Kottke TE, Trapp MA. Implementing Nurse-Based Screening Systems for Breast and Cervical Cancer. Mayo Clinic Proc (in press).

16. Miller BA, Kolonel LN, Bernstein L, et al (eds), Racial/Ethnic Patterns of Cancer in the United States 1988–1992. Seer Monograph. Publication No. 96-4104. Bethesda, MD: National Cancer Institute, 1996.

17. Paisano R, Cobb N (eds). Cancer Mortality Among American Indians and Alaska Natives in the United States: Regional Differences in Indian Health, 1989–1993. IHS Publication No. 97-615-23. Rockville, MD: Indian Health Service, 1997.

18. Burke W, Daly M, Garber J, et al. Recommendations for follow-up care of individuals with an inherited predisposition to cancer. II. BRCA1 and BRCA2. JAMA 1997;277:997–1003.

19. Thune I, Brenn T, Lund E, Gaard M. Physical activity and the risk of breast cancer. N Engl J Med 1997;336: 1269–1275.

20. Huang Z, Hankinson SE, Colditz GA, et al. Dual effects of weight and weight gain on breast cancer risk. JAMA 1997;278:1407–1411.

21. Grodstein F, Stampfer MJ, Colditz GA, et al. Postmenopausal hormone therapy and mortality. N Engl J Med 1997;366:1769–1775.

22. Fletcher SW, O'Malley MS, Bunce LA. Physicians' abilities to detect lumps in silicone breast models. JAMA 1985;253:2224–2228.

23. Col NF, Eckman MH, Karas RH, et al. Patient-specific decisions about hormone replacement therapy in postmenopausal women. JAMA 1997;277:1140–1147.

24. Indian Health Service. Trends in Indian Health, 1996. Rockville, MD: U.S. Department of Health and Human Services, 1996;Charts 4.6 and 4.7.

25. Brinton LA, Schairer C. Postmenopausal hormone replacement therapy: time for a reappraisal? N Engl J Med 1997;336:1821–1822.

26. McGinnis JM, Lee PR. *Healthy People 2000* at mid decade. JAMA 1995;273:1123–1129.

Part X
Psychiatric Disorders

Chapter 33
Depression and Suicide

Michael Biernoff

Depression is an illness commonly seen in a primary care practice setting. Because of its association with significant disability, the added risk for suicide, and its generally good response to treatment, adequate diagnosis and treatment of depression are important. In a National Comorbidity Survey,[1] depression was identified as the most common mental disorder, with 17% of the adult population in the United States experiencing depression in the course of their lives and approximately 10% of people experiencing depression in a given 12-month period. It has been estimated that depression and its associated dysfunction cost the U.S. economy $16–44 billion per year.

Although complaints or symptoms related to depression are common in a primary care setting (studies of the occurrence of depression in primary care outpatient settings have shown an 8.4–9.7% prevalence[2]), the diagnosis of depression is often missed. When it is made, treatment is often inadequate.

In Indian country, depression is probably at least as common as in a non-Indian setting. Its linkage to substance abuse and cultural considerations in assessment and treatment further complicate its identification and management and make appropriate diagnosis and treatment all the more critical.

Epidemiology

No nationwide epidemiologic studies have been done on the prevalence of depression among American Indians. The information available is limited to specific small studies involving individual communities, with little consistency between studies. The National Center for American Indian/Alaska Native Mental Health Research, affiliated with the University of Colorado in Denver, has been most active in carrying out epidemiologic research on mental disorders in American Indian/Alaska Native populations. Significant additions to the epidemiologic

knowledge base are anticipated in the near future. Although overall there is evidence to support higher prevalence rates among Indians for some mental disorders, such as depression,[3, 4] there is tremendous variation from one Indian community to another. One must be cautious in generalizing data from one community or population to other Indian communities and populations. (There is some indication that another mood disorder, bipolar disorder, has a lower prevalence in Indian populations.) Factors that are associated with an increased prevalence of depression are certainly found in American Indian communities. Poverty, displacement, and the relative lack of viable roles and jobs contribute to an increased incidence and prevalence of depression and suicide. The frequent experience of traumatic death and loss may be expected to adversely affect children and other community members. Child abuse and alcohol abuse may also contribute to higher rates of depression, both for those immediately and secondarily affected. Certain chronic medical conditions, including diabetes, which have a higher prevalence in some Indian communities, are also associated with higher rates of depression. Since the early 1990s, there has been much discussion of a possible long-term impact of the many generations of deprivation, loss, and forced dependence that American Indians have sustained in their contact with the non-Indian world. Such historic trauma may also contribute to the burden of depression and other ills in Indian communities.

Suicide is a traumatic event that leaves its mark on survivors and the community. Its finality and subsequent recording as a death statistic usually but does not always ensure that it will be identified and reported. Such assurance may be tempered by the stigma often associated with suicide, resulting in underreporting. As with depression, suicide rates vary tremendously from one community to another. Some communities have suicide rates several times higher than those of neighboring non-Indian communities. (The national annual age-adjusted suicide rate [1991–1993] was 11 per 100,000; for American Indians and Alaska Natives, it was 16 per 100,000.[5]) Other Indian communities experience suicide rates significantly lower than those of neighboring non-Indian communities. Given concerns about labeling Indian communities, one must be especially cautious in generalizing suicide rates derived from one community or population to others.

Some characteristics of American Indian suicide are a frequent association with alcohol use and a relatively higher incidence among adolescents and young adults,[6, 7] which diminishes with age (a pattern opposite the national trend). The suicide rate for American Indians and Alaska Natives ages 15–24 years (1991–1993) was 31.7.[5] The U.S. all races suicide rate for ages 15–24 years (1992) was 13.0.[5] Because most Indian communities are small, a single suicide tends to have a tremendous impact on the community. A cluster phenomenon of multiple suicides in a brief period may occur.

Suicide gestures and attempts are much more common than completed suicides, as is true in the general population, and they typically involve a different set of individuals. (As a rule of thumb, it has been estimated that suicide gestures and attempts occur 10 times as often as completed suicide.) The epidemiologic data on such behavior is in some ways more difficult to capture accurately, primarily because of underreporting. Suicide gestures and attempts are usually made by younger individuals, with women being reported more often than men. Such suicidal behavior tends to be impulsive and associated with alcohol use.

Clinical Presentation

Depression presents in different ways. Many patients with depression actually appear the way that might be expected: looking depressed and tearful, with downcast eyes, a sad voice, and slow movements and speech. Many other patients with depression may not appear with such typical presentation, and health care providers must be sensitive to other manifestations of depression. Depression always occurs within a cultural context, and this context may influence the presentation of depression. In Indian populations, for example, in which the psychiatric concept of depression may not traditionally exist, a patient may not associate particular symptoms with depression. Somatic symptoms may predominate, and the patient may deny feelings of "depression." Although such somatic symptoms usually include "vegetative" signs (such as slowed movements, fatigue, depressed affect, sleep disorder, loss of appetite), aches and pains or anxiety symptoms, such as restlessness, may predominate.

Depression may be reflected in decreased performance of daily activities, including chores or reduced involvement in social activities, and such change in performance and activities may be identified as a presenting symptom. As with non-Indian populations, depression is reported more often in women. Alcohol abuse is associated with depression in men and women and in fact, may mask depression, in which case the symptoms of alcohol abuse predominate. A large percentage of "dual diagnosis" cases involve alcohol abuse and depression.

Depressed children may present differently from adults. Not only are children less likely to verbalize feelings of depression, they also may exhibit more somatic symptoms and more "acting-out" behavior, such as school problems, conduct problems, and anxiety.

Depression in the elderly is common and may present primarily with nonspecific somatic complaints. Of special importance is the frequent confusion of depression in the elderly with degenerative cognitive changes. Depression may mimic some of the changes seen in degenerative cognitive disorders (e.g., psychomotor retardation and poor concentration), but depression usually responds well to treatment, thus underscoring the importance of appropriate and accurate assessment and treatment.

Usually, suicide gestures and attempts are readily identified as such. Sometimes, gestures and attempts are denied, especially if significant time has elapsed since the act or if it occurred "under the influence," and the patient is now sober. If there is any question about suicidal intent, the provider should always inquire. Sometimes, suicidal behavioral is masked and not readily apparent. It is suspected that a number of lethal single motor vehicle accidents involving single occupants are suicidal acts.

Assessment

The *Diagnostic and Statistical Manual of Mental Disorders,* 4th Edition (*DSM-IV*)[8] published by the American Psychiatric Association, which contains the standard diagnostic criteria used in psychiatry, defines a major depressive episode as including a series of symptoms, such as depressed mood, loss of interest or pleasure, significant weight change, sleep disorder, fatigue or loss of energy, psychomotor agitation or retardation, feelings of worthlessness or excessive guilt, diminished ability to concentrate, and recurrent thoughts of death or suicide. At least five of these symptoms, including a depressed mood or loss of interest or pleasure, must be present for at least 2 weeks and must cause significant distress or impairment in functioning. The symptoms are not due to the effects of a substance or due to a general medical condition. The provider should refer to the *DSM-IV* itself for complete details.

This section focuses on the assessment of major depressive disorders among American Indians. Such disorders are the source of much suffering and disability and are associated with a higher risk for suicide. Other types of mood disorders, including bipolar mood disorder, are not addressed here. The provider should refer to the

DSM-IV for diagnostic criteria for other mood disorders and to standard psychiatric references[9] for treatment guidelines. Practitioners rely heavily on the mental status examination as an assessment tool, in conjunction with established diagnostic criteria. The assessment of mental disorder in American Indians is hampered by the fact that, with only a few small exceptions, neither the elements of the standard mental status examination nor the diagnostic criteria were standardized on this population. Thus, their use with these populations must be approached with some caution.

In the assessment of depression in American Indians, attention to the vegetative signs may be most useful. Other signs, such as feelings of excessive guilt, may not be present because guilt feelings may not be a common expression within the culture. On the other hand, a significant cultural issue (such as decrease in social interactions) may be identified as a significant symptom of depression. Bereavement is commonly encountered in patients, and although it may involve significant disability, usually for proscribed periods, it should not be confused with depression unless it is unusually prolonged and meets the other criteria for severe depression. In some American Indian cultures, the experience of hearing voices of deceased family members may be culturally appropriate. It is usually associated with bereavement and does not represent acute psychosis unless accompanied by other signs and symptoms indicative of severe disorder. Depression in patients with alcohol abuse must be carefully assessed because depression may be an alcohol-related symptom that may resolve after alcohol withdrawal, although remission may not occur fully for 30–60 days. Other causes of depression or conditions associated with depression, including diabetes, thyroid disorder, and medication side effect or interaction, must be ruled out.

When assessing depression, the provider must always consider the issue of dangerousness. As part of the formal assessment, the patient should always be asked about suicidal feelings. Providers are often not comfortable asking about suicidal feelings, but the question must be broached. It turns out that patients usually do not have difficulty responding to this inquiry, and there is no evidence that such inquiry leads to suicidal acts. The question can be asked in terms of "suicide," "feelings of hurting oneself," "self-harm," or other terms suitable to and clearly understood by the patient. Although risk for suicide is not always easy to ascertain, risk factors include previous attempts, concrete plans, alcohol use, availability of lethal weapons, being male, inability to control suicidal feelings, and social isolation. As a rule of thumb, if the provider thinks the patient is at high risk, he or she should consider a safe and supervised environment for the patient, which may include hospitalization.

As part of the assessment of depression, it is critical that the provider elicit the patient's perspective of what is wrong. This is especially critical in a cross-cultural setting, in which expectations and understandings may differ. Providers may learn things they had never anticipated. Such inquiry also facilitates the establishment of rapport, which is essential to the assessment itself and subsequent interventions. Good bedside manner is a prerequisite to successful patient care in a primary care setting, whether providers are working with Indian or non-Indian patients. The provider must show qualities of respect, caring, concern, and warmth. A calm, quiet demeanor should be encouraged, and a brusque, loud, demanding manner should be discouraged. Eye contact or the lack of eye contact is probably less important than ensuring a respectful, unintrusive interaction.

In some American Indian populations, an Indian language may be a primary language, and English may be a secondary language or may not be spoken by the patient. Translation and interpretation may be required. Depending on the circumstances, this service can be provided by family members, other workers, or individuals with a specific role as translator and interpreter. The provider should be aware of some of the limitations in the use of translator or interpreter services. Equivalent words and concepts may not exist in different languages. Different languages may conceptualize things quite differently. In the mental health arena, in which feelings, thoughts, and emotions are so important, translation or interpretation may be especially difficult. Although providers often rely on family members to provide the translation or interpretation, they may bring their own biases. Other workers, although fluent in the Indian language, may not know the specific terminology or concepts being translated and interpreted. Although they are often unavailable, experienced and trained translators or interpreters are preferred.

Treatment

Treatment of depression follows a thorough and accurate assessment. If depression is severe or suicidal ideation is present, an immediate decision is whether to hospitalize. Sometimes, the decision to hospitalize is easy, given the severity of symptoms and the absence of alternate resources. At other times, it is a difficult decision and depends on the provider's clinical judgment and comfort level in managing depression and suicidal behavior as well as available resources, including family support. Regarding suicidal ideation, the decision usually turns on the assessment of lethality, as described above, as described in the preceding section, and the presence or absence of a safe and secure environment. Acute suicidal ideation most typically resolves over a matter of hours, and so the safety issue is most critical in this period.

Severe or psychotic depression without suicidal ideation may also lead to consideration of hospitalization, given the severe disability and dysfunction that usually accompany this condition and that may include risk to life.

Depression secondary to medical illness and caused by drug side effects or interactions must also be treated immediately. The treatment of choice is usually to address and correct the underlying causal factors.

When patients present in immediate social or personal crisis, typically marked by psychological agitation with or without suicidal ideation, crisis intervention techniques may be quite effective in reducing the expressed emotion and resolving the crisis. Such interventions may be provided by trained behavioral health staff, although with some training and experience, a primary care provider with enough time could certainly provide such interventions. The principles of crisis intervention and its techniques are described in standard psychiatric references. Effective crisis intervention usually entails bringing the relevant parties together in a neutral environment, reviewing the events leading up to the crisis and the crisis itself with a more controlled expression of emotion, exploring alternate solutions and ways to resolve the crisis, and obtaining some commitment to follow up. The goal is to see the patient return to the level of functioning before the crisis.

In the usual outpatient primary care setting, the most common presentation of depression does not require hospitalization. As emphasized in the section on assessment, it is critical to gain an understanding from the perspective of the patient (and of significant others, if available) of what is wrong. Such an understanding becomes a framework for treatment. For example, if the patient understands the condition in terms of somatic or physical dysfunction, it may be most effective to address treatment through such a metaphor. If causality is attributed to social conflict, addressing this issue may be the most effective pathway to treatment.

Not all depressed patients require or are candidates for antidepressant medication. The decision to prescribe antidepressant medication should be based on a consideration of the type and severity of depression. Major depression presenting with marked vegetative signs (slowed movements, fatigue, depressed affect, sleep disorder, loss of appetite) tends to respond very well to antidepressant medication, and antidepressant medication should be considered in such cases. Mild forms of depression and normal bereavement may not respond as clearly to antidepressant medication, and other verbal, cognitive or behavioral, and social therapies should be considered. In any case, whether antidepressant medication is prescribed, the accompanying primary and secondary psychological and social issues must be addressed. The primary care provider may be in a good position to address such issues effectively, especially when the patient is well known to the provider. Identification of life stressors, including social conflict, is often not difficult, and the introduction of stress reduction techniques and

mutual problem solving and planning can be quite helpful and effective.

When considering the use of antidepressant medication, it is important to take time to discuss the medication with the patient and with significant others, if available. Medication should be presented in the manner most acceptable and understandable to the patient. A clear and concise review of the symptoms and signs and reason for the diagnosis is helpful. A brief discussion of the biological model of depression and medication's mechanism of action (in terms of redressing a chemical imbalance) is usually well received. Anticipated response (a lessening of the weighed-down feeling), target symptoms (the vegetative symptoms), and possible side effects should all be reviewed. The anticipated delay in antidepressant effect (almost 2 weeks) should be mentioned, and the importance of regular daily dosing should be stressed.

In selecting an antidepressant, it is important to know if the patient has previously taken antidepressant medication and the response to such medication. If the patient reports a clear-cut positive response, consider restarting the same medication and continuing at the previously effective dose. If the patient has not taken antidepressant medication previously, and there are otherwise no contraindications, consider beginning with a member of the selective serotonin reuptake inhibitor (SSRI) class. SSRIs are now considered the treatment of choice for most major depressions. The tricyclic antidepressant class (imipramine, amitriptyline, nortriptyline), although very effective, is associated with a number of unpleasant side effects and is usually considered a secondary choice.

Initial starting dose is typically fluoxetine 20 mg daily, sertraline 50 mg daily, or paroxetine 20 mg daily. (When prescribing fluoxetine, warn patients to take the medication in the morning to avoid evening and night agitation as a side effect.) After an initial 1- to 3-week period, the dose may be increased. Most patients seem to respond to a dose of fluoxetine 20 mg per day, sertraline 50–100 mg per day, or paroxetine 20–30 mg per day. If the patient does not respond within the usual dose range, consider increasing the dose, and then, if no response, switching to a tricyclic antidepressant. Refer to a standard drug reference guide, such as drug information handbooks, *Physician's Desk Reference*, or Micromedex (Micromedex, Inc., Englewood, CO) software program, for full details, including contraindications, side effects, and drug interactions (e.g., serious adverse interaction with monoamine oxidase inhibitors).

Many practitioners have reported that American Indian patients have often responded to lower doses of tricyclic antidepressants than non-Indians have required for similar antidepressant effect. It is noteworthy that primary care physicians have tended to undertreat depression by underdosing and treating for an insufficient length of time.[10]

When prescribing antidepressant medication, dispense less than a lethal dose at a time. (SSRIs are considerably safer than tricyclic antidepressants in this regard.) Always provide the patient a return appointment, and when starting antidepressant medication, make the return appointment within a week if possible. Give the patient instructions about contacting help if problems arise before the next scheduled appointment.

Major depression may be a one-time event or may recur. It is usually recommended that, with a first episode of clear-cut major depression, antidepressant medication be continued for at least a 6- to 9-month period. It can be explained to the patient that while the symptoms are being controlled by medication, the patient can work on strengthening coping skills, which can provide some protection against depression when the medication is discontinued. Recurrent depression may need to be treated for longer periods, with close follow-up once medication is discontinued. For severe depression with psychotic features, neuroleptic medication may need to be added to the antidepressant medication to achieve control of the psychotic features.

Psychiatric consultation and referral should be sought in treating complicated and atypical depression and depression not responding to the usual treatments. Psychiatric consultation and referral should also be sought in cases presenting a diagnostic or treatment quandary and in cases requiring hospitalization. The primary care provider should ideally have on-site psychiatric consultation available or at least access to a psychiatrist by telephone. It is advisable to develop and maintain protocols outlining access to psychiatric services, including hospitalization.

The primary care provider treating depression should develop an overall treatment plan. Medication alone is insufficient. Other components of the treatment plan should include exercise, stress management and coping skills, and effective lifestyle changes. Social support and activities, spiritual involvement, and other cultural considerations must also be addressed. The treatment plan should be developed together with the patient (and significant others, if possible) and be readily understood and supported by the patient. It should make sense and fit within the patient's cultural context. For example, in Indian communities with a vital extended family system, ways of using the supports such a system can offer should be addressed. Much of the treatment plan involves support for the patient and patient education. In the treatment of depression, any concomitant or predisposing factors must be treated, such as alcohol abuse, panic disorder and anxiety, and posttraumatic stress disorder and other sequelae of trauma.

Some or occasionally all aspects of the treatment plan could be carried out by the primary care provider, but usually other providers should be involved as part of a treatment team. Other providers may be in mental health, social service, and substance abuse programs. Each of these providers has specific expertise that can be used to address major components of the overall treatment plan. The primary care provider should have contacts in these programs and know how to use these services. As with psychiatric services, it is useful to have protocols in place that address access and referral to these programs. With other providers involved in carrying out aspects of the treatment plan, it becomes important to coordinate services and to have some mechanism for communicating with one another. The principles of case management are helpful in carrying out such coordination of care.

Traditional healing is alive and well in many Indian communities. Its forms vary tremendously from one community to another. Many Indian people rely on a variety of healing traditions, including indigenous, charismatic Christian, and other traditions. Such healing can be extremely powerful and effective, and the primary care provider should learn to support traditional healing practices, which can complement the practices of the primary care provider. In a traditional cultural context, healing a depression may include certain actions and healing practices, often involving family and other community members, which can provide an antidepressant effect. The primary care provider can convey support for such practices with respectful (not probing) inquiry and encouragement that acknowledges value in traditional practices. Patients are usually good about setting limits on information that can be shared. Such an approach also helps to establish the doctor-patient rapport so essential in treatment.

Prevention

Following a public health model, the best antidote to depression and suicide is prevention. A prevention perspective is a natural fit for most Indian communities and is usually readily understood and supported. Health care agencies and communities should commit to offering a variety of general health-education activities and targeted prevention and early intervention activities. In Indian country, encouraging a strong sense of Indian identity and pride has been well received and effective. One example is the Gathering of Native Americans curriculum, a community empowerment model, developed with the support of the National Center for Substance Abuse Prevention. Parenting classes with at-risk mothers, Head Start screening and intervention, and therapeutic recreation groups with at-risk adolescents have been effective. The Jicarilla Apache Tribe in New Mexico has embarked on a community-wide adolescent suicide-prevention project, which has reported success in significantly reducing adolescent suicide behavior.

The primary care provider can play a significant role in identifying and treating depression in individual patients. As a public health practitioner taking a broad perspective, the provider can play a leadership role in identifying and addressing factors in the community that may contribute to or be associated with depression and suicide.

Points to Remember

- Depression is commonly seen in a primary care practice setting. Look for it. It may be masked.
- Depression is a treatable illness.
- Understand depression from the patient's perspective. Consider cultural factors.
- Assess lethality.
- Formulate a holistic treatment plan. Be sure to address psychosocial issues. Never use medication alone.
- Antidepressant medication works. Use a sufficient dose and treat for an adequate period.
- Become an advocate for community prevention and early intervention activities.

References

1. Kessler RC, McGonayle KA, Zhao S, et al. Results from the National Comorbidity Study. Lifetime and 12-month prevalence of DSM-III-R psychiatric disorders in the United States. Arch Gen Psychiatry 1994;51:8–19.
2. Depression Guideline Panel. Depression in Primary Care (Vol 1). Detection and Diagnosis, Technical Report No. 5. Rockville, MD: U.S. Department of Health and Human Services, Public Health Service, 1993.
3. Manson SM, Walker RD, Kivlahan DR. Psychiatric assessment and treatment of American Indians and Alaska Natives. Hosp Community Psychiatry 1987;38:165–173.
4. Thompson JW, Walker RD, Silk-Walker P. Psychiatric Care of American Indians and Alaska Natives. In AC Gaw (ed), Culture, Ethnicity, and Mental Illness. Washington, DC: American Psychiatric Press, 1992.
5. Indian Health Service. Trends in Indian Health, 1996. Rockville, MD: U.S. Department of Health and Human Services, IHS, 1996.
6. May PA. Suicide and self-destruction among American Indian youths. Am Indian Alsk Native Ment Health Res 1987;1:52–69.
7. Thompson JW, Walker RD. Adolescent suicide among American Indians and Alaska Natives. Psychiatric Annals 1990;20:128–133.
8. American Psychiatric Association, Committee on Nomenclature and Statistics. Diagnostic and Statistical Manual of Mental Disorders (4th ed). Washington, DC: American Psychiatric Association, 1994.
9. Gabbard GO (ed). Treatment of Psychiatric Disorders

(2nd ed) (Vols 1, 2). Washington, DC: American Psychiatric Press, 1995.
10. Wells KB, Katon W, Rogers B, Camp P. Results from the medical outcomes study. Use of minor tranquilizers and antidepressant medications by depressed outpatients. Am J Psychiatry 1994;151:694–700.

Suggested Readings

American Indian/Alaska Native Suicide Task Force Report. Albuquerque, NM: American Indian/Alaska Native Task Force, April 1996.

American Psychiatric Association, Committee on Nomenclature and Statistics. Diagnostic and Statistical Manual of Mental Disorder (4th ed). Washington, DC: American Psychiatric Association, 1994.

Depression Guideline Panel. Depression in Primary Care (Vol 1). Detection and Diagnosis, Technical Report No. 5. Rockville, MD: U.S. Department of Health and Human Services, Public Health Service, 1993.

Depression Guideline Panel. Depression in Primary Care (Vol 2). Detection and Diagnosis, Technical Report No. 5. Rockville, MD: U.S. Department of Health and Human Services, Public Health Service, 1993.

Gabbard GO (ed), Treatment of Psychiatric Disorders (2nd ed) (Vols 1, 2). Washington, DC: American Psychiatric Press, 1995.

Indian Health Service. Trends in Indian Health, 1996. Rockville, MD: U.S. Department of Health and Human Services, IHS, 1996.

Kessler RC, McGonayle KA, Zhao S, et al. Results from the National Comorbidity Study. Lifetime and 12-month prevalence of DSM-III-R psychiatric disorders in the United States. Arch Gen Psychiatry 1994;51:8–19.

LaFramboise TD. American Indian mental health policy. Am Psychol 1988;43:388–397.

Manson SM, Walker RD, Kivlahan DR. Psychiatric assessment and treatment of American Indians and Alaska Natives. Hosp Community Psychiatry 1987;38:165–173.

May PA. Suicide and self-destruction among American Indian youths. Am Indian Alsk Native Ment Health Res 1987;1:52–69.

Thompson JW, Walker RD. Adolescent suicide among American Indians and Alaska Natives. Psychiatric Ann 1990;20:128–133.

Thompson JW, Walker RD, Silk-Walker P. Psychiatric Care of American Indians and Alaska Natives. In AC Gaw (ed). Culture, Ethnicity, and Mental Illness. Washington, DC: American Psychiatric Press, 1992.

Wells KB, Katon W, Rogers B, Camp P. Results from the medical outcomes study. Use of minor tranquilizers and antidepressant medications by depressed outpatients. Am J Psychiatry 1994;151:694–700.

Chapter 34
Alcohol and Solvent Abuse

Mario Cruz

Native American alcohol and other substance use and abuse are highly complex multivariate phenomena marked by tribal and individual variation. More than 500 tribes are presently recognized by the federal government, with populations ranging from less than 100 to more than 100,000.[1] There are more than 200 different tribal dialects and languages.[1] More than half of all Native Americans reside in urban communities.[1, 2] Native Americans have large family households (average 4.6 members), a young median age (22.4 years), and the highest birth rate of all ethnic groups in the United States. One of every four Native American households is headed by a single working mother, and fewer than one-third of all Native Americans hold a high school degree (and only 7% hold college degrees).[3] These statistics paint a picture of an ethnic group with access to few economic and social resources. Although alcohol and substance abuse disorders affect all ethnic and socioeconomic groups, the most profound and negative consequences occur at more disturbing rates among the less fortunate economically.

In 1987, the death rate for Native Americans was 25.9 per 100,000 (compared with 6 per 100,000 for all Americans).[4] The average life expectancy for Native Americans is roughly 6 years less than that of the general population.[2] Alcoholism is a significant contributor to these alarming statistics. The alcohol-related mortality rate in Native Americans is reported to be 4.3 times that of the general population.[2] Five of the 10 major causes of death among Native Americans may be related to alcohol.[1, 5, 6]

Another serious problem facing the Native American population is the use of solvents as euphoriants by child, adolescent, and young adult populations. On average, solvent abuse is twice as prevalent in Native American populations as in the general U.S. population.[1] Solvent abuse has dramatic effects on cognitive, perceptual, and motor function as well as social and physiologic development. The use of alcohol and other substances may lead to social isolation, affective disturbances, and a higher potential for suicide.

Native American Aboriginal Use of Alcohol

The statistics related to alcohol and solvent abuse among Native American people are of concern, but significant positive changes appear to be afoot. The rates of alcohol-related mortality and accidental injury deaths have fallen significantly since the 1970s. An awakening sense of pride among Native American people portends further decreases in alcohol and substance abuse rates, a trend that is already occurring in many areas. In addition, some tribes are approaching alcohol use and abuse as a public health issue and developing political and social initiatives to curb the problem. Alcohol and solvent abuse among Native American people is a serious problem, affecting the physical, mental, and social aspects of Native Americans, but Native American communities have begun their own effective interventions.

Contrary to public opinion, not all Native American tribes were naive to the effects of alcohol before European contact.[7] Before this contact, the use of alcoholic beverages was primarily confined to Native American tribes in the Southwest, but there was scattered use in other parts of the country. Southwestern tribes were influenced by their mesoamerican ancestors, the Mayan Indians. They produced *balche*, a wine made from honey and balche bark. The Mayan use of alcohol is thought to have influenced the drinking complexes of the Aztec and Northern Mexican tribes. More than 40 different alcoholic beverages were made in Mexico from a variety of plant substances such as honey, palm sap, wild plum, and pineapple. The Aztec developed intricate ceremonies and social rules governing the proper use of alcohol. Its use was clearly prescribed for religious purposes and not for secular and social purposes.

The diffusion of the Mayan and Aztec influences spread northward, reaching as far as the Pima, Papago, and Apache tribes. Other southwestern tribes known to have produced and used alcoholic beverages before European contact are the Coahuiltecan of southern Texas, the Yuman of western Arizona, and the Rio Grande River and Zuni Pueblo tribes of New Mexico. Native American tribes located in California, the Great Basin (Utah and Nevada), the northwestern United States and Alaska, the north and southeast United States, and the Great Plains had no knowledge of alcohol until their contact with whites.

Aboriginal use of alcohol generally did not involve excessive drunkenness but controlled and supervised use, often in highly ritualized occasions. Furthermore, accounts of Native Americans' initial encounters with alcoholic beverages did not describe reckless or uninhibited behavior. It was with ongoing European contact that the use of alcohol assumed more destructive characteristics.

Genetics, Flushing, and the Firewater Myth

In the *Diagnostic and Statistical Manual of Mental Disorders,* 4th Edition (*DSM-IV*), individuals with chronic social, occupational, and physical problems related to persistent alcohol use are defined as having either alcohol dependence or abuse. A 1980–1985 community study conducted in the United States revealed that approximately 8% of the general adult population were alcohol dependent and 5% had abused alcohol at some time in their lives.[8]

Alcohol dependence often has a familial pattern, and at least some of this transmission can be traced to genetic factors, as shown in twin adoption studies comparing the relative risk for alcohol dependence in monozygotic and dizygotic twins. Yet, genetic factors explain only a portion of the risk, whereas a substantial proportion of the risk is attributed to psychological, environmental, and social factors.

Along with the controversy about the degree to which genes contribute to the evolution of alcohol disorders, two myths have permeated the public's view of alcohol in relationship to specific ethnic groups: flushing and the firewater myth.

The "alcohol flushing response" was reported as a cutaneous vasodilatation reaction after moderate alcohol ingestion, resulting in visible reddening of the face and the upper chest, acute drowsiness, and increased heart rate.[9] The time between ingestion and the flushing response has been hypothesized to be related to the risk for acquiring an alcohol-related disorder. Fast flushing (flushing occurring within 15 minutes of alcohol ingestion) reportedly lowers the risk for acquiring

alcohol-related disorders due to its associated dysphoric reaction.[9]

The flushing response is thought to be a consequence of elevated acetaldehyde serum levels. Flushing reportedly occurs in individuals who have at least one inactive ALDH2*2 allele (mitochondrial aldehyde dehydrogenase).[9–11] In this scenario, the flushing response is a consequence of alcohol breaking down to acetaldehyde by alcohol dehydrogenase (ADH) and a subsequent slower-than-normal oxidation of acetaldehyde due to the inactive ALDH2*2. This results in elevated serum acetaldehyde levels. The circulating acetaldehyde facilitates the release of catecholamines from the adrenal medulla and sympathetic nerve endings, resulting in the alcohol-related flush.

Genotype and phenotype data support the association of the ALDH2*2 allele with a low risk of developing alcoholism. The allele frequency of the mutant ALDH2*2 in Chinese alcoholics (~8%) is less than that in healthy controls (30–31%).[9] Similarly, the frequency of ALDH2-inactive phenotypes is only 2.3% in Japanese alcoholics compared to 40% in the general population.[9] Contrary to the predictions based on genotype, the relationship of flushing to reduced drinking is only marginal and varies from study to study. Increasingly accessible genotyping methods have revealed more flushing subtypes; some associated with a heightened risk for alcoholism in ways that could not be explained by the acetaldehyde hypothesis. For example, 18% of white subjects who reported occasional fast "flushing" also reported problem drinking in themselves or their parents.[9] When 1,225 Japanese were assessed for their flushing frequency (defined as "always," "sometimes," and "never"), some unexpected findings were observed. The "sometimes" flushing men were 1.7 times more likely than the "never" flushers and three times more likely than the "always" flushers to abuse alcohol. Results for Japanese women in the study revealed that "sometimes" flushers had a 2.8 times greater risk than the "never" flushers and a 7.8 times greater risk to abuse alcohol than the "always" flushers.

Complicating the relationship between flushing and alcohol-related disorders further, there is no empiric evidence that flushing per se is aversive. In fact, although high levels of acetaldehyde are aversive to drinking alcohol, low levels have been reported to be reinforcing.[9] Clinically, this is seen in alcoholics seeking the use of disulfiram to achieve what is known as the "Antabuse high."

In Native Americans, the evidence weighs against a flushing response to alcohol. In one clinical study of a small sample of Sioux and Navajo, no evidence for a flushing response was found. Additionally, in a postmortem study of Native Americans, liver biopsies revealed that the sample was homozygous for the active ALDH2*1 allele.[10]

It is clear that the relationship between alcohol abuse and the "flushing" response is more complex than previously thought and does not always correlate with a reduced incidence of alcohol-related disorders.

Another myth perpetuated for centuries is the "firewater" myth—that is, that Native Americans possess an inherent inability to tolerate alcohol's effect. The term was first used in the seventeenth century.[7] The myth gained scientific popularity in the 1970s, when Fenna et al. found that whites metabolized alcohol significantly faster than did Native Americans.[1] Bennion and Li later found no difference between whites and Native Americans in rate of alcohol metabolism.[1] Additionally, some studies comparing prevalence of active and inactive alleles of ADH and ALDH2 show no consistent differences between the two groups.[10, 11] In summary, although genes contribute to the risk of developing alcohol-related disorders, there appear to be more substantial risks associated with familial, social, and environmental factors.

Native American Alcoholism: Two Theories

From a sociocultural perspective, controversy continues about the devastating impact of alcohol use on Native American tribes. Two competing theories remain from the 1970s, the structural-functionalist theory of anomie and the aboriginal social pathology theory.[1] The theory of anomie maintains that many Native American tribes are mourning the loss of a historic tradition and are reacting to the stresses of acculturation, including the demand to integrate and identify with mainstream society. Structurally, the historic events contributing to this situation include forced relocation of tribes from traditional homelands, the breakup of families, constant harassment from soldiers and settlers, nomadic hunter-gatherer tribes forcibly turned into farmers, and government-fostered subsistence dependence. The "reservation system failed to provide a well-defined set of social roles, and this in turn fostered a condition in which many Native Americans attempt to assert their 'Indianness' by turning the firewater myth into a self-fulfilling prophecy."[1] Functionally, structural aspects of the anomie theory foster the conditions necessary for increasing cultural and individual tension with few constructive outlets. Alcoholism then can be seen as learned through negative reinforcement. By becoming associated with the avoidance of anomic situations, alcohol and its personal, pleasurable effects and rewards positively reinforce its continued use.

An alternative theory is aboriginal social pathology, which proposes that social pathology present before the introduction of alcohol into their cultures can explain alcohol's subsequent destructive effect. There has been limited empiric research to validate either theory. Additional research is necessary to understand the social variables that perpetuate this problem.

Epidemiology

The use and effect of alcohol on Native American tribes is far from uniform. Such factors as social norms, economic status, and educational customs affect attitudes toward alcohol use and the prevalence of alcohol-related problems. These factors can vary tremendously, even between tribes in geographic proximity. Not surprisingly, some tribes on the whole drink moderately and have few alcohol-related problems; some tribes drink heavily and therefore have many alcohol-related problems.[12] One encouraging fact is that the age-adjusted alcoholism death rates for Native Americans and Alaska Natives decreased by 63% between 1973 and 1988[12] (Figure 34-1). The historic course and use of alcohol by Native American men is very similar to the general population in that the highest use occurs in men ages 16–29 years, with use diminishing after the age of 35–40 years.[4] Present estimates are that 30–50% of middle-aged Native American men who abstain are former moderate or heavy drinkers.[1, 4] Additionally, abstinence is quite common among Native American women and adults older than age 30 years.[4]

This positive epidemiologic data must be tempered by more disturbing reports of the youthful Native American population. In one study on school achievement[4] in Native American youth, poor school achievement was found to be linked to weekly to daily alcohol abuse among poor school achievers. It has been hypothesized that alcohol abuse may contribute to the high absentee rates for Native American youth in many schools (up to 40%) and the low high school graduation rate (33%).[4]

In terms of alcohol-related hospitalizations, Indian Health Service (IHS) discharge rates for nondependent abuse of alcohol and for alcoholic liver disease are both 3.4 times greater than the national average rates. The IHS discharge rate for alcoholic psychosis is four times greater than the national average.[1]

Much of our epidemiologic data refers to Native Americans from reservations. Few data have been gathered on the 50% of Native Americans living in urban centers. What we do know is that urban Native Americans are approximately three times more likely to drink two or more times daily than their rural counterparts (16.2% vs. 5.8%).[4] Incarcerated Native American youth in major urban centers began drinking at an earlier age than other incarcerated youth, had more binge drinking episodes, and more illegal drug use.[13]

Identification of Alcohol-Related Disorders and Medical Complications

Individuals who have severe social, occupational, or physical impairments related to alcohol use generally meet *DSM-IV* criteria for alcohol abuse or dependence.[8]

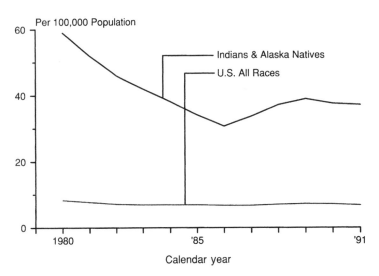

Figure 34-1. The age-adjusted alcoholism death rate for American Indians and Alaska Natives has decreased 37% since 1979–1981. In 1990–1992, it was 37.2 deaths per 100,000 population, or 5.5 times the 1991 U.S. all races rate of 6.8. Reprinted with permission from Indian Health Service. Trends in Indian Health, 1996. Washington, DC: U.S. Department of Health and Human Services, Indian Health Service, Office of Planning, Evaluation, and Legislation, Division of Program Statistics, 1997.

These individuals are predisposed to poor dietary status, cigarette smoking, abuse of other licit and illicit substances, comorbid psychiatric disturbances and death from numerous medical causes, including hypothermia related to cold exposure, cirrhosis of the liver, cerebrovascular accidents, cardiomyopathy, gastrointestinal bleeds, and malignant neoplasms, to name just a few. Alcoholics also have high morbidity rates from low-grade hypertension, intracerebral and subarachnoid hemorrhages[14] and other cardiovascular diseases; cortical diseases, such as generalized cortical dementia and specific corpus callosal[15] and cerebellar defects, transient confusional states or severe memory impairment related to B vitamin deficiencies, acute intoxication, or withdrawal; peripheral neuropathies, evidenced by muscular weakness, paresthesias, and decreased peripheral sensation; and gastrointestinal ulcerative disease and pancreatitis. These disorders typically occur in late middle age for heavy-drinking men and earlier in heavy-drinking women.[8, 16] Although women may generally begin drinking later in life than men, they progress to developing alcohol abuse or dependence more rapidly. That women experience the adverse consequences of heavy drinking faster than their male counterparts is thought to occur because women tend to develop higher blood alcohol concentrations than men do at a given dose of alcohol per kilogram because of their lower percentage of body water, higher percentage of body fat, and slower metabolism of alcohol.[8, 15]

Most patients with alcohol-related disorders rarely present themselves to health care providers for alcohol treatment.[4] Generally, the health care provider must determine it as an issue through a formal interview and physical examination. The interview should include the following CAGE questionnaire, which has been shown to have high validity and reliability in outpatient clinical settings.[16]

1. Have you ever felt you should **C**ut down on your drinking?
2. Have people **A**nnoyed you by criticizing your drinking?
3. Have you ever felt bad or **G**uilty about your drinking?
4. Have you ever had a drink first thing in the morning to steady your nerves or to get rid of a hangover (e.g., **E**ye-opener)?

Answering yes to all these questions indicates an alcohol-related disorder.

The physical examination may show symptoms of one of the illnesses described earlier in this section. Supporting evidence on the physical examination includes resting or unintentional hand tremor, unsteady gait with a history of falls (particularly in the elderly),[16] and insomnia and erectile dysfunction. If the patient is male and has a long history of alcohol dependence, he may present with decreased testicular size and feminization effects. Patients with alcohol withdrawal may present with nausea, vomiting, elevated blood pressure, tachycardia, gastritis, hematemesis, dry mouth, puffy blotchy complexion, and mild peripheral edema.[8]

It is also important to do a brief mental status examination. Patients may show attentional or short-term memory impairments, disorientation, and visual and at times auditory hallucinations. These changes are generally transient and are related to the effects of either acute alcohol intoxication or alcohol withdrawal. Problems with short-term memory associated with confabulation and disturbances in judgment can portend more serious chronic cortical dysfunction, however, such as alcoholic dementia or alcoholic amnestic disorder.

Associated laboratory findings follow.[8, 17] The most common elevated laboratory value in chronic heavy drinkers is gamma-glutamyltransferase (GGT). At least 70% of individuals with a high GGT level are heavy drinkers. Mean corpuscular volume (MCV) may be high normal in heavy drinkers because of liver dysfunction, B vitamin deficiencies, and alcohol's direct inhibiting effect on erythropoiesis. Other less specific laboratory findings are elevated liver enzymes, elevated lipid levels, and high normal uric acid levels.

In terms of treatment, there is a good success rate for individuals who are high functioning (e.g., employed, with a stable family and financial situation). Individuals with these characteristics have a 1-year abstinence rate after treatment of 65%.[2, 8] For individuals without these characteristics, success is no greater than natural non-treatment outcomes of 20%.[1, 8, 18] Treatment consists of coping skills training to identify high-risk behaviors and situations for drinking and taking actions to reduce the risk by using self-help groups, such as Alcoholics Anonymous, and at times, medication. No empirically based studies have been done on treatment outcomes for Native Americans. Native Americans do tend to have a higher treatment dropout rate than most other ethnic groups.[1, 2, 19, 20]

Although lithium and carbamazepine (Tegretol) have been shown to have mild effects on reducing craving for alcohol, they are not considered pharmacotherapeutic mainstays for alcohol abstention. Presently, two medications appear to show promise in this area. Naltrexone at doses of 50 mg/day appeared to differentially prevent relapse among subjects who "sampled" an initial alcoholic drink.[17] This is a common occurrence with alcoholics. Naltrexone also reduced the number of days on which alcohol was consumed and increased the time to relapse to heavy drinking. The "sampling" effect is thought to occur through blocking conditioned neuroendocrine changes to environmental cues that were previously paired with alcohol consumption. Acamprosate, the second medication, is an analogue of homocysteine acid, which is the structural analogue of L-glutamic acid. It meets criteria for an endogenous ligand that is active at the N-methyl-D-aspartate receptor. Acamprosate appears to lower neuronal excitability by reducing the postsynaptic efficacy of excitatory amino acid neurotransmitters.[21] In one 48-week randomized, double-blinded, placebo-controlled study, subjects who took acamprosate showed a higher continuous abstinence rate with fewer side effects than did the placebo-treated group.

Solvent Abuse

As troubling as alcohol use and abuse is among Native American youth, solvent abuse can be more troubling and life threatening. The earliest published reference to solvent abuse, glue sniffing, was made in 1959 and concerned the arrest of a number of children in Tucson, Arizona.[22, 23] Beauvais et al.[24] found that inhalants were among the first drugs used by Native American youth, even preceding the first time drunk.[2] Adolescents who are solvent abusers tend to come from homes marked by family turmoil, insufficient warmth and caring, poor communication, and a lack of respect.[22] The worst combination appears to be parents who model regular drug use and fail to provide a nurturing, supportive environment.

Three types of solvent users have been identified. There are (1) the experimental user, who uses solvents a few times and then rejects further use; (2) the recreational user, who uses solvents as a vehicle to socialization; and (3) the retreatist, who uses solvents in isolation and who appears to have other psychological disturbances.[1]

Solvent abuse has been associated with suicide attempts in the young[25] and death from cardiac arrhythmias, cardiac arrest, and suffocation as a consequence of laryngospasm.[1] A range of solvents have been reported to be abused: gasoline, antifreeze, butane gas, glues, paint thinner and stripper, correction fluid, lighter fuels, adhesives, sealants, acetone, ether, hair lacquer, nail polish remover, dyes, metal polish, cement, chloroform, and cleaning fluid.[22, 26]

The initial intoxicant experience appears to be marked by mild excitement and euphoria. Self-control and the will to direct behavior are rapidly lost at this stage, as is muscular coordination and orientation. Delusions of perception gradually give way to hallucinations, followed by stupor and unconsciousness.[22] Although most organ effects of these intoxicants appear to be transient, some are chronic, such as the permanent encephalopathies and cerebellar dysfunctions from gasoline sniffing. Other transient organ effects are type I renal tubular acidosis, chemical hepatitis, hematopoietic dysfunction, cardiac arrhythmias, pulmonary damage, and sensorimotor neuropathy.[22]

Telltale signs of solvent abusers are a strong smell of chemicals about a person and suspicious stains on skin areas of the mouth, nose, and hands. Treatment consists of abstention from solvents, evaluation and treatment for underlying psychiatric disturbances, and evaluation of the home situation by the local Child Protective Service for possible placement outside the home. From a social perspective, there is evidence that strong peer sanctions against the use of solvents and low peer encouragement of solvent use are strong preventive forces against chronic use.[1] Therefore, peer-generated sanctions against solvent use through education about the deleterious effects of chronic use may be effective in limiting recreational use.

Summary

Although alcohol and substance abuse is a national health problem, the impact is greatest among the underprivileged. Native American populations as a whole are one of the most impoverished groups in our nation. Coupled with dominant culture–enforced estrangement from cultural norms and lands, these factors provide all the necessary ingredients for the use of alcohol and drugs to momentarily quell group and individual tension. These tension-reduction tools carry their own destructive consequences of excessive use, including escalation of the harsh alcohol- and substance abuse–promoting demographics described in this chapter.

There is significant promise for a brighter future, as discussed previously in this chapter. The rates of substance abuse–related disorders in Native American women and adults older than 35 years remain low, and the rates of complication from alcohol use are significantly falling. With the introduction and acceptance of pharmacotherapeutic and psychotherapeutic treatments geared toward symptom remission, if not cure, and successful community interventions, the future for Native American tribes can be bright.

References

1. Young TJ. Substance use and abuse among Native Americans. Clin Psychol Rev 1988;8:125–138.
2. Gurnee CG, Vigil DE, Krill-Smith S, Crowley TJ. Substance abuse among American Indians in an urban treatment program. Am Indian Alask Native Ment Health Res 1990;3:17–26.
3. Barthwell AG. Cultural Considerations in the Management of Addictive Disease. In NS Miller, MS Gold, DE Smith (eds), Manual of Therapeutics for Addictions. New York: Wiley-Liss, 1997;246–254.
4. Myers HF, Kagawa-Singer M, Kumanyika SK, et al. Panel III: Behavioral risk factors related to chronic diseases in ethnic minorities. Health Psychol 1995;14:613–621.
5. Young TJ. Alcoholism prevention among Native American youth. Child Psychiatry Hum Dev 1993;24:41–47.
6. Booth BM, Blow FC, Cook CAL, et al. Age and ethnicity among hospitalized alcoholics: a nationwide study. Alcohol Clin Exp Res 1992;16:1029–1034.
7. Abbott PJ. American Indian and Alaska Native aboriginal use of alcohol in the United States. Am Indian Alsk Native Ment Health Res 1996;7:1–13.
8. Frances A, Pincus HA. Diagnostic and Statistical Manual of Mental Disorders (4th ed). Washington, DC: American Psychiatric Association, 1994.
9. Chao HM. Alcohol and the mystique of flushing. Alcohol Clin Exp Res 1995;19:104–109.
10. Rex DK, Bosron WF, Smialek JE, Li TK. Alcohol and aldehyde dehydrogenase isoenzymes in North American Indians. Alcohol Clin Exp Res 1985;9:147–152.
11. Wall TL, Garcia-Andrade C, Thomasson HR, et al. Alcohol dehydrogenase polymorphisms in Native Americans: identification of the ADH2*3 allele. Alcohol Alcohol 1997;32:129–132.
12. Secretary, U.S. Department of Health and Human Services. Eighth Special Report to the U.S. Congress on Alcohol and Health. 1993;28.
13. Morris RE, Harrison EA, Knox GW, et al. Health risk behavioral survey from 39 juvenile correctional facilities in the United States. J Adolesc Health 1995;17:334–344.
14. Juvela S. Prevalence of risk factors in spontaneous intracerebral hemorrhage and aneurysmal subarachnoid hemorrhage. Arch Neurol 1996;53:734–774.
15. Hommer D, Momenan R, Rawlings R, et al. Decreased corpus callosum size among alcoholic women. Arch Neurol 1996;53:359–366.
16. Fink A, Hays RD, Moore AA, Beck JC. Alcohol-related problems in older persons: determinants, consequences, and screening. Arch Intern Med 1996;156:1150–1156.
17. O'Malley SS, Jaffe AJ, Chang G, et al. Six-month follow-up of Naltrexone and psychotherapy for alcohol dependence. Arch Gen Psychiatry 1996;53:217–222.
18. Vaillant GE. A long-term follow-up of male alcohol abuse. Arch Gen Psychiatry 1996;53:243–254.
19. Westermeyer J, Peake E. Ten-year follow-up of alcoholic Native Americans in Minnesota. Am J Psychiatry 1983;140:189–194.
20. Flores PJ. Alcoholism treatment and the relationship of Native American cultural values to recovery. International J Addictions 1985–86;20:1707–1726.
21. Sass H, Soyka M, Mann K, Zieglgansberger W. Relapse prevention by acamprosate: results from a placebo-controlled study on alcohol dependence. Arch Gen Psychiatry 1996;53:673–680.
22. O'Connor DJ. A profile of solvent abuse in school children. J Child Psychol Psychiatry 1979;20:365–268.
23. Hershey CO, Miller S. Solvent abuse: a shift to adults. International J Addictions 1982;17:1085–1089.
24. Beauvais F, Oetting ER, Edwards RW. Trends in drug use of Indian adolescents living on reservations. Am J Drug Alcohol Abuse 1985;11:220–229.
25. Kirmayer LJ, Malus M, Boothroyd LJ. Suicide attempts among Inuit youth: a risk community survey of prevalence and risk factors. Acta Psychiatr Scand 1996;94:8–17.
26. Channer KS, Stanley S. Persistent visual hallucinations secondary to chronic solvent encephalopathy: case report and review of the literature. J Neurol Neurosurg Psychiatry 1983;46:83–86.

Chapter 35

Cross-cultural Aspects of Mental Health and Culture-Bound Illnesses

Yvette Roubideaux

Primary care providers working in Indian health facilities are commonly involved in the initial diagnosis and management of mental health disorders because many Indian mental health programs cannot meet the need for services in the communities they serve.[1] Primary care providers, who are trained from a Western medical perspective, often encounter mental health problems in their Native American patients that are influenced by the patient's traditional beliefs and culture. These mental health problems may be variations of disorders that are familiar to the provider, or they may be illnesses that are unique to the specific tribe or culture of the patient, which are commonly referred to as *culture-bound illnesses*.[2]

It is important for primary care providers to understand the cross-cultural aspects of mental illness in Native American patients so that they can effectively evaluate and manage these disorders. Providers should understand the differences between Western and traditional Indian perspectives in the role of culture in mental health and how these perspectives may influence the types of mental disorders they see in Native American patients. This chapter illustrates the cross-cultural aspects of mental health from the two perspectives and provides recommendations on the evaluation and management of mental health disorders in Native American patients.

Role of Culture in Mental Health: Western versus Traditional Indian Perspectives

From a Western medical perspective, mental health is generally viewed as separate from physical health. Mental health disorders are diagnosed and treated primarily by mental health professionals, such as psychiatrists and psychologists, who are trained to diagnose and treat these disorders separately from other providers who care for the patient's physical health. Often, mental health professionals practice in separate areas or buildings away from

other professionals who are trained to care for the patient's physical complaints. When primary care providers discover symptoms of mental illness in their patients, they often refer these patients to mental health professionals for further care. Although efforts are being made to train primary care providers to broaden their care of patients to include mental illness, the distinction between mental and physical health remains in Western medical training.

From a traditional Indian perspective, mental and physical health are not separate, and in fact, are closely connected. Health is generally defined as a balance of mind, body, and spirit, and illness results when there is an imbalance in any of these areas. Traditional Indian medicine providers, such as medicine men or healers, understand illness from this perspective and in the context of their particular culture or tribe. Traditional Indian medicines and ceremonies are often used to restore this balance of health. The traditional Indian perspective does not separate mental and physical health.

These differing perspectives influence the role of culture in the diagnosis and classification of mental illness. From a Western perspective, mental health professionals assign diagnoses to patients based on an international classification system found in the *Diagnostic and Statistical Manual of Mental Disorders*, 4th Edition (*DSM-IV*).[3] The diagnoses are based on groups of symptoms that define specific disorders, which are assumed to exist across cultures. Groups of symptoms that do not fit into the usual categories and are thought to be unique to certain cultures are classified as "culture-bound illnesses" and are placed in a glossary at the end of *DSM-IV*. In the literature on the role of culture in mental illness, various authors disagree on the classification and terminology of diseases that seem to be influenced or related to the culture of the individual patient.[2, 4–6] As a result, the mental health field has attempted to address the role of culture in *DSM-IV* by including an appendix that outlines a way to evaluate and report the impact of a patient's culture on his or her mental health diagnoses. This "cultural formulation" is clearly separated from the usual diagnostic categories.

From a traditional Indian perspective, the role of culture in the diagnosis of mental illness is fundamental because cultural beliefs often explain the etiology of symptoms and illness. Traditional healers in each tribe or community often diagnose illness based on both the symptoms of the patient and an understanding of the potential etiology of these symptoms, which is usually based in the beliefs of their culture or tribe. For example, in some tribes, illness may be caused by not following traditional ways, witchcraft or hexes by others, something done to or by the patient, or a significant event, such as the death of a relative. These illnesses are often given names in the language of that particular tribe, and these names are often used in the community to refer to patients with these conditions. Traditional healers may have specific medicines or ceremonies to treat each condition, and many treatments have been used by traditional healers for generations.

It is important for the provider to note that these perspectives are generalizations and that the perspectives of individual Native American patients may vary greatly, depending on the extent of their beliefs in their traditional culture. Native Americans are a diverse group of individuals, with a spectrum of beliefs that includes very traditional patients, patients with a combination of traditional and Western beliefs, and patients who are very acculturated into Western society and have little or no knowledge of their traditional culture. Native American patients from different tribes or regions of the country may not share the same beliefs. Because of this spectrum of beliefs, the types of mental illnesses in Native American patients can vary greatly. Native American patients with symptoms of mental illness can present with typical Western disorders, illnesses similar to Western disorders that have different names in the patient's tribal language, illnesses with some atypical symptoms or etiologies with a cultural basis, or culture-bound illnesses.

For example, depression is a common mental illness found in all cultures, and many Native American patients are found to be depressed by their Western medical providers. For some patients, their symptoms fit the *DSM-IV* classification of depression. In some tribes, the symptoms typical of depression have a name in the tribal language, such as *wacinko*, found in the Oglala Sioux culture, which describes a condition similar to reactive depression.[7] In other tribes, the symptoms of depression may be accompanied by unusual symptoms, such as visions or hallucinations of a dead relative, as is seen in some members of the Hopi tribe during periods of mourning.[7] In cases such as these, the cause of the depression is linked to a specific etiology, such as the death of a relative. In some tribes, the depressive symptoms are a part of

unique conditions, such as the spirit sickness of the Salish tribe[8] or the ghost illness of the Navajo tribe.[9] These conditions are caused by the death of a relative and, in their most extreme form, may lead to the patient's own death. Although depressive symptoms are present in all these conditions, the role of culture is much more prominent in the Indian-identified conditions, with their own cultural names, meanings, and types of symptoms. Some of these illnesses may not respond to the usual Western treatments for depression and may require traditional Indian medicines or ceremonies to cure.

It is therefore not surprising that a primary care provider trained in Western medicine may have difficulty evaluating and managing mental illness in Native American patients. Some patients may present with symptoms that fit the provider's Western concept of illness, such as depression, but the patient may refer to these symptoms with a different name or present with some atypical symptoms. Some patients may present with symptoms that do not fit Western disease classifications, and the provider may actually be dealing with a unique culture-bound illness. In addition, because some of these mental health problems may be linked to causes or etiologies related to cultural beliefs, they might be more effectively treated by a traditional healer. Therefore, the primary care provider must learn about the cross-cultural aspects of mental health disorders in Native American patients to effectively evaluate and manage these illnesses.

Approach to the Native American Patient: Evaluation and Management

Primary care providers can use a variety of strategies to help evaluate and manage mental illness in their Native American patients. The provider must first learn as much as possible about the traditional and cultural beliefs of the local community or tribe. Ideally, Indian health facilities provide an orientation to all new employees on the predominant cultural beliefs and traditions of their patient population, but many facilities do not have this type of orientation available. In these cases, the primary care provider must learn about the local culture from more experienced providers, ancillary and support staff, and community members. The facility staff may know of a local traditional healer who is willing to speak with new providers. Often, the behavioral health or mental health department in the facility is also familiar with the local culture. Even though most providers can learn this information over time on their own, it is preferable to have a formal orientation to the culture and traditional beliefs of the local culture. Providers should encourage their facility directors to develop this type of orientation for all employees.

It is also important for primary care providers to recognize that they were trained from a Western medical perspective and that their patients may have a completely different perspective on illness, as detailed in the previous section. A common mistake of new Indian health providers is to ignore or minimize the role of culture in their patient's medical and mental health problems, even though the patient may mention that he or she believes his or her illness has a cultural cause. If a provider reacts in a judgmental or negative manner, the patient may lose confidence and trust in the provider and may not return to that provider in the future. Providers must be aware of the role of culture in their patient's health problems, so that they can react in a nonjudgmental manner and gain the confidence of their patients.

Primary care providers must also learn to recognize when culture may have a role in their patients' symptoms. Although the patient may mention his or her beliefs about the role of culture in his or her symptoms, most patients do not offer this information unless asked. The primary care provider must therefore recognize when a patient's symptoms seem unusual or do not fit usual patterns of illness. If the provider has taken the time to learn about local patterns of illness, he or she may recognize specific symptoms of culture-bound illnesses. The primary care provider may also consider the role of culture with patients who have symptoms of mental illness that are not responding to the usual Western treatments. Once the provider suspects that culture may have a role in the patient's symptoms, it is important for the provider to discuss this with the patient and to ask appropriate questions in a nonjudgmental manner. If the provider has previously established trust with this patient, then the conversation is usually quite helpful.

Published guidelines in the mental health and medical literature detail how to ask patients about their cultural beliefs and how these beliefs may influence their health. The *DSM-IV* contains an "Outline for Cultural Formulation," which describes a systematic way to review the "cultural identity of the individual, cultural explanations of the individual's illness, cultural factors related to psychosocial environment and levels of functioning, cultural elements of the relationship between the individual and the clinician, and an overall cultural assessment for diagnosis and care."[3] An example of using this formulation in the psychiatric diagnosis of a Native American patient is listed in the references.[10] Primary care providers may not have the time during routine clinic visits to develop such an extensive evaluation.

Another author has developed a framework of questions about spirituality that a primary care physician can ask patients, organizing them into a mnemonic called *SPIRIT*[11] (*s*piritual belief system, *p*ersonal spirituality, *i*ntegration with spiritual community, *r*itualized practices and restrictions, *i*mplications for medical care, *t*erminal events planning). (For further discussion of the specific questions related to this mnemonic, please refer to Table 6-2.) This mnemonic helps the primary care provider to remember what types of questions to ask about the patient's culture and spirituality during the medical history; it is not meant to be completed in one office visit. The provider is encouraged to gather this type of information over time or when it is particularly relevant to the care of the patient.

Both guidelines encourage providers to ask the patient about his or her cultural beliefs and how these beliefs may affect his or her health. When caring for Native American patients, the primary care provider can ask about the degree to which the patient believes in and follows his or her traditional culture and whether he or she thinks that his or her symptoms are related to his or her cultural beliefs. Asking patients what they think might be causing their symptoms gives them an opportunity to mention culturally relevant causes. The provider can clarify these beliefs with further questions and discuss potential treatments that address these beliefs.

Management of mental illness in Native Americans may involve both Western and traditional Indian therapies. For the patients who are more acculturated, Western treatments, such as counseling and psychoactive drugs, may be the only types of treatments needed. If the patient believes that his or her traditional culture plays a role in his or her symptoms, then traditional Indian treatments may be needed in addition to, or instead of, Western treatments. Of course, the primary care provider cannot provide traditional Indian treatments but can help patients by referring them to appropriate resources. Traditional healers from the patient's tribe or mental health programs and treatment centers that provide traditional approaches to treatment of mental disorders can be used. An example of integrating the local culture into mental health services is provided in the references.[12] Primary care providers may need to do some extra homework to find these resources, but knowledge of these resources is necessary to help patients return to a state of good mental health. More experienced providers and community members can usually recommend resources for traditional Indian healing in the local community.

Summary and Key Points

Primary care providers working in Indian health must understand the cross-cultural aspects of mental health in their Native American patients to effectively evaluate and manage their symptoms of mental illness. In some cases, these patients have symptoms typical of Western mental disorders and respond to Western treatments. Some Native American patients have symptoms that are influenced by their traditional cultural beliefs, however, and these patients may require traditional Indian treatments in addition to the usual therapy. Less commonly, patients may present with symptoms that are unique to their own culture (culture-bound illnesses) and that require traditional Indian medicines or ceremonies.

Primary providers can effectively evaluate and manage symptoms of mental illness that are influenced by the patient's culture by doing the following:

- Recognizing Western and traditional Indian perspectives of mental illness
- Learning about the role of culture in mental disorders, including culture-bound illnesses, in the local tribal community
- Learning how to recognize when culture may have a role in an individual patient's symptoms
- Learning how to evaluate an individual patient's perspective on the role of his or her cultural beliefs in his or her symptoms
- Learning how to refer patients to local resources that provide traditional Indian treatments, such as traditional healers or mental health services and treatment programs that include traditional Indian treatment methods
- Encouraging Indian health facilities to orient new providers on the culture and beliefs of the local community or tribes

References

1. Walker RD, Lambert MD, Walker PS, Kivlahan DR. Treatment implications of comorbid psychopathology in American Indians and Alaska Natives. Cult Med Psychiatry 1993;16:555–572.
2. Levine RE, Gaw AC. Culture-bound syndromes. Psychiatr Clin North Am 1995;18:523–536.
3. American Psychiatric Association. Diagnostic and Statistical Manual of Mental Disorders (4th ed). Washington, DC: American Psychiatric Association, 1994.
4. Hahn RA. Culture-bound syndromes unbound. Soc Sci Med 1985;21:165–171.
5. Simons RC, Hughes CC. The Culture-Bound Syndromes. Dordrecht, Holland: Reidel, 1985;3–38.
6. Prince R, Tcheng-Laroche F. Culture-bound syndromes and international disease classifications. Cult Med Psychiatry 1987;11:3–19.
7. O'Nell TD. Psychiatric investigations among American Indians and Alaska Natives: a critical review. Cult Med Psychiatry 1989;13:51–87.
8. Grossman DC, Putsch RW, Inui TS. The meaning of death to adolescents in an American Indian community. Fam Med 1993;25:593–597.
9. Putsch RW. Ghost illness: a cross-cultural experience with the expression of a non-Western tradition in clinical practice. Am Indian Alsk Native Ment Health Res 1988;2:6–26.
10. Fleming CM. Cultural formulation of psychiatric diagnosis. Case no. 01. An American Indian woman suffering from depression, alcoholism and childhood trauma. Cult Med Psychiatry 1996;20:145–154.
11. Maugans TA. The spiritual history. Arch Fam Med 1996;5:11–16.
12. Guilmet GM, Whited DL. Cultural lessons for clinical mental health practice in the Puyallup tribal community. Am Indian Alsk Native Ment Health Res 1987;1:32–49.

Part XI
Pediatric and Adolescent Diseases

Chapter 36
Injury Prevention

David C. Grossman

Injuries were the third leading cause of death to American Indians (AIs) and Alaska Natives (ANs) residing in Indian Health Service (IHS) areas and the fourth leading cause of morbidity and hospitalizations for all ages in 1994. Injuries are the leading cause of death for AIs and ANs ages 1–44 years. The overall age-adjusted injury mortality rates are three to four times higher than those of the general U.S. population, thereby making injury control an urgent priority for the IHS and tribes.[1–3] The control of injuries involves interventions at each phase: prevention, acute care, and rehabilitation. This chapter focuses on prevention strategies that physicians and midlevel providers can use in the office and the community.

There is considerable variation in the incidence of specific types of injuries between IHS areas.[4] The lowest rate of unintentional injury deaths is in the California area (37 per 100,000 population) and the highest is in the Alaska area (143 per 100,000). Rates of individual mechanisms of injury also vary considerably and are influenced by many factors. For example, the rate of motor vehicle deaths is much lower in Alaska than in the Navajo or Aberdeen, South Dakota, areas. Because of the high degree of variation, prevention activities must be tailored to the local epidemiology of injury. This information can be obtained from the National Center for Injury Prevention and Control at the Centers for Disease Control and Prevention or the IHS Injury Prevention Program.

Health care providers involved in the prevention of injury must carefully consider the compatibility of local cultural beliefs with approaches to injury prevention, especially in the communication of information. European and American cultural approaches to injury prevention depend heavily on the communication of information about the magnitude of risk reduction achieved with certain behaviors. Certain tribal cultures may associate individual risk assessment by clinicians with the hastening of injury or illness. For example, the counseling of a traditional Navajo mother about the use of car seats should be framed in terms of broad protective value ("It saves babies' lives") rather than the elevated risk associated with individual nonuse ("Your infant may die or be seriously injured if you don't use this seat"). Some tribal cultures are particularly sensitive to the impact of death-related thinking and prefer not to engage in conversation on this subject.

The main approaches to injury prevention are education and persuasion, legislation, and environmental (physical and social) changes.[5, 6] Most often, clinicians try to educate and persuade their patients to adopt preventive measures. In the pediatric office setting, the effectiveness of this clinical activity in changing behavior has been demonstrated in the prevention of some types of injuries; most of these evaluations have focused on the promotion of car safety seats. Much less is known about the effectiveness of injury prevention counseling in adult clinical settings. Ideally, clinicians' advice is reinforced in a consistent manner in other settings (e.g., public health nurses, media, police) to maximize its potency.

Clinicians working in IHS or tribal health programs also should be aware of the activities of the injury prevention specialists in their area. Centered in the environmental health program, these specialists are very active in the promotion of community-based programs to prevent injury. Each IHS area has an injury prevention specialist, and many areas have additional personnel working at local levels on these projects.[7, 8] The program is sustained by a fellowship training program for active IHS and tribal employees interested in developing skills to promote injury prevention and evaluate the effect of interventions. Both clinicians and nonclinicians have participated in the fellowship, and some have developed highly sophisticated projects as a part of the fellowship.

The following sections address specific strategies that clinicians in AI and AN settings may use to promote injury prevention both from the office and at the community level.

Motor Vehicle–Related Injuries

Injuries from motor vehicle crashes constitute the single biggest cause of death among Native Americans younger than age 45 years. Because of the highly rural environment in which many Native Americans live and the higher rates of behavioral risk factors associated with occupant injuries, Native Americans are at substantially higher risk of these types of injuries.[9, 10] The vast proportion of individuals who die from motor vehicle collisions are vehicle occupants. The remainder are pedestrians, bicyclists, and motorcyclists. Physicians and other providers may have great influence on reducing occupant injuries by targeting two key behaviors with their patients: alcohol use while driving and use of seat belts or car seats. Addressing alcohol use among patients is a well-recognized need for clinicians working with Native Americans, but the magnitude of the association between intoxication and crash injuries requires clinicians to be aggressive by testing for the presence of alcohol and initiating early intervention in the emergency department and hospital. Brief interventions by clinicians may be highly cost-effective for drinkers who are not already dependent on alcohol. These have been proved to be efficacious in numerous randomized controlled trials.[5] They may be particularly effective with younger drivers after a first-time incident of drunk driving.

Clinicians can use clinical encounters to spend time discussing occupant safety measures and the use of restraints while traveling in motor vehicles. There is some evidence from pediatric studies that patients respond positively to office-based interventions to promote restraint use. Rather than using a purely risk-based approach to counseling (e.g., "It has been shown that seat belts reduce the risk of serious injury and death by approximately 40%"), providers may obtain a more positive response to specific examples and stories of how seat belts have saved lives. Specific practices of belt use should be emphasized, for example, noting that seat belts are a supplemental restraint device and should always be used, regardless of the presence of an airbag. The high rate of child car seat misuse requires efforts from clinicians and community health personnel to assist parents with proper car seat use. In tribes that use traditional cradle boards for children, special crash tests have shown that the cradle board is not an effective safety device to protect infants; their use in cars should be strongly discouraged. Finally, the placement of passengers in the rear of pickup trucks is associated with a high risk of injury and also should be strongly discouraged. The IHS area injury specialists may be of special assistance in these efforts.

Efforts to promote occupant safety can be potentiated by collaborative efforts with community health, police personnel, and tribal councils to plan health promotion and legal interventions to reduce drunk driving and boost the rate of seat-belt use. On many reservations, state laws on the use of seat belts and driver intoxication are not enforced because of respect for the legal autonomy of Indian nations. Some tribes have instituted their own legal statutes to address these issues, but many have not. Clinicians can help to serve as advocates and advisors to tribal councils as they begin to address the passage and enforcement of injury control measures.[11]

Pedestrian injuries are disproportionately high on many Indian reservations. Important risk factors include the high exposure of pedestrians to rural roads without sidewalks, alcohol use by pedestrians, and the lack of lighting on rural roads.[12] Potentially successful interventions will likely require environmental improvements in the walking environment of pedestrians and reducing the likelihood that intoxicated pedestrians are walking along roadways. Some successful interventions for the prevention of all types of crash injuries in Indian communities have tracked the location of pedestrian collisions and devised specific interventions where clusters appear to occur.

Bicycle injuries claim a disproportionate number of children as victims. Most who die of bicycle-related injuries die of a head injury. Approximately 90% of fatally injured bicyclists have been struck by motor vehicles. Bicycle helmets have been shown to lead to a reduction of serious brain injuries by 85%, among the most effective of any type of preventive measure. Rates of bicycle helmet use have been shown to be boosted by several measures, such as laws mandating usage (accompanied by enforcement) and community-based campaigns promoting voluntary helmet use (using clinicians as key purveyors of safety messages). Many communities have successfully promoted helmets by providing economic incentives to families and by providing discount coupons or free helmets from clinical sites. Given the high level of effectiveness of helmets, their promotion must be a priority for clinicians and injury control personnel in Native communities.

Fire- and Burn-Related Injuries

The risk of injury and death from burns and fire are disproportionately high among Native Americans. The key independent risk factors associated with house fires are the presence of smokers and alcohol-impaired persons in the household, residence in a mobile home structure, and the absence of a smoke detector. Probable additional risk factors present in many Native American households are the use of open fires for cooking and heating and the use of portable fuel-based heaters. Clinicians are in an excellent position to influence many of these risk factors in their daily encounters with patients. Smoking cessation is an independently worthy goal, but an intermediate goal that would likely lead to a reduction in burn risk is to avoid smoking indoors, thus decreasing the likelihood that a smoker, especially if intoxicated, would fall asleep in a chair or in bed. Smoke detectors are widely prevalent in most communities, but many are not functional due to intentional disarming or battery failure. Efforts to boost the use and maintenance of functional smoke detectors are a continuing priority for injury control specialists.[13] Community-based programs that distribute free smoke detectors have led to a substantial decrease in morbidity and mortality from house fires.

The most common mechanism of nonfatal burns is scalding liquids. These result from high water temperatures in hot water heaters and from the spill of beverages and food. Many states require hot water heaters to have a preset temperature of no more than 120°F to prevent scald burns, especially to children, but some do not, and many adults raise the thermostat to higher temperatures. Clinicians treating children and the elderly must emphasize the importance of these measures to reduce scald burns. No currently available strategies have proved successful in reducing other types of scald burns.

Drowning

Rates of drowning are also disproportionately high among Native Americans, both in coastal and inland regions. One mechanism of drowning in the general population, pool drownings, are probably unusual in AI communities. Extrapolation of risk factor studies in the general population may not be completely useful for Native Americans living on reservations because of the distinctly different environments, but several probable risk factors likely are shared by AI and AN populations. These include the use of alcohol on boats or near open water, poor swimming abilities, and lifejacket nonuse. Little is known about the efficacy of any intervention that is specifically aimed at drowning prevention, but there is some evidence that swimming lessons strengthen the swimming skills of preschool children. Clinicians working in areas adjacent to open waters and rivers should strongly urge patients to acquire and use personal flotation devices when boating; children without swimming skills should use them while swimming. Some AN communities have successfully promoted the use of float coats, for flotation and warmth, among Native fishermen on rivers. Early reports suggest that this promotional campaign may be leading to a significant decrease in the rate of drowning in these areas.

Other Native communities have instituted swimming lessons using portable pools as a preventive measure. Until further evidence is available, this is a worthwhile strategy that clinicians should be promoting in their communities.

Firearm Injuries

Firearm injuries are either intentional (resulting from assault or suicide attempt) or unintentional (accidental). Although Native Americans have generally higher rates of intentional injury deaths than the general population, the rates of firearm-related deaths are only approximately 0.7 times the general U.S. rate. Firearm involvement in homicides and suicides is also lower than the general U.S. rate. Despite lower absolute rates, clinicians must be aware that the presence of a firearm in the household elevates the risk of both homicide and suicide in the household, independent of other risk factors. The prevalence of long guns (rifles and shotguns) in Native American households is thought to be high in certain areas because of the reliance on guns for hunting. The prevalence of household handguns in Native American communities is unknown.

Clinicians can help to prevent firearm injuries by informing patients of the potential risks in a culturally acceptable manner. Clearly, removing guns from the household leads to the greatest risk reduction. During clinical encounters with patients who are actively suicidal or who have been domestic assault victims, the clinical staff should inquire about the presence of firearms in the home. In these cases, all efforts should be made to remove the weapons, with assistance from the police. Patients wishing to maintain possession of firearms should be counseled on proper storage techniques to prevent unauthorized access to the weapons by children, adolescents, or other high-risk family members. Probably the most cost-effective storage measure for rifles and shotguns is using a trigger lock and then locking the rifle in a cabinet or safe. Trigger locks are widely available and can be purchased for $10–15. For handguns, several options are available. These include the handgun lockbox, a small safe with a push-button combination that allows quick access without a key. These devices are particularly attractive to patients who keep a handgun for protection, but they are relatively expensive. Trigger locks are a cheaper method, but they do not conceal the gun from view nor do they allow quick access. Some trigger locks can be defeated by children.

Summary

In summary, injuries are the leading cause of death for children and young adults living in Native American communities. Many effective prevention strategies exist and can be used in both clinic and community settings. Prevention counseling is culturally challenging and requires knowledge of local belief systems and epidemiology. Many successful injury-prevention projects have been implemented in Native American communities, but further progress requires more active involvement of clinicians who have contact with patients on a daily basis.

References

1. Baker SP, O'Neill B, Ginsburg MJ, Li G. The Injury Fact Book (2nd ed). New York: Oxford University Press, 1992.
2. Berger LR, Kitzes J. Injuries to children in a Native American community. Pediatrics 1989;84:152–156.
3. Sugarman JR, Grossman DC. Trauma among American Indians in an urban county. Pub Health Rep 1996;111: 321–327.
4. Wallace LJD, Kirk ML, Houston B, et al. Injury Mortality Atlas of Indian Health Service Areas, 1979–1987. Atlanta: Centers for Disease Control and Prevention, 1993.
5. Rivara FP, Grossman DC, Cummings P. Injury prevention [first of two parts]. N Engl J Med 1997;338:543–548.
6. Rivara FP, Grossman DC, Cummings P. Injury prevention [second of two parts]. N Engl J Med 1997;338: 613–618.
7. Smith RJ. IHS fellows program aimed at lowering injuries, deaths of Indians, Alaska Natives. Pub Health Rep 1988;103:204.
8. Robertson LS. Community injury control programs of the Indian Health Service: an early assessment. Pub Health Rep 1986;101:632–637.
9. Grossman DC, Sugarman JR, Fox C, Moran J. Motor-vehicle crash-injury risk factors among American Indians. Accid Anal Prev 1997;29:313–319.
10. Mahoney MC. Fatal motor vehicle traffic accidents among Native Americans. Am J Prev Med 1991;7: 112–116.
11. Centers for Disease Control and Prevention. Safety belt use and motor vehicle related injuries: Navajo nation, 1988–91. MMWR Morb Mortal Wkly Rep 1992;41: 705–708.
12. Gallaher MM, Fleming DW, Berger LR, Sewell CM. Pedestrian and hypothermia deaths among Native Americans in New Mexico: between bar and home. JAMA 1992;267:1345–1348.
13. Kuklinski DM, Berger LR, Weaver JR. Smoke detector nuisance alarms: a field study in a Native American community. NFPA J 1996;Sept/Oct:65–72.

Chapter 37
Fetal Alcohol Syndrome

David Kessler

Alcohol is a known teratogen, and it has a dose-related effect on the developing fetus. The spectrum of defects is wide, with some infants severely affected and others much more subtly so. *Fetal alcohol syndrome* (FAS) is the term used to describe children who meet certain criteria; it is the most dramatic pattern of malformation related to maternal alcohol abuse. The term *fetal alcohol effect* was popular for children who met only some of the criteria for FAS. It has fallen out of favor because many of the nonspecific effects of alcohol are associated with other risk factors as well. Instead, *suspected fetal alcohol effects* or *in utero alcohol exposure* is used to describe a child with developmental disabilities that may be related to maternal alcohol consumption.

The minimal criteria for diagnosing FAS include the following:

- Central nervous system involvement; such as developmental delays, intellectual deficits, microencephaly, or neurologic abnormalities (e.g., ptosis, low tone, and poor suck)
- Characteristic craniofacial abnormalities with at least two of the following signs: micro-ophthalmia, short palpebral fissures, poorly developed philtrum, thin upper lip, flat nasal bridge, short upturned nose
- Prenatal or postnatal growth delay (i.e., weight, length, or head circumference below the tenth percentile)

Many other less specific malformations present in most children with FAS. These include cardiovascular anomalies (ventricular septal defect, atrial septal defect, coarctation of the aorta), skeletal abnormalities (flexion contractions at the elbows, congenital hip dislocations, camptodactyly, tapering terminal phalanges with hyperplastic nails, foot position defects, altered palmar crease pattern), and other defects (cleft lip or palate, myopia, strabismus, dental malocclusion, renal anomalies, hearing loss). The behavior of children with FAS is often

characteristic: Infants tend to be irritable and restless, to cry excessively, or to have disturbed sleep patterns. Their poor suck leads to feeding difficulties, and failure to thrive is common. Older children may be hyperactive and have attention deficits, language dysfunction, and perceptual problems. Adolescents often have problems with judgment, resulting in maladaptive behaviors.[1] Their average IQ is low (though there is a wide range), and they tend to do poorly in academic subjects (especially mathematics).

The variability in the effects of alcohol is thought to be due to differences in blood alcohol concentration at critical stages of fetal development and to differences in tissue susceptibility.[2] The amount of alcohol consumed, as well as the timing, duration, and rate of its use are some of the variables of maternal alcohol consumption that affect the fetus. The brain is probably most vulnerable in the third trimester because this is the time of its most rapid growth and organization. Some problems reflect permanent damage and thus persist; others represent delays in development and diminish with time. There is little doubt that some children exposed to alcohol show only some of the signs of FAS rather than the entire constellation of signs. However, there is no way to confirm or deny this possibility at present. There are many other causes of the developmental delay and other defects found in FAS. It may be difficult, for example, to differentiate between the effects of alcohol and the effects of anticonvulsant therapy, or of neglect and deprivation. For all these reasons, it is extremely important that the diagnosis of FAS be made by a physician experienced in making this diagnosis, preferably a dysmorphologist. It is clearly not useful if every child of an alcoholic mother is automatically labeled as having FAS.

In regard to FAS among Native Americans, the clinical features of FAS are identical to those seen in other racial groups.[3] Although some Indians have broad faces with relatively low nasal bridges, these features rarely cause confusion in making the diagnosis, even in new-borns. It is often believed that the incidence of FAS is higher among Native Americans than the general population. In fact, there are large variations in incidence among different tribes, and all figures must be approached with some caution. The stereotype of the "drunken Indian," along with unreliable criteria and very questionable diagnoses, make some investigations worthless. There may be an ascertainment bias even in the better community-wide screening, records, follow-up, and diagnosis in various Indian communities. The most reliable surveys show an incidence of FAS of 1–2 per 1,000 among the Navajo and pueblo groups (JM Aase, personal communication), which is identical to that in the general U.S. population. The Plains Indians do appear to have an incidence 7–10 times higher than average; one study estimated it at 10.3 per 1,000 births. It is therefore crucial to assess the rate in a specific tribe rather than using estimates in other groups.

FAS cannot be treated after the fact. Working with affected children can be extremely frustrating and difficult. Recommendations for the management of such children include early intervention services; education of parents and the entire family; frequent developmental, behavioral, and neurologic evaluations; and comprehensive medical attention. Management of the environment seems to have better results than specific treatment of the child; for example, limiting distractions, providing consistent schedules and surroundings, giving positive reinforcement, and disciplining immediately.

FAS is completely preventable. The full-blown syndrome has not been seen in babies born to women who drink less than 30 ml absolute alcohol per day. No safe level of alcohol consumption among pregnant women has been established, however, hence the recommendation for complete abstinence. Whenever drinking stops, the chances of having a healthy baby improve. Several studies have shown that babies born to mothers who reduce their drinking before the third trimester have fewer problems than do those born to women who drink throughout the pregnancy. When drinking ceases, the direct toxic effects of alcohol diminish, maternal nutrition tends to improve, and an opportunity is provided for fetal catch-up growth and healing. Recommendations for helping pregnant women to quit drinking include education (e.g., on the effects of alcohol on the fetus), accentuating the positive (e.g., increased chances of a healthy baby, feeling better when not drinking), avoiding criticism that could raise anxiety and lead to increased alcohol intake, assistance with social and emotional problems, and referral for specialized alcohol treatment if indicated. Incarceration of chronic drinkers for the duration of their pregnancy is advocated by some, but this entails treading a legal slippery slope that is being challenged at several levels of the judicial system. In general, it has been found that the personal relationship between the high-risk mother and the individual trying to help seems to be the most important factor in achieving abstinence. Attention to tribe-specific cultural factors that relate to childbearing and alcohol use is crucial. Public health measures are extremely important in attempts to prevent FAS. It is essential to educate health care providers, social service workers, community health representatives, teachers, and counselors about the effects of alcohol use by women. Attempting to define a subpopulation at high risk has great importance because it allows concentration of resources directed at this group.

The rates of alcohol use during pregnancy are rising throughout the country.[4] In 1995, 16% of pregnant women admitted to drinking at least once in the previous month, whereas in 1991, the rate was 12%. Rates of frequent drinking in the two study periods (defined as consumption of an average of 7 or more drinks per week or five or more drinks on at least one occasion), were 3.5% and 0.8%, respectively. The economic cost of treating only the medical complications of FAS has been estimated at approximately $350 million per year; this does not include educational costs, nor does it begin to estimate pain and suffering. Clearly, much work remains to be done in preventing this syndrome.

References

1. Streissguth AP, Aase JM, Clarren SK, et al. Fetal alcohol syndrome in adolescents and adults. JAMA 1991;265:1961–1967.
2. Phillips D, Henderson GI, Schenker S. Pathogenesis of fetal alcohol syndrome. Alcohol Health Res World 1989;13:219–223.
3. Aase JM. The fetal alcohol syndrome in American Indians: a high risk group. Neurobehav Toxicol Teratol 1981;3:153–155.
4. Centers for Disease Control and Prevention. Alcohol consumption among pregnant and childbearing-aged women. MMWR Morb Mortal Wkly Rep 1997;46:346.

Part XII
Nutrition

Chapter 38
Nutritional Problems

Nicolette I. Teufel

In the United States, nutritional problems are defined relative to the dietary recommendations developed for Americans in the 1990s by the U.S. Department of Agriculture (USDA), the U.S. Department of Health and Human Services (USDHHS), and the National Research Council (NRC). The Food Guide Pyramid, developed by the USDA and the USDHHS, and the recommended dietary allowances (RDAs), developed by the NRC, are tools to guide food choices to meet or exceed the nutritional needs of healthy people. Relative to these guidelines, the primary nutritional problems among Native Americans at the end of the twentieth century are these:

- Energy (calorie) intake exceeding energy needs
- High total fat intake (more than 30% of total caloric intake)
- High intake of alcohol (> 2 drinks/day or 14 drinks/week
- Low intake of dietary fiber (<20 g/day)
- Low intake of iron (<10 mg/day)
- Low intake of calcium (<1,200 mg/day)
- Low intake of vitamin A (<800 µg retinal equivalent mg/day)
- Low intake of vitamin C (<60 mg/day)

Intake of protein and other nutrients is generally adequate (75% or more of the RDAs).

Epidemiology of Food Behaviors and Nutrient Intake of Native Americans

Medical reports and surveys conducted from the 1860s to 1940 indicated that undernutrition was the primary nutritional problem of Native Americans.[1–6] Although the severity of the problem had eased by the mid-1900s, selected accounts of stunted growth, kwashiorkor (protein-calorie malnutrition), and marasmus (calorie malnutrition) in remote reservation locations continued through the 1970s.[7–10] By the 1960s, reports of overnutrition, specifically energy (calories), and subsequent obesity began to escalate.[11–15] By the mid-1980s and through the 1990s, diet and anthropometric studies conducted in tribes across the country indicated that the proportion of excessive energy and fat intake relative to the RDAs and rates of obesity are higher among Native Americans than among other U.S. populations.[16–21] In some cases, these studies revealed that although energy intake is high, nutrient quality is low, which contributes to deficiencies in iron, calcium, and some vitamins.[22–28]

Nutritional reports have been coupled with observations of low levels of physical activity and low energy requirements. This trend toward a more sedentary lifestyle reflects employment in jobs that are not physically demanding, absence of community recreation facilities, and increased reliance on a cash economy and labor-saving technology. These changes reduce the need to walk long distances, chop wood, and maintain traditional subsistence practices, such as farming, hunting, fishing, and gathering.

With the advent of social and technological change, all U.S. populations have been confronted with the health consequences of overnutrition, poor nutrient density, and inactivity. For Native Americans, particularly those relocated to reservations, this process of cultural change has been unique. Abrupt lifestyle changes have often occurred in isolation, separate from mainstream America, and were coupled with the threat of starvation and extinction. Shifts in traditional subsistence activities led to periods of undernutrition and starvation that today affect cultural perspectives of appropriate body size and food restriction and reinforce food as a symbol of strength and survival.[29, 30] Federal food assistance programs, both historically (e.g., military rations) and currently (e.g., the Women, Infants and Children's Program, the USDA Food Commodity Program, and the USDA Food Stamp Program), have

Table 38-1. Factors Influencing Native American Food Choices and Nutrient Intakes

Income level relative to household size
Access to food stores, including
    Proximity to stores
    Access to reliable transportation
Food stores vary from trading posts and small local convenience stores that carry predominantly canned foods, soft drinks, prepackaged snack foods, and other items having a long shelf life to supermarkets offering a wide selection of fresh and frozen foods, as well as "designer foods" (e.g., low-fat and low-sugar selections)
Reliance on food assistance programs, such as
    Supplemental Food Program for Women, Infants, and Children (WIC)
    United States Department of Agriculture (USDA) Food Commodity Program
    USDA Food Stamp Program
    Tribal feeding and food assistance programs
Availability of cooking facilities, which is influenced by
    Access to electricity and gas to maintain a functional oven and range
    Reliance on wood cooking stoves
    Access and use of other appliances (hot plate, microwave)
Availability of reliable refrigeration
Adherence to traditional food practices, including
    Use and availability of wild food sources
    Use of and familiarity with traditional food preparation techniques
    Use of and familiarity with traditional food preservation techniques
Cultural food preferences and ideas of "healthy" foods
Historic experience with food insecurity, undernutrition, and starvation, which influences cultural perspectives of appropriate body size and food restriction
Quality and taste of water supply, which influences sugared beverage consumption
Impact of local nutrition education and intervention programs

encouraged rapid acceptance of non-Native foods. High mineral content and the general poor taste of some reservation and rural water supplies contribute to the frequent use of sugar beverage powders to cover the taste of the water and, more recently, to the high consumption of soda drinks.[31] Most important, many Native Americans lack the social and economic power to change the environmental conditions that support poor nutrition and inactivity.

At the end of the twentieth century, nutrient intake of Native Americans across the country varies, but notable patterns emerge from nutritional studies and dietary reports. These patterns reflect an adaptation to food insecurity and loss of traditional resources and an emphasis on adequate energy and protein intake. In the twentieth cen-

tury, the following food choices and cooking practices have increasingly influenced Native American nutrient intake:

1. Meat and other high-protein foods, such as beans, have social importance and often take precedence over fruits and vegetables.
2. Foods are fried to enhance flavor, to use fat products (e.g., salt pork, lard, and butter) provided through historic and contemporary food assistance programs, and to continue a familiar style of cooking over a fire or range (baking is generally not a daily method of food preparation and often is done in groups or for special occasions, or both).
3. Reliance on wild plant and animal foods has decreased because the biodensity of reservation lands, a fraction of traditional occupation areas, cannot meet the needs of concentrated settlements.
4. Potatoes have gained importance as an inexpensive way to achieve satiation.
5. Purchase and intake of foods having a short shelf life, such as fresh fruits and vegetables, is low, thus reducing the risk of food waste through rapid food spoilage.

A wide range of economic, social, cultural, and geographic factors influence the variability of Native American food choices and nutrient intake. The presence and incidence of nutritional problems vary by tribe and may vary within tribes, depending on inter- and intratribal variability of these factors. The information in Table 38-1 is provided to heighten awareness of the range of factors that influence Native American dietary patterns.

Epidemiology of Nutritional Problems among Native Americans

Inactivity and several of the food behaviors documented in current reports of Native American diet (i.e., high frequency of meat and fried food consumption and low frequency of fruit and vegetable consumption) have been identified as risk factors for chronic and degenerative diseases and for complications in pregnancy. Table 38-2 is based on studies of nutritional epidemiology in Native and non-Native populations and the findings and recommendations of the NRC,[32] the USDA, and USDHHS,[33] and it identifies diet-disease associations noted for the primary nutritional problems reported for Native Americans. (For a more comprehensive discussion of the epidemiology, clinical presentation, and diagnosis of these diseases in Native Americans, see Chapters 25–29 in this volume.)

Indian Health Service (IHS) statistics clearly demonstrate an association between disease rates and excessive energy and fat intake, low fiber intake, inadequate intake of select nutrients, and physical inactivity.[34–38] Diet and activity have been implicated in the etiology of at least four of the 10 leading causes of adult mortality and morbidity among Native Americans: cardiovascular disease, specific cancers, cirrhosis of the liver, and non–insulin-

Table 38-2. Diet-Disease Associations

Diet	Diseases	Diet	Diseases
Energy intake > energy needs	Atherosclerotic cardiovascular disease Hypertension Non–insulin-dependent diabetes mellitus Breast cancer Endometrial cancer Intestinal cancer Gallbladder disease Preeclampsia Eclampsia		Hepatitis virus B infection Fetal alcohol syndrome Impaired fetal growth Reduced fertility Increased susceptibility to infection
		Dietary fiber intake <20 g/day	Atherosclerotic cardiovascular disease Hypertension Non–insulin-dependent diabetes mellitus Constipation Breast cancer Stomach cancer Colorectal cancer
Total fat intake >30% of total kcals	Breast cancer Ovarian cancer Prostate cancer Colorectal cancer Hypertension	Iron intake <10 mg/day	Anemia
Total alcohol intake >2 drinks/day or 14 drinks/wk	Atherosclerotic cardiovascular disease Hypertension Renal disease Cirrhosis of the liver Oropharyngeal cancer Laryngeal cancer Esophageal cancer Liver cancer Pancreatic cancer Colorectal cancer Breast cancer Osteoporosis Anemia Malnutrition, especially deficiencies of thiamine, folate, and vitamin C Hypoglycemia Hyperuricemia Gout Peripheral neuropathy Wernicke's encephalopathy	Calcium intake <1,200 mg/day Vitamin A intake <800 µg RE/day Vitamin C intake <60 mg/day	Dental caries Osteoporosis Night blindness Xerophthalmia Keratomalacia Increased susceptibility to infection Breast cancer Cervical cancer Esophageal cancer Lung cancer Colorectal cancer Epithelial cancer Skin cancer Scurvy Esophageal cancer Lung cancer Stomach cancer Pancreatic cancer Cervical cancer Increased susceptibility to viral infections

RE = retinal equivalent.

dependent diabetes mellitus.[35, 36, 39, 40] Of the 12 leading reasons cited by IHS for clinical nutrition patient contacts (Table 38-3), eight involved consultation related to excessive consumption of energy, fat, or alcohol; low physical activity; and inadequate consumption of nutrient-dense foods.[36] The remaining categories may have involved similar consultation topics, but the exact reason for the referral is less clear.

Obesity: Precursor to Chronic Disease

Obesity is a major health problem in the United States. In the 1990s, more than 33% of adults of all races are obese.[41] In some Native American communities, more than 65% of adults are obese.[42, 43] Obesity is a precursor

to several disease states, increasing risk of morbidity and mortality attributed to diabetes mellitus, hypertension, dyslipidemia, cardiovascular disease, complications in pregnancy, and some cancers.

Obesity is often used interchangeably with *overweight*, but the terms have separate physiologic definitions. Obesity is defined as an excessive amount of body fat. Obesity criteria are sex specific and relative to total body composition; a diagnosis of obesity is appropriate when adipose tissue is 20% or more of total body composition in males and 30% or more in females. Accurate, direct measurement of obesity requires sophisticated techniques that are often expensive and require special equipment. These techniques (e.g., hydrostatic weighing, bioelectric impedance, dual-energy x-ray absorptiometry) involve measuring body density and assessing the

Table 38-3. Leading Reasons for Clinical Nutrition Patient or Client Contacts (Fiscal Year 1992)[a]

Reason	Percentage
General nutrition[b]	39.0
Diabetes[c]	26.3
Weight control[c]	8.2
Prenatal	6.4
Alcohol related[c]	3.7
Cardiovascular disease[c]	3.1
Breast-feeding	2.4
Undernutrition	1.8
Gestational diabetes[c]	1.7
Renal disease[c]	1.4
Anemia[c]	1.0
Hypertension[c]	1.0
All other	6.0

[a]Figures indicate percent of total nutrition contacts for all Indian Health Service units.[36]
[b]No information was provided to clarify the "general nutrition" category or to define how a contact was recorded if a client had more than one nutritional problem.
[c]Consultation is required about excessive consumption of energy, fat, or alcohol; low physical activity; and inadequate consumption of nutrient-dense foods.

relative contribution of water, fat, and fat-free mass to total body composition. Indirect methods of assessing body composition include measures of subcutaneous fat and relative weight for height. A variety of skinfold sites and combinations of skinfold measurements have been proposed to calculate the percentage of body fat.[44] In this context, a simple two-site formula is used. Valid measures of subcutaneous fat require skill and familiarity with the techniques as well as substantial practice; reference to manuals describing techniques and consultation with experts in the field of body composition are strongly recommended.[44, 45]

Adverse effects of obesity are linked to the pattern of fat deposition. *Central* or *abdominal obesity* refers to a disproportionate fat accumulation in the trunk; *peripheral obesity* is associated with excessive fat deposition in the hips, thighs, and upper arms. As a population, Native Americans exhibit a high prevalence of central obesity. Central obesity is strongly associated with insulin resistance, glucose intolerance, high blood pressure, and dyslipidemia.

Pattern of fat deposition is estimated using a waist-hip circumference ratio (WHR). Central obesity is defined in men as a WHR greater than 0.95 and in women as a WHR greater than 0.80.[46, 47] Peripheral obesity is defined as a WHR below these values. Estimates of percentage of body fat using measures of subcutaneous fat should include a comparable number of measures taken from the trunk and the limbs (legs or arms). This approach pre-

vents distinct patterns of fat deposition from skewing the estimate of percentage of body fat.

Overweight is excessive weight for height, defined by a body mass index (BMI) of weight (kg)/height^2 (m). Based on the assumption that excessive fat accumulation and body weight are highly correlated, BMI is frequently used as an indirect measure of obesity. *Overweight* for both men and women is defined as having a BMI greater than 25.[48] In this context, a general guideline of 27 is suggested to accommodate potential population variation in fat-free mass density. A BMI greater than 30 can be used as an indirect indicator of obesity.[48] Another technique used for assessing appropriate weight for height is to make a comparison with the 1983 Metropolitan Life Insurance Company desirable height and weight tables.[49] *Overweight* is defined as more than 120% of desirable weight for height.[49]

Nutritional Assessment and Diagnosis

Evaluation of nutritional status is generally based on a minimum of two assessment methods. The four most frequently used methods are (1) anthropometric indices, (2) physical examination, (3) biochemical tests, and (4) record of food intake behaviors.[50]

Anthropometric indices provide a measure of protein and fat reserves and of developmental progress. Anthropometric measures and indices are compared to population standards to assess degree of under- or overnutrition. Ethnicity or racial variation influence population standards. Native American–specific standards (e.g., height-weight charts, growth curves, and mid-arm muscle skeletal mass) do not exist. The heterogeneity of Native American morphology and ancestry precludes the development of useful reference standards. Limited reports suggest distinct morphologic trends in Native American populations. For example, high mineral content or bone density and a high muscle-to-bone-mass ratio[51] could influence measures of weight and body composition in Native Americans.[52] A high prevalence of central or abdominal body fat deposition could influence indirect measures (e.g., skinfold measurements) of total body composition.[20, 53, 54] Such morphologic trends suggest that anthropometric measures and indices should be used in conjunction with other nutritional assessment methods and that indirect measures of body fat and muscle mass should be interpreted with caution. Using a higher baseline acknowledges the potential morphologic variability.

Most physical signs of malnutrition are nonspecific— that is, they are not related to a single nutrient deficiency or excess. Physical signs tend to be most useful for recognizing severe malnutrition. Early clinical signs of malnutrition are often nonspecific (e.g., fatigue, apathy, irritability) or lacking, so they are useless diagnostically.

As with other measures of nutritional status, physical signs should be used in conjunction with other assessment techniques.

Biomedical tests can be used to identify nutritional problems, particularly in preclinical stages, and to monitor adherence to therapeutic interventions. Biochemical evaluation of nutritional status provides greater precision, sensitivity, and specificity than do anthropometric measures, physical examination, and records of food behavior but offers little insight into the circumstances promoting malnutrition. When available, biochemical assessment at baseline and at periodic follow-ups is recommended to assess the extent of malnutrition and the effectiveness of interventions. In the collection and interpretation of biochemical information, attention to the overall clinical picture is important (i.e., fasting vs. postprandial conditions and hydration status can artificially inflate or deflate test results). For example, dehydration falsely increases serum albumin and hematocrit levels, making an accurate evaluation impossible. Depending on the test, some laboratory measures of nutritional status can be expensive (e.g., those requiring unusual specimen matrices or handling procedures) or may be unavailable, except in research settings. Quality nutritional testing may not be available to all physicians; in such cases, reliance on a combination of less invasive methods is acceptable.

Records of food behaviors can include a dietary history or one or more 24-hour dietary recalls. A dietary history provides qualitative, rather than quantitative, information about usual food habits. Clients are asked about the number and type of meals they usually eat, how often they consume various foods (e.g., green and yellow vegetables, fruits, meats, eggs, fried foods, cereals), their food preferences and avoidances, food allergies, preferred food preparation techniques (e.g., frying, broiling, boiling), and seasonal variations. Inquiry about wild food consumption (game meats and wild plants) and traditional food processing techniques (alkali-processed corn meal and smoking, curing, pickling, or salting meats and fish) should be incorporated into dietary histories collected from most Native American clients. Alkali (wood ash or lime) processing of corn improves digestibility, absorption, and utilization of available nutrients (e.g., niacin and protein); intensifies color and flavor; and contributes potassium and calcium to the diet (NI Teufel, ethnographic field notes collected with Black Seminole of Coahuila, Mexico, 1992–1994).[55–57] Salt-, brine-, and smoke-cured foods have been associated with an increased risk of stomach cancer.[58, 59] These food behaviors may not be specific to clients in reservations or rural areas. Clients living in urban areas may receive wild or traditionally prepared foods as gifts, or they may regularly return to rural homelands to obtain these foods.

Table 38-4 provides examples of directed, concise dietary assessment questions to assist in evaluating a client's risk for nutrition-related chronic disease.

Table 38-4. Disease-Specific Diet History Questions

Disease	Questions for Diet History
Anemia	How often do you drink alcohol?
	How much alcohol do you drink at one time?
	Do you eat beef or mutton? If yes, how many times in a day?
	How often do you eat dark green, leafy vegetables such as spinach?
	Do you eat dark green wild plant foods?
	How often do you eat oranges, grapefruits, or lemons?*
Cancer	See Coronary artery disease below. Also:
	Do you eat white or dark bread?
	Do you eat breakfast cereal? If yes, what type?
	How often do you eat grilled or barbecued foods?
	How often do you eat smoked, salted, or pickled foods?
	How often do you eat fruit?
	How often do you eat vegetables other than potatoes?
Coronary artery disease	What do you usually eat for breakfast?
	Do you add margarine, butter, or gravy to your foods?
	How often do you eat away from home (fast food or restaurants)?
	Do you remove the skin and fat from chicken and meat before cooking?
	Do you drink milk? If yes, what type?
	How often do you eat fruits and vegetables?
Diabetes mellitus	Do you add sugar to your coffee or tea?
	What do you drink during the day when you are thirsty?
	Do you frequently eat dessert or other sweets?
	How many meals do you eat each day?
Hypertension	Do you add salt to your food?
	Do you eat salted snacks? sunflower seeds?
	How often do you eat away from home (fast food or restaurants)?
	Do you eat canned vegetables?
	How often do you eat bacon? sausage? ham? hot dogs? canned meat? jerky?
	How often do you drink milk?
Osteoporosis	Do you drink milk? If yes, how often?
	How much coffee, tea, cola, or caffeinated soda do you drink?
	Do you take a calcium supplement?
	How often do you eat cheese? cottage cheese?
Renal disease	Do you use salt or salt substitute?
	How often do you eat beef or mutton?
	Do you drink milk? If yes, how often?
	Do you eat fruits or vegetables? If yes, what types?

*Vitamin C enhances iron absorption.
Source: Adapted from CA Thomson. Clinical Nutrition. In H Greene (ed), Clinical Medicine (2nd ed). St. Louis: Mosby, 1998.

Dietary Therapy

Physician-prescribed and self-prescribed nutrient supplementation is prevalent throughout the United States. Concerns about the growing dependence on nutrient supplementation suggest that users have become complacent about their nutritional status and take little responsibility for their food choices. The nutritional problems most often reported in Native American communities can be treated effectively with diet therapy and behavior modification and generally do not require chemical intervention. Potentially, diet therapy can have a greater impact on Native American health than nutrient supplementation. As clients are taught and supported in developing healthy food habits, these behaviors are observed and shared by family and other community members. Building the community information base on healthy food choices is an effective prevention strategy and may reduce the incidence of disease risk.

Table 38-5 provides recommendations for dietary intervention for the primary nutritional problems reported in Native Americans. Recommendations are based on reports of Native American food behaviors and preferences and on successful intervention strategies.[20, 31, 60–62]

Table 38-5. Diet Therapy for Specific Nutritional Problems

Nutritional Problem	Diet Therapy

Energy intake exceeds energy needs	Reduce consumption of fried foods.
	Increase use of nonfrying cooking methods:
	    Boiled eggs rather than fried eggs
	    Baked and broiled meats rather than fried meats
	    Remove fat and skin from meat prior to cooking
	    Baked or boiled potatoes rather than fried potatoes
	Replace high-sugar beverages with water and sugar-free beverages.
	Avoid adding butter or margarine to vegetables when cooking or serving.
	Reduce the size of entree servings.
	Experiment with low-fat food choices:
	    Skim and 1% milk
	    Low-fat salad dressings (replace salad dressings with lemon juice)
	    Low-fat cheeses (replace cheddar and longhorn cheese with low-fat varieties, such as
	       mozzarella)
	    Remove the skin from chicken or turkey
	Increase intake of high-fiber foods to promote satiation:
	    Increase consumption of fruits and vegetables (especially raw)
	    Cook beans without adding fat
	    Try cereals with ≥ 5 g fiber per serving
	    Try whole-grain breads
	Discuss and encourage low-energy, low-fat restaurant and fast food choices:
	    Grilled chicken breast sandwich rather than a burger
	    No mayonnaise
	    Single burger rather than a multiple-patty burger
	    No cheese added to the sandwich
	    No french fries
	Increase level of physical activity.
	    Encourage walking for short-distance errands and visiting.
	    Walk, play outside sports (e.g., basketball, baseball), or work out with friends or family
	       members.

High total fat intake (>30% of kcals)	Reduce consumption of fried foods.
	Increase use of nonfrying cooking methods:
	    Boiled eggs rather than fried eggs
	    Baked and broiled meats rather than fried meats
	    Remove fat and skin from meat before cooking
	    Baked or boiled potatoes rather than fried potatoes
	Reduce consumption of meat, vegetable, and milk gravies.
	Reduce consumption of luncheon meats, bacon, sausage, and canned meat.
	Reduce intake of high-fat breads (e.g., fried bread, tortillas* made with fat, and pastries).
	Experiment with low-fat food choices:

Nutritional Problem	Diet Therapy
	Skim and 1% milk
	Low-fat salad dressings (replace salad dressings with lemon juice)
	Low-fat cheeses (replace cheddar and longhorn cheese with low-fat varieties, such as mozzarella)
	Remove the skin from chicken or turkey
	Increase intake of high-fiber foods to promote satiation:
	Increase consumption of fruits and vegetables (especially raw)
	Cook beans without adding fat
	Try cereals with ≥5 g fiber per serving
	Try whole-grain breads
	Discuss and encourage low-energy, low-fat restaurant and fast food choices (same as for Energy intake exceeds energy needs).
	Increase level of physical activity (same as for Energy intake exceeds energy needs).
High intake of alcohol	The metabolism of alcohol increases the need for certain nutrients. Inflammation of the stomach, pancreas, and intestine leads to the malabsorption of certain nutrients. Patient should increase intake of nutrient-dense foods, particularly foods high in the B vitamins, folate, and vitamin C. Nutrient-dense foods that are often available and preferred: citrus fruits and juices, potatoes with skins, green peppers, wild and domestic berries, tomatoes, chili peppers, all types of beans, organ meats, spinach and other wild and domestic greens, fish, sweet potatoes and yams, red meat, and cabbage (as coleslaw or cooked).
	Refer to an alcohol or behavioral health counselor.
Low intake of dietary fiber	Increase intake of fruits and vegetables to five servings per day.
	High-fiber fruits that are often available and preferred: apples, apricots, oranges, pears, strawberries, and all domestic and wild berries, cactus fruits, plums, and prunes.
	High-fiber vegetables that are often available and preferred: all types of beans (preferably boiled with no or little added fat), carrots, green peas, spinach, and other wild and domestic berries, leafy greens, and all types of squash. All vegetables should be baked, boiled, steamed, or roasted with no or little added fat.
	Increase intake of whole grains to six servings per day.
	High-fiber grain products often available and preferred: oatmeal, corn (including popcorn with no or little added fat), bran flakes, and other high-fiber cereals.
Low intake of iron	Increase intake of dietary sources of iron to two servings or more per day.
	High iron foods often available and preferred: organ meats, red meat, fish, poultry, iron-fortified cooked and cold cereals, red meat, raisins, all types of beans, molasses, and dark leafy wild and domestic greens.
Low intake of calcium	Increase intake of dietary sources of calcium to two or more servings per day. High-calcium foods that are often available and preferred: cheese (particularly low-fat varieties, such as mozzarella and cottage cheese), canned sardines and salmon with bones, dark leafy wild and domestic greens, foods made with ash, or lime-processed corn.
	If appropriate, encourage sucking bones.
	Reduce caffeine intake.
	Prevalence of lactose intolerance is high in many Native American communities; if milk products are well tolerated, encourage intake of skim and 1% milk. If milk products are not tolerable (lactose intolerance), calcium supplementation may be necessary (1,000 mg/day).
Low intake of vitamin A	Increase intake of foods high in vitamin A to two or more servings per day. Foods high in vitamin A that are often available and preferred: apricots (dried and fresh), beef liver, fish liver oil, cantaloupe, carrots (raw or cooked), mixed vegetables, squash (including pumpkin), spinach and other domestic and wild dark leafy greens, sweet potatoes, chili peppers, peaches, tomatoes, and watermelon.
Low intake of vitamin C	Increase intake of foods high in vitamin C to two or more servings per day. Foods high in vitamin C that are often available and preferred: cabbage (raw or cooked), citrus fruits and juices (include lemons and lemonade), green peppers, chili peppers, spinach and other wild and domestic greens, wild and domestic berries, cantaloupe and other melons, potatoes with skins, tomatoes (fresh, cooked, and juice), and vegetable juice.

*Many Native Americans make flour tortillas without added fat. Inquire as to the ingredients in homemade tortillas and encourage the production and consumption of no-fat tortillas.

It is *strongly* recommended that one or more family members (even children 3 years of age) accompany the client during any nutritional consultation sessions. Eating is a social event, and in Native American cultures, food continues to be a strong symbol of generosity. Food behavior modification is more successful and effective when some or all members of the client's social network experiment, support, and participate in these new and perhaps unfamiliar food choices and food preparation techniques. A client who fears disrupting the patterns of his or her household or who hesitates to draw undue attention to him- or herself often does not try any of the dietary recommendations.

Conclusions

Across the United States, Native American food choices are quite variable. In general, meat or other high-protein staples, such as beans, often prepared with added fat, are prominent in the diet. In many communities, access to and familiarity with a variety of fresh fruits and vegetables are low. The cost of produce, when locally available, may drive households to spend limited funds on more highly valued protein foods. The extent to which an individual household or community follows this general pattern is influenced by a variety of economic, geographic, and cultural factors.

Reports of Native American nutrient intake have not been systematic and do not adequately represent the heterogeneity of the population. Since the 1980s, reported nutrient intake of Native Americans compared to the RDAs indicate that the primary nutritional problems are energy (calorie) intakes exceeding energy needs, high intake of total fat (and in some sectors of the population, alcohol), and low intake of dietary fiber, iron, calcium, and vitamins A and C.

Guidelines for identifying and treating these conditions are provided. Treatment recommendations stress behavior modification by reinforcing healthy food practices, especially those grounded in traditional beliefs and behaviors, gradually introducing new food choices and cooking styles, and including family members in any discussions of dietary change. The importance of eating as a social event and of food as a symbol of generosity and a source of strength are perhaps best exemplified in Native American culture. To provide dietary advice or counseling outside the social and cultural environment is largely fruitless.

Summary Points

- Meat and other high-protein foods (e.g., beans) are an important part of the Native American diet.
- Under economic constraints, meat, beans, and potatoes are generally purchased instead of fruits, vegetables, and whole grains.

- The Native American diet tends to be high in protein and fat and low in fiber, iron, calcium, and vitamins A and C.
- The extent to which a household follows these dietary patterns is influenced by economic conditions, location (rural vs. urban), adherence to traditional food practices and beliefs, and impact of local nutrition education programs.
- Treatment should be oriented to the family and the household and should build on existing healthy contemporary and traditional food behaviors.

References

1. Dodd TH. Report of US Agent for the Navajoes, Bosque Redondo, NM. Report to the Commissioner of Indian Affairs. U.S. Government Printing Office, 1866.
2. Hoffman WJ. Miscellaneous Ethnographic Observations of Indians Inhabiting Nevada, California, and Arizona. In FV Hayden (ed), 10th Annual Report of the U.S. Geological and Geographical Survey of the Territories. Washington, DC: Government Printing Office, 1878;461–478.
3. Hrdlicka A. Notes on the Pima of Arizona. American Anthropologist 1906;8:39–46.
4. Moore PE, Kruse HD, Tisdall FF, Corrigan RS. Medical survey of nutrition among the northern Manitoba Indian. Can Med Assoc J 1946;54:223–233.
5. Shanklin H. Report of US Agent for the Wichita, Leased District Indian Territory. Report to the Commissioner of Indian Affairs. Washington, DC: U.S. Government Printing Office, 1866.
6. Vivian RP, McMillan C, Moore PE, et al. The nutrition and health of the James Bay Indian. Can Med Assoc J 1948;59:505–518.
7. Lukaczer M. School breakfasts and Indian children's health. J Am Indian Edu 1976;15:7–12.
8. Moore WM, Silverberg MM, Read MS (eds). Nutrition, Growth and Development of North American Indian Children. DHEW (NIH) Publication No. 72-26. Washington, DC: U.S. Department of Health, Education, and Welfare, National Institutes of Health, 1972.
9. Van Duzen J, Carter J, John PH, et al. Protein and calorie malnutrition among preschool Navajo Indian children. Am J Clin Nutr 1969;22:1362–1370.
10. Van Duzen J, Carter J, John PH, et al. Protein and calorie malnutrition among preschool Navajo Indian children: a follow-up. Am J Clin Nutr 1976;29:657–662.
11. Draper HH. Dietary Habits and Nutritional Status of Eskimos. In PL White, N Selvey (eds), Nutrition in Transition: Proceedings of Western Hemisphere Nutrition Congress V. Monroe, WI: American Medical Association, 1978.
12. Joos SK. Diet, obesity and diabetes mellitus among the Florida Seminole Indians. Florida Scientist 1980;43:148–152.
13. Lee ET, Anderson PS, Bryan J, et al. Diabetes, parental diabetes, and obesity in Oklahoma Indians. Diabetes Care 1985;8:107–113.

14. Mayberry RH, Lindeman RD. A survey of chronic disease and diet in Seminole Indians in Oklahoma. Am J Clin Nutr 1963;13:127–134.

15. Tompkins RA. A cross-sectional study of height, weight, and triceps skinfold measurements of Cherokee Indian youths ages 13–17. Ph.D. diss., University of Tennessee—Knoxville, 1980.

16. Bell RA, Shaw HA, Dignan MB. Dietary intake of Lumbee Indian women in Robeson County, North Carolina. J Am Diet Assoc 1995;95:1426–1428.

17. Broussard BA, Johnson A, Himes JH, et al. Prevalence of obesity in American Indians and Alaska Natives. Am J Clin Nutr 1991;53(suppl):1535–1542.

18. Gruber E, Anderson MM, Ponton L, DiClimente R. Overweight and obesity in Native-American adolescents: comparing nonreservation youths with African-American and Caucasian peers. Am J Prev Med 1995;11:306–310.

19. Hall TR, Hickey ME, Young TB. Evidence for recent increases in obesity and non-insulin dependent diabetes mellitus in a Navajo community. Am J Hum Biol 1992;4:547–553.

20. Teufel NI, Dufour DL. Patterns of food use and nutrient intake of obese and non-obese Hualapai Indian women of Arizona. J Am Diet Assoc 1990;90:1229–1235.

21. Young TK. The Health of Native Americans: Towards a Biocultural Epidemiology. New York: Oxford University Press, 1994.

22. Calloway DH, Gibbs JC. Food patterns and food assistance programs in the Cocopah Indian community. Ecology of Food and Nutrition 1976;5:183–196.

23. Dustrude AM. Nutrient intake of selected non-reservation Native Americans residing in southwest Oregon. Master's thesis, Oregon State University, 1981.

24. Harland BF, Smith SA, Ellis R, et al. Comparison of the nutrient intakes of blacks, Siouan Indians, and whites in Columbus County, North Carolina. J Am Diet Assoc 1992;92:348–350.

25. Nobmann ED, Byers T, Lanier AP, et al. The diet of Alaska Native adults: 1987–1988. Am J Clin Nutr 1992;55:1024–1032.

26. Shephard RJ, Rode A. Health Consequences of "Modernization": Evidence from Circumpolar Peoples. New York: Cambridge University Press, 1996.

27. Story M, Tompkins RA, Bass MA, Wakefield LM. Anthropometric measurements and dietary intakes of Cherokee Indian teenagers in North Carolina. J Am Diet Assoc 1986;86:1555–1560.

28. Thouez JP, Rannou A, Foggin P. The other face of development: Native population, health status and indicators of malnutrition: the case of the Cree and Inuit of Northern Quebec. Soc Sci Med 1989;29:965–974.

29. Gittelsohn J, Harris SB, Thorne-Lyman AL, et al. Body image concepts differ by age and sex in an Ojibway-Cree community in Canada. J Nutr 1996;126:2990–3000.

30. Teufel NI. Skinny women don't make good wives: cultural conflicts and the failure of weight-loss programs. Presented at the Ninety-First Annual Meeting of the American Anthropological Association, Washington, DC, December 1992.

31. Teufel NI, Ritenbaugh CK. Development of a primary prevention program: insight gained in the Zuni Diabetes Prevention Program. Clin Pediatr 1998;37:131–142.

32. National Research Council. Recommended Dietary Allowances (10th ed). Washington, DC: National Academy Press, 1989.

33. U.S. Department of Agriculture/U.S. Department of Health and Human Services. Nutrition and Your Health: Dietary Guidelines for Americans (4th ed). Home and Garden Bulletin No. 232. Washington, DC: USDA, USDHHS, 1995.

34. Buckley DI, McPherson RS, North CQ, Becker TM. Dietary micronutrients and cervical dysplasia in Southwestern American Indian women. Nutr Cancer 1992;17:179–185.

35. Byers T. Nutrition and cancer among American Indians and Alaska Natives. Cancer 1996;78:1612–1616.

36. Indian Health Service. Trends in Indian Health: 1994. Rockville, MD: U.S. Department of Health and Human Services, Public Health Service, IHS, Office of Planning, Education, and Legislation, and Division of Program Statistics, 1994.

37. Reid JM, Fullmer SD, Pettigrew KD, et al. Nutrient intake of Pima Indian women: relationships to diabetes mellitus and gallbladder disease. Am J Clin Nutr 1971;24:1281–1289.

38. Rhoades ER, Hammond J, Welty TK, et al. The Indian burden of illness and future health interventions. Public Health Rep 1987;102:361–368.

39. Jackson MY. Nutrition in American Indian health: past, present, and future. J Am Diet Assoc 1986;86:1561–1565.

40. Teufel NI. Nutrient-health associations in the historic and contemporary diets of Southwest Native Americans. J Nutritional Environmental Med 1996;6:179–189.

41. Solomon CG, Manson JE. Obesity and mortality: a review of the epidemiologic data. Am J Clin Nutr 1997;66(suppl):1044–1050.

42. Gohdes D. Diabetes in North American Indians and Alaska Natives. In National Diabetes Data Group (ed), Diabetes in America (2nd ed). NIH Publication No. 95-1468. Washington, DC: National Institute of Diabetes and Digestive and Kidney Diseases, National Institutes of Health, 1995.

43. White LL, Ballew C, Gilbert TJ, et al. Weight, body image, and weight control practices of Navajo Indians: findings from the Navajo Health and Nutrition Survey. J Nutr 1997;127(suppl 10):2094–2098.

44. Norgan NG. Anthropometric Assessment of Body Fat and Fatness. In JH Himes (ed), Anthropometric Assessment of Nutritional Status. New York: Wiley-Liss, 1991;197–212.

45. Lohman TG, Roche AF, Martorell R (eds), Anthropometric Standardization Reference Manual. Champaign, IL: Human Kinetics Books, 1988.

46. Bray GA. An Approach to the Classification and Evaluation of Obesity. In P Bjorntorp, BN Brodoff (eds), Obesity. Philadelphia: Lippincott, 1992;294–308.

47. Bjorntorp P. Classification of obese patients and complications related to the distribution of surplus fat. Am J Clin Nutr 1987;45:1120–1125.

48. National Heart, Lung, and Blood Institute. Clinical

Guidelines on the Identification, Evalution, and Treatment of Overweight and Obesity in Adults. Bethesda, MD: National Institute of Health, 1998.

49. Metropolitan Life Insurance Company. 1983 Height and Weight Tables. Statistical Bulletin, Metropolitan Insurance Company 1984;64:2–9.

50. Thomson C, Ritenbaugh C, Kerwin JP, DeBell R. Preventive and Therapeutic Nutrition Handbook. New York: Chapman & Hall, 1996.

51. Rode A, Shephard RJ. Prediction of body fat content in an Inuit community. Am J Hum Biol 1994;6:249–254.

52. Stolarczyk LM, Heyward VH, Hicks VL, Baumgartner RN. Predictive accuracy of bioelectrical impedance in estimating body composition of Native American women. Am J Clin Nutr 1994;59:964–970.

53. Johnston FE, Schell LM. Anthropometric Variation of Native American Children and Adults. In WS Laughlin, GB Harper (eds), The First Americans: Origins, Affinities, and Adaptations. New York: Wenner Gren Foundation, 1979.

54. Szathmary EJE, Holt N. Hyperglycemia in Dogrib Indians of the Northwest Territories, Canada: Association with age and a centripetal distribution of body fat. Hum Biol 1983;55:493–515.

55. Calloway DH, Giauque RD, Costa FW. The superior mineral content of some American Indian foods in comparison to federally donated counterpart commodities. Ecol Food Nutr 1974;3:203–211.

56. Katz SH, Hediger ML, Valleroy LA. Traditional maize processing techniques in the New World. Science 1974;184:765–773.

57. Kuhnlein HV, Calloway DH, Harland BF. Composition of traditional Hopi foods. J Am Diet Assoc 1979;75:37–41.

58. Williams GM, Wynder EL. Diet and Cancer: A Synopsis of Causes and Prevention Strategies. In RR Watson, SI Mufti (eds), Nutrition and Cancer. New York: CRC Press, 1996;1–12.

59. World Cancer Research Fund and the American Institute for Cancer Research. Food, Nutrition and the Prevention of Cancer: A Global Perspective. Washington, DC: American Institute for Cancer Research, 1997.

60. Szathmary EJE, Ritenbaugh C, Goodby CSM. Dietary change and plasma glucose levels in an American Indian population undergoing cultural transition. Soc Sci Med 1987;24:791–804.

61. Teufel NI. Alcohol consumption and its effect on the dietary patterns of Hualapai Indian women. Med Anthropol 1994;16:79–97.

62. Wein EE, Freeman MM. Inuvialuit food use and food preferences in Aklavik, Northwest Territories, Canada. Arctic Medi Res 1992;51:159–172.

Suggested Reading

Brackenridge BP, Warshaw H. The Healthy Eating Food Guide for Diabetes: A Nutrition Education Tool for Native Americans. Handbook and Resource Guide for Health Care Providers. Albuquerque, NM: Indian Health Service Diabetes Program, September 1995.

Broussard BA, Johnson A, Himes JH, et al. Prevalence of obesity in American Indians and Alaska Natives. Am J Clin Nutr 1991;53(suppl):1535–1542.

Friedman L, Fleming NF, Roberts DH, Hyman SE. Source Book of Substance Abuse and Addiction. Baltimore: Williams & Wilkins, 1996.

Gittelsohn J, Harris SB, Thorne-Lyman AL, et al. Body image concepts differ by age and sex in an Ojibway-Cree community in Canada. J Nutr 1996;126:2990–3000.

Jackson MY. Nutrition in American Indian health: past, present, and future. J Am Diet Assoc 1986;86:1561–1565.

Teufel NI. Nutrient-health associations in the historic and contemporary diets of Southwest Native Americans. J Nutr Environmental Med 1996;67:179–189.

World Cancer Research Fund and the American Institute for Cancer Research. Food, Nutrition and the Prevention of Cancer: A Global Perspective. Washington, DC: American Institute for Cancer Research, 1997.

Part XIII
Neurology

ther a state nor divided up into counties. Hendrie et al.[27] modified the MMSE for use in a Cree population. Any instrument used to measure cognitive state that does not have demonstrated reliability and validity in AI and AN populations should be used with caution. If the diagnosis is in question, an alternative method of cognitive assessment is neuropsychological testing. This testing method may also be used to assess the progression of disease and to identify an affective component.

Mental illness in the AI and AN population may not be characterized in the same manner as in Western society. Causes and treatments may be very different. To assist in the determination of the AI or AN patient's view of etiology, the patient can be asked what he or she perceives to be the cause of illness. Depression is the most frequent mental illness diagnosis in mental health facilities serving AIs of all ages.[28] The Indian Depression Schedule is a diagnostic instrument that unites the AI and the Western psychiatric viewpoints.[29]

Ethics

Western biomedical ethics is grounded in the consideration of several principles: autonomy, confidentiality, beneficence, honesty, and social justice. The desired outcome in ethical decision making is balance of these principles for the individual, the community, and society as a whole. The Omnibus Reconciliation Act of 1987 and the Patient Self-Determination Act of 1991 were enacted to protect patient rights. The desire for treatment and the extent of aggressive treatment, including resuscitation and intubation, are included in the determination of patient rights. AI and AN cultural beliefs may conflict with the approach of the mandated patient protection law. In some cultures, the open discussion of death and dying is not as accepted as in Western society. Speaking of death may be interpreted as willing it on oneself. It is part of the health provider's responsibility to "do no harm." From the cultural viewpoint, the consequences of transgressing the taboo (i.e., speaking of death) may harm the patient in physical or emotional ways. Self-determination, the very reason for these laws, is subjugated if the patient is not willing to participate fully in a discussion that contradicts his or her values and beliefs. The Western principles of ethics can be applied to AI and AN elders but only with a collaborative, partnered, and fully informed approach that takes into account the cultural values of the individual.

Recommendations for the Clinical Interaction

Most AI and AN tribes, villages, and groups share broad, general values but have specific and differing beliefs. The implementation of the following recommendations must be accompanied by vigilant attention to avoiding stereotypes. As an attending physician for family medicine residents, I have found that when residents return from a seminar addressing multiculturalism, they apply the specific recommendations to all AIs, regardless of tribal affiliation. The provider must learn the attitudes, beliefs, and behaviors of the specific AI or AN tribal group he or she serves.

Non-Indian health providers are being evaluated, just as they are evaluating the population they serve. Most likely, the population being served has a stereotype of Western-trained providers. Providers may be viewed suspiciously and critiqued through the filter of the patient's culture. The psychiatrist Louise Jilek-Aall, who practiced among a Canadian First Nations group, related the observation of a young First Nation member, "The white man has two ways of getting rid of Indians who make trouble for him: He puts them in prison or in the mental hospital. Stay away from the mental hospital! If you go to prison, you always know how much time you have to do; but you never know when they will let you out of the mental hospital."[30] Other likely stereotypes of non-Indian providers are their insensitive nature, greed, feelings of superiority to others, lack of modesty, untrustworthiness, intrusiveness, and assumption that all people are like them. If difficulty develops in the patient-provider interaction, these preconceived notions may be at the root of it and should be addressed.

The culture of Western medicine comes with its own set of values and beliefs. The values of Western medicine may be in direct conflict with the provider's own culture and with the culture of those being served. Be aware of personal cultural values and of how these values might affect medical decisions. Your own attitudes, values, and beliefs may conflict with those of the new culture in which you find yourself. Be willing to come in with an open mind, and be ready to listen, learn, and adjust while remaining true to yourself. You must be able to sort out the three cultural systems, determine which values are operating and when they are operating, and bring forth that which is best for the health care of AI and AN elders. Any encounter between the physician and patient should embody confidentiality, respect, honesty, polite conduct, compassion, equality, and friendliness. This is especially true for AI elder patients. This seems to be such a simple, obvious recommendation, but to actually implement it on a daily basis is not easy, particularly when one is already behind three patients. Be prepared to adjust your approach to the culture being served.

Attitude is critical. The Western physician relies heavily on the importance of scientifically proved methods and treatments, and anything short of it may not be an acceptable alternative to therapy. What happens, then, when one encounters a population whose healing methods are not "scientifically valid"? Should this preclude the use of this form of therapy? The two extremes of the spectrum would answer with a resounding yes and no.

The self-righteous attitude of those who answer yes markedly diminishes any effective relationship that may have developed between health provider and patient. On the other hand, to answer no without taking into account the patient's cultural awareness and acceptance of the scientifically unproved therapy may likewise damage the professional relationship. The key is learning about, recognizing, and incorporating into health care decisions the physician's personal attitude and beliefs and the patient's values and beliefs.

Effective communication is key to encouraging patient acceptance of the prescription and subsequent action. The patient must thoroughly understand the disease process and the recommendations for treatment. The provider must deliver the explanation so that the patient can understand it in his or her own terms. Communication is enhanced among AI and AN elders if the following recommendations are considered:

- Give the patient enough time to answer, and allow a few seconds after the patient's last thought. To interrupt a thought or not allow time for full completion of the thought is disrespectful.
- Provide specific information on what organs are affected, how they are affected, and what the changes mean for everyday life.
- Do not assume that the patient's lack of questions is confirmation of his or her understanding.
- Use the lifestyle of the patient to assist in presenting your explanation. If the patient butchers animals (sheep, deer, bear, moose), take this opportunity to apply the knowledge of animal anatomy to the patient's understanding of his or her own anatomy and disease.
- Tailor the medical explanation to the educational level of the individual. This means taking more time in getting to know the patient, but the outcome is greatly enhanced.
- Ask if the patient would like the input of nuclear and extended family members and who should be present. Depending on the degree of acculturation, extended family members' opinions are valued.
- Determine gender concerns. From the cultural point of view, determine which topics can be discussed with men or women providers, with a family group, or with the individual only. Does it make a difference when and what part of the physical examination can be done by either gender?
- Patients' rights are compromised if an interpreter is not provided when necessary. Ask whether the patient would like an interpreter even if the patient speaks English. Several variables affecting the comfort zone of an interpreter are his or her level of medical knowledge, gender concerns on sensitive topics, interpretation for family members, and language fluency.

- Ask about other traditional healing practices if they are applicable to the outcome, but do not be offended if patients are not forthcoming in their answers about this very private issue.

Just as much time should be devoted to learning about the culture as is spent updating medical skills. The scope of excellent medical care includes the delivery of knowledge that is acceptable to AI and AN elders.

In establishing rapport with patients, nonverbal communication is just as critical as verbal communication. The broad categories to consider are space proximity, body language (i.e., the manner in which a person sits or stands), dress, gestures, and where the patient and family members sit. Although these variables should be considered with all patient populations, the provider must determine what differences may exist for AI and AN elders.

Patient compliance is the measure of the ability of the patient to fulfill the provider prescription, whether it is taking medications, exercising, making dietary changes, or incorporating preventive measures into the patient's lifestyle. Cautious interpretation of noncompliance is essential when serving AI and AN cultures. The actions of a patient who is labeled noncompliant should be analyzed through the lens of the patient's culture. Your recommendation may have been embarrassing for the patient or the family member, traditional cultural events may have prohibited the recommended action, or family concerns may take precedence over clinic appointments. The determination of patient expectations minimizes the likelihood of noncompliance. Several crucial questions can be posed:

- How can I help you?
- Are there other people whom you think would be helpful in your care?
- Am I helping you the way you expected me to?
- Is there more that I can do for you?

Patience, perseverance, self-education, and developing a trust relationship are important in establishing good relationships with your AI and AN patients.

Conclusion

The AI and AN elder population is growing rapidly. As in the general U.S. geriatric population, preparing to meet the service needs of the increasing prevalence of chronic disease, rehabilitation, long-term care, and mental illness is important. If the delivery of health care in populations with non-Western cultural values, beliefs, and behaviors is not incorporated into the formula, the health outcome will not be optimal.

References

1. Dorland's Medical Dictionary (28th ed). Philadelphia: Saunders, 1994.
2. Dinges NG, Trimble JE, Manson SM, et al. Counseling and Psychotherapy with AI/AN. In Marsell A, Pedersen P (eds), Cross Cultural Counseling and Psychotherapy. Elmsford, NY: Pergamon, 1981;243–276.
3. Klein BT. Reference Encyclopedia of the American Indian (6th ed). West Nyack, NY: Todd Publications, 1993.
4. Statistical Abstract of the U.S. 1995. National Data Book (115th ed). Washington, DC: U.S. Department of Commerce, Economics, and Statistics Administration, Bureau of Census, 1995.
5. National Indian Council on Aging. American Indian Elderly: A National Profile. Albuquerque, NM: NICOA, 1981.
6. Heath SW, Ornelas R, Marquart C. A work group action plan for AI/AN elders. Q J International Inst Aging 1994;4:14–19.
7. McCabe M. Long term care and the Navajo elder. Journal of Long Term Home Health Care, The Pride Institute Journal 1995;14:11–18.
8. Stone RI. Rural Caregiving: Implications for the Aging Network. The Future of Aging in Rural America: Proceedings of a National Symposium. Chevy Chase, MD: Project Hope, 1991;51–64.
9. Kramer JB. Serving American Indian elders in cities: an invisible minority. BOLD 1994;4:20–23.
10. McCabe M, Cuellar J. Aging and Health: American Indian/Alaska Native Elders (2nd ed). SGEC Working Paper Series, Ethnogeriatric Reviews, No. 6. Palo Alto, CA: Stanford Geriatric Education Center, 1994;5–7.
11. John R. The State of Research on American Indian Elders' Health, Income, Security, and Social Support Networks. In Minority Elders: Longevity, Economics, and Health, Building a Public Policy Base. Washington, DC: Gerontological Society of America, 1991;38–50.
12. Indian Health Service. Trends in Indian Health, 1996. Statistical Review of Native North Americans. Washington, DC: U.S. Department of Health and Human Services, Indian Health Service, Office of Planning, Evaluation, and Legislation, Division of Program Statistics, 1997.
13. Reddy MA (ed). Statistical Record of Native North Americans. Detroit: Gale Research, 1993.
14. Navajo Office on Aging and The Northern Arizona Regional Gerontology Institute. Report on Navajo Elder Abuse. A Study Conducted in Oljato Chapter. Window Rock, AZ: Navajo Office on Aging, and Flagstaff, AZ: Northern Arizona University, The Northern Arizona Regional Gerontology Institute, 1986;1–24.
15. Folstein MF, Folstein S, McHugh PR. Mini-Mental State: a practical method for grading the cognitive state of patients for the clinician. J Psych Res 1975;12:189–198.
16. Murden RA, McRae T, Kaner S, et al. Mini-Mental State Exam scores vary with education in blacks and whites. J Am Geriatr Soc 1991;39:149–155.
17. Fillenbaum G, Heyman A, Williams K, et al. Sensitivity and specificity of standardized screens of cognitive impairment and dementia among elderly black and white community residents. J Clin Epidemiol (mdBiol) 1990;43:651–660.
18. Escobar JL, Burnam A, Karno M, et al. Use of the Mini-Mental State Examination (MMSE) in a community population of mixed ethnicity—cultural and linguistic artifacts. J Nerv Ment Dis 1986;174:607–614.
19. Mungas D, Marshall SC, Weldon M, et al. Age and education correction of Mini-Mental State Examination for English- and Spanish-speaking elderly. Neurology 1996;46:700–706.
20. Liu HC, Teng EL, Lin KN, et al. Performance on a dementia screening test in relation to demographic variables. Arch Neurol 1994;51:910–915.
21. Bassett SS, Folstein M. Cognitive impairment and functional disability in the absence of psychiatric diagnosis. Psychol Med 1991;21:77–84.
22. Rocca WA, Bonaiuto S, Lippi A, et al. Prevalence of clinically diagnosed Alzheimer's disease and other dementing disorders: a door-to-door survey in Appignanao, Macerata Province, Italy. Neurology 1990;40:626–631.
23. Friedl W, Schmidt R, Stronegger WJ, et al. Mini Mental State Examination: influence of sociodemographic, environmental and behavioral factors, and vascular risk factors. Clin Epidemiol 1996;49:73–78.
24. Tangolos EG, Smith GE, Ivnik RJ, et al. The Mini-Mental State Examination in general medical practice: clinical utility and acceptance. Mayo Clin Proc 1996;71:829–837.
25. Tombaugh TN, McIntyre NJ, et al. The Mini-Mental State Examination: a comprehensive review. J Am Geriatr Soc 1992;40:922–935.
26. Bird HR, Canino G, Stipec M et al. Use of the Mini-Mental State Examination in a probability sample of a Hispanic population. J Nerv Ment Dis 1987;175:731–737.
27. Hendrie HC, Hall KS, Pillay N, et al. Alzheimer's disease is rare in Cree. Int Psychogeriatr 1993;5:5–14.
28. Manson SM, Shore JH, Bloom JD, et al. The Depressive Experience in American Indian Communities: A Challenge for Psychiatric Theory and Diagnosis. In A Kleinman, YB Good (eds), Culture and Depression. Berkeley, CA: University of California Press, 1985;331–368.
29. Baron AE, Manson SM, Ackerson LM, et al. Depressive Symptomatology in Older American Indians with Chronic Disease: Some Psychometric Considerations. In CC Attkisson, JM Zich (eds), Depression in Primary Care: Screening and Detection. New York: Routledge, 1990.
30. Jilek-Aall L. The Western psychiatrist and his non-Western clientele. Can Psychiatric Assoc J 1976;21:353–359.

Part XVI
Podiatry

Chapter 43

Care of the Foot and Ankle, with Special Reference to Diabetes

Eugene Dannels

This is a quick reference to the primary care provider for commonly encountered conditions of the lower extremities. Early recognition of lower-extremity pathology with prompt, appropriate treatment or referral is essential in obtaining optimal response and maximal recovery.[1] Delay in starting therapy, overly aggressive therapy, and incorrect therapy are frequently due to failure to fully recognize the presenting pathology. Because knowledge of lower-extremity anatomy is necessary, a review is presented in the section on physical examination.

All Native American people have some risk of developing diabetes mellitus or of presenting with previously undiagnosed diabetes mellitus. Diagnosis and treatment of foot problems are presented with frequent reference to diabetes.

History and Physical Examination

History

Taking a history for foot and ankle complaints requires thorough questioning. Patient perceptions of disease are often distorted by diabetic sensory neuropathy or by chronic or episodic alcohol abuse. The time of onset of symptoms, progression of symptoms, and description of location and degree of pain may not correspond positively to clinical findings.

Physical Examination

Physical examination requires a basic knowledge of external, internal, and radiographic anatomy of the foot and ankle. Footwear and socks should be examined for foreign bodies, wear, stains from body fluids, and identifying odors. The entire lower extremity must be examined for skin color, skin lesions, edema, symmetry, deformities, and hygiene. Lower-extremity odors pro-

vide insight about personal hygiene, mycotic infections, aerobic and anaerobic bacterial infections, and tissue necrosis.

Visually, the integumentary and musculoskeletal systems can be examined at the same time. Bony prominences may be accompanied by blisters, calluses or preulcers, or ulcers. Ecchymosis, cyanosis, erythema, and atypical pigmentation may be noted. Areas where osseous or tendinous anatomy are obscured by edema can be identified. Abrasions, punctures, lacerations, and maceration can be seen as breaks in the skin. Distribution of hair and condition of toenails can be seen.

Touching the lower extremity reveals differences in skin temperature to correlate with visual findings. Joint range of motion and the presence or absence of crepitus or pain can be assessed. Edema can be pitting or nonpitting. Raised lesions and masses can be evaluated for adherence to underlying structures. Ulcers and lacerations can be assessed for depth and involvement of underlying structures. Subluxing or ruptured tendons and dislocated joints can be palpated.

Sensation is easily tested with the Semmes-Weinstein 5.07 monofilament, which is used to evaluate the presence or absence of protective sensation in the feet (Figure 43-1).[2] Failure to perceive the 5.07 monofilament in any part of the foot indicates that repetitive or sustained pressure in small amounts can result in soft tissue injury, such as ulceration, with little or no pain. This method of testing is especially important to document the diabetic patient's baseline ability to protect his or her feet. Diabetic patients frequently complain of numbness, burning, or tingling, especially in their toes, although their monofilament examinations continue to show that the 5.07 monofilament can be felt. These individuals usually develop a loss in protective sensation within 1 year. Regular testing for protective threshold identifies new sensory deficits and allows prompt institution of appropriate preventative measures. Reflex testing, muscle strength testing, and other sensory

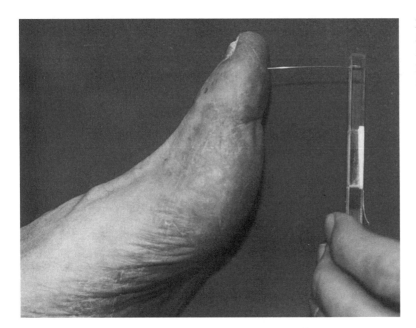

Figure 43-1. Semmes-Weinstein 5.07 monofilament being applied in perpedicular manner to the plantar aspect of the hallux or great toe.

testing may be performed. Locations and description of pain or tenderness must be documented.

The basic arterial examination for circulation in the foot requires that the dorsalis pedis artery, on top of the foot, and the posterior tibial artery, behind the medial ankle, are palpated. The location of the dorsalis pedis artery is quite variable, whereas the location of the posterior tibial artery is consistent. Both can be hidden from palpation by edema. Documentation as palpable or not palpable is adequate. Attempts to grade pulses (i.e., bounding, normal, barely palpable, or absent) are subjective and not quantifiable but may be helpful. Handheld Doppler with stethoscope-type listening devices or speakers are helpful in locating pulses (Figure 43-2). With Dopplers, pulses are heard as monophasic, biphasic, or triphasic, when present. Doppler reliability varies with the model, condition, and battery strength.

Radiographic Evaluation

Radiographic evaluation and interpretation can be a challenge. Standing or weightbearing radiographs of the dorsoplantar and lateral foot should be taken when pathology allows. Repeat radiographics are then consistent and show functional relationships of bones. Oblique foot and most ankle radiographs are nonweightbearing. If comparison radiographs would be helpful in diagnosis but past radiographs are not available, it may be helpful to take comparison radiographs of the opposite foot or ankle. This is especially useful in children. Standing radiographs should not be attempted if patients, staff, or equipment may be placed at risk of injury or damage.

Foot and Ankle Emergencies

Gas Gangrene

Diagnosis

Gas gangrene is most commonly encountered in Native Americans when an immunocompromised individual, such as a diabetic, is infected through an existing ulcer, open wound, or puncture. These infections are serious and require immediate surgical intervention. Individuals are generally very ill, with flulike symptoms of fever, chills, nausea, and joint and muscle aches. The individual's foot is generally very painful, red, hot, and swollen and may be crepitant. Onset and progression of symptoms is rapid. Gas infections can advance very rapidly along tendons and fascial planes into the leg, resulting in calf or leg involvement. The white cell count is generally quite high, as is the systemic temperature. Radiographs may reveal gas bubbles, which appear as dark spots. Three views should be taken to assist with problems of superimposition of the many bones and joints.

Treatment

The patient with gas gangrene must be admitted to the hospital. Tetanus status must be current. Immediate referral to a qualified surgical podiatrist, surgeon, or orthopedist for surgical debridement is necessary. Antibiotic therapy and intravenous fluid support should be started in consultation with the surgical specialist. Cultures from wounds may be misleading because of the difficulty in isolating the pathogenic organism through an existing polymicrobial contaminated wound. Blood cultures and intraoperative cultures

Figure 43-2. Handheld Doppler vascular testing devices with speakers assist in locating arteries, documenting arterial status, and aid in teaching patients about arterial health and disease.

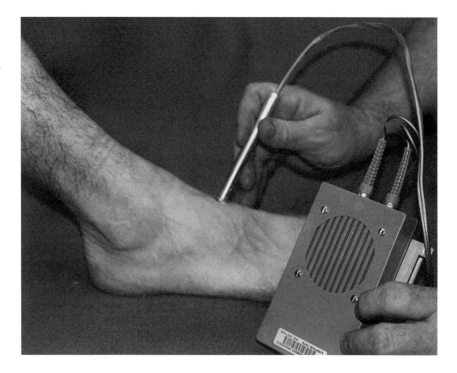

are more reliable. The patient should be kept nonweight-bearing and encouraged not to move his or her foot and leg because movement can spread the infection. Splinting should be used rather than casting. Delayed surgical intervention may result in limb loss.

Compartment Syndrome

Diagnosis

A crush injury or significant fractures can result in abnormally high pressure within the myofascial compartments of the patient's foot or leg. A severe burn can create abnormally high pressures beneath the stiff, thickened skin. Individuals may complain of progressive pain, described as tightness or deep pain not relieved by medication. Patients may be anxious, with elevated blood pressure, heart rate, and respiratory rate. The primary findings in the extremity may be pain and tense edema with progressive pallor, pulselessness, and numbness.

Treatment

Because diagnosis is very difficult, a high index of suspicion is needed. Pressure measurements may be performed if an appropriate device is available. The appropriate surgical podiatrist, surgeon, or orthopedist must be consulted immediately. Surgical release of the fascia or, in burns, the eschar, must be done as soon as possible to prevent necrosis of the deep tissues. The patient must be kept nonweightbearing and the pain

treated. Radiographs are helpful to rule out fractures, dislocations, and gas gangrene.

Post-traumatic Neurovascular Compromise

Diagnosis

Fractures and dislocations can result in nerves and blood vessels becoming stretched, transected, or compressed by malpositioned bones. Pain may seem disproportionate. The involved foot and ankle may demonstrate severe deformity. Knowledge of normal local anatomy is essential.

Treatment

Immediate consultation and referral to the appropriate surgical podiatrist or orthopedist is required. Reduction of the deformity or release of the compression is needed. Delays result in irreversible damage to nerves or vessels. Nonweightbearing and immobilization are required. Relocation or reduction attempted by untrained individuals can result in damage to the neurovascular structures.

Diabetic Charcot Fractures

Diabetic Charcot fractures are unique because they are difficult to diagnose and difficult to treat.[3] Misdiagnosis of Charcot joint disease as osteomyelitis often results in unnecessary hospitalization and delay in providing appropriate care. A seemingly minor foot sprain with no radiographic changes can progress to fragmentation, dislocation, and dissolution of bones and joints of the foot and ankle in diabetic patients. This degeneration may be rapid (over a few weeks) or may linger as vague symptoms of pain, localized increased temperatures, and edema for several months before showing radiographic changes. Rockerbottom foot is an example of disabling Charcot joint disease in which the cuneiform bone is displaced plantarly, often resulting in ulceration. All bones and joints of the foot and ankle can be affected.

A high index of suspicion is needed, as is a preventive approach. In diabetic patients, even minor foot sprains should be immobilized, and protective weightbearing should be started. Radiographs should be repeated in 4–8 weeks, depending on resolution or progression of symptoms. Continued local tenderness, edema, or increased temperature suggest unresolved problems and the need to continue treatment while evaluating other possible diagnoses. Referral to a podiatrist or consultation with a podiatrist is recommended when diagnosis is unclear.

Ulcerations

Wound Care Concepts

All ulcers and wounds are not the same. However, ulcerations and open surgical wounds of the feet share basic requirements for healing. Healthy, well-nourished, normally hydrated individuals heal better than poorly controlled diabetic individuals.

Patient and family compliance is a critical factor in wound healing. Obesity, loss of vision, decreased flexibility, and loss of dexterity for the patient or family member caregiver can preclude compliance in home ulcer care. Native languages may not translate accurately into seemingly basic wound care instructions involving time, order, priority, urgency, or even color. Transportation, telephones, housing, electricity, and food cannot be assumed to be consistently available. All of these affect compliance.

Diabetic individuals with ulcerations or open foot wounds almost always have some loss of protective sensation and some level of arterial insufficiency. Inadequate or reduced arterial profusion can be localized to the tip of a toe secondary to thrombosed vessels, or can involve significant occlusion of one or all of the major arteries entering the lower extremity. Ulcers and wounds cannot heal without adequate local blood flow.

Pressure on a wound in a sensate person causes pain and tissue necrosis if the pressure impairs the blood flow to the wound. In a diabetic individual with sensory neuropathy, there is a reduced or absent pain response to this same injurious pressure. Excessive pressure can result from standing, walking, sitting, or lying without protective redistribution of pressure away from the ulcer or wound. Tight bandages, heavy bed coverings, elastic or tight footwear or socks can create pressure. Ulcers and wounds cannot heal without protection from injurious pressure.

Necrotic or devitalized tissue in a wound or ulcer creates an enhanced environment for infection and inflammation. Conservative sharp débridement is the most expedient method for debris removal. Sensate individuals require anesthesia. Local anesthetic does not work in areas of inflammation or infection.

Infections must be treated. Undiagnosed osteomyelitis or deep soft tissue infections will delay or prevent healing of involved foot wounds or ulcers. Leakage of synovial fluid from disrupted joint capsules or tendon sheaths can delay healing even without infection.

More than 150 manufacturers market greater than 1,000 wound care dressings and topical agents. These products are effective only after the basic requirements for wound healing have been met as previously described.

The concept of moist wound healing has gained broad acceptance and fostered the development of specialized dressing materials and topical agents. Dressings divided into categories based on materials include: transparent films, polymeric foams, hydrogels, hydrocolloids, alginates, collagens, hydrofibers, hydropolymers, superabsorbents, and combinations. The volume of choices can be overwhelming. Sterile gauze dressings are still acceptable if a podiatrist or other wound-care-knowledgeable provider is not available.

Topical wound care agents are less confusing. Agents cleanse, reduce bacterial growth, débride, hydrate, absorb exudate, or add growth factor. Sterile Ringer's lactate, or normal saline are inexpensive, available, and not cytotoxic for irrigating ulcers and wounds. There are more than 50 wound cleansing sprays or liquids available. Antibacterials include silver sulfadiazine (Silvadene); polymyxin B sulfate and bacitracin zinc (Polysporin); bacitracin; and polymyxin B sulfate, bacitracin zinc, and neomycin (Neosporin). Débriding agents include papain-urea (Accuzyme), Santyl, fibrinolysin and desoxyribonuclease (Elase), and papain-urea-chlorophyllin copper complex sodium (Panafil).

Topical wound care agents such as Curasol gel and Dermagran gel help maintain a moist wound environment in ulcers or wounds prone toward drying. Agents such as calcium alginate (Sorbsan) and collagen calcium alginate (Fibracol) absorb large volumes of exudate. Another agent useful in difficult to heal wounds is becaplermin (Regranex) gel 0.01%. The only recombinant platelet-derived growth factor available, becaplermin has been approved by the U.S. Food and Drug Administration for treatment of diabetic foot ulcers.

Diabetic Neuropathic Ulcers

Diagnosis

Diabetic neuropathic ulcers occur in patients with diabetes mellitus when protective sensation is markedly decreased and when pressure is applied to a localized area of skin.[4] Generally, these occur over a bony prominence. Common areas are the tips and tops of toes, the knuckle areas between toes, under the metatarsal heads, under the big toe, under the base of the fifth metatarsal, on the sides of the first and fifth metatarsal heads, and at the heel.

Ulcers may appear as calluses or corns with hematomas beneath them. Sometimes they present as blisters and sometimes they are deep holes, with exposed tendon or bone. Seldom is pain a complaint unless the ulcer is infected or involves a fracture, as with Charcot fractures. Uninfected ulcers can cause increased foot temperature because increased blood flow is needed to heal the ulcer. Infected ulcers may not cause warm feet because the patient may not mount an adequate inflammatory response. Similarly, edema can be the result of something other than the ulcer. Ulcer bases usually appear red and vascular.

Swab cultures of ulcers are not helpful because they typically yield polymicrobial colonies. Most ulcers are not infected. Swab cultures may result in antibiotic therapy for uninfected ulcers or inappropriate broad-spectrum antibiotic therapy. Oral temperatures, white cell counts, and radiographs are helpful in determining whether an infection exists. Systemic complaints may be present with infected ulcers.

Treatment

Uninfected neuropathic ulcers are best treated with local wound care and total protection from pressure. Irrigating the ulcer or cleansing with normal saline or Ringer's lactate reduces bacterial counts, thereby reducing the risk of infection. The use of foot soaks and whirlpools is controversial. Total-contact casts are of great benefit if applied by an experienced provider and if the patient is reliable and has easy access to a specialist if complications arise.[5, 6] A more benign alternative is a posterior sugar-tong splint and crutches with at least daily dressing changes at home. Healing sandals can be fabricated using postoperative shoes and sheet orthotic material. These are less effective in reducing pressure, but they permit walking. There is much controversy about the best dressing for each circumstance. Frequent cleaning with noncytotoxic liquids and sterile dressings are a safe start. Patients with neuropathic foot ulcers should be referred to the podiatrist. Debridement should only be attempted by primary care providers with documented training and experience. Recurrence can be prevented through shoe therapy or reconstructive surgery.[7, 8]

Ischemic Ulcers

Diagnosis

Ischemic ulcers tend to be painful and do not usually have rapid onset. Skin is often dark, stiff, and dystrophic. Pulses are not palpable and may be monophasic when evaluated with Doppler handheld vascular testing devices.

If bleeding occurs, it is not robust. Ulcer bases are generally dry and often black. Ischemic ulcers can occur in otherwise vascular feet, especially in the toes, if digital arteries become occluded. When dry and not infected, these ulcers may demarcate and produce a mummified portion, which can be treated nonacutely.

Treatment

The first goal is to prevent additional injury to the foot. Constriction from dressings, stockings, and footwear should be avoided. Sheets and blankets can cause ischemia if too tight or heavy. Sitting or reclining with unprotected heels against the bed, chair, or floor can cause injury. Foam heel protectors and open-toed post-surgical shoes can provide immediate relief. Foot cradles can hold covers away from toes in bed. Antibiotic ointment and a dry sterile dressing can moisten tissue, but care must be taken to avoid maceration, which can result in additional tissue loss. Referral for baseline vascular evaluation is needed. Ulcers that are malodorous, mushy with necrosis, or soupy with liquefied tissue may require antibiotic therapy, but more urgently they require debridement to limit maceration necrosis of adjacent tissue. Vascular reconstruction is not always possible or successful. Partial leg amputations are sometimes required.

Infected Ulcers

Diagnosis

Infected ulcers may have a benign appearance with minimal localized or systemic reaction, as with a chronic osteomyelitis. In contrast, ulcers may be malodorous, draining, and painful. The foot or leg may be hot, red, and swollen. The patient may have fever, chills, nausea, and uncontrolled diabetes. White cell counts may be normal or elevated. Radiographs may show gas, bone erosion from osteomyelitis, or fluid from abscess formation. Malodorous ulcers may be infected or may be filled with necrotic decomposing tissue.

Treatment

Diabetic individuals with infected lower-extremity ulcers must be admitted to the hospital. Local wound care should include irrigation with normal saline or Ringer's lactate and application of absorptive dry sterile dressings. The patient is kept nonweightbearing to prevent mechanical spreading of infection. The patient should be hydrated using intravenous fluids. Electrolytes and blood sugars should be evaluated and stabilized. Because the risk of amputation is present, nearly all cases of infected diabetic ulcers should be admitted to the hospital. If there is any question about the presence of osteomyelitis, abscess, or necrotic or undermined tissue, the patient should be immediately referred to a surgical podiatrist, orthopedist, or surgeon for debridement. Appropriate antibiotic therapy is best based on intraoperative deep-tissue cultures.

Venous Stasis Ulcers

Diagnosis

Most frequently located in the supramalleolar areas of the legs, these ulcers are moist with granulating bases and normal sensation. Left untreated, they can completely encircle the leg. Edema is always present, and fluid leakage from the ulcer is profound. Infection is almost never a problem, and bone is rarely involved. Neuropathic ulcers and ischemic ulcers are rarely found in this location. Ulcerations are sensate, wet, and associated with edema.

Treatment

Resolution of the ulcer occurs through maintaining a clean wound and controlling edema. Elevation of the patient's feet above his or her heart is necessary but not adequate. Compression can be applied with dry dressings and flexible bandages (Ace), but it is impossible to maintain consistent pressure. A calamine gelatin zinc oxide–impregnated bandage may be used to prevent additional edema and promote ulcer healing. Several other commercial products attempt to provide a positive healing environment for the ulcer and consistent, appropriate compression for the edema. Draining ulcers require more frequent dressing changes. Once resolved, graded compression stockings discourage recurrence. Recalcitrant ulcers may require surgical ligation of perforating veins.

Punctures, Lacerations, and Foreign Bodies

Diagnosis

Diabetic foot infections in Native Americans are most often related to neuropathic ulcerations, but puncture wounds, lacerations, or foreign bodies are associated with most other diabetic foot infections. Diabetic sensory neuropathy and alcohol-induced amnesia can make the circumstance and time of injury unclear.

Inoculation of deep structures with debris or bacteria may result in deep infections. Organic material, such as wood, pine needles, cactus spines, and animal hair, are not visible on radiographs but often result in infections. Fragments of shoe or sock are sometimes implanted with puncture or laceration wounds, are not evident on radiographs, and are often associated with infections.

Puncture and laceration injuries to bone, joint, and tendon are often not diagnosed. Lacerations often transect tendons in front of the ankle or leg, on top of the foot or toes, and in the Achilles tendon area. Lacerated tendons often retract, leaving no evidence of injury. Transected nerves blend with the color of fascia. Unless a bone defect or fragment is evident on radiographs, bone or joint injury may not be recognized.

The time of the injury and the level of contamination must be determined. A sensory examination must be documented before injecting local anesthetics. Arterial status must be documented. Muscle and tendon function of the injured extremity should be compared to the uninjured extremity. Radiographs should be taken. Tetanus prophylaxis status must be determined.

Treatment

Tetanus status must be updated. Radiographs are read and findings documented. Local anesthetic may be injected proximal to the injury before cleaning and inspecting the wound. Eye protection should be used when irrigating the wound with normal saline or Ringer's lactate.

Unnecessary manipulation of tissue with forceps or hemostats will cause additional tissue necrosis. Transected tendons should be referred to a surgical specialist. Wounds can be enlarged to permit retrieval of foreign material, but it is not prudent to dissect into deep tissues where sensitive structures may be injured.

Glass is difficult to see if not colored and can be broken in the wound if aggressive instrumentation is attempted. Copious irrigation should be done. Wounds greater than 6 hours old or contaminated with debris should be packed open and oral antibiotics prescribed. No wound should be closed under tension.

Injuries involving nerves, arteries, tendons, or bones must be immobilized in a splint and protected from weightbearing. For patients with normal sensation, dressing changes may be painful. All punctures and lacerations should be rechecked in 3–5 days. Injuries involving bones or joints should be evaluated radiographically in approximately 3 weeks to rule out fractures or osteomyelitis.

Infections

Cellulitis

Diagnosis

The patient's lower extremity presents with erythema, edema, pain, and localized increased temperature. There may be intact uninjured skin or a history of trauma, puncture wound, ulceration, maceration, dermatitis, or ingrown toenail. The white cell count and erythrocyte sedimentation rate may be elevated. Radiographs may be unremarkable. The patient may be febrile and present with flulike symptoms or may have only local symptoms.

Superficial swab cultures of ulcers are not helpful because they are frequently polymicrobial and do not contain pathogens. Blood cultures, if indicated and when positive, may help to identify a pathogenic organism.

Attempts to aspirate organisms directly from inflamed soft tissue in the absence of a septic joint or well-defined abscess are not indicated.

Treatment

In the absence of necrotic tissue, abscess, osteomyelitis, or joint sepsis, the patient should be protected from additional stress to the infected limb and provided with appropriate antibiotic therapy. Consultation with a pharmacist about local patterns of bacterial sensitivity and resistance is recommended. The decision to hospitalize rather than treat on an outpatient basis must be made based on the degree of involvement of the extremity, the overall health of the patient, and access-to-care factors, such as distance, weather, and availability of reliable transportation.

All septic individuals should be admitted to the hospital. All immunocompromised individuals, such as diabetic patients, also should be admitted. Hospitalized patients should be kept nonweightbearing to reduce the spread of infection along fascial planes. Lower-extremity elevation and splint immobilization are recommended unless there is arterial compromise.

Abscess

Diagnosis

An abscess may form with or without an open wound because callus may cover ulcers and puncture wounds may become indistinct. Cellulitis may be very localized or diffuse. There is generally localized pain and tense edema, frequently with shiny skin overlying the abscess. White cell counts and erythrocyte sedimentation rates are elevated. Radiographs show fluid levels as dark areas that are visible when three views of the involved foot are compared or when radiographs of the involved and uninvolved foot are compared.

Fluid can be aspirated from the abscess for Gram's stain, culture, and sensitivity. The site should be prepared with povidone-iodine (Betadine), cleaned with alcohol, and allowed to dry. Local anesthetics may be ineffective because of the infection.

Treatment

An abscess should be treated like cellulitis, except that the abscess must be opened and drained of exudate and debrided of necrotic tissue. Because surgery is needed, appropriate prompt referral to a surgical podiatrist, orthopedist, or surgeon must be done at the time of diagnosis.

Joint Sepsis

Diagnosis

Joint sepsis must be differentiated from inflammatory arthritis, degenerative arthritis, and Charcot joint disease. There may be a history of a puncture wound or an existing ulceration close to the joint involved. Presentation is similar to an abscess, except that the infection is contained in a joint. Radiographs may show distention of the joint. In the absence of an entry point for bacteria, joint sepsis is not likely to occur. Systemic response may be mild unless there is cellulitis or an open wound. Attempts to aspirate fluid from joints in the foot or ankle should be deferred to someone with appropriate training and experience.

Treatment

Because joints are relatively avascular, an infection can quickly develop into osteomyelitis. Joint sepsis cannot be treated solely with antibiotics. All suspected or diagnosed cases of joint sepsis must be hospitalized and referred promptly to the appropriate surgical specialist.

Osteomyelitis

Diagnosis

Bone infection or osteomyelitis can occur through direct inoculation (as in a puncture wound), as a result of an adjacent ulceration (as occurs in diabetic individuals), or through hematogenous spread. Charcot joint disease can be confused with osteomyelitis clinically and radiographically. Although rare, osteomyelitis from tuberculosis or fungus can mimic bone tumors both radiographically and clinically. Definitive diagnosis can be made only through positive bone cultures and positive histologic findings. Erosion of bone seen on current radiographs when compared to past radiographs suggests osteomyelitis if positively correlated with clinical findings. Expensive examinations, such as magnetic resonance imaging, computed tomography scans, or technetium or gallium scans, may suggest but not confirm a diagnosis of osteomyelitis. Exposed, contaminated bone is presumed to be infected.

Treatment

All cases should be referred promptly. Biopsies and bone cultures must be done intraoperatively to select appropriate antibiotics. Patients should be kept nonweightbearing until evaluated by a surgical podiatrist, orthopedist, or surgeon.

Gas Gangrene

See Gas Gangrene under Foot and Ankle Emergencies.

Toenails

Fungal or Mycotic Toenails

Diagnosis

Fungal toenails present as thick, brittle, yellow or white nails with thick, crumbly debris under the nail and a distinctive odor. The fungus generally attacks and undermines the free edge of the nail until the nail is no longer connected to the nail bed.

Treatment

Treatment is aimed at removing the loose nail and debris using toenail nippers. This prevents further undermining caused by the loose nail catching on socks or sheets. Topical antifungal creams or solutions can be applied to the nail and nail bed to moisten and to contain the spread. Care should be taken to not spread fungus to uninfected nails with the nail nippers. Fungus in toenails can spread to the feet, causing tinea pedis, and can spread to other family members. Showers and bathtubs may be cleaned with bleach to prevent spread of fungus to other family members. Clean, dry socks should be changed at least daily. Shoes should be dry, clean, and rotated. If athletic shoes are washed, care must be taken to watch for shrinkage, especially in patients with sensory neuropathy or vascular compromise. New oral antifungal agents are marketed, but none have proved to be consistently effective in completely resolving and preventing recurrence of mycotic toenail infections.[9] Debridement rather than nail avulsion is recommended for primary care providers because avulsion can damage the nail matrix, and avulsed nails regrow. Nail avulsions with destruction of the root or matrix can be done by the podiatrist.

Partial Toenail Avulsions

Diagnosis

Partial toenail avulsions may occur with crushing injuries or when the tip of the nail gets caught on another object. There is frequently bleeding and pain when the involved toenail is touched. With crush injuries, there is risk of fracture of the distal phalanx; therefore, radiographs should be taken.

Treatment

With tearing or crush injuries, the nail bed should be cleaned with a mild detergent, diluted hydrogen peroxide, or diluted povidone-iodine solution. Free, unattached nail should be removed using toenail nippers, taking care not to pry the nail against the matrix area, which would further deform the new nail. If the patient requires anesthesia, 1% or 2% plain lidocaine may be injected between the base and head of the proximal phalanx of the toe in a ring block to anesthetize all four nerves entering the toe. Under no circumstances should anesthetic be injected into the tip of the toe or into the nail bed because this causes unnecessary additional trauma and does not provide adequate anesthesia. The torn nail bed may be sutured. A nonstick dressing (e.g., Adaptic) makes dressing changes less painful and is appreciated by the patient. Antibiotics are not required unless there is infection or an open frac-

ture. The nail bed should be cleaned with soap and water and antibacterial ointment applied daily. The new nail regrows in approximately 6 months but may be deformed. If the primary care provider does not routinely do nail surgery, a prompt referral to podiatry is appropriate. Fractures of the distal tuft are usually absorbed or coalesce and do not require buddy taping or splinting.

Ingrown Toenails

Diagnosis

Ingrown toenails can be extremely painful for individuals with normal protective sensation. They occur because of the shape of the nail, the manner in which the nail has been cut, and the type of pressure applied to the nail. Once the nail breaks the skin, an infection may occur, with erythema, edema, increased local temperature, and drainage. A pyogenic granuloma or proud flesh often forms at the site of ingrowth. The toenail is treated by the body as a foreign object.

Treatment

The portion of the toenail causing injury to the toe must be removed. If only the end corner of a toenail is involved, a sharp nail nipper is sometimes used to cut diagonally through the offending corner to remove the triangular piece of nail. Anesthetic is not generally needed for this. If the entire side of the toenail is causing pressure, the toe should be anesthetized as previously described in Treatment under Partial Toenail Avulsions. Then the toe should be gently scrubbed. Sterile technique and sterile instruments should be used. Scissors are not appropriate for this procedure because they cause unnecessary damage to the nail bed and matrix. Cleaning with mild soap and water daily and applying sterile dry dressings for several days facilitates healing. Most infected nail margins respond to removal of the piece of offending nail and topical cleaning with a week of oral antibiotics. Cephalexin, 500 mg, or dicloxacillin, 500 mg, generally works well. If infection persists, cultures should be done and radiographs should be taken to rule out osteomyelitis or joint sepsis. Recurrent cases should be referred to a podiatrist for permanent destruction of the involved portion of the nail matrix.

Thickened Toenails

Diagnosis

A thickened toenail occurs secondary to repeated trauma to the matrix area at the base of the nail. These nails are hard, sometimes discolored, and uniform in consistency. Thickened toenails can cause subungual ulceration or ulceration of adjacent toes in diabetic, neuropathic individuals.

Treatment

Patients or family members can use nail files or emery boards to sand the top layers off the nails. Nail removal is not recommended.

Subungual Hematomas

Diagnosis

Subungual hematoma occurs with trauma to the top of the nail. A dark spot of red, blue, purple, or brown is evident beneath the nail with rounded margins, consistent with a past or present fluid level. In neuropathic individuals, there may be no patient history of trauma.

Treatment

Frequently, no treatment is needed. The hematoma will move forward with nail growth to disappear off the distal end of the toe. If pressure under the nail causes excessive discomfort, the nail can be punctured with a heated sterile steel needle. Care should be taken not to cause injury with the needle.

Heel Pain: Plantar Fasciitis

Diagnosis

Radiographs are not indicated for diagnosis or treatment for most heel pain patients. A thorough history and physical examination permit diagnosis of most cases with the chief complaint of heel pain. Radiographs are mandatory if any of the following are suspected: fracture, foreign body, osteomyelitis, dislocation, bone tumor, or cyst.

Plantar fasciitis is by far the most common reason for heel pain. Pain is recurrent or progressive, relieved by rest, and exacerbated by standing after resting. Pain may be very localized or diffuse on the plantar aspect of the heel. After the patient starts walking, pain sometimes subsides. Edema may or may not be present. Side compression or squeezing the heel between the palms of the hand does not elicit pain, as it often does with fractures. Radiographs are not helpful or indicated because the presence or absence of a spur does not correlate with the presence or absence of heel pain.

Treatment

Treatment can begin with a nonsteroidal anti-inflammatory agent, ice to the bottom of the involved heel or heels, and rest from unnecessary activity. Injections of anesthetic and steroid without addressing the underlying problem provide only temporary relief. Athletic footwear or walking shoes provide some support. Over-the-counter arch supports provide generic support. Referral to podiatry for evaluation and treatment should be done in resistant cases. Surgery is seldom required. Weight loss or change in style of footwear is frequently needed. Stretching the Achilles tendon also helps to reduce tension on the plantar fascia.

Pediatrics

Heel Pain: Calcaneal Apophysitis

Diagnosis

Heel pain in an 8- to 14-year-old child affecting the posterior calcaneus at the attachments of the Achilles tendon and the plantar fascia in one or both feet is most likely *calcaneal apophysitis*. Mild edema and mild localized increases in temperature with focal tenderness at the posterior-inferior calcaneus or on dorsiflexion of the patient's foot strongly suggests this diagnosis. Radiographs may be helpful if trauma suggests a calcaneal fracture, although these are rare in children. Radiographs may be helpful if there is concern about infection or foreign bodies. Radiographs must be interpreted with caution because the calcaneal apophysis is sometimes misread as fractured.

Treatment

In severe cases, a below-the-knee cast for 4–6 weeks is recommended, starting with slight plantarflexion of the foot. Less severe cases may be treated with 0.25-in. firm heel lifts inside the shoe, ice to the heels, and crutches. Referral to a podiatrist for evaluation and treatment of the predisposing pathology is recommended if the patient does not respond.

Arch Pain

Diagnosis

Arch pain is often secondary to pes planus or flexible flat foot. If there is a painful hard bump in the apex of the medial arch, the problem is probably an enlarged or extranavicular bone. Flexible flat foot and accessory navicular bones are confirmed radiographically.

Treatment

Flexible flat foot should be treated by a podiatrist, with orthotics or arch supports. Accessory or enlarged navicular bones may need to be surgically corrected by a podiatrist to restore the proper function of the posterior tibial muscle, which attaches to the navicular bone and normally supports the arch. Extranavicular bones are common among some Native American people.

Salter-Harris Fractures

Diagnosis

Salter-Harris fractures involve the growth plates and are unique to children.[10]

Any child presenting with pain localized to a bone or joint after trauma should have radiographs. Special attention must be paid to the growth plates of the bones. Salter I fractures may not be evident radiographically and may be diagnosed because of the location of the tenderness along the growth plate.

Treatment

All Salter-Harris fractures should be immobilized in a well-padded splint, and the child should be kept non-weightbearing with crutches. Ice reduces edema and pain. All these fractures should be referred to a podiatrist or orthopedist with experience in pediatric surgery because some of these may require surgical reduction and fixation. Attempts to reduce these fractures by an inexperienced provider can injure the growth plate further and lead to premature closure or angulational deformities.

Summary

Knowing when to treat and when to refer is critical to providing good care to patients with foot and ankle disease. Referral differs greatly throughout the facilities in which Native American people are cared for by primary care providers. In some facilities, podiatry, surgery, orthopedics, and physical therapy are available. In other facilities, one or more of these may be available only via telephone and a long patient transport.

Rapid and accurate diagnosis of foot and ankle disease is not something taught in most primary care programs. With experience and the availability of specialists, most primary care providers can become comfortable and competent at recognizing the abundance and variety of lower-extremity pathology seen in Native American health care facilities. The ability to treat each pathology described depends on the individual provider, the support staff, the physical plant, and proximity to specialists. Every Indian health care facility should have access to the services of a board-certified or board-qualified podiatric surgeon.

Acknowledgements

Special thanks to two of the first Indian health podiatrists, Dr. Charles Markham and Dr. James Konieczny, for their insight and support in writing this chapter.

References

1. Dannels EG. Prevention of Complications of Partial Foot Amputations in American Indian Diabetics. In Harkless LB, Dessis KJ (eds), The Diabetic Foot Clin Pod Med and Surg 1987;4:503–516.
2. Birke JA, Sims DS. Plantar sensory threshold in the ulcerative foot. Lepr Rev 1986;57:261–267.
3. Sanders LJ, Frykberg RG. Diabetic Neuropathic Osteoarthropathy: The Charcot Foot. In RG Frykbert (eds), The High Risk Foot in Diabetes Mellitus. New York: Churchill Livingstone, 1991;297–338.
4. Brand PW. Management of the insensitive limb. Phys Ther 1979;59:8–12.
5. Coleman WC, Brand PW, Birke JA. The total contact case, a therapy for plantar ulceration on insensitive feet. J Am Podiatr Med Assoc 1984;74:548.
6. Burnett O. Total Contact Cast. In Harkless LB, Dennis KJ (eds), The Diabetic Foot Clin Pod Med and Surg 1987;4:471.
7. Dannels EG. A preventive metatarsal osteotomy for healing pre-ulcers in American Indian diabetics. J Am Podiatr Med Assoc 1986;76:33.
8. Dannels E. Neuropathic foot ulcer prevention in diabetic American Indians with hallux limitus. J Am Podiatr Med Assoc 1989;79:447.
9. Joseph WS. Oral treatment options for onychomycosis. J Am Podiatr Med Assoc 1997;87:520.
10. Salter RB, Harris WR. Injuries involving the epiphyseal plate. J Bone Joint Surg Am 1963;45:587.

Part XVII
Dentistry

Chapter 44
Dental Problems

John F. Neale

The primary care physician frequently receives little formal training in the diagnosis and treatment of dental diseases, yet he or she is often the first health care professional to see a patient with a dental problem. Additionally, oral diseases have almost universal prevalence among Native Americans; individuals rarely, if ever, go unaffected by one of the oral diseases throughout their lifetime. The World Health Organization (WHO) has estimated that the oral cavity can be affected by up to 265 categories of diseases or conditions. Most prevalent among these are conditions affecting the teeth and those affecting the periodontium, the supporting structures of the teeth. The vast majority of dental services provided to Native Americans are directed toward the treatment and prevention of caries and periodontitis. Of equal or greater public health importance, due to the devastating effects of the disease, are the prevention and treatment of oral cancer. This chapter provides an overview of three oral conditions with great public health significance among Native Americans and reviews strategies for their prevention, diagnosis, and treatment. This should aid the primary care physician in recognizing dental problems in their early stages, providing preventive and curative therapy when indicated, and making appropriate referrals to dental professionals for definitive care when necessary.

Dental Caries

Epidemiology

Because of oral health status surveys conducted by the Indian Health Service (IHS) in 1984 and 1991, much is currently known about the distribution of caries among Native Americans. Far less is known about the determinants of this disease entity in this population.

Dental caries rates in populations are measured using the DMF index, which counts the number of decayed teeth

(D), teeth missing due to tooth decay (M), and filled (F) teeth (T) or tooth surfaces (S). It measures the total lifetime caries experience of individuals and accounts for both treated and untreated disease. Because the index is cumulative, the number of both DMFT and DMFS increases with age.

In the general population of the United States, the prevalence of dental caries has been declining since the 1970s. In 1987, as measured in the National Institute of Dental Research (NIDR) Dental Caries Prevalence Survey, 50% of U.S. children ages 5–17 years had never had a cavity in their permanent teeth, compared with only 37% in 1980. Additionally, the DMFS was 3 for urban children in this age group, 3.2 for rural children, and 3.4 for minorities. By contrast, in the 1991 IHS Oral Health Status Survey, only 35% of Native American children ages 5–17 were free of caries, the DMFS for the age group was 5, and a much larger proportion of Native American children had a DMFS of 7 or higher (28%) than did the U.S. children in the 1987 survey (17%).[1] The trends are similar among adults. Native American adults in 1991 averaged 2.3 decayed teeth, compared with only 0.6 in the U.S. population in a 1985 NIDR Oral Health Survey of U.S. Employed Adults, a difference of more than three times.

Etiology, Clinical Presentation, Diagnostics, Prevention, and Therapy

Dental caries is the disease process that leads to the destruction of the tooth surface, commonly known as *cavities*. Multiple factors must be present for the caries process to progress: a susceptible tooth surface, cariogenic bacteria, and a substrate or diet containing fermentable carbohydrate or sugar. Enamel destruction is caused by the effects of organic acids on the inorganic crystalline hydroxyapatite component of the enamel. The organic acids are produced by microorganisms as metabolic by-products of the fermentation of carbohydrates and sugars. These microorganisms colonize the tooth surface by producing a soft, sticky film known as *plaque* that holds both the microorganisms and the organic acids in tight proximity to the tooth surface. Specific microorganisms are known to play important roles in the pathogenesis of dental caries. *Mutans streptococci* are the primary organisms associated with coronal caries, although *Lactobacillus* species are associated with the further development of coronal carious lesions. *Actinomyces* species, on the other hand, are associated with root surface caries.

Baby bottle tooth decay (BBTD), also known as *nursing bottle caries* and *bottle mouth*, is a unique pattern of severe tooth decay seen in infants and young children. The decay pattern begins with the primary maxillary incisors followed by the cuspids and primary molars, in order of eruption. Mandibular incisors are seldom involved, except in the most severe cases. BBTD is caused by many behaviors, such as giving a child a bottle containing carbohydrates at bedtime, bottle-feeding past the age of 12 months, the use of pacifiers dipped in sweeteners such as honey, and prolonged, at-will breast-feeding.[2] *Early childhood caries* (ECC) is a broader term that describes dental decay in preschool-age children from any source and includes BBTD. In 1988, Ripa[3] reviewed the prevalence of BBTD in the United States and other Western countries. He found a prevalence of this condition in these countries of 5% or less. By contrast, the 1983–1984 IHS Oral Health Status survey showed a prevalence of BBTD of 52%,[4] and Kelly and Bruerd,[5] in 1987, found the prevalence in Native American populations to have a mean of 53%, with a range of 17–85%. The 1991 IHS survey revealed a prevalence of 51.7%, which was only 0.3% less than the 1984 rate. Unpublished data from some IHS programs have shown prevalence of more than 90%.

BBTD/ECC can be a devastating condition for the young child. The numerous, large carious lesions associated with this condition cause chronic pain for the child and place the child at significant risk of developing odontogenic infections, leading to fascial cellulitis, fascial space infections, and similar sequelae. The treatment of severe cases of ECC in the young, precooperative child often requires treatment in the operating room to restore or extract teeth as needed. Cook et al.[6] found the mean cost of treating nursing caries in the Choctaw Indian Head Start program in Mississippi to be $2,141.75 for cases requiring operating room treatment. With medical inflation, this cost is significantly higher today.

Prevention of BBTD/ECC has been an ongoing effort for more than 10 years in IHS dental programs. A BBTD prevention program based on community-level education and training of parents and caregivers in 12 Native American communities led to a reduction in the prevalence of BBTD from 57% in 1986 to 43% in 1990.[7] By 1995,

however, it was clear that this reduction was not maintained unless the full intervention program continued. In the five sites that continued the full program, the prevalence had fallen to 38%, but in the seven sites that discontinued the program, the net reduction was only 13% over the 8 years of the program. Staff turnover was the primary reason for stopping the program. The authors concluded that the BBTD intervention program was effective but that it must become institutionalized for continuing success.[8]

Although the American Academy of Pediatric Dentistry recommends that children receive their first dental examination by age 1 year, this occurs infrequently in Native American populations. Patient visit data from the Uintah and Ouray Service Unit of the IHS for fiscal year 1996 revealed that only 11 of 200 children younger than age 36 months received dental care. IHS programs that have a pediatric dentist on staff may have higher use by this age group. In comparison, by the time a child first visits a dentist, he or she may have had seven or more medical appointments for well-child examinations and immunizations.[9] Dental evaluation by the primary care physician is therefore an important part of the physical examination of the infant and young child.[9]

Dental evaluation of the infant and young child for BBTD/ECC is a simple procedure. The primary care practitioner lifts the child's upper lip to examine the maxillary anterior teeth for signs of caries and the labial aspect of the maxillary gingiva and alveolar mucosa for evidence of dental infection. Dental caries can appear as opaque white-spot lesions, usually at or near the gum line, in its earliest form. Later, brown cavitations may appear. In its most severe form, there may be complete loss of the tooth crown. The latter is frequently accompanied by a swollen area or draining sinus tract, often called a "gum boil," on the gingiva or alveolar mucosa near the apex of the root of the affected tooth. Any of these signs of caries or odontogenic infection should generate a referral to a dentist. Besides providing a referral, the primary care physician can provide fluoride supplements in areas where the water is deficient in fluoride and can reinforce the following simple prevention messages on appropriate feeding habits:

1. Wean the baby from the bottle by 1 year of age.
2. Never put a baby to bed with a bottle.
3. Do not let a child have continuous access to a bottle during the day.
4. Do not share food or utensils with the child.

It is currently recognized that dental caries is an infectious and transmissible disease. It can be managed medically, by reducing or eliminating the causative organism, as well as surgically, by extracting the carious tooth or removing carious tooth structure and repairing the damage with a dental restoration. Currently, the best predictor of a person's risk of developing new carious lesions is the presence of current or past carious lesions. This risk can be diminished by reducing the patient's levels of *M. streptococci* through elimination of active carious lesions by extractions or restorations and the use of chemotherapeutic agents, such as chlorhexidine gluconate and topical fluorides, to reduce bacterial populations.

M. streptococci requires the presence of a stable surface, such as a tooth, to colonize the oral cavity. Oral mucosa, the surface of which is continuously being renewed, cannot be colonized. Therefore, before the first tooth erupts into the oral cavity, an infant's mouth is free of *M. streptococci*. The child appears to acquire *M. streptococci* during a discrete window of infectivity, which Caufield et al.[10] demonstrated to occur between 9 months and 44 months of age, with a median of 26 months. Because of their very high caries rate, Native American children are thought to fall into the earlier portion of this range. The child's mother appears to be the caregiver most often responsible for transmitting the bacteria to the child. If the transmission of *M. streptococci* from caregiver to child can be prevented until the child has established stable oral flora, then that transmission may be prevented altogether. Therefore, the child's risk of ever developing dental caries is greatly diminished.

During prenatal visits, the primary care physician should briefly assess the mother's oral health or make a referral to a dentist. It is currently thought that the transmission of *M. streptococci* to the unborn child may be prevented or delayed if the mother's oral health is improved before the birth. This includes treating any active, cavitated carious lesions and attempting to reduce the mother's *M. streptococci* counts through the use of chemotherapeutic agents before the child enters the window of infectivity.

As stated earlier, *Actinomyces* species are also associated with the development of root caries. Root caries is a disease associated with aging because it is often with increasing age that recession of the gingiva and periodontium leaves the root surfaces of the teeth exposed and susceptible to carious attack. The 1985 NIDR Oral Health Survey of U.S. Employed Adults revealed that 63% of men and 53% of women in older populations had at least one root surface lesion. Root surface caries was not specifically measured in the 1984 or 1991 IHS Oral Health Surveys, so a comparison with the Native American population is not available.

Beyond age, few variables have been consistently associated with the formation of root caries. One risk factor that does appear to be associated, at least empirically, is the presence of xerostomia (dry mouth), which is a side effect of many medications used in aging populations. Saliva is the oral cavity's principal defense against caries. Minerals in the saliva contribute to the remineralization of the tooth surface, and the buffering capacity of the saliva helps to neutralize the organic acids produced by cariogenic bacteria. The use of topical fluoride applications, such as stannous fluoride gels and fluoride varnishes, seems helpful in preventing root surface caries. Artificial saliva substitutes containing fluoride may also help to prevent these lesions in patients with xerostomia. A preparation of pilocarpine HCl 5-mg tablets is marketed for the specific purpose of stimulating salivary flow in patients with xerostomia who still have salivary function. It is therefore appropriate for primary care physicians to consider referring any older patients who are on chronic medications that can cause xerostomia to a dentist so that salivary flow can be evaluated and appropriate treatment or preventive regimens begun.

At any age, dental caries, left untreated, can progress until it invades the pulp of the tooth. When oral flora penetrate the carious lesion, infection of the dental pulp can lead to the formation of alveolar abscesses. This occurs when the infection progresses beyond the end of the root of the tooth. Such odontogenic infections can progress into facial cellulitis or infections of the fascial spaces of the head, neck, and oropharynx. Patients with these infections often first seek care in the emergency room, where the first medical professional to evaluate and treat them is often a physician. Odontogenic infections are usually mixed infections consisting of gram-negative and gram-positive aerobes and anaerobes. *Bacteroides* and *Streptococcus* species are commonly found in odontogenic infections. In the absence of cultures and sensitivities, penicillin V potassium remains the drug of choice to treat these infections, with a minimum oral dose of 500 mg every 6 hours for the normal adult. Broader-spectrum antibiotics, such as amoxicillin, cephalexin, and amoxicillin/clavulanate potassium, are usually not needed for the primary treatment of odontogenic infections. Therapeutic failures with penicillin V potassium almost always respond to combination therapy with penicillin V potassium/metronidazole (also at a 500-mg dose four times a day) or to therapy with clindamycin at an oral dose of 300 mg four times a day. Once the primary care physician has placed the emergency room patient on the appropriate antibiotic regimen, he or she should refer the patient to a dentist for definitive treatment of the infected tooth.

Periodontal Disease

Epidemiology

The term *periodontal disease* refers to a group of diseases and conditions of the hard and soft tissues that surround and support the teeth, including the gingiva, the periodontal ligament, and the alveolar bone, collectively known as the *periodontium*. The majority of adults exhibit some signs of periodontal disease, and gingival attachment loss has been measured in age groups as young as the early teens. At least five types of periodontal diseases have been identified: (1) adult periodontitis, (2) early-onset or juvenile periodontitis, (3) periodontitis associated with systemic diseases, (4) necrotizing ulcerative periodontitis, and (5) refractory periodontitis.[11] Adult periodontitis is the most common of these, but periodontitis associated with type II diabetes mellitus is increasingly important among Native American populations. Gingivitis, the inflammation of the gums, is a separate but related disease. Gingivitis can occur without progressing to destructive periodontitis, but periodontitis has not been reported to occur without having been preceded by gingivitis. Gingivitis is usually measured by bleeding of the gingiva, whereas periodontitis is frequently measured by the loss of attachment of the gingiva and periodontium from the root surface of the tooth.

Trends in the prevalence of periodontitis are less clear than dental caries trends. The 1985 NIDR Oral Health Survey of U.S. Employed Adults revealed the prevalence of gingivitis, as measured by bleeding, to be 43.5% in the employed sample and 46.8% among the seniors. Attachment loss of 2 mm or greater occurred in 76.6% of the employed and 95.1% of the seniors. This survey also revealed that 17% of U.S. adults ages 35–44 years had advanced periodontal disease, as measured by periodontal attachment loss. In contrast, 21% of Native Americans were found to have advanced periodontal disease in a 1990 WHO study of a community-based sample of Native Americans (Sioux and Navajo).[1] The 1991 IHS Oral Health Status Survey of clinical patients found advanced periodontal disease in 19% of nondiabetic patients and in 34% of diabetic patients.[1] Both the WHO and IHS studies used the Community Periodontal Index of Treatment Needs (CPITN) to assess periodontal condition rather than using attachment loss, as did the NIDR study. The CPITN measures periodontal pocket depth rather than attachment loss. Although the two are correlated, they are not equivalent.

Risk factors associated with the prevalence of periodontal disease include increasing age, poor education, lack of professional dental care, previous periodontal destruction, tobacco use, and diabetes.[12] Periodontal disease has been recognized by the American Diabetes Association as the sixth complication of diabetes mellitus.

In Native Americans, the association between periodontal disease and type 2 diabetes has been closely studied.[13–15] The Pima Indians of the Gila River Indian Community in Arizona have the highest reported incidence and prevalence of type 2 diabetes in the world, with more than 50% of those older than age 35 years affected. Other Native American populations, such as the Navajo, Northern Ute, and Tohono O'odham, also have type 2 diabetes rates much higher than the general U.S. population.

Studies of the Pima Indians have shown that diabetic status, age, and the presence of subgingival calculus are significantly associated with increased prevalence and severity of periodontal disease. Diabetic subjects had an increased risk of destructive periodontal disease, with an odds ratio of 3.43 when bone loss was used to measure periodontal destruction. After adjusting for the effects of demographic variables and several oral health indices, type 2 diabetes remained significantly related to both prevalence and severity of disease in this population.[13] In addition, Shlossman et al.[16] found a twofold-greater risk for severe periodontitis in patients with poorly controlled diabetes.

Etiology, Clinical Presentation, Diagnosis, Prevention, and Therapy

Periodontal disease occurs because of infection with pathogenic plaque bacteria in a susceptible host, leading to metabolic changes that cause pockets, attachment loss, and bone loss. Currently, at least 15 organisms have been closely associated with the development of destructive periodontitis, including *Actinobacillus actinomycetemcomitans*, *Porphyromonas gingivalis*, *Prevotella intermedia*, *Bacteroides intermedius*, *Eikenella corrodens*, and *Fusobacterium nucleatum*. The microflora found in type 2 diabetes patients is similar to that found in nondiabetic patients with chronic adult periodontitis. However, the strains of *P. gingivalis* from diabetic patients have been shown to exhibit more virulence than those from nondiabetic patients. As with dental caries, it has been demonstrated that the bacteria associated with periodontal disease are communicable but are not readily transmissible, with saliva being the major vector for bacterial transmission.[17]

Gingivitis associated with the accumulation of plaque is the most common of the periodontal diseases. It is characterized by redness, edema, enlargement, or bleeding of the gingiva and is often accompanied by pain or tenderness of the gingiva. Periodontitis represents a progression of the inflammation of the gingiva into the other supporting structures of the tooth. Left untreated, periodontitis can lead to a progressive destruction of the periodontal ligament and alveolar bone. This can result in the formation of periodontal pockets, periodontal attachment loss, and, ultimately, loosening and loss of the teeth.

The diagnosis of periodontal disease is entering a new era. Previously, the dentist could diagnose periodontal disease by pocket probing, visual examination, and radiography. However, these methods reveal only periodontal destruction that has already occurred and give little information about the current level of activity of periodontal disease. New methods are being developed to make these determinations,[18] including the following:

- Tests for causative factors, such as plaque bacteria, including bacterial culture, DNA probes, enzyme-linked immunosorbent assay (ELISA), and *n*-benzoyl-DL-arginine-naphthylamide test

- Tests for host susceptibility, such as polymorphonuclear chemotaxis
- Tests for inflammation, tissue damage, or tissue death, such as collagenases, elastase, prostaglandins, and aspartate aminotransferase

To date, not all these tests are available for use in the dental office. Some new diagnostic tools that are currently available include bacterial cultures, DNA probes (through reference laboratories), the test for neutral proteinases, force-controlled and automatic recording periodontal probes, and digital radiology. ELISA tests for the putative organisms are currently available in Europe, and it is hoped that these tests as well as rapid chairside tests using ELISA technology will soon be available in the United States.

As with dental caries, the prevention and treatment of periodontal disease is undergoing a philosophic reevaluation in the dental community. Traditionally, periodontal disease has been treated using a surgical model. This can include scaling and root planing the affected teeth, surgical debridement of the periodontal pockets, and recontouring of the gingiva and alveolar bone to aid in oral hygiene after the site has healed. The medical model for the treatment of periodontal disease, on the other hand, concentrates on strategies to reduce or eliminate the pathologic bacteria and to limit destructive effects of the inflammatory process on the periodontal structures.

The identification of the pathogenic bacteria specifically related to periodontal disease has led to the routine use of antibiotics in periodontal therapy. The use of tetracycline-impregnated cord packed into the periodontal pocket has been studied since the late 1980s and has reduced pocket depth and inflammation.[19] Systemic use of doxycycline has been effective in reducing the levels of the putative bacteria in high-risk patients.[20] Chlorhexidine gluconate as a 0.12% oral rinse is effective as a broad-spectrum antiplaque agent and as an irrigant in the ultrasonic debridement of periodontal pockets. To date, no resistance has developed to the antibacterial effects of chlorhexidine.

It has also been shown that the progression of periodontal disease can be slowed by blocking the inflammatory pathways that play a role in the destruction of periodontal tissues. Clinical trials with flurbiprofen, naproxen, and ketoprofen indicate that it is possible to slow periodontal disease progression by using these nonsteroidal anti-inflammatory drugs. Animal studies also show that chemically modified tetracycline can inhibit collagenase and thereby slow disease progression.[19] Many studies show that the surgical and nonsurgical treatment of periodontal disease yield comparable long-term results.[21, 22]

Oral Cancer

Epidemiology

Oral carcinomas, including cancers of the lips, tongue, floor of mouth, palate, gingiva, buccal mucosa, and oral pharynx, account for approximately 3% of all cancers in the United States. Approximately 85% of these cancers occur on the tongue, oropharynx, lips, and floor of mouth. Because most oral cancers are advanced when diagnosed, they have a very low survival rate, with almost half of all patients dying within 5 years of diagnosis. The death rate would be even higher if cancers of the lip, which are most frequently localized when diagnosed, were excluded. Silverman and Gorsky[23] determined that more than 79% of oropharyngeal cancers showed regional lymph node metastases at the time of diagnosis and that 73% of cancers of the tongue were already advanced when discovered.

The risk of developing oral cancer is directly associated with age; the average age at diagnosis is 60–65 years. The use of tobacco in any form increases the risk of oral cancer, and this risk is increased further by heavy alcohol use.

Although oral cancer has been rare among Native Americans in the past, the relationship between the use of smokeless tobacco and oral cancer is of concern in this population. Many studies have shown that smokeless tobacco use among Native Americans, especially Native American children and adolescents, is significantly higher than among other Americans. Wolfe and Carlos[24] found that, among Navajo adolescents ages 14–19 years, 75.4% of males and 49% of females used smokeless tobacco. More than 25% of the users had leukoplakia, a potential precursor to oral cancer. In a survey of sixth, ninth, and eleventh graders in the state of Washington, Hall and Dexter[25] found that 34% of Native American males and 20% of females were current users of smokeless tobacco compared with 20% and 4%, respectively, of their non-Native counterparts. Bruerd[26] reported prevalence of regular smokeless tobacco use among Native American school children ranging from 18% in kindergartners through sixth graders to 55.9% among ninth and tenth graders. Smokeless tobacco use has been observed in Native American children as young as 4 years of age. In general, Native American smokeless tobacco use begins at an earlier age than in non-Native Americans, has a similar prevalence among males and females, and has a higher overall prevalence than in non-Native Americans.

Clinical Presentation, Prevention, and Control

The vast majority of cancers of the oral cavity are squamous cell carcinomas. The clinical presentation of the lesions varies by the sites at which they occur. Cancers of the lip usually begin as small areas of thickening, induration, ulceration, or irregularity of the vermilion border to one side of the midline. As it enlarges, the lesion can produce a craterlike defect. Carcinoma of the tongue usually presents as a painless mass or ulcer on the lateral border or ventral surface of the tongue. Carcinoma of the floor of the mouth typically presents as an indurated ulcer to one side of the midline. Cancer of the buccal or labial mucosa is the type most commonly associated with the use of smokeless tobacco. These lesions commonly begin as areas of leukoplakia, which are white patches or plaques on the mucosal surface that do not rub off. The surface of the leukoplakia often appears thickened and wrinkled when compared to normal adjacent mucosa. If the leukoplakia contains granular pinkish gray or red areas, these areas may represent carcinoma in situ or even invasive carcinoma. Any such areas should be biopsied.

Prevention programs that lead to a reduction in the use of tobacco products, especially smokeless tobacco, are important in the prevention and control of oral cancers. Early detection through regular periodic examinations of the oral cavity is also important. Patients who use tobacco products should have at least an annual oral examination for the early detection of premalignant or malignant lesions. The primary care physician can either do these examinations for their patients who use tobacco or refer these patients to a dentist. In the IHS service population, fewer than 30% of Native Americans visit the dentist annually, so the primary care physician can play an important role in the prevention and early detection of this disease.

Conclusion

Dental diseases, especially caries and periodontal disease, occur at much higher rates in the Native American population than in the U.S. all races population. The use of smokeless tobacco, a major risk factor in the development of oral cancer, is much more prevalent among Native Americans than in the general U.S. population. The primary care physician is frequently the first allied medical professional to see patients with dental problems. The ability to recognize these conditions; to provide preventive, supportive, and therapeutic care; and to know when to make appropriate referrals to a dentist are very important when providing services to Native American populations.

Summary Points

- Dental caries occurs among Native American populations at significantly higher rates than among the U.S. general population. BBTD/ECC, a particularly devastating presentation of dental caries, is pandemic among Native American children.

- Periodontal disease affects a large proportion of Native American adults and has been measured in children as young as the early teens. The prevalence of periodontal disease among Native Americans with type 2 diabetes is double the prevalence in the U.S. general population, and diabetes is increasing among Native American populations.
- Oral cancer is closely associated with the use of smokeless tobacco. Native American adolescents tend to use smokeless tobacco at much higher rates than their non-Native counterparts, and they tend to begin the use of the products at much younger ages.

References

1. Niendorff W. The Oral Health of Native Americans: A Chart Book of Recent Findings, Trends and Regional Differences. Albuquerque, NM: Indian Health Service, Dental Field Support and Program Development, August 1994.
2. Ripa LW. Nursing habits and dental decay in infants: "nursing bottle caries." J Dent Child 1978;45:274–275.
3. Ripa LW. Nursing caries: a comprehensive review. Pediatr Dent 1988;10:268–282.
4. Niendorff W, Collins R. Oral health status of Native Americans, selected findings from a survey of dental patients conducted in FY 1983–84 by the Indian Health Service. Paper presented at the annual meeting of the American Public Health Association, Las Vegas, Nevada, October 1986.
5. Kelly M, Bruerd B. The prevalence of baby bottle tooth decay among two Native American populations. J Public Health Dent 1987;47:94–97.
6. Cook HW, Duncan WK, De Ball S, Berg B. The cost of nursing caries in a Native American Head Start population. J Clin Pediatr Dent 1994;18:139–142.
7. Bruerd B, Jones C, Krise D. Preventing baby bottle tooth decay and early childhood caries among AI/AN infants and children. IHS Primary Care Provider 1997;22:37–39.
8. Bruerd B, Jones C. Preventing baby bottle tooth decay: eight year results. Public Health Rep 1996;111:63–65.
9. Park BZ, Kinney MB, Steffensen JEM. Putting teeth into your physical exam. Part I. Children and adolescents. J Fam Pract 1992;35:459–462.
10. Caufield PW, Cutter GR, Dasanayake AP. Initial acquisition of *Mutans streptococci* by infants: evidence for a discrete window of infectivity. J Dent Res 1993;72:37–45.
11. American Academy of Periodontology. Proceedings of the World Workshop in Clinical Periodontics. Chicago: American Academy of Periodontology, 1989.
12. Fox CH. New considerations in the prevalence of periodontal disease. Curr Opin Dent 1992;2:5–11.
13. Emrich LJ, Shlossman M, Genco RJ. Periodontal disease in non–insulin-dependent diabetes mellitus. J Periodontol 1991;62:123–131.

14. Shlossman M, Knowler WC, Pettitt DJ, Genco RJ. Type 2 diabetes mellitus and periodontal disease. J Am Dent Assoc 1990;121:532–536.

15. Nelson RG, Shlossman M, Budding LM, et al. Periodontal disease and NIDDM in Pima Indians. Diabetes Care 1990;13:836–840.

16. Shlossman M, Nelson RG, Arevalo A. Periodontal disease: a complication of diabetes. J Dent Res 1989;68:381.

17. Greenstein G, Lamster I. Bacterial transmission in periodontal diseases: a critical review. J Periodontol 1997; 68:421–431.

18. Jeffcoat MK. Current concepts in periodontal disease testing. J Am Dent Assoc 1994;125:1071–1078.

19. Williams RC, Beck JD, Offenbacker SN. The impact of new technologies to diagnose and treat periodontal disease. A look to the future. J Clin Periodontol 1996;23: 299–305.

20. Kulkarni GV, Lee WK, Aitken S, et al. A randomized, placebo-controlled trial of doxycycline: effect on the microflora of recurrent periodontitis lesions in high risk patients. J Periodontol 1991;62:197–202.

21. Forabosco A, Galetti R, Spinato S, et al. A comparative study of a surgical method and scaling and root planing using the Odontoson. J Clin Periodontol 1996;23: 611–614.

22. Antczak-Bouckoms A, Joshipura K, Burdick E, Tullock JF. Meta-analysis of surgical versus non-surgical methods of treatment for periodontal disease. J Clin Periodontol 1993;20:259–268.

23. Silverman S, Gorsky M. Epidemiologic and demographic update in oral cancer: California and national data: 1973–1985. J Am Dent Assoc 1990;120:495–499.

24. Wolfe MD, Carlos JP. Oral health effects of smokeless tobacco use in Navajo Indian adolescents. Community Dent Oral Epidemiol 1987;15:230–235.

25. Hall RL, Dexter D. Smokeless tobacco use and attitudes towards smokeless tobacco among Native Americans and other adolescents in the northwest. Am J Public Health 1998;78:1586–1588.

26. Bruerd B. Smokeless tobacco use among Native American school children. Public Health Rep 1990;105: 196–201.

Part XVIII
Pulmonary

Chapter 45
Pulmonary Diseases

Amitabha Karmakar, Sardar Ijlal Babar,
and Linda S. Snyder

Respiratory disorders cause significant disability and death in Native Americans.[1, 2] Although statistics are limited, certain respiratory diseases stand out as major health problems for Native Americans.[3] The occurrence and manifestations of pulmonary diseases in Native Americans differ from those of the general U.S. population. American Indians have increased rates of infectious lung diseases and lower rates of smoking-related diseases than does the general population.

This chapter focuses on five common pulmonary disorders health care providers encounter when caring for Native American adults in an ambulatory care setting: pneumonia (excluding tuberculosis), chronic obstructive pulmonary disease (COPD), asthma, lung cancer, and obstructive sleep apnea (OSA) syndrome. The clinical presentation, diagnosis, and therapeutic options of each are discussed.

Mortality Rates Associated with Specific Respiratory Diseases

Comparing mortality rates for selected pulmonary diseases in Native Americans and in the general U.S. population reveals valuable information for clinicians.[1] Pneumonia was the leading cause of respiratory deaths among American Indians for the period 1984–1988. Between 1980 and 1986, pneumonia accounted for 97% of respiratory deaths of those younger than age 44 years.[3] For 1990–1991, although COPD was the fourth leading cause of death for all Americans, it was the ninth leading cause of death for Native Americans. COPD is a leading cause of hospitalization, however, ranking above both tuberculosis and lung cancer.[3] Asthma is also an important respiratory disease in Native Americans. Asthma, along with respiratory allergy and hay fever, was the tenth most common reason for ambulatory visits by American Indians in 1987.[1] The low over-

all occurrence of lung cancer in American Indians compared with that in U.S. whites has been documented in a number of studies.[1] Although the mortality from lung cancer is still low among American Indians, the rate may be increasing. Compared with the general population, obesity is more prevalent in Native Americans, placing them at risk for obesity-related respiratory morbidity, such as OSA syndrome.[1] Diagnosis and treatment of these pulmonary diseases are an important part of health care for Native American adults.

Smoking

The prevalence of smoking varies widely among the American Indian tribes. One study confirmed the high prevalence of cigarette smoking among northern plains Indians and low rates among southwestern Indians.[1] The difference in tobacco use among various Indian groups may explain some of the differences observed in rates of lung cancer and cardiovascular disease. Some surveys have also noted a high prevalence of smoking among American Indian adolescents.[4]

Pneumonia

Pneumonia is the sixth leading cause of death of Native Americans of all ages. The clinical presentation of community-acquired pneumonia (CAP) in Native Americans is similar to that in the general population and varies with the cause of the pneumonia and the patient's age and clinical condition. Individuals at risk for CAP include those with coexisting medical conditions, such as diabetes mellitus, COPD, congestive heart failure, and chronic alcohol abuse, and the elderly (older than age 65 years). The history is very important in assessment of predisposing factors, such as an immunocompromising disease, COPD, or alcoholism. The patient often presents with a recent upper respiratory tract

Table 45-1. Epidemiologic Factors and Specific Pathogens in Community-Acquired Pneumonia

Factor	Common Pathogen
Chronic obstructive pulmonary disease and smoking	*Haemophilus influenzae, Streptococcus pneumoniae, Moraxella catarrhalis*
Alcoholism	Oral anaerobes, gram-negative bacilli, *S. pneumoniae*
Nursing home resident	*S. pneumoniae*, gram-negative bacilli, *H. influenzae*
Influenza	Influenza virus, *S. pneumoniae, Staphylococcus aureus*
Exposure to potable water	*Legionella* species
Poor dental hygiene	Oral anaerobes
Travel	Endemic mycoses (e.g., coccidioidomycosis)

Table 45-2. Guidelines for Empiric Initial Therapy in Adults with Community-Acquired Pneumonia (CAP)[a]

Outpatient pneumonia without comorbidity and age <60 yrs
  Macrolide[b] or tetracycline[c]
Outpatient pneumonia with comorbidity or age >60 yrs, or both
  Second-generation cephalosporin or trimethoprim-sulfamethoxazole or beta-lactam/beta-lactamase inhibitor; with or without macrolide
Hospitalized patient with CAP
  Second- or third-generation cephalosporin or beta-lactam, beta-lactamase inhibitor with or without macrolide
Hospitalized patient with severe CAP
  Macrolide plus third-generation cephalosporin with antipseudomonal activity; aminoglycoside should be added during initial therapy, until exclusion of *Pseudomonas aeruginosa*

[a]Consider geographic variability in prevalence of high-level penicillin-resistant *Streptococcus pneumoniae*.
[b]Newer macrolides should be considered in smokers to treat *Haemophilus influenzae*.
[c]Some isolates of *S. pneumoniae* are resistant to tetracycline.
Source: Adapted from MS Niederman, JB Bass, GD Campbell, et al. Guidelines for the initial management of adults with community-acquired pneumonia. Am Rev Respir Dis 1993;148:1418.

infection and then develops chills, fever, cough with purulent sputum, and sometimes pleuritic chest pain. Elderly or immunocompromised patients may present without a fever, however, with a change in eating habits or mental function, and with a paucity of respiratory symptoms. Physical examination may reveal bronchial breath sounds, dullness to percussion, or crackles on auscultation. However, the physical examination may be entirely normal.

The pathogens that cause CAP are *Streptococcus pneumonia, Haemophilus influenzae*, respiratory viruses, *Legionella pneumophila*, and occasionally gram-negative bacilli. Only 30–60% of patients have a specific causative pathogen identified, which highlights the point that empiric therapy is necessary for most patients with CAP. Clinical studies have shown that the etiology of the pneumonia cannot be accurately predicted by clinical, laboratory, or radiographic parameters.[5] Once a patient is suspected of having CAP, however, a number of diagnostic studies are helpful in determining whether the patient should be hospitalized.

Although there are no set "admission criteria" to establish when a patient with CAP should be hospitalized, several studies of CAP have identified factors associated with a complicated course and higher mortality. These include advanced age (older than 65 years), coexisting medical conditions, chronic alcohol abuse, postsplenectomy state, altered mental status, systolic blood pressure less than 90 mm Hg, temperature higher than 101°F, respiratory rate greater than 30 breaths per minute, white blood cell count less than 4,000 or more than 30,000, renal dysfunction, hypoxemia, unfavorable chest radiographic patterns (multilobar infiltrates, effusions, cavities), and evidence of severe infection (metabolic acidosis or end-organ involvement).

Once CAP is suspected, a number of diagnostic studies can be useful. The chest radiograph is useful not only to diagnose the pneumonia but also to reveal effusions or cavities that may predict a complicated course. Blood cultures are very useful in hospitalized patients with CAP and may be positive up to 30% of the time. Routine chemistries and blood counts can stratify patients with regard to risk, noting extremes of white blood cell counts, renal dysfunction, or electrolyte abnormalities. The differential diagnosis of a patient with CAP includes venous thromboembolism, malignancy, unusual pulmonary infections (fungal, tuberculosis), or congestive heart failure.

Therapy is usually empiric and based on the likelihood of certain pathogens being found in a given patient population (Tables 45-1 and 45-2). Studies have shown a high incidence of pneumococcal and *Haemophilus* infections in Native American patients; therefore, these pathogens must be considered in the treatment of CAP.[1] The mortality rate from pneumococcal pneumonia in Native Americans is also significantly higher than that for the general U.S. population. In Native American patients with severe CAP, *L. pneumophila* and gram-negative bacilli must also be treated.

The high incidence and morbidity of pneumococcal infections in Native American adults highlights the importance of administration of the pneumococcal vaccine to high-risk individuals and those older than age 65 years.

Chronic Obstructive Pulmonary Disease

The prevalence of COPD in the United States is rising. COPD is the fourth leading cause of death in the general U.S. population. In 1987, a survey of approximately 6,500 American Indians and Alaska Natives revealed the prevalence of COPD for American Indian men to be 2.4% and 1.4% for women.[1] These prevalence rates are lower than corresponding estimates in the general U.S. population. In addition, mortality rates from COPD among American Indians were approximately two-thirds of the rate for the general U.S. population. These differences appear to be due primarily to differing rates of smoking in the two populations. However, COPD is an important disease to recognize and treat in Native Americans because it is a leading cause of hospitalization (above both tuberculosis and lung cancer) and the ninth leading cause of death.

COPD embraces a heterogeneous group of syndromes characterized by abnormal tests of expiratory flow rates. Cigarette smoking has been solidly established as the most significant risk factor for COPD. Important clinical features of COPD include a history of chronic cough, sputum production, dyspnea, or wheezing. Patients with COPD have usually been smoking at least 20 cigarettes daily for 20 or more years before symptoms develop. Physical examination may reveal slowed expiration and wheezing on forced expiration. As obstruction progresses, hyperinflation becomes evident and the anteroposterior diameter of the chest increases, producing a "barrel chest." Patients often use accessory muscles of respiration and "pursed-lip" breathing to prevent premature closing of airways during expiration. Breath sounds are decreased, expiration is prolonged, and heart tones are distant. Coarse crackles can be heard at the bases, and wheezes are frequently heard, especially on forced expiration. The differential diagnosis of chronic airflow obstruction includes bronchiolitis obliterans, bronchiectasis, chronic upper-airway obstruction, and foreign body aspiration.

The elements needed to diagnose COPD include a complete history and physical examination that suggest the diagnosis of COPD, a chest radiograph, and spirometry. Two important values obtained from spirometry tests are the FEV_1, the average flow during the first second of the breathing maneuver, and the forced vital capacity (FVC), or the total amount of air exhaled. The definition of airways obstruction for clinical purposes is a low FEV_1 to FVC ratio (expressed as a percent). An FEV_1 to FVC of less than 70% is abnormally low and indicates obstructive airways disease. Discussion of abnormal spirometry results can prompt patients to quit smoking. Arterial blood gases, lung volumes, and diffusing capacity for carbon monoxide may be needed to stage the severity of the disease or exclude other pulmonary disorders.

The main goals of therapy for COPD patients are to prevent disease progression, reverse exacerbations, and optimize pulmonary function and quality of life. The majority of patients with COPD are (or were) cigarette smokers. Therefore, primary prevention includes discouraging smoking and assistance in smoking cessation options. Smoking cessation slows the rate of decline in FEV_1.

Pharmacologic therapy for mild COPD includes anticholinergic bronchodilators, beta$_2$-adrenergic agonists, theophylline, corticosteroids, and supplemental oxygen.[6] The anticholinergic bronchodilator, ipratropium, is commonly used in COPD patients and has been found to produce superior bronchodilation compared with standard doses of beta$_2$-adrenergic agonists in many COPD patients. The current recommended dose is 40 mg (two puffs) four times daily; however, four puffs four times daily can be used for maximal bronchodilation. The beta$_2$-adrenergic agonists, such as albuterol, metaproterenol, and terbutaline, are widely used in the management of COPD. Inhaled beta$_2$-agonists have the most rapid onset of action of available bronchodilators. Some studies have shown an additive effect when beta$_2$-agonists are used in conjunction with ipratropium. If symptoms are progressive, sustained-release theophylline can be added.

Corticosteroids are widely used in the treatment of COPD, although their efficacy is controversial. A number of studies have documented that objective improvement with corticosteroids in COPD is seen in only 10–20% of patients. However, it is not possible to clinically predict which patients will respond to a course of corticosteroids. A trial of 2 weeks of oral corticosteroids can be used in patients whose symptoms are progressive and debilitating. However, if objective, significant improvement (FEV_1 increase above 20% or 200 cc) does not occur, the steroids should be stopped. If improvement occurs, corticosteroids should be weaned off or to a low daily dose or alternate-day dose. Inhaled steroids can be used to aid in the tapering of the oral corticosteroids. Supplemental oxygen has been proved beneficial in treatment of patients with chronic hypoxemic COPD. Two large, randomized, controlled oxygen trials conducted in the 1980s in patients with COPD have shown improved survival with oxygen administration. Patients with a room air Po_2 of 55 mm Hg or less or of 55–60 mm Hg with evidence of cor pulmonale or polycythemia are candidates for long-term oxygen therapy.

Asthma

Reports by clinicians in the 1960s and 1970s suggested that asthma was rare in Native Americans. Preliminary work from the Strong Heart Study showed that the prevalence and correlates of asthma in American Indian adults are similar to those of the North American cohort.[7] In addition, allergy and hay fever were the tenth most common reasons for ambulatory visits by Native

Americans in 1987. One survey of children in New Mexico showed that asthma was more common than previously realized.[8] Nationwide mortality data show rates of mortality from asthma to be comparable in Native Americans to those of the general population. Taken together, this information suggests that asthma may be more common than previously suspected and is likely to be encountered in Native American patients in an ambulatory care setting.

The Expert Panel Report for the diagnosis and management of asthma, published in April 1997, is an excellent resource for treatment guidelines in Native American patients.[9] The new asthma paradigm highlights three important points: (1) airway inflammation is central to the disease, (2) bronchospasm or airway reactivity may be the only symptom, and (3) clinicians should treat the disease and ameliorate symptoms as needed.

The typical presenting symptoms of asthma are cough, wheezing, shortness of breath, or chest tightness. The diagnosis of asthma requires episodic symptoms of airflow obstruction, at least partially reversible airflow obstruction, and the exclusion of alternative diagnoses that present in a similar fashion. Establishing a diagnosis of asthma includes a detailed medical history focusing on pulmonary and exercise-induced symptoms as well as an atopy or allergy evaluation. The physical examination should focus on the upper respiratory tract and chest, searching for clues such as rhinitis, nasal polyps, and wheezing on expiration. The differential diagnosis of wheezing, dyspnea, and cough is broad and includes parenchymal lung disease, bronchitis, endobronchial lesions (including malignancy), and cardiac disorders. It is crucial to obtain spirometry to assess lung function and reversibility.

Asthma therapy has five goals: (1) prevent chronic and troublesome symptoms, (2) maintain near "normal" pulmonary function, (3) prevent recurrent exacerbations, (4) minimize the need for emergency department visits or hospitalizations, and (5) provide optimal pharmacologic therapy with minimal side effects. Several important management principles underlie clinical practice:

1. Persistent asthma is best controlled with daily long-term anti-inflammatory therapy.
2. A stepwise approach to pharmacologic therapy is best.
3. Regular follow-up visits are essential.
4. Education of patients is crucial for optimizing pharmacologic therapy and compliance.

Drug therapy for asthma can be divided into drugs that control the disease (corticosteroids, theophylline, long-acting beta$_2$ agonist, leukotriene inhibitors, nedocromil and cromolyn) and those that relieve symptoms (short-acting beta$_2$ agonists, anticholinergic agents, and systemic corticosteroids). In mild asthma, quick relief with short-acting beta agonists used as needed according to symptoms is adequate. However, daily beta$_2$-agonist use or increasing use indicates the need for additional or increased doses of a controller medication (e.g., an inhaled anti-inflammatory agent). In moderate asthma (i.e., symptoms occur daily, exacerbations affect activity, and patients use daily beta$_2$ agonists), long-term control is needed. This often requires medium-dose inhaled steroids plus theophylline or long-acting beta agonists. Severe, persistent asthma generally requires high doses of inhaled steroids and a long-acting bronchodilator, occasionally supplemented by low doses of systemic corticosteroids.

In summary, anti-inflammatory therapy is central to asthma care. Inhaled steroids are the primary anti-inflammatory agent used and must be used with spacers to minimize side effects and enhance compliance. Short-acting bronchodilators are used for symptom relief, and success is achieved when the patient uses them only infrequently. Long-acting bronchodilators may be used to reduce steroid doses. In every asthma patient, objective measurement of lung function with spirometry or peak flow meters is necessary to make treatment decisions. Finally, education and written treatment plans are key to the success of a treatment program.

Lung Cancer

Lung cancer is a disease of almost epidemic proportion: There are approximately 170,000 new cases annually, resulting in 150,000 deaths. The frequency and mortality rate for bronchogenic cancer is not uniform among Native American groups.[2] The mortality rate for bronchogenic cancer among Native Americans of the Southwest is significantly lower than in the north central states. These differences are likely to be associated with higher smoking rates in the northern regions than in the Southwest. Although mortality from lung cancer is uncommon among American Indians, the rate may be increasing. From 1958 to 1982, mortality rates for lung cancer in New Mexico increased 104% among American Indian men and 163% among American Indian women, at least in part related to uranium mining exposure.[2, 10] Thus, clinicians caring for American Indians are likely to encounter this disease in their practice.

Lung cancer may be suspected on the basis of the history, physical examination, and radiographic tests.[11] A firm diagnosis of lung cancer is made with cytologic or histopathologic confirmation of the disease. Physicians should have a high index of suspicion for lung cancer in patients who have a history of cigarette smoking or who were exposed to asbestos, uranium mining, or radon gas. Symptoms can be due to the primary tumor, intrathoracic spread, distant metastases, or a paraneoplastic syndrome. Signs and symptoms of the primary tumor include hemoptysis, dyspnea, cough, or wheezing, often due to endobronchial obstruction. The presence of dysphagia, hoarseness, superior vena cava syndrome, or Horner's syndrome should alert clinicians to intrathoracic spread of lung cancer. The common sites of metastases of lung cancer are lymph nodes, liver, bone, brain, and adrenal glands, and patients may present with symptoms of specific organ involvement. A paraneoplastic syndrome may present with symptoms of a peripheral motor or sensory neuropathy, weakness, confusion, or ataxia. Many patients are asymptomatic and are brought to medical attention because of an abnormal chest radiograph taken for another problem.

The primary diagnostic procedure for the detection of lung cancer is a chest radiograph. Chest radiography is 70–88% accurate in the overall detection of lung cancer; it is less accurate in the detection of hilar or mediastinal adenopathy. The chest radiograph is often the first imaging procedure performed when lung cancer is suspected, but chest computed tomography (CT) is an extremely valuable procedure and is crucial in this evaluation. It allows precise location of the lesion, its relationship to nearby structures, and the status of the pulmonary hila, mediastinum, chest wall, liver, and adrenal glands. The chest CT also serves as a valuable "road map" to guide the pulmonologist at the time of bronchoscopy. The procedures available to secure the diagnosis of lung cancer include bronchoscopy, transthoracic needle aspiration, lymph node biopsy, and mediastinoscopy. The choice of procedure is usually based on the location and size of the lesion and the patient's overall clinical status.

The differential diagnosis of a lung mass is broad and includes indolent fungal or mycobacterial infections, inflammatory lung diseases, vasculitides, and metastatic disease to the lung.

Therapeutic options for patients depend on accurate staging of lung cancer, as determined by the various diagnostic procedures. Routine tests should include a chest CT with contrast (including the upper abdomen to examine the liver and adrenal glands) and laboratory tests, including calcium, liver and renal panel, and complete blood count. In general, bone or liver scans are not obtained in the asymptomatic patient with non–small cell lung cancer. A careful history and physical is crucial; if patients have signs or symptoms suggestive of tumor spread, further testing is required. The therapeutic alternatives (surgical therapy, chemotherapy or radiation therapy) are based on the tumor type and stage, the patient's clinical condition, and the patient's ability to withstand a surgical procedure.

In summary, the goals of diagnostic testing in patients with suspected lung cancer are to establish the diagnosis and determine the stage of the disease so that appropriate therapy can be initiated. The number of Native Americans at risk for lung cancer seems to be increasing due to cigarette smoking and uranium mining exposure, so

clinicians must have a high index of suspicion for this disease.

Obstructive Sleep Apnea Syndrome

OSA is considered an important disorder in Native Americans, being closely related to obesity. Although no prevalence data are available for Native Americans, OSA affects 2–4% of middle-aged men and 1–2% of middle-aged women in the general U.S. population. OSA leads to sleep disruption as well as cardiopulmonary morbidity and occupational disability; thus, it is an important disorder to diagnose and treat.[12]

Risk factors predisposing to OSA include male sex, increasing age, alcohol use, obesity, sedative-hypnotic use, hypothyroidism, and acromegaly. Craniofacial anomalies, such as micrognathia and retrognathia, also increase the risk of developing OSA. Native American patients who present with any of these risk factors and suggestive clinical symptoms should be specifically questioned about possible OSA.

Pathophysiologically, sleep apnea occurs due to collapse of the upper airway lumen during sleep. Normally, the upper airway lumen remains open during sleep because the negative intraluminal pressure is balanced by increasing tone in the dilating musculature of the oropharynx. Therefore, even in normal subjects, the muscle tone decreases and upper-airway resistance increases during sleep. The upper airway of patients with OSA is abnormally narrow, even during wakefulness. Thus, the loss of muscle tone that normally occurs during sleep produces significant occlusion of the upper airway in patients with OSA.

The three cardinal symptoms of OSA are snoring, witnessed apneic episodes, and daytime hypersomnolence. Most patients present with complaints of loud snoring followed by apneic episodes, which are terminated by the patient waking up, gasping for air. In many cases, this history is only obtained from the patient's bed partner and is crucial to considering the diagnosis of OSA. Excessive daytime sleepiness is also an important presenting complaint, with severe examples characterized by falling asleep while driving or during conversations. Other common complaints that should alert the health care provider to possible OSA include abnormal motor activity during sleep, diminished cognitive function, impotence, morning headaches, congestive heart failure, hypertension, and cardiac arrhythmias.

On physical examination, most patients are obese, with a short, thick neck. In fact, neck circumference correlates better with OSA than does body mass index. It is important to examine the nose to ensure patency of the nares. Evidence of retro- or micrognathia should be documented. Typical findings on examination of the oropharynx include a large tongue, enlarged tonsils, thickened uvula, or a long and redundant palate producing a narrow oropharynx. Patients should be carefully evaluated for the presence of cardiovascular disease, such as hypertension, congestive heart failure, or arrhythmias, because these are often associated with OSA.

The definitive diagnostic method for OSA is a polysomnographic (PSG) evaluation. It involves simultaneous measurements of the electroencephalogram, electro-oculogram, chin and leg electromyograms, electrocardiogram, airflow, respiratory effort, and oximetry. PSG is performed only at specialized sleep centers. Overnight oximetry has been used as a screening tool in some circumstances, but it is fairly insensitive. A negative overnight oximetry study does not rule out OSA because not all patients have sharp, periodic drops in oxygen saturation.

Once the diagnosis of OSA is made, it is important to identify associated medical conditions that might be correctable, such as hypothyroidism, acromegaly, or alcohol or sedative use. The presence of obesity should be noted because weight loss can produce significant benefits in some patients. Preventing the patient from sleeping on his or her back ("positional therapy") may be helpful because OSA is generally more severe in the supine position.

The mainstay of therapy of OSA is nasal continuous positive airway pressure (CPAP). CPAP acts as a "pneumatic splint," preventing closure of the upper airway. Although CPAP is very effective, patient compliance is poor because of various side effects associated with this therapy. These include dryness of the nose and mouth, mask discomfort, claustrophobia, noise, pressure sores around the nose, and rhinitis. Surgical therapy may be helpful in some cases. Tracheostomy is extremely effective because it bypasses the site of obstruction, but frequent episodes of bronchitis or tracheitis and cosmetic concerns coupled with the advent of nasal CPAP have made this an infrequently used therapy. Uvulopalatopharyngoplasty is a less radical surgical procedure that involves resection of the uvula, portions of the soft palate, and redundant pharyngeal tissue. However, only approximately 50% of patients who undergo this procedure experience a significant reduction in apneic events. Other procedures, such as mandibular advancement, may be considered in patients with severe retrognathia. Few drugs are of significant benefit in OSA. Protriptyline, a nonsedating tricyclic antidepressant, reduces the amount of rapid eye movement sleep, the sleep stage in which apneic events are most pronounced. However, no significant decrease in apneic episodes has been observed. Medroxyprogesterone is a central respiratory stimulant that is used mainly for the obesity-hypoventilation syndrome and is not useful for OSA. In summary, OSA is an important disorder to consider in Native Americans, and a sleep history should be obtained in all individuals with risk factors.

Summary Points

- American Indians have increased rates of infectious lung diseases compared with the general U.S. population. Bacterial pathogens of importance are *S. pneumoniae* and *H. influenzae*.
- The pneumococcal vaccine should be administered to high-risk individuals and those older than age 65 years.
- Primary prevention of COPD includes active discouragement of smoking and assistance for patients with smoking cessation options.
- Objective measurement of spirometry is essential to diagnose COPD; if abnormal, it can prompt patients to quit smoking.
- Corticosteroids for COPD patients should be used sparingly because they have significant side effects and are effective in only 10–20% of patients.
- The new paradigm emphasizes asthma as an inflammatory disease of the airways, and anti-inflammatory therapy is central to treatment.
- Inhaled steroids are the primary anti-inflammatory agent used in chronic asthma.
- Objective measurements of lung function with spirometry or peak flow meters is necessary to make treatment decisions in asthma.
- Patient education about asthma and the need for chronic anti-inflammatory therapy is crucial to successful treatment.
- Lung cancer survival rates are related to the stage of the disease, histology of the cancer, and overall condition of the patient. Early diagnosis and smoking cessation are major factors that enhance survival of lung cancer patients.
- Risk factors for OSA include obesity, hypertension, and alcohol use. Health care providers must ask specific questions about snoring, apnea, and daytime hypersomnolence in these patients.

References

1. NHLBI Working Group. Respiratory diseases disproportionately affecting minorities. Chest 1995;108:1380–1392.
2. Coultas DB, Gong H, Grad R, et al. Respiratory diseases in minorities of the United States. Am J Respir Crit Care Med 1993;149(suppl):93–131.
3. Rhoades ER. The major respiratory diseases of American Indians. Am Rev Respir Dis 1990;141:595–600.
4. Blum RW, Harmon B, Harris L, et al. American Indian-Alaska Native youth health. JAMA 1992;267:1637–1644.
5. Niederman MS, Bass JB, Campbell GD, et al. Guidelines for the initial management of adults with community-acquired pneumonia. Am Rev Respir Dis 1993;148:1418–1426.
6. Ferguson GT, Cherniack RM. Management of chronic

obstructive pulmonary disease. N Engl J Med 1993;
328:1017–1022.

7. Welty TK, Lee ET, Yeh J, et al. Cardiovascular disease
risk factors among American Indians: the Strong Heart
Study. Am J Epidemiol 1995;142:269–287.

8. Clark D, Gollub R, Green WF, et al. Asthma in Jemez
Pueblo schoolchildren. Am J Respir Crit Care Med
1995;151:1625–1627.

9. Expert Panel Report 2. Guidelines for the Diagnosis
and Management of Asthma. Publication No. 97-4051.
Baltimore: National Institutes of Health, 1997.

10. Roswe RJ, Deddens JA, Salvan A, Schnorr TM. Mortality among Navajo uranium miners. Am J Public
Health 1995;85:535–540.

11. Karsell PR, McDougall JC. Diagnostic tests for lung
cancer. Mayo Clin Proc 1993;68:288–296.

12. Bootzin RR, Quan SF, Bamford CR, et al. Sleep disorders. Compr Ther 1995;21:401–406.

Part XIX
Gastrointestinal

Chapter 46
Cholelithiasis

William W. Lunt and Richard E. Sampliner

Western medicine is a relatively new concept in some Native American cultures. In the early 1950s, the U.S. Public Health Service took over the responsibility for administering and delivering Native American health care. It has been recognized that several diseases occur with increased frequency among Native Americans, including obesity, diabetes, renal disease, and gallbladder disease.

Population-based studies of Native Americans demonstrated significantly higher prevalence of gallbladder disease compared to the Framingham, Massachusetts data.[1, 2] The tribes reported to have high prevalence include the Pima and Apache of the Southwest; the Arapaho, Shoshone, and Sioux tribes of the northern plains; the Chippewa of northern Minnesota[1]; the Micmac of Nova Scotia[3]; the Cree-Ojibwa Indians of northern Manitoba and Ontario, Canada[4]; as well as Alaska Natives.[5] The highest rates of cholelithiasis occur among the Pima Indians of southern Arizona. In women, the prevalence is 73% in the age group 25–34 years, and it remains high in older individuals.[6] Gallbladder disease in this group of Native Americans is characterized by an early age of onset, a higher incidence in women than men, and increased incidence with age in both sexes.[6] Possible risk factors for gallbladder disease in Native Americans have been studied. Although the association with parity is controversial, there appears to be no association between gallbladder disease and diabetes, serum cholesterol levels, and obesity in contrast to the Framingham findings.[1, 6, 7]

Pathogenesis and Natural History

In whites, 75% of gallstones are cholesterol stones. In Native Americans, gallstones are nearly exclusively cholesterol in composition.[8] Cholesterol gallstones result from precipitation of supersaturated cholesterol bile with subsequent formation of microliths. These small stones continue to grow until clinically detected.[9]

This cholesterol-laden lithogenic bile appears to predominate in Native American women, in whom there is an increased incidence of stone formation at puberty.[6, 9] There is also a 15% higher bile saturation in women than men.[9] At birth, bile cholesterol saturation is relatively low, but during pubertal growth and development, the relative bile cholesterol content rises to a point at which, in many subjects, cholesterol precipitation can occur rapidly, leading to cholesterol stone formation. The lag time between the appearance of such lithogenic bile and the appearance of gallstones averages 8 years.[9]

There is presently no data for Native Americans, but a study of predominantly white men demonstrates a plateauing risk of developing symptoms from asymptomatic gallstones of 10% at 5 years, 15% at 10 years, and 18% at 15 and 20 years from stone detection. If a patient remained asymptomatic after 20 years, he was unlikely to develop complications.[10] In comparison, Native Americans have more aggressive cholesterol stone formation with earlier age of onset, so an increased risk of developing symptoms from silent stones can be anticipated.

The overall death rate in Pima Indians with gallstones is nearly double those without gallstones. The death rate attributed to malignancies in those with gallbladder disease is 6.6 times higher than those lacking gallbladder disease.[11] The mortality rates for noncancerous gallbladder disease in Native Americans are almost five times the rates for whites.[1] The risk of developing gallbladder cancer or dying from complications of gallstones is still low enough to not recommend prophylactic cholecystectomy for asymptomatic gallstones.

Recognition and Evaluation

Most patients with gallstones have no symptoms. Symptomatic gallstones are identified by the characteristic upper abdominal pain known as biliary "colic" (Table

Table 46-1. Findings Associated with Gallstones

Symptoms
  Constant epigastric or right upper quadrant pain for
    >30 mins
  Nausea and vomiting
  Pain referred to the back or shoulders
Signs
  Fever
  Epigastric or right upper quadrant tenderness
  Leukocytosis
  Elevated liver tests (especially bilirubin and alkaline
    phosphatase)
  Gallstones on abdominal ultrasound

Table 46-2. Complications of Gallstones

Cholecystitis
Common bile duct obstruction
Ascending cholangitis
Gallstone pancreatitis
Gallbladder cancer
Increased noncancer mortality

46-1). It is usually a sudden, severe, steady ache in the epigastrium or right upper quadrant lasting longer than 30 minutes and then gradually disappearing over 30–60 minutes. At times, a dull ache or soreness may persist for up to 24 hours. These episodes of pain occur intermittently, separated by pain-free intervals of days to years.[12, 13]

Evaluation of patients with symptomatic gallstones should include a history of biliary pain that may or may not be exacerbated by a heavy meal. There may be referred pain to the right shoulder, and nausea and vomiting frequently accompany these episodes.[13] Pregnancy is important to exclude, and pregnancy tests should be obtained when appropriate. On physical examination, epigastric or right upper quadrant tenderness is present, and a distended gallbladder is rarely felt.

Biliary pain is caused by gallstones that intermittently obstruct the cystic duct or common bile duct (Table 46-2). If this obstruction is prolonged, mild elevation of bilirubin may be seen. Persistently high bilirubin with an elevated alkaline phosphatase suggests common duct stones. Mild elevation of serum transaminases may also occur. If there is transient obstruction of the pancreatic duct by a common duct stone, the amylase level may be elevated. The presence of fever and chills suggests a complication such as cholecystitis, ascending cholangitis, or pancreatitis. These complications are preceded by biliary pain in 90% of cases.[13]

Radiologic Diagnosis

When patients present with abdominal pain, the first radiologic test performed is usually the plain abdominal x-ray. This is rarely useful for cholelithiasis because only 15–20% of gallstones contain enough calcium to be radiopaque.[14]

Ultrasound is the diagnostic modality of choice to evaluate gallbladder disease because of its high sensitivity and specificity, accessibility, and low cost. With ultrasound, the gallbladder is easily visualized, and stones as small as 2

mm in diameter can be detected, with characteristic acoustic shadowing. Biliary sludge can also be visualized, appearing as echogenic material without acoustic shadows that shift with change in patient position.[14]

Ultrasonographic signs of cholecystitis include gallbladder wall thickening greater than 2 mm, air within the gallbladder wall, fluid surrounding the gallbladder, and right upper quadrant pain during the examination.[14] Ultrasound scans may also indicate common bile duct dilation and common or intrahepatic ductal dilatation, and rarely pancreatic duct ectasia. These findings indicate a distal ductal obstruction, most commonly from gallstones.

Nuclear medicine examinations use technetium-99m-iminodiacetic acid derivatives (HIDA/DIDA), which are rapidly removed from the blood, accumulated in the liver, and excreted into the bile. HIDA scans also have very high sensitivity and specificity for diagnosing cystic duct obstruction but are difficult to obtain, expensive to administer, and, if significant cholestasis is present, may not be diagnostic. In a patient with abdominal pain, a normal scan virtually rules out the diagnosis of acute cholecystitis.

Gallstones may also be diagnosed using oral cholecystography, but this technique has largely been replaced by ultrasound. Although computed tomography scans of the abdomen can visualize some gallstones and may detect dilated bile ducts, they are rarely used as a primary diagnostic tool for gallbladder disease.

Therapy

No specific therapy is necessary for asymptomatic gallstones. Because the cumulative risk of developing symptoms is only 2–4% per year, there is no advantage to prophylactic cholecystectomy. Treatment is considered appropriate in patients with symptoms from gallstones and in individuals who have developed complications, such as cholecystitis, ascending cholangitis, or gallstone pancreatitis. Laparoscopic cholecystectomy surgery is the therapy of choice. It is a minimally invasive approach to remove the gallbladder with only a 1% mortality. Most centers perform this surgery on outpatients, and many patients return to work within 1 week. In experienced surgical hands, there is less than a 5% risk of complication requiring conversion to an open cholecystectomy.[12, 15]

If patients are not operative candidates, medical therapy with oral bile acids may be effective. The first bile acid used to dissolve gallstones was chenodeoxycholic acid, but due to its side effects of diarrhea and reversible hepatic toxicity, it has fallen out of favor. More recently, ursodeoxycholic acid, which does not induce diarrhea or elevate serum transaminases, is now the bile acid of choice.[13]

Factors for successful gallstone dissolution with ursodeoxycholic acid depend on stone size and composition and a functioning gallbladder. Ideal candidates have predominantly cholesterol stones, which most Native Americans have, with stone size greater than 1.5 cm. Success in these ideal candidates is 60–70% over 2 years, but approximately 50% redevelop stones over a 5-year period.[13] Intermittent or long-term dissolution therapy is therefore required.

Extracorporeal shock-wave lithotripsy is rarely performed. This treatment uses high-energy sound waves to fracture stones. Again, small cholesterol stones are ideal, and patients are usually placed on ursodeoxycholic acid to dissolve the small fragments. Complications are usually seen when fragments are passed, and biliary pain is common.

Summary Points

- The incidence and the morbidity and mortality from gallstones is extremely high in Native Americans.
- Gallstones occur predominantly in Native American women in their 20s and 30s. There may be coincidence with parity, but serum cholesterol level, diabetes, and obesity are not associated with gallstone formation.
- Cholesterol stones predominate.
- Gallstones and their complications are recognized by classic symptoms of biliary "colic," manifested by steady epigastric or right upper quadrant pain lasting more than 30 minutes.
- Laboratory data obtained should include transaminase levels, alkaline phosphatase, bilirubin, and amylase.
- Abdominal ultrasound is the primary test to evaluate biliary stones in gallbladder disease.
- Gallbladder disease recognition, diagnosis, evaluation, and treatment is the same as for other populations.
- Observation for silent gallstones and surgery or medical therapy for symptomatic gallstones is recommended.

References

1. Morris DL, Buechley RW, Key CR, Morgan MV. Gallbladder disease and gallbladder cancer among American Indians in tricultural New Mexico. Cancer 1978;42:2472–2477.
2. Comess LJ, Bennett PH, Burch TA. Clinical gallbladder disease in Pima Indians. Its high prevalence in contrast to Framingham, Massachusetts. N Engl J Med 1967;277:894-898.
3. Williams CN, Johnston JL, Weldon KLM. Prevalence of gallstones and gallbladder disease in Canadian Micmac Indian women. Can Med Assoc J 1977;117:758–760.
4. Young TK, Roche BA. Factors associated with clinical gallbladder disease in a Canadian Indian population. Clin Invest Med 1990;13:55–59.
5. Welty TK. Health implications of obesity in American Indians and Alaska Natives. Am J Clin Nutr 1991;153(suppl):1616–1620.
6. Sampliner RE, Bennett PH, Comess LJ, et al. Gallbladder disease in Pima Indians. Demonstration of high prevalence and early onset by cholecystography. N Engl J Med 1970;283:1358–1364.
7. Thistle JL, Eckhart KL, Nensel RE, et al. Prevalence of gallbladder disease among Chippewa Indians. Mayo Clin Proc 1971;46:603–608.
8. Diehl AK, Schwesinger WH, Holleman DR, et al. Gallstone characteristics in Mexican Americans and non-Hispanic whites. Dig Dis Sci 1994;39:2223–2228.
9. Bennion LJ, Knowler WC, Mott DM, et al. Development of lithogenic bile during puberty in Pima Indians. N Engl J Med 1979;300:873.
10. Gracie WA, Ransohoff DF. The natural history of silent gallstones: the innocent gallstone is not a myth. N Engl J Med 1982;307:798.
11. Grimaldi CH, Nelson RG, Pettitt DJ, et al. Increased mortality with gallstone disease: results of a 20-year population-based survey in Pima Indians. Ann Intern Med 1993;118:185–190.
12. Johnston DE, Kaplan MM. Pathogenesis and treatment of gallstones. N Engl J Med 1993;328:412–421.
13. Shaffer EA, Bayles TM (eds). Cholelithiasis. Current Therapy in Gastroenterology and Liver Disease (4th ed). St. Louis: Mosby, 1994;607–610.
14. Greenberger NJ, Isselbacher KJ. Harrison's Principles of Internal Medicine (13th ed, Vol 2). New York: McGraw-Hill, 1994;1504–1516.
15. Lee SP, Kuver R, Yamada T (eds), Gallstones. Textbook of Gastroenterology (2nd ed, Vol 2). Philadelphia: Lippincott, 1995;2187–2212.

Index

Note: Page numbers followed by *f* indicate figures; page numbers followed by *t* indicate tables.